The Wills Eye Manual

Office and Emergency Room Diagnosis
and Treatment of Eye Disease

EIGHTH EDITION

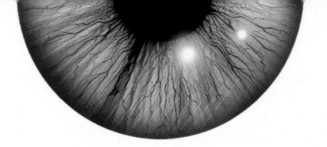

The Wills Eye Manual

Office and Emergency Room Diagnosis and Treatment of Eye Disease

EIGHTH EDITION

Text Editors

Kalla A. Gervasio • **Travis J. Peck**

Multimedia Editors

Cherie A. Fathy • **Meera D. Sivalingam**

Founding Editors

Mark A. Friedberg • **Christopher J. Rapuano**

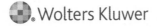. Wolters Kluwer

Philadelphia • Baltimore • New York • London
Buenos Aires • Hong Kong • Sydney • Tokyo

Acquisitions Editor: Chris Teja
Development Editor: Eric McDermott
Senior Editorial Coordinator: Emily Buccieri
Editorial Assistant: Maribeth Wood
Marketing Manager: Kirsten Watrud
Production Project Manager: Kirstin Johnson
Design Coordinator: Stephen Druding
Manufacturing Coordinator: Beth Welsh
Prepress Vendor: TNQ Technologies
Cover Photo Credit: Christopher J. Rapuano, M.D.

Eighth edition
Copyright © 2022 Wolters Kluwer.

Seventh Edition © 2017 Wolters Kluwer
Sixth Edition, © 2012 by Lippincott Williams & Wilkins, a Wolters Kluwer business
Fifth Edition © 2008 Lippincott Williams & Wilkins, a Wolters Kluwer business
Fourth Edition © 2004, by Lippincott Williams & Wilkins, a Wolters Kluwer business
Third Edition, © 1999 by Lippincott Williams & Wilkins
Second Edition, © 1994 by Lippincott-Raven Publishers
First Edition, © 1990 by J.B. Lippincott Company

9 8 7 6 5 4 3 2 1

Printed in Mexico

Library of Congress Cataloging-in-Publication Data

ISBN-13: 978-1-9751-6075-3

Cataloging in Publication data available on request from publisher.

shop.lww.com

QUADM0922

Contributors

CONTRIBUTORS TO THE EIGHTH EDITION

Michael D. Abendroth, M.D., M.B.A.
Dilru C. Amarasekera, M.D.
Cherie A. Fathy, M.D., M.P.H.
Ollya V. Fromal, M.D.
Kalla A. Gervasio, M.D.
Michele D. Markovitz, M.D.
Douglas R. Matsunaga, M.D.
Kyle B. McKey, M.D.
Austin R. Meeker, M.D.
Rakhi Melvani, M.D.
Erin E. Nichols, M.D.
Samir N. Patel, M.D.
Travis J. Peck, M.D.
Marisa A. Schoen, M.D.
Vikram A. Shankar, M.D.
Meera D. Sivalingam, M.D.
Joshua H. Uhr, M.D.
Connie M. Wu, M.D.

CONTRIBUTORS TO THE SEVENTH EDITION

Murtaza K. Adam, M.D.
Faheem Ahmed, M.D.
Blair Armstrong, M.D.
Michael N. Cohen, M.D.
Nathan Cutler, M.D.
Brenton Finklea, M.D.
Alison Huggins, M.D.
Marta McKeague, M.D.
Nina Ni, M.D.
Jinali Patel, M.D.
Priya Sharma, M.D.
Christine Talamini, M.D.
Alice L. Williams, M.D.
Michelle Wilson, M.D.

CONTRIBUTORS TO THE SIXTH EDITION

Fatima K. Ahmad, M.D.
Christopher J. Brady, M.D.
Adam T. Gerstenblith, M.D.
Meg R. Gerstenblith, M.D.
Katherine G. Gold, M.D.
Sebastian B. Heersink, M.D.

Suzanne K. Jadico, M.D.
Brandon B. Johnson, M.D.
Jennifer H. Kim, M.D.
Amanda E. Matthews, M.D.
Melissa D. Neuwelt, M.D.
Anne M. Nguyen, M.D.
Linda H. Ohsie, M.D.
Kristina Yi-Hwa Pao, M.D.
Michael P. Rabinowitz, M.D.
Mindy R. Rabinowitz, M.D.
Vikram J. Setlur, M.D.
Gary Shienbaum, M.D.
Eileen Wang, M.D.
Douglas M. Wisner, M.D.

CONTRIBUTORS TO THE FIFTH EDITION

Text Contributors

Paul S. Baker, M.D.
Shaleen L. Belani, M.D.
Shawn Chhabra, M.D.
John M. Cropsey, M.D.
Emily A. DeCarlo, M.D.
Justis P. Ehlers, M.D.
Gregory L. Fenton, M.D.
David Fintak, M.D.
Robert E. Fintelmann, M.D.
Nicole R. Fram, M.D.
Susan M. Gordon, M.D.
Omesh P. Gupta, M.D., M.B.A.
Eliza N. Hoskins, M.D.
Dara Khalatbari, M.D.
Bhairavi V. Kharod, M.D.
Matthew R. Kirk, M.D.
Andrew Lam, M.D.
Katherine A. Lane, M.D.
Michael A. Malstrom, M.D.
Chrishonda C. McCoy, M.D.
Jesse B. McKey, M.D.
Maria P. McNeill, M.D.
Joselitio S. Navaleza, M.D.
Avni H. Patel, M.D.
Chirag P. Shah, M.D., M.P.H.
Heather N. Shelsta, M.D.
Bradley T. Smith, M.D.
Vikas Tewari, M.D.
Garth J. Willis, M.D.
Allison P. Young, M.D.

Photo Contributors

Elizabeth L. Affel, M.S., R.D.M.S.
Robert S. Bailey, Jr., M.D.
William E. Benson, M.D.
Jurij R. Bilyk, M.D.
Elisabeth J. Cohen, M.D.
Justis P. Ehlers, M.D.
Alan R. Forman, M.D.
Scott M. Goldstein, M.D.
Kammi B. Gunton, M.D.
Becky Killian
Donelson R. Manley, M.D.
Julia Monsonego, C.R.A.
Christopher J. Rapuano, M.D.
Peter J. Savino, M.D.
Bruce M. Schnall, M.D.
Robert C. Sergott, M.D.
Chirag P. Shah, M.D., M.P.H.
Heather N. Shelsta, M.D.
Carol L. Shields, M.D.
Jerry A. Shields, M.D.
George L. Spaeth, M.D.
William Tasman, M.D.

Medical Illustrator

Paul Schiffmacher

CONTRIBUTORS TO THE FOURTH EDITION

Seema Aggarwal, M.D.
Edward H. Bedrossian, Jr., M.D.
Brian C. Bigler, M.D.
Vatinee Y. Bunya, M.D.
Christine Buono, M.D.
Jacqueline R. Carrasco, M.D.
Sandra Y. Cho, M.D.
Carolyn A. Cutney, M.D.
Brian D. Dudenhoefer, M.D.
John A. Epstein, M.D.
Colleen P. Halfpenny, M.D.
ThucAnh T. Ho, M.D.
Stephen S. Hwang, M.D.
Kunal D. Kantikar, M.D.
Derek Y. Kunimoto, M.D.
R. Gary Lane, M.D.
Henry C. Lee, M.D.
Mimi Liu, M.D.
Mary S. Makar, M.D.
Anson T. Miedel, M.D.
Parveen K. Nagra, M.D.
Michael A. Negrey, M.D.

Heather A. Nesti, M.D.
Vasudha A. Panday, M.D.
Nicholas A. Pefkaros, M.D.
Robert Sambursky, M.D.
Daniel E. Shapiro, M.D.
Derrick W. Shindler, M.D.

CONTRIBUTORS TO THE THIRD EDITION

Christine W. Chung, M.D.
Brian P. Connolly, M.D.
Vincent A. Deramo, M.D.
Kammi B. Gunton, M.D.
Mark R. Miller, M.D.
Ralph E. Oursler III, M.D.
Mark F. Pyfer, M.D.
Douglas J. Rhee, M.D.
Jay C. Rudd, M.D.
Brian M. Sucheski, M.D.

Medical Illustrator

Marlon Maus, M.D.

CONTRIBUTORS TO THE SECOND EDITION

Mark C. Austin, M.D.
Jerry R. Blair, M.D.
Benjamin Chang, M.D.
Mary Ellen Cullom, M.D.
R. Douglas Cullom, Jr., M.D.
Jack Dugan, M.D.
Forest J. Ellis, M.D.
C. Byron Faulkner, M.D.
Mary Elizabeth Gallivan, M.D.
J. William Harbour, M.D.
Paul M. Herring, M.D.
Allen C. Ho, M.D.
Carol J. Hoffman, M.D.
Thomas I. Margolis, M.D.
Mark L. Mayo, M.D.
Michele A. Miano, M.D.
Wynne A. Morley, M.D.
Timothy J. O'Brien, M.D.
Florentino E. Palmon, M.D.
William B. Phillips, M.D.
Tony Pruthi, M.D.
Carl D. Regillo, M.D.
Scott H. Smith, M.D.
Mark R. Stokes, M.D.
Janine G. Tabas, M.D.

John R. Trible, M.D.
Christopher Williams, M.D.

Medical Illustrator

Neal H. Atebara, M.D.

**CONTRIBUTORS TO THE FIRST
EDITION**

Melissa M. Brown, M.D.
Catharine J. Crockett, M.D.
Bret L. Fisher, M.D.

Patrick M. Flaharty, M.D.
Mark A. Friedberg, M.D.
James T. Handa, M.D.
Victor A. Holmes, M.D.
Bruce J. Keyser, M.D.
Ronald L. McKey, M.D.
Christopher J. Rapuano, M.D.
Paul A. Raskauskas, M.D.
Eric P. Suan, M.D.

Medical Illustrator

Marlon Maus, M.D.

Consultants

CORNEA

Consultants

Brandon D. Ayres, M.D.
Brad H. Feldman, M.D.
Brenton D. Finklea, M.D.
Beeran B. Meghpara, M.D.
Parveen K. Nagra, M.D.
Irving M. Raber, M.D.
Christopher J. Rapuano, M.D
Zeba A. Syed, M.D.

GLAUCOMA

Major Consultants

Natasha N. Kolomeyer, M.D.
Reza Razeghinejad, M.D.
Aakriti G. Shukla, M.D.

Consultants

Scott J. Fudemberg, M.D.
L. Jay Katz, M.D.
Daniel Lee, M.D.
Anand V. Mantravadi, M.D.
Marlene R. Moster, M.D.
Michael J. Pro, M.D.

NEURO-OPHTHALMOLOGY

Consultants

Adam A. Debusk, D.O.
Mark L. Moster, M.D.
Robert C. Sergott, M.D.

OCULOPLASTICS

Major Consultant

Jurij R. Bilyk, M.D.

Consultants

Blair K. Armstrong, M.D.
Jacqueline R. Carrasco, M.D.
Scott M. Goldstein, M.D.
Alison B. Huggins Watson, M.D.
Robert B. Penne, M.D.
Michael P. Rabinowitz, M.D.
Sathyadeepak Ramesh, M.D.
Mary A. Stefanyszyn, M.D.

ONCOLOGY

Consultant

Carol L. Shields, M.D.

PEDIATRICS

Consultants

Alex V. Levin, M.D.
Jade M. Price, M.D.
Bruce M. Schnall, M.D.
Barry N. Wasserman, M.D.
Yoshihiro Yonekawa, M.D.

RETINA

Major Consultants

William E. Benson, M.D.
Sunir J. Garg, M.D.
Omesh P. Gupta, M.D., M.B.A.
Allen C. Ho, M.D.
Jason Hsu, M.D.
Carl D. Regillo, M.D.
James F. Vander, M.D.

Consultants

Julia A. Haller, M.D.
Richard S. Kaiser, M.D.
Marc J. Spirn, M.D.

UVEITIS

Consultants

James P. Dunn, M.D.
Sunir J. Garg, M.D.

GENERAL OPHTHALMOLOGY

Major Consultant

Bruce J. Markovitz, M.D.

Consultants

Elizabeth N. Derham, M.D.
Brad H. Feldman, M.D.
Christina B. McGowan, M.D.

FELLOW CONSULTANTS

Shaza N. Al-Holou, M.D.
Michael J. Ammar, M.D.
John C. Anhalt, M.D.
Jordan D. Deaner, M.D.
Maya Eiger-Moscovich, M.D.
Jason S. Flamendorf, M.D.
Zachary C. Landis, M.D.
Lindsay A. Machen, M.D.
Ravi R. Pandit, M.D., M.P.H.
Luv G. Patel, M.D.
Archana Srinivasan, M.D.
Matthew R. Starr, M.D.
Michael E. Sulewski, Jr., M.D.
Neil R. Vadhar, M.D.
David Xu, M.D.

Foreword

Over a decade ago, in Vientiane with the Orbis Flying Eye Hospital, I was examining patients with a small group of Southeast Asian ophthalmologists from Laos, Cambodia, Vietnam, Thailand, and Myanmar. A middle-aged lady came in with a dense vitritis, and I could see through the haze with an indirect ophthalmoscope to an active macula-threatening toxoplasmosis lesion in the posterior pole. We started reviewing antibiotics available in that part of the world, and to help the discussion, I sent out to the bus where we had stashed a box of latest-edition Wills Eye Manuals. As we paged through the book's section on toxoplasmosis, I became aware of a flurry of hushed whispers in the room, and looked up questioningly at my interpreter to find out what all the fuss was about. "It's your book," he explained, "Everyone is excited to see it. Once they saw a Xeroxed copy of it in Bangkok."

How proud I was to tell the thrilled group that we had an actual copy of the *The Wills Eye Manual* for each of them, brought all the way from Philadelphia! Their palpable delight was a special reciprocal gift.

That pride finds its echo today as I peruse this new edition of what has become a standard work in the Eye Canon, the best-selling book in our field worldwide, compiled originally from a sheaf of famously helpful notes assembled by two Wills residents, Chris Rapuano and Marc Friedberg. That remarkable pocket compendium, shared with their fellow trainees for reference as they worked in the clinics and emergency room, grew into the first manual, published in 1990. Thirty years later, it retains its immediacy and clinical relevance, despite many iterations and changes, most recently to adapt it to online access including expanded video resources – and of course the reason for this is that it is still authored by Wills residents, who know what frontline patient care demands: ready, conveniently available, concise, accurate, and up-to-date information!

This foreword would not be complete without a grateful acknowledgement of the two giants no longer with us, whose editorial skills anchored the book for its previous three decades: Dr. William Tasman and Dr. Edward Jaeger. Peerless and indefatigable proofreaders and advisors, their mentorship and support have been key to the success and reach of the manual. May this new edition of *The Wills Eye Manual* serve as a special salute not only to the Wills Residency that these tremendous academicians served so ably, but also to the legacy of their irreplaceable editorial pen, wise counsel, clinical acumen, and unmatchable collegiality.

Julia A. Haller MD
Ophthalmologist-in-Chief
Wills Eye Hospital

THE WILLS EYE MANUAL EDITORS

First Edition, 1990:
Editors: Mark A. Friedberg, M.D. and Christopher J. Rapuano, M.D.

Second Edition, 1994:
Editors: R. Douglas Cullom, Jr., M.D. and Benjamin Chang, M.D.

Third Edition, 1999:
Editors: Douglas J. Rhee, M.D. and Mark F. Pyfer, M.D.

Fourth Edition, 2004:
Editors: Derek Y. Kunimoto, M.D., Kunal D. Kanitkar, M.D., and Mary S. Makar, M.D.

Fifth Edition, 2008:
Editors: Justis P. Ehlers, M.D. and Chirag P. Shah, M.D.

Associate Editors: Gregory L. Fenton, M.D., Eliza N. Hoskins, M.D., and Heather N. Shelsta, M.D.

Sixth Edition, 2012:
Editors: Adam T. Gerstenblith, M.D. and Michael P. Rabinowitz, M.D.

Associate Editors: Behin I. Barahimi, M.D. and Christopher M. Fecarotta, M.D.

Seventh Edition, 2017:
Editors: Nika Bagheri, M.D. and Brynn N. Wajda, M.D.

Multimedia Editors: Charles M. Calvo, M.D. and Alia K. Durrani, M.D.

Eighth Edition, 2022:
Editors: Kalla A. Gervasio, M.D. and Travis J. Peck, M.D.

Multimedia Editors: Cherie A. Fathy, M.D., M.P.H., and Meera D. Sivalingam, M.D.

Preface

It is our sincere pleasure to present the eighth edition of *The Wills Eye Manual*. This edition arises from the foundation laid by all preceding contributors and, as in years past, would not have been possible without the collaborative efforts, teamwork, and never-satisfied mentality of the Wills Eye residents, fellows, and faculty. Our hope is for readers to find within this text the most up-to-date information and collective clinical recommendations regarding the office and emergency room evaluation, diagnosis, management, and treatment of ophthalmic disease.

The eighth edition includes the results of major clinical trials since the last edition. Changing trends in the workup, categorization, and treatment of various ophthalmic specialties including trauma, oculoplastics, cornea, pediatrics, neuro-ophthalmology, uveitis, and retinal disease are reflected in this current edition. We are proud to share our updated multimedia component of *The Wills Eye Manual*, including an electronic database of various clinical conditions and the addition of new office and emergency room procedures. While incorporating current medical and technological trends, we strived to maintain the original goals of the founding editors, namely to provide a streamlined, concise, and readily accessible resource for healthcare providers approaching patients in need of eye care.

We hope you continue to utilize the eighth edition of *The Wills Eye Manual* and find it to be a convenient, easy-to-use guide for the management of ophthalmic disease.

Kalla A. Gervasio, M.D.

Travis J. Peck, M.D.

Cherie A. Fathy, M.D., M.P.H.,

Meera D. Sivalingam, M.D.

Preface to the First Edition

Our goal has been to produce a concise book, providing essential diagnostic tips and specific therapeutic information pertaining to eye disease. We realized the need for this book while managing emergency room patients at one of the largest and busiest eye hospitals in the country. Until now, reliable information could only be obtained in unwieldy textbooks or inaccessible journals.

As residents at Wills Eye Hospital, we have benefited from the input of some of the world-renowned ophthalmic experts in writing this book. More importantly, we are aware of the questions that the ophthalmology resident, the attending ophthalmologist, and the emergency room physician (not trained in ophthalmology) want answered immediately.

The book is written for the eye care provider who, in the midst of evaluating an eye problem, needs quick access to additional information. We try to be as specific as possible, describing the therapeutic modalities used at our institution. Many of these recommendations are, therefore, not the only manner in which to treat a particular disorder, but indicate personal preference. They are guidelines, not rules.

Because of the forever changing wealth of ophthalmic knowledge, omissions and errors are possible, particularly with regard to management. Drug dosages have been checked carefully, but the physician is urged to check the *Physicians' Desk Reference* or *Facts* and *Comparisons* when prescribing unfamiliar medications. Not all contraindications and side effects are described.

We feel this book will make a welcome companion to the many physicians involved with treating eye problems. It is everything you wanted to know and nothing more.

Christopher J. Rapuano, M.D.

Mark A. Friedberg, M.D.

Contents

Video List

The accompanying ebook includes embedded videos, found in their respective sections as listed below. Each is narrated with audio. Details on how to access the ebook are found in the inside front cover.

▶ **3.8. VIDEO:** Eyelid Laceration Repair

▶ **3.10. VIDEO:** Canthotomy and Cantholysis

▶ **3.11. VIDEO:** Relative Afferent Pupillary Defect

▶ **3.14. VIDEO:** Cyanoacrylate Corneal Glue

▶ **4.11. VIDEO:** Corneal Culture Procedure

▶ **10.5. VIDEO:** Third Cranial Nerve Palsy

▶ **10.7. VIDEO:** Fourth Cranial Nerve Palsy

▶ **10.8. VIDEO:** Sixth Cranial Nerve Palsy

▶ **10.11. VIDEO:** Ocular Myasthenia

▶ **10.13. VIDEO:** Internuclear Ophthalmoplegia

▶ **11.3. VIDEO:** B-scan Ultrasound Tutorial

▶ **11.13. VIDEO:** B-scan Ultrasound Tutorial

▶ **11.27. VIDEO:** B-scan Ultrasound Tutorial

▶ **14.8. VIDEO:** B-scan Ultrasound Tutorial

▶ **Appendix A.7. VIDEO:** Probe and Irrigation

▶ **Appendix A.11. VIDEO:** Intravitreal injection

▶ **Appendix A.11. VIDEO:** Intravitreal Tap and Inject

▶ **Appendix A.13. VIDEO:** Anterior Chamber Paracentesis

Chapter 1

Differential Diagnosis of Ocular Symptoms

BURNING

More Common. Blepharitis, meibomitis, dry eye syndrome, conjunctivitis.

Less Common. Inflamed pterygium or pinguecula, episcleritis, superior limbic keratoconjunctivitis, ocular toxicity (medication, makeup, contact lens solutions), contact lens–related problems.

CROSSED EYES IN CHILDREN

See 8.4, ESODEVIATIONS (eyes turned in), or 8.5, EXODEVIATIONS (eyes turned out).

DECREASED VISION

1. Monocular
   - Acute

Painless. Retinal artery or vein occlusion, ophthalmic artery occlusion, ischemic optic neuropathy, giant cell arteritis, vitreous hemorrhage, retinal detachment, sudden discovery of preexisting unilateral visual loss.

Painful. Corneal lesion (abrasion, ulcer), uveitis, dry eye syndrome, acute angle-closure glaucoma, endophthalmitis, corneal hydrops, optic neuritis (pain with eye movement; however, ~10% of cases are painless).

   - **Transient** (vision returns to normal within 24 hours)

Painless. Amaurosis fugax, optic disc drusen, impending central retinal vein occlusion (CRVO), ocular ischemic syndrome, orthostatic hypotension.

Painful. Migraine, dry eye syndrome, superficial punctate keratopathy.

2. Binocular
   - Acute and/or transient

Painless. Stroke (homonymous hemianopsia), vertebrobasilar insufficiency, ciliary spasm or ciliary body rotation, papilledema.

Painful. Migraine, dry eye syndrome, superficial punctate keratopathy, pituitary apoplexy, papilledema (may have headache).

3. Monocular/binocular
   - **Chronic**

Painless. Refractive error, cataract, open angle glaucoma, chronic angle-closure glaucoma, corneal scar, optic neuropathy, dry eye syndrome, chronic retinal disease (e.g., diabetic retinopathy, age-related macular degeneration [AMD]).

Painful. Dry eye syndrome, superficial punctate keratopathy.

4. Posttraumatic visual loss: Corneal irregularity, hyphema, ruptured globe, traumatic cataract, commotio retinae, retinal detachment, retinal or vitreous hemorrhage, lens dislocation, traumatic optic neuropathy, cranial neuropathies, central nervous system (CNS) injury, sympathetic ophthalmia (rare).

 NOTE: Although a diagnosis of exclusion, remember to consider nonphysiologic vision loss.

DISCHARGE

See "RED EYE" in this chapter.

DISTORTION OF VISION

More Common. Refractive error including astigmatism (e.g., from anterior segment surgery, periorbital or eyelid edema/mass [e.g., chalazion, orbital trauma]), macular disease (e.g., central serous chorioretinopathy, macular edema, and

1

AMD), corneal irregularity (e.g., keratoconus, epithelial basement membrane dystrophy), corneal opacity, intoxication (e.g., ethanol, methanol).

Less Common. Pellucid marginal degeneration, post–refractive surgery corneal ectasia, topical eye drops (e.g., miotics, cycloplegics), retinal detachment, migraine (transient), hypotony, pharmacologic (anticholinergic medications), and nonphysiologic.

DOUBLE VISION (DIPLOPIA)

1. **Monocular** (diplopia remains when the uninvolved eye is occluded)

More Common. Refractive error, incorrect spectacle alignment, corneal opacity or irregularity including keratoconus, cataract, iris defects (e.g., iridectomy), dry eye syndrome, superficial punctate keratopathy.

Less Common. Dislocated natural lens or lens implant, macular disease, CNS causes (rare), nonphysiologic.

2. **Binocular** (diplopia eliminated when either eye is occluded)
   - **Typically intermittent:** Myasthenia gravis, intermittent decompensation of an existing phoria.
   - **Constant:** Isolated sixth, third, or fourth cranial nerve palsy; orbital disease (e.g., thyroid eye disease, carotid cavernous sinus fistula); cavernous sinus syndrome; status-post ocular surgery (e.g., residual anesthesia, displaced muscle, muscle surgery, restriction from scleral buckle, severe aniseikonia after refractive surgery); status-post trauma (e.g., orbital wall fracture with extraocular muscle entrapment, orbital edema); convergence/divergence insufficiency; internuclear ophthalmoplegia; vertebrobasilar artery insufficiency; other CNS lesions; spectacle problem.

DRY EYES

See 4.3, DRY EYE SYNDROME.

EYELASH LOSS

Trauma, burn, cutaneous neoplasm (e.g., sebaceous carcinoma), eyelid infection or inflammation, radiation, chronic skin disease (e.g., alopecia areata), trichotillomania.

EYELID CRUSTING

More Common. Blepharitis, meibomitis, conjunctivitis.

Less Common. Canaliculitis, nasolacrimal duct obstruction, dacryocystitis.

EYELID DROOPING (PTOSIS)

See 6.1, PTOSIS.

EYELID SWELLING

1. **Associated with inflammation** (usually erythematous and tender to palpation).

More Common. Hordeolum, blepharitis, conjunctivitis, preseptal or orbital cellulitis, trauma, contact dermatitis, herpes simplex or varicella zoster dermatitis.

Less Common. Ectropion, corneal pathology, urticaria or angioedema, insect bite, dacryoadenitis, erysipelas, eyelid or lacrimal gland mass, autoimmunities (e.g., discoid lupus, dermatomyositis).

2. **Noninflammatory:** Chalazion; prolapse of orbital fat; eyelid or lacrimal gland mass; foreign body; cardiac, renal, or thyroid disease; superior vena cava syndrome; festoons.

EYELID TWITCH

Orbicularis myokymia (related to fatigue, excess caffeine, medication, or stress), corneal or conjunctival irritation, dry eye syndrome, blepharospasm (bilateral), hemifacial spasm, Tourette syndrome, tic douloureux, albinism/congenital glaucoma (photosensitivity).

INABILITY TO COMPLETELY CLOSE EYELIDS (LAGOPHTHALMOS)

Severe proptosis, ectropion or eyelid laxity, severe chemosis, eyelid scarring, eyelid retractor muscle scarring, seventh cranial nerve palsy, status-post botulinum toxin injections, after facial cosmetic or reconstructive surgery, thyroid eye disease.

EYES "BULGING" (PROPTOSIS)

See 7.1, ORBITAL DISEASE.

EYES "JUMPING" (OSCILLOPSIA)

Acquired nystagmus, internuclear ophthalmoplegia, myasthenia gravis, vestibular function loss, opsoclonus/ocular flutter, superior oblique myokymia, various CNS disorders.

FLASHES OF LIGHT

More Common. Posterior vitreous detachment, retinal break or detachment, migraine, rapid eye movement (particularly in darkness), oculodigital stimulation, dysphotopsias from an intraocular lens.

Less Common. Retinitis/uveitis (e.g., white dot syndromes), CNS (particularly occipital lobe) disorders, vestibulobasilar artery insufficiency, optic neuropathies, entoptic phenomena, drug-related, hallucinations, iatrogenic (e.g., after laser photocoagulation).

FLOATERS

See "Spots in Front of the Eyes" in this chapter.

FOREIGN BODY SENSATION

Dry eye syndrome, blepharitis, conjunctivitis, trichiasis, corneal or conjunctival abnormality (e.g., abrasion, erosion, foreign body, loose/broken suture, exposed suture tail/tube/buckle/hardware, conjunctival cyst, recurrent corneal erosion, superficial punctate keratopathy), contact lens–related problem, episcleritis, pterygium, pinguecula, postoperative.

GLARE

Cataract, pseudophakia, posterior capsular opacity, corneal edema or opacity, pharmacologic dilation, altered pupillary structure or response, status-post refractive surgery, posterior vitreous detachment.

HALLUCINATIONS (FORMED IMAGES)

Posterior vitreous detachment, retinal or choroidal detachment, optic neuropathies, blindness or bilateral eye patching (i.e., Charles Bonnet syndrome), psychosis, parietotemporal lesions, other CNS causes, medications.

HALOS AROUND LIGHTS

Cataract, pseudophakia, posterior capsular opacity, corneal edema from acute angle-closure glaucoma or other causes (e.g., Fuchs dystrophy, aphakic or pseudophakic bullous keratopathy, contact lens overwear), corneal dystrophies, corneal opacity, status-post refractive surgery, discharge, dry eye syndrome, superficial punctate keratopathy, pigment dispersion syndrome, vitreous opacities, drugs (e.g., digitalis, chloroquine).

HEADACHE

See 10.26, Headache.

ITCHY EYES

Conjunctivitis (especially allergic, atopic, and viral), blepharitis, dry eye syndrome, contact dermatitis, giant papillary conjunctivitis, contact lens–related problems.

LIGHT SENSITIVITY (PHOTOPHOBIA)

1. **Abnormal eye examination**

More Common. Corneal abnormality (e.g., abrasion, ulcer, edema), anterior uveitis.

Less Common. Conjunctivitis (mild photophobia), posterior uveitis, scleritis, albinism, aniridia, total color blindness, mydriasis of any etiology (e.g., pharmacologic, traumatic), congenital glaucoma.

2. **Normal eye examination:** Migraine, meningitis, concussion, retrobulbar optic neuritis, subarachnoid hemorrhage, trigeminal neuralgia, lightly pigmented irides.

NIGHT BLINDNESS

More Common. Refractive error (especially undercorrected myopia), advanced glaucoma or optic atrophy, miosis (especially pharmacologic), retinitis pigmentosa, congenital stationary night blindness, after panretinal photocoagulation, drugs (e.g., phenothiazines, chloroquine, quinine).

Less Common. Vitamin A deficiency, gyrate atrophy, choroideremia.

PAIN

1. **Ocular:**
   - Typically mild to moderate: Dry eye syndrome, blepharitis, infectious conjunctivitis, episcleritis, inflamed pinguecula or pterygium, foreign body (corneal or conjunctival), superficial punctate keratopathy, superior limbic keratoconjunctivitis, ocular medication toxicity, contact lens–related problem, postoperative, ocular ischemic syndrome, eye strain from uncorrected refractive error (asthenopia).
   - Typically moderate to severe: Corneal disorder (e.g., abrasion, erosion, infiltrate/ulcer, chemical injury, ultraviolet burn), trauma, anterior uveitis, scleritis, endophthalmitis, acute angle-closure glaucoma.
2. **Periorbital:** Trauma, hordeolum, preseptal cellulitis, dacryocystitis, dermatitis (e.g., contact, chemical, varicella zoster, or herpes simplex), referred pain (e.g., dental, sinus), giant cell arteritis, trigeminal neuralgia.
3. **Orbital:** Trauma, sinusitis, orbital cellulitis, idiopathic orbital inflammatory syndrome, orbital tumor or mass, optic neuritis, acute dacryoadenitis, migraine or cluster headache, microvascular cranial nerve palsy, postherpetic neuralgia.
4. **Asthenopia:** Uncorrected refractive error, phoria or tropia, convergence insufficiency, accommodative spasm, pharmacologic (miotics).

RED EYE

1. **Adnexal causes:** Trichiasis, distichiasis, floppy eyelid syndrome, entropion or ectropion, lagophthalmos, blepharitis, meibomitis, acne rosacea, dacryocystitis, canaliculitis.
2. **Conjunctival causes:** Ophthalmia neonatorum (in infants), conjunctivitis (infectious, chemical, allergic, atopic, vernal, medication toxicity), subconjunctival hemorrhage, inflamed pinguecula, superior limbic keratoconjunctivitis, giant papillary conjunctivitis, conjunctival foreign body, symblepharon and associated etiologies (e.g., mucous membrane pemphigoid, Stevens–Johnson syndrome, toxic epidermal necrolysis), conjunctival neoplasia.
3. **Corneal causes:** Infectious or inflammatory keratitis, contact lens–related problems (see 4.20, CONTACT LENS–RELATED PROBLEMS), corneal foreign body, recurrent corneal erosion, pterygium, neurotrophic keratopathy, medicamentosa, chemical or ultraviolet burn.
4. **Other:** Trauma, postoperative, dry eye syndrome, anterior uveitis, episcleritis, scleritis, endophthalmitis, pharmacologic (e.g., prostaglandin analogs), angle-closure glaucoma, carotid–cavernous fistula (corkscrew conjunctival vessels), cluster headache.

"SPOTS" IN FRONT OF THE EYES

1. **Transient:** Migraine.
2. **Persistent:**

More Common. Vitreous syneresis, posterior vitreous detachment, vitreous hemorrhage, intermediate or posterior uveitis.

Less Common. Hyphema/microhyphema, retinal break or detachment, corneal opacity, or foreign body.

 NOTE: Some patients are referring to a blind spot in their visual field caused by a retinal, optic nerve, or CNS disorder.

TEARING

1. **Adults**
   - **Pain present:** Corneal abnormality (e.g., abrasion, erosion, foreign body or rust ring, edema), anterior uveitis, eyelash or eyelid disorder (e.g., trichiasis, entropion), conjunctival foreign body, dacryocystitis, canaliculitis, trauma.
   - **Minimal/no pain:** Dry eye syndrome, blepharitis, nasolacrimal duct obstruction, punctal occlusion, lacrimal sac mass, ectropion, conjunctivitis (especially allergic and toxic), crocodile tears (congenital or seventh cranial nerve palsy), emotional state.
2. **Children:** Nasolacrimal duct obstruction, congenital glaucoma, corneal or conjunctival foreign body, other irritative disorder.

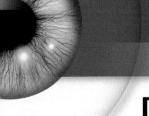

Chapter 2

Differential Diagnosis of Ocular Signs

ANTERIOR CHAMBER/ANTERIOR CHAMBER ANGLE

Hyphema

Trauma, iatrogenic (e.g., intraocular surgery or laser), iris neovascularization, blood dyscrasia or clotting disorder (e.g., hemophilia), anticoagulation, herpes simplex or zoster iridocyclitis, Fuchs heterochromic iridocyclitis, intraocular tumor (e.g., juvenile xanthogranuloma, retinoblastoma, angioma).

Hypopyon

Infectious keratitis, severe anterior uveitis (e.g., HLA-B27 associated, Behçet disease), endophthalmitis, contaminant during intraocular surgery (i.e., toxic anterior segment syndrome), retained lens particle, intraocular foreign body, intraocular tumor necrosis (e.g., pseudohypopyon from retinoblastoma), tight contact lens, severe inflammatory reaction from a recurrent corneal erosion, drugs (e.g., rifampin).

Blood in Schlemm Canal on Gonioscopy

Iatrogenic (compression of episcleral vessels by a gonioprism), Sturge–Weber syndrome, arteriovenous fistula (e.g., carotid–cavernous sinus fistula [c-c fistula]), superior vena cava obstruction, hypotony.

CORNEA/CONJUNCTIVAL FINDINGS

Conjunctival Swelling (Chemosis)

Allergy, ocular or periocular inflammation, postoperative, drugs, venous congestion (e.g., c-c fistula), angioneurotic edema, myxedema.

Conjunctival/Corneal Dryness (Keratoconjunctivitis Sicca)

Exposure (e.g., lagophthalmos, proptosis, poor blink reflex), Sjögren syndrome, vitamin A deficiency, mucous membrane pemphigoid, postcicatricial conjunctivitis, Stevens–Johnson syndrome, radiation, chronic dacryoadenitis.

Corneal Crystals

See 4.14, CRYSTALLINE KERATOPATHY.

Corneal Edema

1. **Congenital:** Birth trauma (e.g., forceps injury), congenital glaucoma, congenital hereditary endothelial dystrophy (bilateral), posterior polymorphous corneal dystrophy (PPCD).
2. **Acquired:** Trauma, chemical injury, contact lens overwear, acute increase in intraocular pressure (e.g., angle-closure glaucoma), corneal hydrops (decompensated keratoconus), herpes simplex or zoster keratitis, uveitis, postoperative edema, aphakic or pseudophakic bullous keratopathy, Fuchs endothelial dystrophy, failed corneal graft, iridocorneal endothelial (ICE) syndrome, PPCD.

Corneal Opacification in Infancy

Birth trauma (e.g., forceps injury), infectious keratitis, metabolic abnormalities (bilateral; e.g., mucopolysaccharidoses), anterior segment dysgenesis (e.g., Peters anomaly, sclerocornea), edema (e.g., congenital glaucoma), congenital hereditary endothelial or stromal dystrophy (bilateral), PPCD, corneal dermoid.

Dilated Episcleral Vessels (Without Ocular Irritation or Pain)

Underlying uveal neoplasm, arteriovenous fistula (e.g., c-c fistula), polycythemia vera, leukemia, ophthalmic vein or cavernous sinus thrombosis, extravascular blockage of ophthalmic or orbital venous outflow.

5

Enlarged Corneal Nerves

Multiple endocrine neoplasia type 2 (i.e., medullary thyroid carcinoma and pheochromocytoma), neurofibromatosis, acanthamoeba keratitis, keratoconus, failed corneal graft, Fuchs endothelial dystrophy, PPCD, multiple myeloma, Refsum syndrome, Riley–Day dysautonomia, trauma, congenital glaucoma, leprosy, ichthyosis, idiopathic, normal variant.

Follicles on the Conjunctiva

See 5.1, ACUTE CONJUNCTIVITIS and 5.2, CHRONIC CONJUNCTIVITIS.

Membranous Conjunctivitis

Classic teaching is that membrane removal is difficult and causes bleeding. Streptococci, pneumococci, *Corynebacterium diphtheriae*, herpes simplex, chemical injury, ligneous conjunctivitis, ocular vaccinia, rarely epidemic keratoconjunctivitis or Stevens–Johnson syndrome (more often causes pseudomembranous conjunctivitis).

Pseudomembranous Conjunctivitis

Classic teaching is that pseudomembrane removal is easy and does not cause bleeding. All the causes of membranous conjunctivitis listed above, gonococci, staphylococci, chlamydia (especially in newborns), mucous membrane pemphigoid, superior limbic keratoconjunctivitis.

Pannus (Superficial Vascular Invasion of the Cornea)

Hypoxia from contact lens tightness or overwear, staphylococcal hypersensitivity, phlyctenule, ocular rosacea, herpes simplex or zoster keratitis, chlamydia (trachoma and inclusion conjunctivitis), chemical injury, superior limbic keratoconjunctivitis (micropannus), vernal keratoconjunctivitis, mucous membrane pemphigoid, aniridia, molluscum contagiosum, leprosy.

Papillae on the Conjunctiva

See 5.1, Acute Conjunctivitis and 5.2, Chronic Conjunctivitis.

Pigmentation/Discoloration of the Conjunctiva

Complexion-associated melanosis (perilimbal), primary acquired melanosis, nevus, melanoma, ocular and oculodermal melanocytosis (blue–gray, not conjunctival but episcleral), Addison disease, pregnancy, radiation, jaundice, resolving subconjunctival hemorrhage, conjunctival or subconjunctival foreign body, pharmacologic (e.g., chlorpromazine, topical epinephrine), cosmetic (e.g., mascara/makeup deposits, tattoo).

Symblepharon (Fusion of the Palpebral and Bulbar Conjunctiva)

Mucous membrane pemphigoid, Stevens–Johnson syndrome, chemical injury, trauma, epidemic keratoconjunctivitis, atopic conjunctivitis, chronic conjunctivitis, radiation, drugs, congenital, iatrogenic (e.g., postsurgical).

Verticillata (Whorl-Like Opacity in the Corneal Epithelium)

Amiodarone, chloroquine, atovaquone, Fabry disease and carrier state, phenothiazines, indomethacin, topical Rho kinase inhibitors (e.g., netarsudil, ripasudil).

EYELID ABNORMALITIES

Eyelid Edema

See "EYELID SWELLING" in Chapter 1, Differential Diagnosis of Ocular Symptoms.

Eyelid Lesion

See 6.11, MALIGNANT TUMORS OF THE EYELID.

Ptosis and Pseudoptosis

See 6.1, PTOSIS.

FUNDUS FINDINGS

Bone Spicules (Widespread Pigment Clumping)

See 11.28, RETINITIS PIGMENTOSA AND INHERITED CHORIORETINAL DYSTROPHIES.

Bull's-Eye Macular Lesion

Age-related macular degeneration (AMD), Stargardt disease or fundus flavimaculatus, albinism, cone dystrophy, rod–cone dystrophy, chloroquine or hydroxychloroquine retinopathy, adult-onset foveomacular vitelliform dystrophy, Spielmeyer–Vogt syndrome, central areolar choroidal dystrophy.

See 11.32, CHLOROQUINE/HYDROXYCHLOROQUINE TOXICITY.

Choroidal Folds

Orbital or choroidal tumor, posterior scleritis, idiopathic orbital inflammatory syndrome, hypotony, thyroid eye disease, retinal detachment, marked hyperopia, scleral laceration, papilledema, postoperative.

Choroidal Neovascularization (Gray–Green Membrane or Blood Deep to the Retina)

More Common. AMD, polypoidal choroidal vasculopathy, ocular histoplasmosis syndrome, high myopia, angioid streaks, choroidal rupture (trauma).

Less Common. Optic nerve head drusen, tumors, retinal scarring after laser photocoagulation, posterior uveitis (e.g., Vogt–Koyanagi–Harada disease, multifocal choroiditis, serpiginous choroiditis), idiopathic.

Cotton–Wool Spots

See 11.5, COTTON–WOOL SPOT.

Embolus

See 10.22, TRANSIENT VISUAL LOSS/AMAUROSIS FUGAX; 11.6, CENTRAL RETINAL ARTERY OCCLUSION; 11.7, BRANCH RETINAL ARTERY OCCLUSION; 11.33, CRYSTALLINE RETINOPATHY.

- Platelet–fibrin (dull gray and elongated): Carotid disease, less commonly cardiac.
- Cholesterol (sparkling yellow, usually at an arterial bifurcation): Carotid disease.
- Calcium (dull white, typically around or on the disc): Cardiac disease.
- Cardiac myxoma (common in young patients, particularly in the left eye; often occludes the ophthalmic or retrobulbar central retinal artery and is not visualized).
- Talc and cornstarch (small, yellow–white glistening particles in macular arterioles; may produce peripheral retinal neovascularization): Intravenous drug use.
- Lipid or air (often see cotton–wool spots rather than emboli): Chest trauma (Purtscher retinopathy) and fracture of long bones.
- Others (tumors, parasites, other foreign bodies).

Macular Exudates

More Common. Diabetes, choroidal neovascular membrane, hypertension.

Less Common. Macroaneurysm, Coats disease (children), peripheral retinal capillary hemangioma, retinal vein occlusion, papilledema, radiation retinopathy.

Normal Fundus With Decreased Vision

Retrobulbar optic neuritis, other optic neuropathy (infiltrative, toxic [e.g., alcohol, tobacco], Leber hereditary optic neuropathy), amblyopia, Stargardt disease or fundus flavimaculatus, cone degeneration, rod monochromatism, cancer-associated retinopathy (CAR), melanoma-associated retinopathy (MAR), nonphysiologic visual loss.

Optociliary Shunt Vessels on the Disc

Orbital or intracranial tumor (especially meningioma), optic nerve glioma, prior central retinal vein occlusion, chronic papilledema (e.g., pseudotumor cerebri), chronic open angle glaucoma.

Retinal Neovascularization

1. **Posterior pole:** Diabetes, prior central retinal vein or artery occlusion.
2. **Peripheral:** Sickle cell retinopathy, prior branch retinal vein occlusion, diabetes, sarcoidosis, syphilis, ocular ischemic syndrome (carotid occlusive disease), pars planitis, Coats disease, retinopathy of prematurity, embolization from i.v. drug abuse (e.g., talc retinopathy), chronic uveitis, leukemia, anemia, Eales disease, familial exudative vitreoretinopathy.

Roth Spots (Retinal Hemorrhages With White Centers)

More Common. Diabetes, leukemia, septic chorioretinitis (e.g., from bacterial endocarditis).

Less Common. Pernicious anemia (and rarely other forms of anemia), sickle cell disease, scurvy, systemic lupus erythematosus, other connective tissue diseases.

Sheathing of Retinal Veins (Periphlebitis)

More Common. Syphilis, sarcoidosis, pars planitis, sickle cell disease.

Less Common. Tuberculosis, multiple sclerosis, Eales disease, viral retinitis (e.g., herpes virus, human immunodeficiency virus), Behçet disease, fungal retinitis, bacteremia.

2

Tumor

See 11.36, CHOROIDAL NEVUS AND MALIGNANT MELANOMA OF THE CHOROID.

INTRAOCULAR PRESSURE

Acute Increase in Intraocular Pressure

Acute angle-closure glaucoma, inflammatory open angle glaucoma, malignant glaucoma, hyphema, glaucomatocyclitic crisis (Posner–Schlossman syndrome), postoperative complications (see "POSTOPERATIVE COMPLICATIONS" in this chapter), suprachoroidal hemorrhage, c-c fistula, spontaneous closure of cyclodialysis cleft, retrobulbar hemorrhage, other orbital disease.

Chronic Increase in Intraocular Pressure

See 9.1, PRIMARY OPEN ANGLE GLAUCOMA, and 9.5, CHRONIC ANGLE-CLOSURE GLAUCOMA.

Decreased Intraocular Pressure (Hypotony)

Ruptured globe, phthisis bulbi, retinal/choroidal detachment, iridocyclitis, severe dehydration, cyclodialysis cleft, ocular ischemia, drugs (e.g., glaucoma medications), postoperative complications (see "POSTOPERATIVE COMPLICATIONS" in this chapter), traumatic ciliary body shutdown.

IRIS

Iris Heterochromia (Irides of Different Colors)

1. **Involved iris is lighter than normal:** Congenital Horner syndrome, most cases of Fuchs heterochromic iridocyclitis, chronic uveitis, juvenile xanthogranuloma, metastatic carcinoma, Waardenburg syndrome.
2. **Involved iris is darker than normal:** Ocular melanocytosis or oculodermal melanocytosis, hemosiderosis, siderosis, retained intraocular foreign body, ocular malignant melanoma, diffuse iris nevus, retinoblastoma, leukemia, lymphoma, ICE syndrome, some cases of Fuchs heterochromic iridocyclitis.

Iris Lesion

1. **Melanotic (brown):** Nevus, melanoma, adenoma, or adenocarcinoma of the iris pigment epithelium.

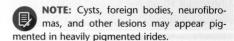
NOTE: Cysts, foreign bodies, neurofibromas, and other lesions may appear pigmented in heavily pigmented irides.

2. **Amelanotic (white, yellow, or orange):** Amelanotic melanoma, inflammatory nodule or granuloma (e.g., sarcoidosis, tuberculosis, leprosy, other granulomatous disease), neurofibroma, patchy hyperemia of syphilis, juvenile xanthogranuloma, medulloepithelioma, foreign body, cyst, leiomyoma, seeding from a posterior segment tumor.

Neovascularization of the Iris

Diabetic retinopathy, ocular ischemic syndrome, prior central or branch retinal vein or artery occlusion, chronic uveitis, chronic retinal detachment, intraocular tumor (e.g., retinoblastoma, melanoma), other retinal vascular disease.

LENS

See Also 13.1, Acquired Cataract.

Dislocated Lens (Ectopia Lentis)

See 13.10, SUBLUXED OR DISLOCATED CRYSTALLINE LENS.

Iridescent Lens Particles

Drugs, hypocalcemia, myotonic dystrophy, hypothyroidism, familial, idiopathic.

Lenticonus

1. Anterior (marked convexity of the anterior lens): Alport syndrome (hereditary nephritis).
2. Posterior (marked concavity of the posterior lens): Usually idiopathic, may be associated with persistent fetal vasculature.

NEUROOPHTHALMIC ABNORMALITIES

Afferent Pupillary Defect

1. **Severe (2+ to 3+):** Optic nerve disease (e.g., ischemic optic neuropathy, optic neuritis, tumor, glaucoma); central retinal artery or vein occlusion; less commonly, a lesion of the optic chiasm or tract; extensive retinal detachment or retinoschisis.
2. **Mild (trace to 1+):** Any of the preceding, amblyopia, dense vitreous hemorrhage, advanced macular degeneration, branch

retinal vein or artery occlusion, less extensive retinal detachment or retinoschisis, or other retinal pathology.

Anisocoria (Pupils of Different Sizes)

See 10.1, ANISOCORIA.

Limitation of Ocular Motility

1. With exophthalmos and resistance to retropulsion: See 7.1, ORBITAL DISEASE.
2. Without exophthalmos or resistance to retropulsion: Isolated third, fourth, or sixth cranial nerve palsy; multiple ocular motor nerve palsies (see 10.10, CAVERNOUS SINUS AND ASSOCIATED SYNDROMES [MULTIPLE OCULAR MOTOR NERVE PALSIES]), myasthenia gravis, chronic progressive external ophthalmoplegia and associated syndromes, orbital blow-out fracture with muscle entrapment, ophthalmoplegic migraine, Duane syndrome, other central nervous system (CNS) disorders.

Optic Disc Atrophy

More Common. Glaucoma; prior central retinal vein or artery occlusion; prior ischemic optic neuropathy; chronic optic neuritis; chronic papilledema; compression of the optic nerve, chiasm, or tract by a tumor or aneurysm; prior traumatic optic neuropathy.

Less Common. Syphilis, retinal degeneration (e.g., retinitis pigmentosa), toxic or metabolic optic neuropathy, Leber hereditary optic atrophy, Leber congenital amaurosis, radiation neuropathy, lysosomal storage disease (e.g., Tay–Sachs disease), other forms of congenital or hereditary optic atrophy (nystagmus almost always present in congenital forms).

Optic Disc Swelling (Edema)

See 10.15, PAPILLEDEMA.

Optociliary Shunt Vessels

See "FUNDUS FINDINGS" in this chapter.

Paradoxical Pupillary Reaction (Pupil Dilates in Light and Constricts in Darkness)

Congenital stationary night blindness, congenital achromatopsia, optic nerve hypoplasia, Leber congenital amaurosis, Best disease, optic neuritis, dominant optic atrophy, albinism, retinitis pigmentosa, rarely amblyopia.

ORBIT

Extraocular Muscle Thickening on Imaging

More Common. Thyroid orbitopathy (often spares tendon), idiopathic orbital inflammatory syndrome (involves tendon).

Less Common. Tumor (e.g., lymphoma, metastasis, or spread of lacrimal gland tumor to muscle), c-c fistula, superior ophthalmic vein thrombosis, cavernous hemangioma (usually appears in the muscle cone without muscle thickening), rhabdomyosarcoma (children).

Lacrimal Gland Lesions

See 7.6, LACRIMAL GLAND MASS/CHRONIC DACRYOADENITIS.

Optic Nerve Lesion (Isolated)

More Common. Optic nerve glioma (especially children), optic nerve meningioma (especially adults).

Less Common. Metastasis, leukemia, idiopathic orbital inflammatory syndrome, sarcoidosis, increased intracranial pressure with secondary optic nerve swelling.

Orbital Lesions/Proptosis

See 7.1, ORBITAL DISEASE.

PEDIATRICS

Leukocoria (White Pupillary Reflex)

See 8.1, LEUKOCORIA.

Nystagmus in Infancy

See ALSO 10.21, NYSTAGMUS.

Congenital nystagmus, spasmus nutans, congenital cataracts, congenital corneal opacities, aniridia, albinism, optic nerve hypoplasia, Leber congenital amaurosis, CNS (thalamic) injury, optic nerve or chiasmal glioma.

POSTOPERATIVE COMPLICATIONS

Shallow Anterior Chamber

1. **Accompanied by increased intraocular pressure:** Pupillary block (acute angle closure) glaucoma, capsular block syndrome, suprachoroidal hemorrhage, malignant glaucoma (aqueous misdirection).

2. **Accompanied by decreased intraocular pressure:** Wound leak, choroidal detachment, overfiltration after glaucoma filtering procedure.

Hypotony

Wound leak, choroidal detachment, cyclodialysis cleft, retinal detachment, ciliary body shutdown, pharmacologic aqueous suppression, overfiltration after glaucoma filtering procedure.

REFRACTIVE PROBLEMS

Progressive Hyperopia

Orbital tumor compressing the posterior globe, elevation of the retina (e.g., subretinal fluid from central serous chorioretinopathy, choroidal thickening from posterior scleritis), presbyopia, hypoglycemia, after radial keratotomy or other refractive surgery.

Progressive Myopia

High (pathologic) myopia, staphyloma and elongation of the globe, diabetes, cataract, corneal ectasia (keratoconus or sequela of corneal refractive surgery), medications (e.g., miotic drops, sulfa drugs, tetracycline), childhood (physiologic).

VISUAL FIELD ABNORMALITIES

Altitudinal Field Defect

More Common. Ischemic optic neuropathy, optic neuritis, hemi- or branch retinal artery or vein occlusion.

Less Common. Glaucoma, optic nerve or chiasmal lesion, optic nerve coloboma.

Arcuate Scotoma

More Common. Glaucoma.

Less Common. Ischemic optic neuropathy (especially nonarteritic), optic disc drusen, high myopia, optic neuritis.

Binasal Field Defect

More Common. Glaucoma, bitemporal retinal disease (e.g., retinitis pigmentosa).

Rare. Bilateral occipital disease, tumor or aneurysm compressing both optic nerves or chiasm, chiasmatic arachnoiditis, nonphysiologic.

Bitemporal Hemianopsia

More Common. Chiasmal lesion (e.g., pituitary adenoma, meningioma, craniopharyngioma, aneurysm, glioma).

Less Common. Tilted optic discs.

Rare. Nasal retinitis pigmentosa.

Blind Spot Enlargement

Papilledema, glaucoma, optic nerve drusen, optic nerve coloboma, myelinated nerve fibers off the disc, drugs, disc with myopic crescent, multiple evanescent white dot syndrome (MEWDS), acute idiopathic blind spot enlargement syndrome (may be on same spectrum as MEWDS).

Central Scotoma

Macular disease, optic neuritis, ischemic optic neuropathy (more typically produces an altitudinal field defect), optic atrophy (e.g., from tumor compressing the nerve, toxic or metabolic disease), rarely an occipital cortex lesion.

Constriction of the Peripheral Fields Leaving a Small Central Field (Tunnel Vision)

Glaucoma, retinitis pigmentosa or other peripheral retinal disorders (e.g., gyrate atrophy), chronic papilledema, sequela of panretinal photocoagulation or cryotherapy, central retinal artery occlusion with cilioretinal artery sparing, bilateral occipital lobe infarction with macular sparing, nonphysiologic visual loss, medications (e.g., phenothiazines), vitamin A deficiency, carcinoma, melanoma, autoimmune-associated retinopathy.

Homonymous Hemianopsia

Temporal, parietal, or occipital lobe lesion of the brain (e.g., stroke and tumor more commonly; aneurysm and trauma less commonly), optic tract or lateral geniculate body lesion, migraine (transiently).

VITREOUS

Vitreous Opacities

Asteroid hyalosis, vitreous hemorrhage, inflammatory cells from vitritis or posterior uveitis, snowball opacities of pars planitis or sarcoidosis, normal vitreous strands from age-related vitreous degeneration, tumor cells, foreign body, hyaloid remnants, synchysis scintillans, rarely amyloidosis, or Whipple disease.

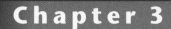

Chapter 3

Trauma

3.1 Chemical Burn

Treatment should be instituted IMMEDIATELY, even before testing vision, unless an open globe is suspected.

> **NOTE:** This includes alkali (e.g., lye, cements, plasters, airbag powder, bleach, ammonia), acids (e.g., battery acid, pool cleaner, vinegar), solvents, detergents, and irritants (e.g., mace).

Emergency Treatment

1. Copious but gentle irrigation using saline or Ringer lactate solution. Tap water can be used in the absence of these solutions and may be more efficacious in inhibiting elevated intracameral pH than normal saline for alkali burns. NEVER use acidic solutions to neutralize alkalis or vice versa as acid–base reactions themselves can generate harmful substrates and cause secondary thermal injuries. An eyelid speculum and topical anesthetic (e.g., proparacaine) may be placed prior to irrigation. Upper and lower fornices must be everted and irrigated. After exclusion of open globe injury, particulate matter should be flushed or manually removed. Manual use of intravenous tubing connected to an irrigation solution best facilitates the irrigation process.

2. Wait 5 to 10 minutes after irrigation is stopped to allow the dilutant to be absorbed; then check the pH in the fornices using litmus paper. Irrigation is continued until neutral pH is achieved (i.e., 7.0 to 7.4). The pH should be read before the litmus paper dries.

> **NOTE:** The volume of irrigation fluid required to reach neutral pH varies with the chemical and with the duration of the chemical exposure. The volume required may range from a few liters to many liters (over 10 L).

3. Conjunctival fornices should be swept with a moistened cotton-tipped applicator to remove any sequestered particles of caustic material and necrotic conjunctiva, especially in the case of a persistently abnormal pH. If there is concern for retained material, double eversion of the eyelids with Desmarres eyelid retractors may be performed to identify and remove particles in the deep fornix.

4. Acidic or basic foreign bodies embedded in the conjunctiva, cornea, sclera, or surrounding tissues may require surgical excision.

MILD TO MODERATE BURNS

Signs

Critical. Corneal epithelial defects range from scattered superficial punctate keratopathy (SPK), to focal epithelial loss, to sloughing of the entire corneal epithelium. No significant areas of perilimbal ischemia are seen (i.e., no blanching of the conjunctival or episcleral vessels).

Other. Focal areas of conjunctival epithelial defect, chemosis, hyperemia, hemorrhages, or a combination of these; mild eyelid edema; mild anterior chamber (AC) reaction; first- and second-degree burns of the periocular skin with or without lash loss.

> **NOTE:** If you suspect a corneal epithelial defect but do not see one with fluorescein staining, repeat the fluorescein application to the eye. Sometimes the defect is slow to take up the dye. If the entire epithelium sloughs off, only Bowman membrane remains, which may take up fluorescein poorly.

Workup

1. History: Time of injury? Specific type of chemical? Time from exposure until irrigation

3

started? Duration, amount, and type of irrigation? Eye protection? Sample of agent, package/label, or material safety data sheets are helpful in identifying and treating the exposing agent.

2. Slit lamp examination with fluorescein staining. Eyelid eversion to search for foreign bodies. Evaluate for and diagram conjunctival and corneal epithelial defects and ulcerations. Check the intraocular pressure (IOP). In the presence of a distorted cornea, IOP may be most accurately measured with a Tono-Pen, pneumotonometer, or rebound tonometer. Gentle palpation may be used if necessary.

Treatment

1. See EMERGENCY TREATMENT above.
2. Consider cycloplegic (e.g., cyclopentolate 1% or 2%, homatropine 5% b.i.d. to t.i.d.) if significant photophobia, pain, or AC inflammation. If limbal ischemia is suspected, avoid phenylephrine because of its vasoconstrictive properties.
3. Frequent (e.g., q1–2h while awake) use of preservative-free artificial tear drops, artificial tear, or antibiotic ointment (e.g., erythromycin, bacitracin) depending on presence and size of corneal and/or conjunctival epithelial defects.
4. Consider topical steroids (e.g., prednisolone acetate 1% q.i.d.) as adjunctive treatment with topical antibiotic (e.g., trimethoprim/polymyxin B or fluoroquinolone drops q.i.d.) for a week even if epithelial defect is present, especially for an alkali injury.
5. Oral pain medication (e.g., acetaminophen with or without codeine) as needed.
6. If IOP is elevated, acetazolamide 250 mg p.o. q.i.d., acetazolamide 500 mg sequel p.o. b.i.d., or methazolamide 25 to 50 mg p.o. b.i.d. or t.i.d. may be given. Electrolytes, especially potassium, should be monitored in patients on these medications. Add a topical beta-blocker (e.g., timolol 0.5% b.i.d.) if additional IOP control is required. Alpha-agonists should be avoided because of their vasoconstrictive properties, especially if limbal ischemia is present.

Follow Up

Initially daily, then every few days until corneal epithelial defect is healed. Topical steroids should be initiated if there is significant inflammation. Monitor for corneal epithelial breakdown, stromal thinning, and infection.

SEVERE BURNS

Signs (in addition to the above)

(See Figure 3.1.1.)

Critical. Pronounced chemosis and conjunctival blanching, corneal edema and opacification, a moderate to severe AC reaction (may not be appreciated if the cornea is opaque).

Other. Increased IOP, second- and third-degree burns of the surrounding skin, and local necrotic retinopathy as a result of direct penetration of alkali through the sclera.

Workup

Same as for mild-to-moderate burns.

Treatment

1. See EMERGENCY TREATMENT above.
2. Hospital admission may be needed for close monitoring of IOP and corneal healing.
3. Debride necrotic tissue containing foreign matter.
4. Cycloplegic (e.g., cyclopentolate 1% or 2% b.i.d. to t.i.d., homatropine 5% b.i.d. to t.i.d., or atropine 1% daily to b.i.d.). Avoid phenylephrine due to vasoconstriction.
5. Topical antibiotic (e.g., trimethoprim/polymyxin B or fluoroquinolone drops q.i.d.; erythromycin or bacitracin ointment q.i.d.

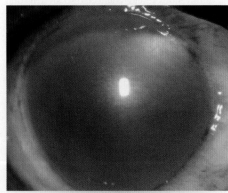

Figure 3.1.1 Alkali burn.

3

to q2h while awake). Caution with cipro-floxacin and large epithelial defects as it can precipitate in the cornea.

6. Topical steroid (e.g., prednisolone acetate 1% or dexamethasone 0.1% q.i.d. to q2h while awake) with concurrent antibiotic coverage even in the presence of an epithelial defect, especially if significant AC or corneal inflammation is present. May use a combination antibiotic/steroid such as tobramycin/dexamethasone drops or ointment q1–2h while awake.

7. IOP-lowering medications as above if the IOP is increased or cannot be determined.

8. Frequent (e.g., q1h while awake) use of preservative-free artificial tears or gel if not using frequent ointments.

9. Oral tetracyclines and vitamin C may also reduce collagenolysis and stromal melting (e.g., doxycycline 100 mg p.o. b.i.d. and vitamin C 1,000 mg p.o. daily).

10. Lysis of conjunctival adhesions b.i.d. by sweeping the fornices may be helpful. If symblepharon begins to form despite attempted lysis, consider using an amniotic membrane ring (e.g., ProKera Plus Ring) or scleral shell to maintain the fornices.

11. In severe cases with large areas of epithelial loss on the bulbar and forniceal conjunctival surfaces, consider suturing a very large amniotic membrane into the fornices.

12. Other considerations:
    - For poorly healing epithelial defects, a therapeutic soft contact lens, collagen shield, amniotic membrane graft (e.g., sutured/glued or self-retained membrane), or tarsorrhaphy may be considered.
    - Ascorbate and citrate for alkali burns has been reported to speed healing time and allow better visual outcome. Administration has been studied intravenously (i.v.), orally (ascorbate 500 to 2,000 mg daily), and topically (ascorbate 10% q1h). Caution in patients with renal compromise secondary to potential renal toxicity.
    - If any melting of the cornea occurs, other collagenase inhibitors may be used (e.g., acetylcysteine 10% to 20% drops q4h while awake).
    - Topical biologic fluids including autologous serum tears, platelet-rich plasma,

umbilical cord serum, and amniotic membrane suspensions may be useful to promote epithelialization.
    - If the melting progresses (or the cornea perforates), consider cyanoacrylate tissue adhesive. An emergency patch graft or corneal transplantation may be necessary; however, the prognosis for grafts is better if performed long after initial injury (over 12 to 18 months).

Follow Up

These patients need to be monitored closely, either as inpatients or daily initially as outpatients. Topical steroids should be tapered after 7 to 14 days, because they can promote corneal melting. If prolonged anti-inflammatory treatment is needed, consider switching to medroxyprogesterone acetate 1% to prevent corneal stromal melting. Long-term use of preservative-free artificial tears q1–6h and lubricating ointments q.h.s. to q.i.d. may be required. A severely dry eye may require a tarsorrhaphy or a conjunctival flap. Conjunctival or limbal stem cell transplantation from the fellow eye may be performed in unilateral injuries that fail to heal within several weeks to several months.

SUPER GLUE (CYANOACRYLATE) INJURY TO THE EYE

 NOTE: Rapid-setting super glues harden quickly on contact with moisture.

Treatment

1. If the eyelids are glued together, they can often be separated with gentle traction. Lashes may need to be cut to separate the eyelids. Misdirected lashes, hardened glue mechanically rubbing the cornea, and glue adherent to the cornea should be carefully removed with fine forceps. Copious irrigation with warm normal saline, warm compresses, or ointment may be used to loosen hardened glue on the eyelids, eyelashes, cornea, or conjunctiva.

2. Epithelial defects are treated as corneal abrasions (see 3.2, CORNEAL ABRASION).

3. Warm compresses q.i.d. may help remove any remaining glue stuck in the lashes that did not require urgent removal.

4. If complete removal of glue is not possible from the eyelid margin, a bandage contact lens may be applied along with topical antibiotic drop therapy until the glue falls off.

Follow Up

Initially daily, then every few days until all corneal epithelial defects are healed.

3.2   Corneal Abrasion

Symptoms

Sharp pain, photophobia, foreign body sensation, tearing, discomfort with blinking, blurred vision, and history of scratching or hitting the eye.

Signs

(See Figure 3.2.1.)

Critical. Epithelial defect that stains with fluorescein; absence of underlying corneal opacification (presence of which indicates infection or inflammation).

Other. Conjunctival injection, swollen eyelid, and mild AC reaction.

Differential Diagnosis

- Recurrent erosion (see 4.2, RECURRENT CORNEAL EROSION).
- Herpes simplex keratitis (see 4.15, HERPES SIMPLEX VIRUS).
- Confluent SPK (see 4.1, SUPERFICIAL PUNCTATE KERATOPATHY).
- Ultraviolet keratopathy (see 4.7, ULTRAVIOLET KERATOPATHY).

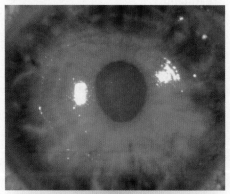

Figure 3.2.1 Corneal abrasion with fluorescein staining.

- Exposure keratopathy (see 4.5, EXPOSURE KERATOPATHY).
- Neurotrophic keratopathy (see 4.6, NEUROTROPHIC KERATOPATHY).
- Chemical burn (see 3.1, CHEMICAL BURN).

Workup

1. Slit lamp examination: Use fluorescein dye, measure the size (e.g., height and width) of the abrasion, and diagram its location. Evaluate for foreign body, infiltrate (underlying corneal opacification), AC reaction, hyphema, corneal laceration, and penetrating trauma.
2. Evert the eyelids to ensure that no foreign body is present, especially in the presence of vertical or linear abrasions.

Treatment

1. Antibiotic
   - Noncontact lens wearer: Antibiotic ointment (e.g., erythromycin, bacitracin, or bacitracin/polymyxin B q2–4h while awake) or antibiotic drops (e.g., polymyxin B/trimethoprim or a fluoroquinolone q.i.d.). Abrasions secondary to fingernails or vegetable matter should be covered with a fluoroquinolone drop (e.g., ofloxacin, moxifloxacin, besifloxacin) or ointment (e.g., ciprofloxacin) at least q.i.d.
   - Contact lens wearer: Must have antipseudomonal coverage (i.e., fluoroquinolone). May use antibiotic ointment or antibiotic drops at least q.i.d.

NOTE: The decision to use drops versus ointment depends on the needs of the patient. Ointments offer better barrier and lubricating function between eyelid and abrasion but tend to blur vision temporarily. They may be used to augment drops at bedtime. We prefer frequent ointments.

2. Cycloplegic agent (e.g., cyclopentolate 1% to 2% b.i.d. or t.i.d.) for traumatic iritis, which may develop 24 to 72 hours after trauma. Avoid steroid use for iritis with epithelial defects because it may impede epithelial healing and increase infection risk. Avoid use of long-acting cycloplegics for small abrasions to allow for faster visual recovery.

3. Patching is rarely necessary and can cause a serious abrasion if not applied properly. Patching should be avoided in all contact lens–related corneal abrasions due to higher risk of infection.

4. Consider a short course of topical nonsteroidal anti-inflammatory drug (NSAID) drops (e.g., ketorolac 0.4% to 0.5% q.i.d. for 3 days) for pain control. Avoid in patients with other ocular surface disease. Oral acetaminophen, NSAIDs, or narcotics (in severe cases) can also be used for pain control.

NOTE: Never prescribe topical anesthetics (e.g., proparacaine, tetracaine) for analgesia, as this may delay epithelial healing and increase infection and ulceration risk.

5. Debride loose or hanging epithelium because it may inhibit healing. A cotton-tipped applicator soaked in topical anesthetic (e.g., proparacaine) or sterile jeweler's forceps (used with caution) may be utilized.

6. Bandage contact lenses may be used to improve comfort and protect the epithelium during healing. Contact lenses are rarely used in the emergency room setting out of concern for patient compliance and follow up. If a bandage contact lens is placed, patients should use prophylactic topical antibiotics (e.g., polymyxin B/trimethoprim or a fluoroquinolone q.i.d.) and should be monitored closely for epithelial healing and contact lens replacement. Do not use for abrasions associated with contact lens wear or if any concern for infection exists.

Follow Up

Noncontact Lens Wearer

1. If patched or given bandage contact lens, the patient should return in 24 hours (or sooner if symptoms worsen) for reevaluation.

2. Central or large corneal abrasion: Return the next day to determine if the epithelial defect is improving. If the abrasion is healing, may see 2 to 3 days later. Instruct patient to return sooner if symptoms worsen. Revisit every 3 to 5 days until healed.

3. Peripheral or small abrasion: Return 2 to 5 days later. Instruct patient to return sooner if symptoms worsen. Revisit every 3 to 5 days until healed.

Contact Lens Wearer

Close follow up until the epithelial defect resolves, and then treat with topical antibiotic (e.g., fluoroquinolone drops) for an additional 1 or 2 days. The patient may resume contact lens wear after the eye feels normal for a week after cessation of a proper medication course. A new contact lens should be used at that time.

3.3 Corneal and Conjunctival Foreign Bodies

Symptoms

Foreign body sensation, tearing, pain, and redness.

Signs

(See Figure 3.3.1.)

Critical. Conjunctival or corneal foreign body with or without a rust ring.

Other. Conjunctival injection, eyelid edema, mild AC reaction, and SPK. A small infiltrate may surround a corneal foreign body; it is usually reactive and sterile. Vertically oriented linear corneal abrasions or SPK may indicate a foreign body under the upper eyelid.

Workup

1. History: Determine the mechanism of injury (e.g., metal striking metal, power tools or weed-whackers, direct pathway with no safety glasses, distance of the patient from the instrument of injury, etc.). Attempt to determine the size, shape, velocity, force, and composition of the object. Always keep in mind the possibility of an intraocular foreign body (IOFB).

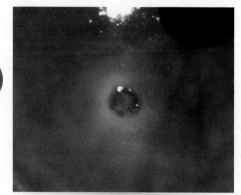

Figure 3.3.1 Corneal metallic foreign body with rust ring.

2. Document visual acuity before any procedure is performed. One or two drops of topical anesthetic may be necessary to facilitate the examination.

3. Slit lamp examination: Locate and assess the depth of the foreign body. Examine closely for possible entry sites (rule out self-sealing lacerations), pupil irregularities, iris tears and transillumination defects (TIDs), lens capsular perforations, lens opacities, hyphema, AC shallowing (or deepening in scleral perforations), and asymmetrically low IOP in the involved eye.

NOTE: There may be multiple foreign bodies with injuries due to power equipment or explosive debris.

If there is no evidence of perforation, evert the eyelids and inspect the fornices for additional foreign bodies. Double everting the upper eyelid with a Desmarres eyelid retractor may be necessary. Carefully inspect conjunctival lacerations to rule out an underlying scleral laceration or perforation. Measure and diagram the dimensions of any corneal or scleral infiltrate and the degree of any AC reaction for monitoring therapy response and progression of possible infection.

NOTE: An infiltrate accompanied by a significant AC reaction, purulent discharge, or extreme conjunctival injection and pain should be cultured to rule out infection, treated aggressively with antibiotics, and followed closely (see 4.11, BACTERIAL KERATITIS).

4. Dilate the eye and examine the posterior segment for possible IOFB (see 3.15, INTRAOCULAR FOREIGN BODY).

5. Consider B-scan ultrasonography, computed tomography (CT) scan of the orbit (axial, coronal, and parasagittal views, 1-mm sections), or ultrasound biomicroscopy (UBM) to exclude an intraocular or intraorbital foreign body. While we prefer a CT scan, a plain film x-ray can also be used to rule out radiodense foreign bodies. Avoid magnetic resonance imaging (MRI) if there is a history of possible metallic foreign body.

Treatment

Corneal Foreign Body (Superficial or Partial Thickness)

1. Apply topical anesthetic (e.g., proparacaine). Remove the corneal foreign body with a foreign body spud or fine forceps such as jeweler's forceps at a slit lamp. Multiple superficial foreign bodies may be more easily removed by irrigation.

NOTE: If there is concern for full-thickness corneal foreign body, exploration and removal should be performed in the operating room.

2. Remove the rust ring as completely as possible on the first visit. This may require an ophthalmic burr **(see Figure 3.3.2)**. It is sometimes safer to leave a deep, central rust ring to allow time for the rust to migrate to

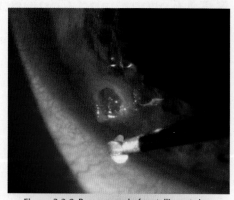

Figure 3.3.2 Burr removal of metallic rust ring.

the corneal surface, at which point it can be removed more easily.

3. Measure and diagram the size of the resultant corneal epithelial defect.

4. Treat as indicated for corneal abrasion (see 3.2, CORNEAL ABRASION).

NOTE: Erythromycin ointment should not be used for residual epithelial defects from corneal foreign bodies as it does not provide strong enough antibiotic coverage.

5. Alert the patient to return as soon as possible if there is any worsening of symptoms.

6. Counsel patient about protective eye wear.

Conjunctival Foreign Body

1. Remove foreign body under topical anesthesia.
   - Multiple or loose superficial foreign bodies can often be removed with saline irrigation.
   - A foreign body can be removed with a cotton-tipped applicator soaked in topical anesthetic or with fine forceps. For deeply embedded foreign bodies, consider pretreatment with a cotton-tipped applicator soaked in phenylephrine 2.5% to reduce conjunctival bleeding.
   - Small, relatively inaccessible, buried subconjunctival foreign bodies may sometimes be left in the eye without harm unless they are infectious or proinflammatory. Occasionally, they will surface with time, at which point they may be removed more easily. Conjunctival excision is sometimes indicated.
   - Check the pH if an associated chemical injury is suspected (e.g., alkali from fireworks). See 3.1, CHEMICAL BURN.

2. Sweep the conjunctival fornices with a cotton-tipped applicator soaked with a topical anesthetic to remove any remaining pieces.

3. See 3.4, CONJUNCTIVAL LACERATION if there is a significant conjunctival laceration.

4. A topical antibiotic (e.g., bacitracin ointment, trimethoprim/polymyxin B drops, or fluoroquinolone drops q.i.d.) may be used.

5. Preservative-free artificial tears may be given as needed for irritation.

Follow Up

1. **Corneal foreign body:** Follow up as with corneal abrasion (see 3.2, CORNEAL ABRASION). If residual rust ring remains, reevaluate in 24 hours.

2. **Conjunctival foreign body:** Follow up as needed, or in 1 week if residual foreign bodies were left in the conjunctiva.

3.4 Conjunctival Laceration

Symptoms

Pain, redness, and/or foreign body sensation, with a history of trauma.

Signs

Fluorescein staining of the conjunctiva. The conjunctiva may be torn and rolled up on itself. Exposed white sclera may be noted. Conjunctival and subconjunctival hemorrhages are often present.

Workup

1. History: Determine the nature of the trauma and whether a ruptured globe or intraocular or intraorbital foreign body may be present. Evaluate the mechanism for possible foreign body involvement, including size, shape, and velocity of object.

2. Complete ocular examination, including careful exploration of the sclera (after topical anesthesia, e.g., proparacaine or viscous lidocaine) in the region of the conjunctival laceration to rule out scleral laceration or subconjunctival foreign body. The entire area of sclera under the conjunctival laceration must be inspected. Since the conjunctiva is mobile, inspect a wide area of the sclera under the laceration. Use a proparacaine-soaked, sterile cotton-tipped applicator to manipulate the conjunctiva. Irrigation with saline may be helpful in removing scattered debris. A Seidel test may be helpful (see APPENDIX 5, SEIDEL TEST TO DETECT A WOUND LEAK). Cellulose surgical

spears may be helpful for detecting vitreous through a wound. Dilated fundus examination, especially evaluating the area underlying the conjunctival injury, must be carefully performed with indirect ophthalmoscopy.

3. Consider a CT scan of the orbit without contrast (axial, coronal, and parasagittal views, 1-mm sections) to exclude an intraocular or intraorbital foreign body. B-scan ultrasound or UBM may be helpful.

4. Exploration of the site in the operating room under general anesthesia may be necessary when a ruptured globe is suspected, especially in children.

Treatment

In case of a ruptured globe or penetrating ocular injury, see 3.14, RUPTURED GLOBE AND PENETRATING OCULAR INJURY. Otherwise,

1. Antibiotic ointment (e.g., erythromycin, bacitracin, or bacitracin/polymyxin B q.i.d.). A pressure patch may rarely be used for the first 24 hours for comfort.

2. Most lacerations will heal without surgical repair. Some large lacerations (≥1 to 1.5 cm) may be sutured with 8-0 polyglactin 910 (e.g., Vicryl) or 6-0 plain gut. When suturing, take care not to bury folds of conjunctiva or incorporate Tenon capsule into the wound. Avoid suturing the plica semilunaris or caruncle to the conjunctiva.

Follow Up

If there is no concomitant ocular damage, patients with large conjunctival lacerations are reexamined within 1 week. Patients with small injuries are seen at longer intervals and instructed to return immediately if symptoms worsen.

3.5 Traumatic Iritis

Symptoms

Dull, aching, or throbbing pain, photophobia, tearing, occasionally floaters, and onset of symptoms usually within 1 to 3 days of trauma.

Signs

Critical. White blood cells (WBCs) and flare in the AC (seen under high-power magnification by focusing into the AC with a small, bright, tangential beam from the slit lamp).

Other. Pain in the traumatized eye when light enters either eye (consensual photophobia); lower (due to ciliary body shock/shutdown) or higher (due to inflammatory debris and/or trabeculitis) IOP than fellow eye; smaller, poorly dilating pupil or larger pupil (often due to iris sphincter tears) in the traumatized eye; perilimbal conjunctival injection; decreased vision.

Differential Diagnosis

- Nongranulomatous anterior uveitis: No history of trauma, or the degree of trauma is not consistent with the level of inflammation. See 12.1, ANTERIOR UVEITIS (IRITIS/IRIDOCYCLITIS).
- Traumatic microhyphema or hyphema: Red blood cells (RBCs) in the AC. See 3.6, HYPHEMA AND MICROHYPHEMA.

- Traumatic corneal abrasion: May have an accompanying sterile AC reaction. See 3.2, CORNEAL ABRASION.
- Traumatic retinal detachment: May produce an AC reaction or demonstrate pigment in the anterior vitreous. See 11.3, RETINAL DETACHMENT.

Workup

Complete ophthalmic examination, including IOP measurement and dilated fundus examination.

Treatment

Cycloplegic agent (e.g., cyclopentolate 1% or 2% b.i.d. to t.i.d.). May use a steroid drop (e.g., prednisolone acetate 0.125% to 1% q.i.d.). Avoid topical steroids if an epithelial defect is present.

Follow Up

1. Recheck in 5 to 7 days.

2. If resolved, discontinue the cycloplegic agent and taper steroid drops if using.

3. Around 1 month after trauma, perform gonioscopy to look for angle recession and indirect ophthalmoscopy with scleral depression to detect retinal breaks or detachment.

3.6 Hyphema and Microhyphema

TRAUMATIC HYPHEMA

Symptoms

Pain, blurred vision, and history of blunt or penetrating trauma.

Signs

(See Figure 3.6.1.)

Clotted or unclotted blood in the AC, usually visible without a slit lamp. A total (100%) hyphema may be black or red. When black, it is called an "8-ball" or "blackball" hyphema, indicating deoxygenated blood; when red, the circulating blood cells may settle with time to become less than a 100% hyphema.

Workup

1. History: Mechanism (including force, velocity, type, and direction) of injury? Protective eyewear? Time of injury? Recent intraocular surgery? Time and extent of visual loss? Maximal visual compromise usually occurs at the time of injury; decreasing vision over time suggests a rebleed or continued bleed (which may cause an IOP rise). Use of anticoagulant medications (e.g., aspirin, NSAIDs, warfarin, or clopidogrel)? Personal or family history of sickle cell disease or trait? Coagulopathy symptoms (e.g., bloody nose blowing, bleeding gums with tooth brushing, easy bruising, bloody stool)?

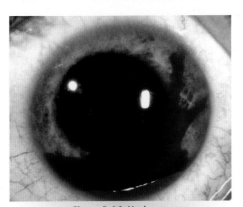

Figure 3.6.1 Hyphema.

2. Ocular examination: First rule out a ruptured globe (see 3.14, RUPTURED GLOBE AND PENETRATING OCULAR INJURY). Evaluate for other traumatic injuries. Document the extent (e.g., measure hyphema height) and location of any clot and blood. Measure the IOP. Perform a dilated retinal evaluation without scleral depression. Consider gentle B-scan ultrasound if the fundus view is poor. Avoid gonioscopy unless intractable increased IOP develops, but if necessary, perform gently. If the view is poor, consider UBM to better evaluate the anterior segment and look for possible lens capsule rupture, IOFB, or other anterior-segment abnormalities.

3. Consider a CT scan of the orbits and brain (axial, coronal, and parasagittal views, 1-mm sections through the orbits) when indicated (e.g., suspected orbital fracture or IOFB, loss of consciousness).

4. Patients should be screened for sickle cell trait or disease (order Sickledex screen; if necessary, may check hemoglobin electrophoresis) as clinically appropriate.

Treatment

Many aspects remain controversial, including whether hospitalization and absolute bed rest are necessary, but an atraumatic upright environment is essential. Consider hospitalization for noncompliant patients, patients with bleeding diathesis or blood dyscrasia, other severe ocular or orbital injuries, and/or concomitant significant IOP elevation and sickle cell trait or disease. Additionally, consider hospitalization and aggressive treatment for children, especially those at risk for amblyopia (e.g., those younger than 7 to 10 years), when a thorough clinical examination is difficult, or when child abuse is suspected.

1. Confine either to bed rest with bathroom privileges or to limited activity. Elevate the head of the bed to allow blood to settle. Discourage strenuous activity, bending, or heavy lifting.

2. Place a rigid shield (metal or clear plastic) over the involved eye at all times. Do not patch because this prevents recognition of sudden visual change in the event of a rebleed.

3

3. Cycloplege the affected eye (e.g., cyclopentolate 1% or 2% b.i.d. to t.i.d., homatropine 5% b.i.d. to t.i.d., or atropine 1% daily to b.i.d.).

4. Avoid antiplatelet/anticoagulant medications (i.e., aspirin-containing products and NSAIDs) unless otherwise medically necessary. Do not abruptly stop daily aspirin regimen without consulting with prescribing physicians.

5. Mild analgesics only (e.g., acetaminophen). Avoid sedatives.

6. Use topical steroids (e.g., prednisolone acetate 1% q.i.d. to q1h) if any suggestion of iritis (e.g., photophobia, deep ache, ciliary flush), evidence of lens capsule rupture, any protein (e.g., fibrin), or definitive WBCs in AC. Taper steroids quickly as soon as signs and symptoms resolve to reduce the likelihood of steroid-induced glaucoma.

NOTE: No definitive evidence exists regarding steroid use in improving outcomes for hyphemas. Use must be balanced with the risks of topical steroids (increased infection potential, increased IOP, cataract). In children, particular caution must be used regarding topical steroids. Children may get rapid rises in IOP, and with prolonged use, there is a risk for cataract. As outlined above, in certain cases, steroids may be beneficial, but steroids should be prescribed in an individualized manner. Children must be monitored closely for increased IOP and should be tapered off steroids as soon as possible.

7. For increased IOP:
   - Non–sickle cell disease or trait (≥30 mm Hg):
     - Start with a beta-blocker (e.g., timolol or levobunolol 0.5% b.i.d.).
     - If IOP is still high, add topical alpha-agonist (e.g., apraclonidine 0.5% or brimonidine 0.1% or 0.2% t.i.d.) or topical carbonic anhydrase inhibitor (e.g., dorzolamide 2% or brinzolamide 1% t.i.d.). Avoid prostaglandin analogues and miotics (may increase inflammation). In children younger than 2 years, topical alpha-agonists are contraindicated.

NOTE: Increased IOP, especially soon after trauma, may be transient, secondary to acute mechanical plugging of the trabecular meshwork. Elevating the patient's head may decrease IOP by causing RBCs to settle inferiorly and clot.

- If topical therapy fails, add acetazolamide (up to 500 mg p.o. q12h for adults, 20 mg/kg/d divided three times per day for children) or mannitol (1 to 2 g/kg i.v. over 45 minutes q24h). If mannitol is necessary to control the IOP, surgical evacuation may be imminent.
- Sickle cell disease or trait (≥24 mm Hg):
  - Start with a beta-blocker (e.g., timolol or levobunolol 0.5% b.i.d.).
  - All other agents must be used with extreme caution: Topical dorzolamide and brinzolamide may reduce aqueous pH and induce increased sickling; topical alpha-agonists (e.g., brimonidine or apraclonidine) may affect iris vasculature; miotics and prostaglandins may promote inflammation.
  - If possible, avoid systemic diuretics because they promote sickling by inducing systemic acidosis and volume contraction. If a carbonic anhydrase inhibitor is necessary, use methazolamide (50 or 100 mg p.o. b.i.d. to t.i.d.) instead of acetazolamide (controversial). If mannitol is necessary to control the IOP, surgical evacuation may be imminent.
  - AC paracentesis may be considered if IOP cannot be safely lowered medically (see APPENDIX 13, ANTERIOR CHAMBER PARACENTESIS). This procedure is typically a temporizing measure when the need for urgent surgical evacuation is anticipated.

8. If hospitalized, use antiemetics p.r.n. for severe nausea or vomiting (e.g., ondansetron 4 or 8 mg q4–8h p.r.n.; if <12 years of age, please refer to the appropriate dosing instructions). **Indications for surgical evacuation of hyphema:**
   - Corneal stromal blood staining, especially in children.
   - Significant visual deterioration.
   - Hyphema that does not decrease to ≤50% by 8 days (to prevent peripheral anterior synechiae).
   - IOP ≥60 mm Hg for ≥48 hours, despite maximal medical therapy (to prevent optic atrophy).
   - IOP ≥25 mm Hg with total hyphema for ≥5 days (to prevent corneal stromal blood staining).

- IOP ≥24 mm Hg for ≥24 hours (or any transient increase in IOP ≥30 mm Hg) in sickle cell trait or disease patients.
- Consider early surgical intervention for children at risk for amblyopia.

NOTE: Previously, systemic aminocaproic acid was used in hospitalized patients to stabilize the clot and to prevent rebleeding. This therapy is rarely used nowadays. Evidence supporting the use of topical antifibrinolytic agents such as aminocaproic acid and tranexamic acid is inconclusive. Some studies suggest that topical antifibrinolytic agents may be useful in reducing the risk of rebleeding but might prolong resolution time. Additionally, aminocaproic acid has been reported to have several adverse side effects; the benefits and risks of antifibrinolytic therapy remain controversial.

Follow Up

1. The patient should be seen daily after initial trauma to check visual acuity, IOP, and for a slit lamp examination. Look for new bleeding (most commonly occurs within the first 5 to 10 days), increased IOP, corneal blood staining, and other intraocular injuries as the blood clears (e.g., iridodialysis; subluxated or dislocated lens, or cataract). Hemolysis, which may appear as bright red fluid, should be distinguished from a rebleed, which forms a new, bright red clot. Rebleeding occurs in 0.4% to 35% of patients, usually 2 to 7 days after trauma. If the IOP is increased, treat as described earlier. Time between visits may be increased once consistent improvement in clinical examination is documented.

2. The patient should be instructed to return immediately if a sudden increase in pain or decrease in vision is noted (which may be symptoms of a rebleed or increased IOP).

3. If a significant rebleed or an intractable IOP increase occurs, hospitalization or surgical evacuation of the blood may be considered.

4. After the initial close follow-up period, the patient may be maintained on a long-acting cycloplegic agent (e.g., atropine 1% daily to b.i.d.) depending on the severity of the condition. Topical steroids may be tapered as the blood, fibrin, and WBCs resolve.

5. Protective glasses or an eye shield should be worn during the day and an eye shield at night.

6. The patient must refrain from strenuous physical activities (including Valsalva maneuvers) for at least 1 week after the initial injury or rebleed. Normal activities may be resumed once the hyphema has resolved and the patient is out of the rebleed time frame.

7. Future outpatient follow up:
   - If hospitalized, see 2 to 3 days after discharge. If not hospitalized, see several days to 1 week after initial daily follow-up period, depending on condition severity (amount of blood, potential for IOP increase, other ocular or orbital injuries).
   - Follow up 4 weeks after trauma for gonioscopy and dilated fundus examination with scleral depression for all patients.
   - Some experts suggest annual follow up because of the potential for development of angle-recession glaucoma.
   - If any complications arise, more frequent follow up is required.
   - If filtering surgery was performed, follow up and activity restrictions are based on the surgeon's specific recommendations.

TRAUMATIC MICROHYPHEMA

Symptoms

See HYPHEMA above.

Signs

Suspended RBCs in the AC (no settled blood or clot), visible with a slit lamp. Sometimes there may be enough suspended RBCs to see a haziness of the AC (e.g., poor visualization of iris details) without a slit lamp; in these cases, the RBCs may eventually settle out as a frank hyphema.

Workup

See HYPHEMA above.

Treatment

1. Most microhyphemas can be treated on an outpatient basis.
2. See treatment for HYPHEMA above.

Follow Up

1. The patient should return on the third day after the initial trauma and again at 1 week. If the IOP is >25 mm Hg at presentation, the patient should be followed daily for 3 consecutive days for pressure monitoring and again at 1 week. Sickle cell patients with initial IOP of ≥24 mm Hg should also be followed daily for 3 consecutive days.
2. Otherwise, see follow up for HYPHEMA above.

NONTRAUMATIC (SPONTANEOUS) AND POSTSURGICAL HYPHEMA OR MICROHYPHEMA

Symptoms

May present with decreased vision or with transient visual loss (intermittent bleeding may cloud vision temporarily).

Etiology of Spontaneous Hyphema or Microhyphema

- Occult trauma: must be excluded; evaluate for child or elder abuse.
- Neovascularization of the iris or angle (e.g., from diabetes, old central retinal vascular occlusion, ocular ischemic syndrome, chronic uveitis).
- Blood dyscrasias and coagulopathies.
- Iris–intraocular lens chafing.
- Herpetic keratouveitis.
- Use of anticoagulants (e.g., ethanol, aspirin, warfarin).

- Other (e.g., Fuchs heterochromic iridocyclitis, iris microaneurysm, leukemia, iris or ciliary body melanoma, retinoblastoma, juvenile xanthogranuloma).

Workup

As for traumatic hyphemas, plus:
1. Gentle gonioscopy initially to evaluate for neovascularization or masses in the angle.
2. Consider the following studies:
   - Prothrombin time (PT)/international normalized ratio (INR), partial thromboplastin time (PTT), complete blood count (CBC) with platelet count, bleeding time, and proteins C and S.
   - UBM to evaluate for possible malpositioning of intraocular lens haptics, ciliary body masses, or other anterior-segment pathology.
   - Fluorescein angiogram of iris.

Treatment

Cycloplegia (see HYPHEMA), limited activity, elevation of head of bed, and avoidance of medically unnecessary antiplatelet/anticoagulant medications (e.g., aspirin and NSAIDs). Recommend protective rigid metal or plastic shield if etiology is unclear. Monitor IOP. Postsurgical hyphemas and microhyphemas are usually self-limited and often require observation only, with close attention to IOP.

REFERENCE
Bansal S, Gunasekeran DV, Ang B, et al. Controversies in the pathophysiology and management of hyphema. *Surv Ophthalmol.* 2016;61(3):297-308.

3.7 Iridodialysis/Cyclodialysis

Definitions

Iridodialysis: Disinsertion of the iris from the scleral spur. Elevated IOP can result from trabecular meshwork damage and/or formation of peripheral anterior synechiae.

Cyclodialysis: Disinsertion of the ciliary body from the scleral spur. Increased uveoscleral outflow occurs initially resulting in hypotony. IOP elevation can later result from closure of a cyclodialysis cleft, leading to glaucoma.

Symptoms

Usually asymptomatic unless glaucoma or hypotony/hypotony maculopathy develop. Large iridodialyses may be associated with monocular diplopia, glare, and photophobia. Both are associated with blunt trauma or penetrating globe injuries. Typically, unilateral.

Signs

(See Figure 3.7.1.)

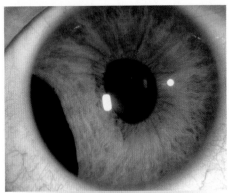

Figure 3.7.1 Iridodialysis.

Critical. Characteristic gonioscopic findings as described above.

Other. Decreased or elevated IOP, glaucomatous optic nerve changes (see 9.1, PRIMARY OPEN ANGLE GLAUCOMA), angle recession, and hypotony syndrome (see 13.11, HYPOTONY SYNDROME). Other signs of trauma include hyphema, cataract, and pupillary irregularities.

Differential Diagnosis

In setting of glaucoma, see 9.1, PRIMARY OPEN ANGLE GLAUCOMA.

Workup

See 9.6, ANGLE-RECESSION GLAUCOMA.

Treatment

1. Sunglasses, contact lenses with an artificial pupil, or surgical correction if large iridodialysis and patient symptomatic.

2. If glaucoma develops, treatment is similar to that for primary open angle glaucoma (see 9.1, PRIMARY OPEN ANGLE GLAUCOMA). Aqueous suppressants are usually first-line therapy. Miotics are generally avoided because they may reopen cyclodialysis clefts, causing hypotony. Strong mydriatics may close clefts, resulting in pressure spikes. Often these spikes are transient and easily controlled with topical therapy, as the meshwork resumes aqueous filtration after several hours.

3. If hypotony syndrome develops due to cyclodialysis clefts, first-line treatment is usually atropine b.i.d. to reapproximate the ciliary body to the sclera and steroids to decrease inflammation. Further surgical treatment is described in Section 13.11, HYPOTONY SYNDROME.

Follow Up

1. See 9.1, PRIMARY OPEN ANGLE GLAUCOMA.

2. Carefully monitor both eyes due to the high incidence of delayed open-angle and steroid-response glaucoma in the traumatized eye and an approximately 50% risk of open-angle glaucoma in the uninvolved eye.

REFERENCES

González-Martín-Moro J, Contreras-Martín I, Muñoz-Negrete FJ, et al. Cyclodialysis: an update. *Int Ophthalmol.* 2017;37:441-457.

Tesluk GC, Spaeth GL. The occurrence of primary open-angle glaucoma in the fellow eye of patients with unilateral angle-cleavage glaucoma. *Ophthalmology.* 1985;92:904-911.

3.8 Eyelid Laceration

Symptoms

Periorbital pain, tearing, bleeding, and history of facial trauma.

Signs

(See Figure 3.8.1.)

Partial- or full-thickness eyelid defect involving the skin and subcutaneous tissues. Superficial lacerations/abrasions may mask a deep laceration, foreign body, or penetrating/perforating injury to the lacrimal drainage system (e.g., punctum, canaliculus, common canaliculus, lacrimal sac), globe, orbit, or cranial vault.

Workup

1. History: Determine the mechanism and timing of injury: bite, foreign body potential, etc.

2. Complete ocular evaluation, including bilateral dilated fundus examination. Ensure there is no injury to the globe, orbital soft tissue

3

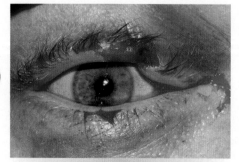

Figure 3.8.1 Marginal eyelid laceration.

(including the optic nerve), or intracranial compartment before attempting eyelid repair.

3. Carefully evert the eyelids and use toothed forceps or cotton-tipped applicators to gently pull open one edge of the wound to determine the depth of penetration. (If foreign body suspected, get imaging described below before extensive wound exploration.)

4. CT scan of brain, orbits, and midface (axial, coronal, and parasagittal views, 1- to 2-mm sections) should be obtained with any history suggestive of penetrating injury or severe blunt trauma to rule out fracture, retained foreign body, ruptured globe, or intracranial injury. If there is any suspicion of deeper injury, obtain imaging *before* eyelid laceration repair. Loss of consciousness mandates a CT of the brain. Depending on the mechanism of injury, the cervical spine may need to be cleared.

5. If laceration is nasal to the punctum, even if not obviously through the canalicular system, punctal dilation and probing with irrigation of the canalicular system should be considered to exclude canalicular involvement **(see Figures 3.8.2** and **3.8.3**; APPENDIX 7, TECHNIQUE FOR DIAGNOSTIC PROBING AND IRRIGATION OF THE LACRIMAL SYSTEM). High suspicion should be maintained for unnoticed canalicular lacerations in the pediatric population, particularly with dog bite injuries.

6. Be suspicious in glancing blunt trauma to the lateral cheek (zygoma). A lateral glancing mechanism may abruptly stretch the medial canthal anatomy, resulting in avulsion of the medial canthal tendon with concomitant canalicular laceration. Canalicular lacerations are often missed with this mechanism because clinical attention is directed laterally to the

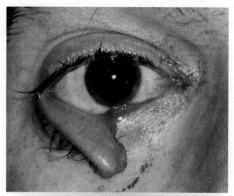

Figure 3.8.2 Canalicular laceration.

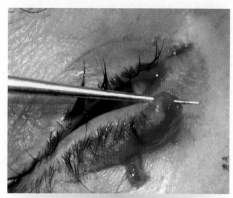

Figure 3.8.3 Canalicular laceration showing exposed tip after probing the punctum.

zygoma and the medial canthal soft tissues often reappose into a normal position, camouflaging the extent of the injury.

NOTE: Dogbites are notorious for causing canalicular lacerations and predominantly occur in young children. Probing should be performed in all such cases, even with lacerations that appear to be superficial. Uncooperative patients should undergo conscious sedation or an examination under anesthesia to thoroughly examine the eyelids, lacrimal drainage system, and globes.

Treatment

1. Consider tetanus prophylaxis (see APPENDIX 2, TETANUS PROPHYLAXIS, for indications).

2. Consider systemic antibiotics for 7 to 10 days if contamination or foreign body is suspected (e.g., amoxicillin/clavulanate [500/125 mg p.o. b.i.d. to t.i.d. or 875/125 mg p.o. b.i.d.], doxycycline [100 mg p.o. b.i.d.], trimethoprim/sulfamethoxazole [80/400 mg or 160/800 mg p.o. daily to b.i.d.], or cephalexin [250 to 500 mg p.o. q.i.d.] [adults]; 25 to 50 mg/kg/d divided into four doses [children]). For human or animal bites, consider penicillin V. If indicated, consider rabies prophylaxis.

 NOTE: In most states, animal bites must be reported to the local Department of Health.

3. Repair eyelid laceration.

   3A. Determine appropriate setting for repair. Indications for operating room repair include the following:

   - Association with ocular or deep adnexal trauma that requires surgery (e.g., ruptured globe or intraorbital foreign body).
   - Involvement of the lacrimal drainage apparatus except when uncomplicated and close to the punctum in a cooperative patient. Note that canalicular laceration repair is not an ophthalmic emergency and can be delayed up to 4 days with no negative effects.
   - Involvement of the levator aponeurosis of the upper eyelid or the superior rectus muscle.
   - Visible orbital fat in an eyelid laceration, indicating penetration of the orbital septum. All such patients require CT imaging and careful documentation of levator and extraocular muscle (EOM) function. Exploration of deeper tissue planes may be necessary.
   - Medial canthal tendon avulsion (exhibits displacement, excessive rounding, or abnormal laxity of the medial canthus).
   - Extensive tissue loss (especially more than one-third of the eyelid) or severe distortion of anatomy.

   3B. Procedure for eyelid laceration repair at the bedside:

NOTE: Eye protection should be worn by all healthcare providers.

- Place a drop of topical anesthetic in each eye. Place a protective scleral shell over the affected eye, and cover the uninvolved eye with a moistened, folded gauze sponge. Clean the area of injury and surrounding skin with copious irrigation and 10% povidone–iodine solution (avoid povidone soap because this irritates the cornea). Isolate the area with surgical drapes.

NOTE: Lacerations from human or animal bites or those with significant contamination risk may require minimal debridement of necrotic tissue. Because of the excellent blood supply to the eyelids, primary repair is usually performed. Alternatively, contaminated wounds may be left open for delayed repair. All attempts should be made to preserve the eyelid skin. However, skin grafting should be considered if significant portions of the skin are necrotic or lost in the initial injury. For primary repair, proceed to the subsequent steps.

- Administer local subcutaneous anesthetic (e.g., 2% lidocaine with epinephrine). Since direct injection of local anesthetic causes tissue distortion and bleeding, use the minimal amount of anesthetic needed or perform field blocks (e.g., supraorbital, infraorbital, and/or anterior ethmoidal nerve blocks).
- If foreign bodies are encountered unexpectedly and appear to penetrate the globe or orbital tissues, do NOT remove. Involvement of the orbit, cavernous sinus, or brain requires an extensive preoperative evaluation and a multidisciplinary approach (e.g., otolaryngology or neurosurgery) and ancillary testing (e.g., angiography).
- Close the laceration as follows.

NONMARGINAL EYELID LACERATION

See bullets above. Then close the skin with interrupted 6-0 absorbable (e.g., plain gut, chromic gut) sutures. Some surgeons prefer using monofilament nonabsorbable material (e.g., nylon, polypropylene) to potentially decrease scarring. Nonabsorbable sutures should be avoided in patients who may not follow up compliantly. Avoid deep sutures within the confines of the orbital rim and never suture the orbital septum. Skin and dermis thickens markedly beyond the orbital rim; in these areas, a layered closure may be indicated to minimize skin tension.

MARGINAL EYELID LACERATION

Key Points

- There are many ways to approach marginal eyelid laceration repair, and we will describe a traditional method. The most important step is reapproximation of the tarsus along its vertical axis to allow for proper eyelid alignment and healing. Reapproximation of the tarsus at the margin alone will not provide structural integrity to the eyelid; the injured tarsus will splay apart, resulting in eyelid notching **(see Figure 3.8.4C)**.

> 📝 **NOTE:** If patient reliability is questionable, use absorbable 6-0 polyglactin sutures (e.g., Vicryl) for every step.

- Be careful to avoid deeper, buried subcutaneous sutures that can incorporate the orbital septum, resulting in eyelid tethering. In general, deep sutures should be avoided in the zone between the tarsus and orbital rim (the vertical lengths of the upper and lower tarsi are approximately 10 mm and 5 mm, respectively).
- Deep tarsal sutures should be lamellar (partial thickness), especially in the upper eyelid, to avoid penetration through the underlying conjunctiva and subsequent corneal irritation/injury.
- If unsure about patient reliability or in patients who will not cooperate for suture removal (e.g., young children, patients with advanced dementia, etc.), use absorbable 6-0 polyglactin suture (e.g., Vicryl) in the eyelid margin instead of nonabsorbable material (e.g., silk).

Procedure Steps

(See Figure 3.8.4.)

a. Place a 6-0 silk suture from gray line to gray line, entering and exiting the gray line 2 mm from the laceration edge. (As already noted, in difficult or unreliable patients, use absorbable suture material only.) Put the suture on traction with a hemostat to ensure good reapproximation of the splayed tarsus and gray line. Leave the suture untied.

> 📝 **NOTE:** This marginal suture provides no structural integrity to the eyelid; its main function is to align the eyelid margin anatomy to ensure a good cosmetic repair.

b. Realign the tarsal edges with interrupted sutures placed through an anterior approach (e.g., 5-0 or 6-0 Vicryl on a spatulated needle). This is the most important structural step in marginal laceration closure. In the upper eyelid, three sutures can usually be placed. In the lower eyelid, two sutures are typically the maximum. A single tarsal suture, in addition to the marginal suture, may be adequate for appropriate tarsal realignment depending on the height of the laceration. *Failure to reapproximate the tarsus along its entire vertical length will result in eyelid splaying and notching.*

c. Tie down and trim the tarsal sutures. Tie down the marginal silk suture leaving long tails.

d. Place and tie another 6-0 silk marginal suture either anterior or posterior to the gray-line suture, again leaving long tails. The posterior suture is often unnecessary, and its absence may decrease the risk of postoperative corneal abrasion. When placing marginal sutures, attempt to realign the normal eyelid anatomy (lash line, meibomian glands, gray line).

e. Use interrupted 6-0 plain gut sutures to close the skin along the length of the laceration. Incorporate the tails of all eyelid margin sutures into the skin suture closest to the eyelid margin to keep tails away from the corneal surface.

f. Final steps:
   - Remove the protective scleral shell.
   - Apply antibiotic ointment (e.g., bacitracin or erythromycin) to the wound t.i.d.
   - Dress the wound and consider oral antibiotics if needed. For lacerations beyond the orbital rim where deeper dermis is encountered, one can apply a topical adhesive (benzoin or Mastisol) and Steri-Strips perpendicular to the axis of the laceration to reinforce the sutures and decrease skin tension. Antibiotic ointment is applied once the strips have been placed.

Follow Up

If nonabsorbable sutures are used (e.g., silk), eyelid margin sutures should be left in place for 5 to 10 days, and other superficial sutures for

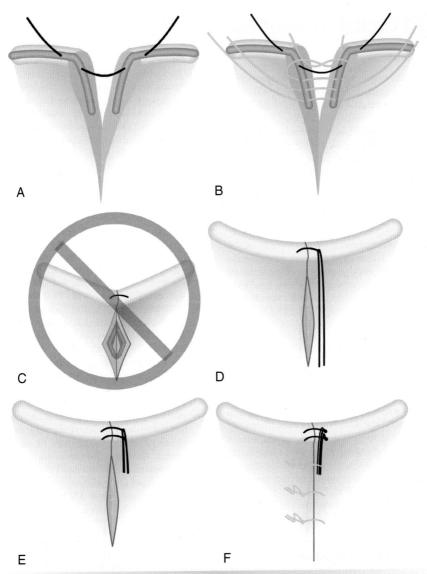

Figure 3.8.4 Marginal eyelid laceration repair, traditional method. **A:** Reapproximate the gray line with a 6-0 silk suture. **B:** The most important step is to realign the tarsal edges with multiple interrupted 5-0 or 6-0 absorbable (e.g., Vicryl) sutures. Take partial-thickness bites. **C:** Failure to realign the tarsus will compromise the integrity of the eyelid, resulting in splaying and notching. **D:** Tie the tarsal and gray line sutures. **E:** Place another marginal 6-0 silk suture. **F:** Suture the skin with interrupted 6-0 plain gut, securing the tails of the marginal sutures.

4 to 7 days. The integrity of an eyelid margin repair is provided by the longer lasting tarsal sutures. Therefore, the eyelid margin sutures can be removed as soon as 5 days postoperatively. If a small notch is present, it can be followed over the ensuing 3 to 6 months to allow for scar maturation. A small eyelid notch will often soften and disappear on its own.

3.9 Orbital Blowout Fracture

Symptoms

Pain with eye movement; local tenderness; eyelid edema; binocular diplopia; crepitus (particularly after nose blowing); and numbness of the cheek, upper lip, and/or teeth. Tearing may be a symptom of nasolacrimal duct obstruction or injury seen with medial buttress, Le Fort II, or nasoethmoidal complex fractures, but this is typically a late complaint. Acute tearing is usually due to ocular irritation (e.g., chemosis, corneal abrasion, iritis).

Signs

Critical. Restricted eye movement (especially in upward gaze, lateral gaze, or both), subcutaneous or conjunctival emphysema, hypesthesia in the distribution of the infraorbital nerve (ipsilateral cheek and upper lip), point tenderness, enophthalmos (may initially be masked by orbital edema and hemorrhage), and hypoglobus.

Other. Epistaxis, eyelid edema, and ecchymosis. Superior rim and orbital roof fractures may manifest hypesthesia in the distribution of the supratrochlear or supraorbital nerve (ipsilateral forehead), ptosis, and step-off deformity along the anterior table of the frontal sinuses (superior orbital rim and glabella). Trismus, malar flattening, and a palpable step-off deformity of the inferior orbital rim are characteristic of tripod (zygomatic complex) fractures. Optic neuropathy may be present secondary to posterior indirect traumatic optic neuropathy (PI-TON) or from a direct mechanism (orbital compartment syndrome [OCS] secondary to retrobulbar hemorrhage, foreign body, etc.; see below).

Differential Diagnosis of Muscle Entrapment in Orbital Fracture

- Orbital edema and hemorrhage with or without a blowout fracture: May have limitation of ocular movement, periorbital swelling, and ecchymosis, but these will markedly improve or completely resolve over 7 to 10 days.
- Cranial nerve palsy: Limitation of ocular movement, but no restriction on forced duction testing. Will have abnormal results on active force generation testing. In cases of suspected traumatic cranial neuropathy, significant skull base and intracranial injury have occurred and CT imaging should be obtained.

- Laceration or direct contusion of EOMs: Often the site of penetrating injury is missed, especially if it occurs in the conjunctival cul-de-sacs. Look carefully for evidence of conjunctival laceration or orbital fat prolapse. Complete EOM laceration usually results in a large angle ocular deviation away from the injured muscle with no ocular movement toward the muscle. CT is often helpful in distinguishing EOM contusion from EOM laceration. On occasion, exploration of the EOM may be necessary under anesthesia.

Workup

1. Complete ophthalmic examination, including visual acuity, motility, IOP, and globe displacement. Check pupils and color vision to rule out TON (see 3.11, TRAUMATIC OPTIC NEUROPATHY). Compare sensation of the affected cheek with that on the contralateral side; palpate the eyelids for crepitus (subcutaneous emphysema); palpate the orbital rim for step-off deformities. Evaluate the globe carefully for an apparent or occult rupture, hyphema or microhyphema, traumatic iritis, and retinal or choroidal damage. A full, dilated examination may be difficult in uncooperative patients with periocular edema but is extremely important in the management of orbital fractures. If eyelid and periocular edema limit the view, special techniques may be necessary (e.g., use of Desmarres eyelid retractors or clean bent paperclips [see **Figure 3.9.1**], lateral cantholysis, examination under general anesthesia).

> **NOTE:** It is of paramount importance to rule out intraocular and optic nerve injury as quickly as possible in ALL patients presenting with suspected orbital fracture.

> **NOTE:** Pediatric patients are particularly at risk for a unique type of blowout injury: the "trapdoor" fracture. Because pediatric bones lack complete calcification, they tend to "greenstick" rather than completely fracture. This results in an initial fracture, herniation of orbital soft tissue (including EOM) through the fracture site, and rapid snapping back of the malleable bone akin to a trapdoor on a spring. Because of the tight

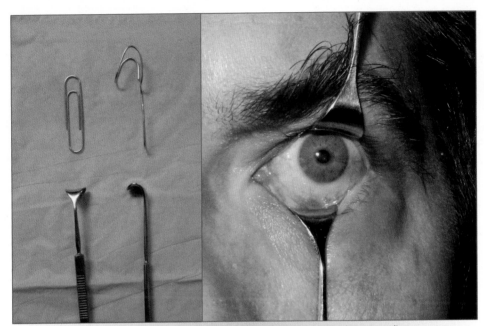

Figure 3.9.1 Eyelid retraction with Desmarres retractors or clean bent paperclips.

reapposition of the fracture edges, the soft tissue trapped within the fracture becomes ischemic. Children with this type of fracture often have a remarkably benign external periocular appearance but significant EOM restriction (usually vertical) on examination; this constellation of findings has been dubbed the "white-eyed blowout fracture" (WEBOF). Children may present with a vague history, allow only a limited ocular examination, and be misdiagnosed as having an intracranial injury (e.g., concussion) leading to delay in management of WEBOF. Be aware of the oculocardiac reflex (nausea or vomiting, bradycardia, syncope, dehydration) that can accompany entrapment. Even in cases where correct orbital imaging is performed, CT evidence of an orbital fracture may be minimal and routinely missed. Careful examination of coronal and parasagittal views is critical in such cases.

In typical (i.e., non-WEBOF) orbital fractures, forced duction testing or testing of the doll's eye reflex may be performed if limitation of eye movement persists beyond 1 week and restriction is suspected. In the early phase, it is often difficult to distinguish soft tissue edema or contusion from soft tissue entrapment in the fracture. SEE APPENDIX 6, FORCED DUCTION TEST AND ACTIVE FORCE GENERATION TEST.

2. CT of the orbit and midface (axial, coronal, and parasagittal views, 1- to 1.5-mm sections, without contrast) is obtained in all cases of suspected orbital fractures. Bone windows are especially helpful in fracture evaluation **(see Figures 3.9.2** and **3.9.3)**, including the narrow, oft-missed WEBOF. Inclusion of the midfacial skeleton is mandatory to rule out zygomatic complex or other midfacial fractures. If there is any history of loss of consciousness, brain imaging is recommended.

NOTE: In the absence of visual symptoms (subjective change in vision, diplopia, periocular pain, photophobia, floaters or flashes), patients with orbital fractures are unlikely to have an ophthalmic condition requiring intervention within 24 hours. However, all patients with orbital fractures should undergo a complete ophthalmic examination within 48 hours of injury. Any patient complaining of blurred vision, severe pain, or other significant visual symptoms should undergo more urgent ophthalmic evaluation.

Treatment

1. Consider broad-spectrum oral antibiotics (e.g., amoxicillin/clavulanate [500/125 mg p.o. b.i.d. to t.i.d. or 875/125 mg p.o. b.i.d.],

doxycycline [100 mg p.o. daily to b.i.d.], trimethoprim/sulfamethoxazole [80/400 mg or 160/800 mg p.o. daily to b.i.d.], or cephalexin [250 to 500 mg p.o. q.i.d.] [adults]) for 7 to 10 days. Antibiotics may be considered if the patient has a history of chronic sinusitis or diabetes or is otherwise immunocompromised. This recommendation is based

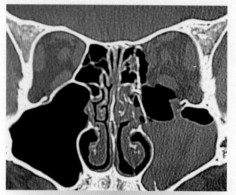

Figure 3.9.2 Computed tomography (CT) of orbital blowout fracture.

on limited, anecdotal evidence. In all other patients, the decision about antibiotic use is left to the treating physician. Prophylactic antibiotics should not be considered mandatory in patients with orbital fractures.

2. Instruct the patient to avoid nose blowing. Forced air into the orbit can lead to OCS and optic neuropathy.

3. Nasal decongestants (e.g., oxymetazoline nasal spray b.i.d.) for 3 days. Use is limited to 3 days to minimize rebound nasal congestion.

4. Apply ice packs to the eyelids for 20 minutes every 1 to 2 hours for the first 24 to 48 hours and attempt a 30-degree inclination when at rest.

5. Consider oral corticosteroids (e.g., methylprednisolone dose pack) if extensive swelling limits examination of ocular motility and globe position. Some experts advise the use of oral antibiotics if corticosteroid therapy is considered, but there are no data to support the effectiveness of such a regimen. Avoid corticosteroids in patients with concomitant traumatic brain injury (TBI).

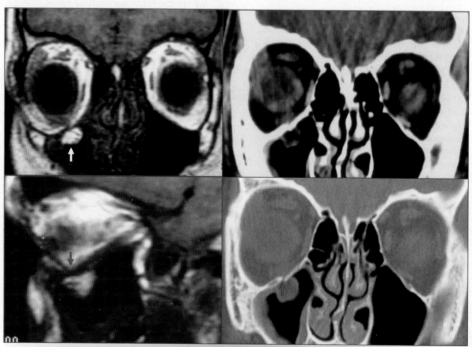

Figure 3.9.3 Coronal and sagittal cuts of a white-eyed blowout fracture (WEBOF) in a patient with an entrapped inferior rectus. White arrow, entrapped orbital soft tissue; red arrows, orbital floor fracture.

6. Neurosurgical consultation is recommended for all fractures involving the orbital roof, frontal sinus, or cribriform plate and for all fractures associated with intracranial hemorrhage. Otolaryngology or oral maxillofacial surgery consultation may be useful for frontal sinus, midfacial, and mandibular fractures.

7. Consider surgical repair based on the following criteria.

> **NOTE:** Orbital fracture repair should be deferred or delayed if there is any evidence of full-thickness globe injury or penetrating trauma. Presence of hyphema or microhyphema typically delays orbital fracture repair for 10 to 14 days.

Immediate Repair (Within 24 to 48 hours)

If there is clinical evidence of muscle entrapment with nonresolving bradycardia, heart block, nausea, vomiting, or syncope (most often encountered in children with WEBOF). Patients with muscle entrapment require urgent orbital exploration to release any incarcerated muscle to decrease the chance of permanent restrictive strabismus from muscle ischemia and fibrosis, as well as to alleviate systemic symptoms from the oculocardiac reflex.

Repair in 1 to 2 Weeks

- Persistent, symptomatic diplopia in primary or downgaze that has not improved over 1 to 2 weeks. CT may show muscle distortion or herniation around fractures. Forced ductions may be useful in identifying bony restriction. Note that diplopia may take more than two weeks to improve or resolve. Some surgeons will wait 6 to 8 weeks before offering surgical repair for persistent diplopia.
- Large orbital floor fractures (>50%) or large combined medial wall and orbital floor fractures that are likely to cause cosmetically unacceptable globe dystopia (enophthalmos and/or hypoglobus) over time. Globe dystopia at initial presentation is indicative of a large fracture. It is also reasonable to wait several months to see if enophthalmos develops before offering repair. There is no clear evidence that early repair is more effective in preventing or reversing globe malposition compared to delayed repair. However, many surgeons prefer early repair simply because dissection planes and abnormal (fractured) bony anatomy are more easily discernable before posttraumatic fibrosis sets in. It may be prudent to avoid early surgery for prevention of possible globe malposition in older patients, patients with significant medical comorbidities, or patients on anticoagulation therapy for significant cardiovascular conditions.

- Complex trauma involving the orbital rim or displacement of the lateral wall and/or the zygomatic arch. Complex fractures of the midface (zygomatic complex, Le Fort II) or skull base (Le Fort III). Nasoethmoidal complex fractures. Superior or superomedial orbital rim fractures involving the frontal sinuses.

Delayed Repair

- Old fractures that have resulted in enophthalmos or hypoglobus can be repaired at any later date.

> **NOTE:** The role of anticoagulation in postoperative or posttrauma patients is debatable. Anecdotal reports have described orbital hemorrhage in patients with orbital and midfacial fractures who were anticoagulated for prophylaxis against deep vein thrombosis (DVT). On the other hand, multiple large studies have also demonstrated an increased risk of DVT and pulmonary embolism (PE) in postoperative patients who are obtunded or cannot ambulate. At the very least, all inpatients with orbital fractures awaiting surgery and all postoperative orbital fracture patients should be placed on intermittent pneumatic compression (IPC) therapy and encouraged to ambulate. In patients at high risk for DVT, including those who are obtunded from concomitant intracranial injury, a detailed discussion with the primary care team regarding anticoagulation should be documented, and the risks for and against such therapy should be discussed in detail with the patient and family.

Follow Up

Patients should be seen at 1 and 2 weeks after trauma to be evaluated for persistent diplopia and/or enophthalmos after the acute orbital edema has resolved. If sinusitis symptoms develop or were present prior to the injury, the patient should be seen within a few days of the

3

injury. Patients should also be monitored for development of associated ocular injuries as indicated (e.g., orbital cellulitis, angle-recession glaucoma, retinal detachment). Gonioscopy and dilated fundus examination with scleral depression is performed about 4 weeks after trauma if a hyphema or microhyphema was present. Warning symptoms of retinal detachment and orbital cellulitis are explained to the patient.

3.10 Traumatic Retrobulbar Hemorrhage (Orbital Hemorrhage)

Symptoms

Pain, decreased vision, inability to open the eyelids due to severe swelling, recent history of trauma or surgery to the eyelids or orbit, and history of anticoagulation. Because the orbit is a bony compartment with firm anterior soft tissue tethering by the orbital septum, any process (blood, pus, air) that rapidly fills the orbit results in a compartment syndrome. As pressure builds within the orbit, ischemia to the optic nerve, globe, and retina occur, potentially resulting in devastating, permanent visual loss. OCS *is an ophthalmic emergency.*

> **NOTE:** Most iatrogenic postoperative orbital hemorrhages evolve within the first 6 hours following surgery.

Signs

(See Figure 3.10.1.)

Critical. Proptosis with resistance to retropulsion, tense ("rock hard") eyelids that are difficult to open, vision loss, afferent pupillary defect, dyschromatopsia, and increased IOP.

Other. Eyelid ecchymosis, diffuse subconjunctival hemorrhage, chemosis, congested conjunctival vessels, evidence of disc swelling from compressive optic neuropathy or retinal vascular occlusion, and limited extraocular motility in any or all fields of gaze.

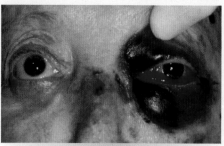

Figure 3.10.1 Retrobulbar hemorrhage.

Differential Diagnosis

- Orbital cellulitis: Fever, proptosis, chemosis, limitation, or pain with eye movement; also may follow trauma, but usually not as acutely. A rapidly expanding orbital abscess may result in OCS, and in such cases, the acute management is the same as that for orbital hemorrhage. See 7.3.1, ORBITAL CELLULITIS.

- Severe orbital emphysema ("tension pneumo-orbit"): Tight orbit, tight eyelids, crepitus, and decreased extraocular motility; may follow orbital fracture with or without nose blowing. See 3.9, ORBITAL BLOWOUT FRACTURE.

- Orbital fracture: Limited extraocular motility, enophthalmos, or proptosis may be present. See 3.9, ORBITAL BLOWOUT FRACTURE.

- Ruptured globe: Subconjunctival edema and hemorrhage may mask a ruptured globe. See 3.14, RUPTURED GLOBE AND PENETRATING OCULAR INJURY.

- High-flow (direct) carotid–cavernous fistula: May follow trauma either acutely or subacutely; most are spontaneous and nontraumatic. Pulsatile exophthalmos, ocular/brow bruit, corkscrew arterialized conjunctival vessels, chemosis, and increased IOP may be seen. Usually unilateral, although bilateral signs from a unilateral fistula may be seen occasionally. See 10.10, CAVERNOUS SINUS AND ASSOCIATED SYNDROMES (MULTIPLE OCULAR MOTOR NERVE PALSIES).

- Varix: Increased proptosis with Valsalva maneuver. Not usually seen acutely after trauma, and in the vast majority of orbital varices, there is no history of trauma or surgery.

- Lymphangioma: Usually in younger patients. May have acute proptosis, ecchymosis, and external ophthalmoplegia after minimal trauma or upper respiratory tract infection. MRI is usually diagnostic.

- Spontaneous retrobulbar hemorrhage: Signs and symptoms are identical to those of traumatic or postoperative hemorrhage. May occur in patients who are chronically anticoagulated or with an underlying coagulopathy from other systemic disease (e.g., hemophilia). Occasionally reported in pregnant women, especially during labor. Typically seen as a subperiosteal hematoma along the orbital roof and may be misdiagnosed as an orbital neoplasm. MRI is helpful in identifying blood-breakdown products (see 14.3, MAGNETIC RESONANCE IMAGING).

Workup

1. Complete ophthalmic examination; check specifically for an afferent pupillary defect, loss of color vision, the degree of tightness of the eyelids, resistance to retropulsion, increased IOP, pulsations of the central retinal artery (often precedes artery occlusion), choroidal folds (sign of globe distortion from severe optic nerve stretching), and optic nerve edema. Note that visual function may span from normal to no light perception.

2. CT scan of the orbit (axial, coronal, and parasagittal views). When vision and/or optic nerve function are threatened, CT should always be delayed until definitive treatment with canthotomy/cantholysis. CT rarely shows a discreet hematoma. Typically, retrobulbar hemorrhage manifests as a diffuse, increased reticular pattern of the intraconal orbital fat. The so-called teardrop or tenting sign may be seen: the optic nerve is at maximum stretch and distorts (tents) the back of the globe into a teardrop shape. This is an ominous radiologic sign, especially if the posterior scleral angle is <130 degrees. The presence of an orbital fracture may help to decompress the orbit and decrease, but not rule out, the possibility of OCS. It is important to remember that patients can still develop OCS and optic neuropathy even with large orbital fractures, as blood may simply fill the adjacent paranasal sinus and then cause an OCS.

> **NOTE:** Retrobulbar hemorrhage with OCS is a clinical diagnosis and does not require imaging. A delay while CT is being obtained may cause further visual compromise. Imaging can be obtained once the OCS has been decompressed and visual function stabilized.

Treatment

The key to effective management of clinically significant retrobulbar hemorrhage with OCS is timely and aggressive soft tissue decompression. The initial goal is to decrease the compression on critical soft tissues, mainly the optic nerve. All patients should be treated utilizing the same guidelines, even if the hemorrhage is thought to have occurred hours or days ago, since it is often impossible to know at what point along the clinical timeline optic neuropathy manifested.

1. If optic neuropathy is present, immediately release orbital pressure with lateral canthotomy and inferior cantholysis **(see Figure 3.10.2 below)**. The procedure can be performed in an office or ER setting with basic instrumentation and local anesthetic injection if possible. Conscious sedation can be used in the ER setting if this does not delay treatment, but is usually unnecessary.

2. If there are no orbital signs and no evidence of ocular ischemia or compressive optic neuropathy but the IOP is increased (e.g., ≥35 mm Hg in a patient with a normal optic nerve, or ≥20 mm Hg in a patient with glaucoma who normally has a lower IOP), the patient is treated in a more stepwise fashion in an effort to reduce the IOP (see below and 9.1, PRIMARY OPEN ANGLE GLAUCOMA).

Canthotomy and Cantholysis

(See Figure 3.10.2.)

The goal of canthotomy and cantholysis is to perform an adequate soft tissue decompression of the orbit by disinserting the lower eyelid from its periosteal attachments. A nonperfused retina infarcts irreversibly in approximately 90 minutes, and a delay of definitive treatment of longer duration may lead to retinal nerve fiber death and permanent vision loss.

> **NOTE:** A canthotomy alone is inadequate treatment. A cantholysis must be performed.

a. Consider subdermal injection of lidocaine 2% with epinephrine (inject away from the eye). Because of the eyelid edema and acidotic local environment, local anesthesia may not be effective. A field block may be used. The patient should be warned that the procedure may be painful, but fortunately in most cases, canthotomy and cantholysis can be performed quickly.

b. Consider placing a hemostat horizontally at the lateral canthus and clamp for 1 minute to

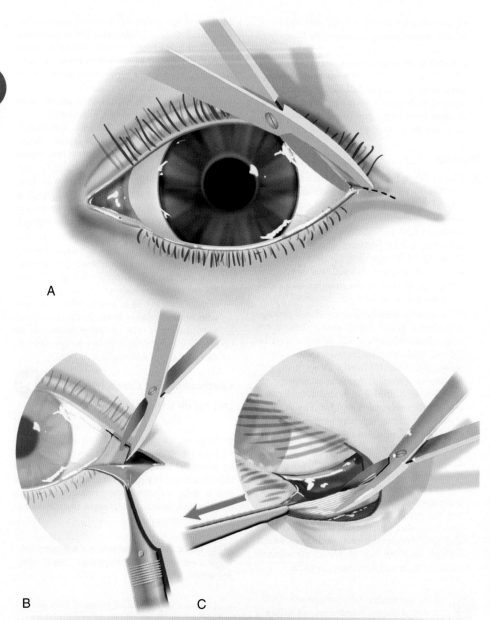

A

B   C

Figure 3.10.2 Lateral canthotomy and cantholysis. **A:** Lateral canthotomy. **B:** Grasp the lateral lower eyelid with toothed forceps. **C:** Pull the eyelid anteriorly. Point the scissors toward the patient's nose, strum the lateral canthal tendon, and cut.

compress the tissue and reduce bleeding (an optional step that should not be performed without good local anesthesia).

c. Only two instruments are needed for canthotomy and cantholysis: A pair of *blunt-tipped* scissors (e.g., Westcott or Stevens) and forceps with *heavy* teeth (e.g., Bishop Harmon or Adson). Avoid sharp-tipped scissors to minimize the chance of globe injury. Delicate forceps (e.g., 0.12-mm Castroviejo) will not provide enough traction to effectively disinsert the eyelid and should not be used.

d. Perform the canthotomy. Place the scissors across the lateral canthus and incise the canthus for about 1-cm full thickness (from conjunctiva to skin). Forceps are not needed for this step. This step simply gains access to the inferior crux of the lateral canthal tendon. It provides little soft tissue decompression.

e. Perform inferior cantholysis. With the toothed forceps, grasp the lower eyelid at the inner edge of the incised canthus. With the patient supine, traction should be directed upward, toward the ceiling. Place the scissors in an open position just beneath the skin, with the tips pointing toward the tip of the nose, and begin to cut. Some advocate "strumming" of the lateral canthal tendon, but this is not essential and sometimes difficult to assess because of tissue edema. As the canthal tendon is released, the eyelid should come completely away from the globe.

> **NOTE:** The cantholysis is critical to decompress the orbit and is done exclusively by feel. Do not visually search for a specific tendon or anatomic landmark.

f. There are several clues to a successful cantholysis. The eyelid should release completely away from the globe. Once the forceps are released, the lateral portion of the eyelid margin should move medially, usually to the lateral aspect of the limbus of the globe. If any eyelid margin still remains in its normal position lateral to the temporal limbus, the cantholysis is incomplete: keep cutting!

g. The incision will bleed; however, cautery is usually unnecessary. Pressure over the bone of the lateral orbital rim (but not on the globe and orbit) for several minutes usually results in good control. However, with the widespread use of anticoagulant and antiplatelet medications (e.g., warfarin, aspirin, clopidogrel) as well as increasing prescription of irreversible anticoagulants (e.g., rivaroxaban, dabigatran, etc.), excessive bleeding can be encountered. In these cases, manual pressure is often inadequate and applying hemostatic aids (e.g., biologic agents such as thrombin and fibrinogen or physical agents such as gelatin, collagen, cellulose) may be necessary. Cautery is effective if available.

h. The results of a successful cantholysis are usually evident within the first 15 minutes. IOP should decrease, and the retina should reperfuse. Cadaver studies have shown a reliable correlation between IOP and intraorbital pressure. A significant decrease in IOP after cantholysis is indicative of a successful orbital soft tissue decompression. Depending on the timing of the cantholysis in relation to the hemorrhage, vision may dramatically improve. Superior cantholysis is usually unnecessary: cadaver studies have not shown a dramatic decrease in intraorbital pressure with superior cantholysis. In addition, superior cantholysis may result in lacrimal gland incision, which can bleed profusely. By far the most common reason for persistent signs of OCS following inferior cantholysis is inadequate cantholysis. Make sure the cantholysis is performed effectively.

3. Close observation is indicated in all cases of retrobulbar hemorrhage, including those that have not yet affected visual function. It is therefore dangerous to assume that a patient with recent injury/surgery, retrobulbar hemorrhage, and normal optic nerve function is stable enough for discharge. In such cases, it is best to follow the patient for 4 to 6 hours with serial examinations in the ER or hospital. If a patient presents with no evidence of OCS 6 or more hours after the initial insult, it is reasonable to discharge the patient with specific instructions (see follow up). For patients presenting with OCS, see NOTE below.

> **NOTE:** The efficacy of inferior cantholysis for OCS is based on the assumption that at the time of the procedure, all active orbital bleeding has tamponaded; this is indeed the case in the majority of retrobulbar hemorrhages. However, if active bleeding persists, the OCS will recur as the blood fills the decompressed orbit. For this reason, it is prudent to monitor patients who present with OCS and optic neuropathy for 12 to 24 hours following cantholysis.

3

4. Anticoagulants (e.g., warfarin) and antiplatelet agents (e.g., aspirin) are often discontinued, if possible, to prevent rebleeding. This decision must be made in conjunction with an internist or cardiologist. Intravenous corticosteroids may be indicated to further decrease soft tissue edema when no TBI is present. Antibiotics may be indicated, depending on the etiology of the hemorrhage. Frequent ice compresses (20 minutes on, 20 minutes off) are important, and their compliant use should be emphasized to the patient and the nursing staff.

5. Medical IOP control as needed (see 9.1, PRIMARY OPEN ANGLE GLAUCOMA and 9.4, ACUTE ANGLE CLOSURE GLAUCOMA for treatment indications/contraindications):

   - Topical IOP-lowering agents such as beta-blockers, alpha-agonists, or carbonic anhydrase inhibitors.
   - Oral carbonic anhydrase inhibitor (e.g., acetazolamide).
   - Hyperosmotic agent (e.g., mannitol).

NOTE: When an OCS exists in a situation where canthotomy/cantholysis cannot immediately be completed, the use of IV mannitol may serve as a temporizing measure and assist in lowering intraocular and intraorbital pressure based on a recent study in which primates were subjected to experimental orbital hemorrhage. However, there should be no systemic or intracranial contraindications to mannitol before administration. *Note that IV mannitol is not a substitute for definitive management of OCS by canthotomy/cantholysis!*

Follow Up

In cases where vision is threatened, monitor the patient closely until stable, with frequent vision and IOP checks.

Any patient with a posttraumatic orbital hemorrhage older than 6 to 8 hours with normal visual function should be instructed in detail on how to serially measure visual function, especially over the first 24 hours, and to return immediately if vision deteriorates. Cantholysis wounds may be left open with application of antibiotic ointment t.i.d. to spontaneously heal, or closed with a secondary canthoplasty 1 to 3 weeks later. If reconstruction of the lateral canthus is indicated, it may be performed as an outpatient procedure under local anesthesia. The inferior canthal tendon is sutured back to the inner aspect of the lateral orbital rim. Interestingly, a significant percentage of eyelids will heal adequately without any surgery. If a residual optic neuropathy is present, the patient should be followed with serial examinations and visual fields. It is not uncommon for visual function to continue to improve over the first 6 months.

REFERENCES

Johnson D, Winterborn A, Kratky V. Efficacy of intravenous mannitol in the management of orbital compartment syndrome: a nonhuman primate model. *Ophthal Plast Reconstr Surg.* 2016;32:187-190.

Murchison AP, Bilyk JR, Savino PJ. Traumatic cranial neuropathies. In: Black EV, Nesi FA, Calvano CJ, Gladstone GJ, Levine MR, eds. *Smith and Nesi's Ophthalmic Plastic and Reconstructive Surgery.* C.V. Mosby; 2021.

3.11 Traumatic Optic Neuropathy

Symptoms

Decreased visual acuity, dyschromatopsia, or visual field defect after a traumatic injury to the eye or periocular area; other trauma symptoms (e.g., pain, periocular edema).

Signs

Critical. A new afferent pupillary defect in a traumatized orbit that cannot be accounted for by previously existing or concomitant ocular pathology.

Other. Decreased color vision in the affected eye, a visual field defect, and other signs of trauma. Acutely, the optic disc appears normal in most cases of posterior indirect TON. In cases of anterior TON, optic disc avulsion may be obvious on funduscopic examination unless obscured by vitreous hemorrhage (VH). Extraocular motility may be compromised in these cases because of associated EOM avulsion or contusion. TON may be associated with intracranial injury.

NOTE: Optic disc pallor usually does not appear for weeks after a traumatic optic nerve injury. If pallor is present immediately after trauma, a preexisting optic neuropathy should be suspected.

Differential Diagnosis of a Traumatic Afferent Pupillary Defect

- Bilateral, asymmetric TON.
- Severe retinal trauma: Retinal abnormality is evident on examination.
- Traumatic, diffuse VH: Obscured view of retina, relative afferent pupillary defect (RAPD) is mild if present.
- Intracranial trauma with asymmetric damage to the prechiasmal optic nerves.

Etiology

TON is typically categorized based on location of injury (anterior or posterior) and mechanism of injury (direct or indirect). Anterior TON is arbitrarily defined as occurring anterior to the entrance of the central retinal artery into the optic nerve. Direct TON is usually due to compression, contusion, and/or laceration of the optic nerve. Indirect TON is typically due to deceleration injury with shearing of the nerve and vascular supply in the optic canal, and much less commonly due to rapid rotation of the globe leading to optic nerve head avulsion.

- Compressive optic neuropathy from orbital hemorrhage: Most common TON. (See 3.10, TRAUMATIC RETROBULBAR HEMORRHAGE.)
- Compressive optic neuropathy from orbital foreign body: A subcategory of direct TON. (See 3.12, INTRAORBITAL FOREIGN BODY.)
- Bony impingement: A posterior direct TON that results from impingement of the apical or intracanalicular optic nerve from a fracture at the orbital apex and/or optic canal. Mechanisms vary widely. Direct bony impingement on the optic canal may result from a skull base fracture that also involves adjacent structures, including the cavernous sinus, with resultant cranial neuropathy **(see Figure 3.11.1)**.

- Optic nerve sheath hematoma: An extremely rare and difficult to diagnose direct or indirect TON. Imaging may show perineural blood in the optic nerve sheath. Often a presumptive diagnosis requiring an abnormal fundus appearance, typically a combination of retinal venous and arterial occlusions (e.g., central retinal artery occlusion, central retinal vein occlusion). Progressive visual loss may occur as the hematoma expands. In most cases, optic nerve sheath hematoma is seen in conjunction with retinal hemorrhages and a subarachnoid intracranial bleed (Terson syndrome).

- Deceleration injury: The second most common form of TON, specifically known as posterior indirect TON, but often simply referred to as TON. The skull (usually the forehead, but can be the midface) hits a static object (e.g., steering wheel, bicycle handlebars, pavement) while the soft tissue within the orbit continues to move forward. Since the optic nerve is tethered at the optic canal, shearing of the nutrient pial vessels may occur with subsequent optic nerve edema within the confined space of the optic canal. A second "shock wave" mechanism may also occur. Cadaver studies have shown that a blow to the frontal bone is transmitted to the optic canal. Visual loss from posterior indirect TON is typically immediate and progresses in fewer than 10% of cases.

- Others (e.g., optic nerve laceration, prechiasmal optic nerve avulsion).

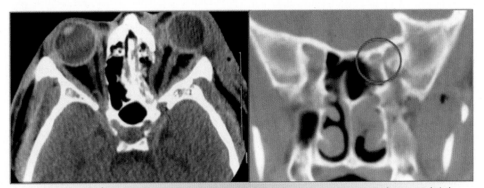

Figure 3.11.1 Computed tomography (CT) of bony impingement of the optic nerve. Red arrow and circle, bone fractures impinging on optic nerve.

Workup

1. History: Mechanism of injury (e.g., deceleration, blow to the forehead)? Loss of consciousness, nausea and/or vomiting, headache, clear nasal discharge (suggestive of cerebrospinal fluid leakage)? Past ocular history including history of amblyopia, strabismus surgery, previous optic neuropathy, retinal detachment, glaucoma, etc.?

2. Complete ocular examination including an assessment of visual acuity and pupils. This may be difficult depending on the patient's mental status, use of sedatives, narcotics, etc.

> **NOTE:** If a bilateral, symmetric TON is present, an RAPD may be absent. Also remember that if an RAPD is present, the patient may have either a unilateral TON or a bilateral asymmetric TON. Do not assume that vision is not compromised in the fellow eye, especially in comatose or sedated patients.

3. Color vision testing in each eye. Checking red desaturation is a useful alternative if Ishihara color plates are not available.

4. Visual fields by confrontation. Formal visual field testing is helpful if available.

5. CT scan of the head and orbit (axial, coronal, and parasagittal views) with thin (i.e., 1 mm) sections through the optic canal and skull base to rule out an intraorbital foreign body or bony impingement on the optic nerve. There may be fractures along the cribriform plate, the sphenoid sinus, and the medial wall of the cavernous sinus. A normal CT in no way rules out posterior indirect TON. Similarly, an optic canal fracture does not mean TON is present.

6. B-scan ultrasound if optic nerve head avulsion is suspected but is obscured clinically by a hyphema, VH, or other media opacity.

Treatment

Depends on the type of TON:

1. Compressive optic neuropathy from orbital hemorrhage: See 3.10, TRAUMATIC RETROBULBAR HEMORRHAGE.

2. Compressive optic neuropathy from orbital foreign body: See 3.12, INTRAORBITAL FOREIGN BODY.

3. Optic nerve sheath hematoma: Optic nerve sheath fenestration may be helpful in the acute stage if optic neuropathy is progressing and no other cause is evident.

4. Optic nerve laceration: No effective treatment.

5. Optic nerve head avulsion: No effective treatment. If external ophthalmoplegia is present, surgical exploration for avulsed EOM may be necessary.

6. Deceleration injury: Effective treatment of posterior indirect TON is, at best, extremely limited. Given the results of the Corticosteroid Randomization After Significant Head Injury (CRASH) study, high-dose corticosteroids should never be offered by ophthalmologists to patients with concomitant TBI or if the TON is older than 8 hours. In the vast majority of cases, we recommend observation alone. If corticosteroids are considered (no evidence of TBI, injury within 8-hour window, no medical comorbidities), the lack of definitive therapeutic evidence and significant side effects must be discussed with the patient and/or family and the primary care team; as a practical matter, this scenario is not frequently encountered. Dosing of methylprednisolone includes a loading dose of 30 mg/kg and then 5.4 mg/kg q6h for 48 hours. Proton-pump inhibitors (e.g., omeprazole) should be given concomitantly. More recently, erythropoietin (EPO) and transcorneal electrical stimulation (TES) have been studied as potential treatments for TON. To date, the evidence is limited by study design, low study power, and lack of randomization and masking. At present, neither modality should be considered standard of care for TON.

7. Bone impingement of the optic canal: Endoscopic optic canal and orbital apex decompression may be offered in select cases, especially if the optic neuropathy is progressive. However, this option should be approached with extreme caution because of the proximity to the cavernous sinus and carotid siphon and possible bony instability of the skull base. The procedure should only be performed by an otolaryngologist and/or neurosurgeon experienced in stereotactic endoscopic sinus and skull base surgery. The patient and/or family should also be informed that there are no definitive data that prove the efficacy of this procedure in TON and that optic canal decompression may result in additional damage to

the intracanalicular optic nerve. On occasion, a transcranial approach for optic canal decompression is indicated, depending on the location of the bone fragments.

Follow Up

Vision, pupillary reaction, and color vision should be evaluated daily for 1 to 2 days in cases of indirect TON where progression is suspected. With a nonprogressive TON, the patient can follow up in weeks to months to assess for spontaneous improvement. If a secondary etiology is causing a TON, follow up depends on the intervention offered and may be more frequent and prolonged. If facial and orbital fracture repair is indicated, it is crucial to document the preoperative visual acuity and visual fields (if possible) and to explain to the patient and family that TON is already present in order to avoid later claims of iatrogenic optic nerve injury. In comatose patients with suspected TON who require facial or orbital fracture repair, the family should be informed that only limited assessment of visual function is possible preoperatively, but significant traumatic visual compromise may have occurred. Always remember that an RAPD may indicate asymmetric, bilateral TON; resist any reassurances to the patient's family of normal contralateral visual function in obtunded or uncooperative patients with an RAPD. Anecdotally, mild to moderate posterior indirect TON may show significant spontaneous improvement over 3 to 6 months in 30% to 60% of patients, while severe initial visual loss seems to carry a worse prognosis.

REFERENCES

Edwards P, Arango M, Balica L, et al. Final results of MRC CRASH, a randomised placebo-controlled trial of intravenous corticosteroid in adults with head injury-outcomes at 6 months. *Lancet.* 2005;365:1957-1959.

Murchison AP, Bilyk JR, Savino PJ. Traumatic cranial neuropathies. In: Black EV, Nesi FA, Calvano CJ, Gladstone GJ, Levine MR, eds. *Smith and Nesi's Ophthalmic Plastic and Reconstructive Surgery.* C.V. Mosby; 2021.

3.12 Intraorbital Foreign Body

Symptoms

Decreased vision, pain, diplopia, or may be asymptomatic. History of trauma, may be remote.

Signs

(See Figures 3.12.1 and 3.12.2.)

Critical. Orbital foreign body identified by clinical examination, radiograph, CT scan, and/or orbital ultrasonography.

Other. A palpable orbital mass, limitation of ocular motility, proptosis, eyelid or conjunctival laceration, erythema, edema, or ecchymosis of eyelids. Presence of an afferent pupillary defect may indicate TON.

Types of Foreign Bodies

1. Poorly tolerated (often lead to inflammation or infection): Organic (e.g., wood or vegetable

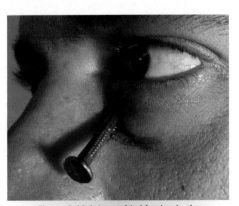

Figure 3.12.1 Intraorbital foreign body.

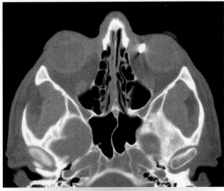

Figure 3.12.2 Computed tomography (CT) of intraorbital foreign body.

3

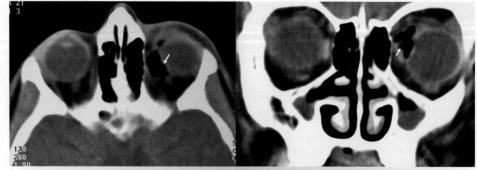

Figure 3.12.3 Axial and coronal computed tomography (CT) of an orbital wooden foreign body, read initially as orbital emphysema. Note the squared-off scleral edge (*arrow*) on the axial image and the "stag horn" appearance (*arrow*) on the coronal image, both suggestive of retained orbital wood.

matter; see **Figure 3.12.3**), chemical (e.g., diesel fuel), and certain retinotoxic metallic foreign bodies (especially copper).

2. Fairly well tolerated (typically produce a chronic low-grade inflammatory reaction): Alloys that are <85% copper (e.g., brass, bronze).

3. Well tolerated (inert materials): Stone, glass, plastic, iron, lead, steel, aluminum, and most other metals and alloys, assuming that they were relatively clean on entry and have a low potential for microbial inoculation.

Workup

1. History: Determine the nature of the injury and the foreign body. Must have high index of suspicion in all trauma. Remember that children are notoriously poor historians.

2. Complete ocular and periorbital examination with special attention to pupillary reaction, IOP, and posterior segment evaluation. Carefully examine for an entry wound: at least 50% of conjunctival entry wounds are missed on clinical examination. Rule out occult globe rupture. Gentle gonioscopy may be needed.

3. CT scan of the orbit and brain (axial, coronal, and parasagittal views, with no larger than 1-mm sections of the orbit) is the initial study of choice regardless of foreign body material to rule out possible metallic foreign body. CT may miss certain materials (e.g., wood may look like air). If wood or vegetative matter is suspected, it is helpful to inform the radiologist in advance. Any lucency within the orbit can then be measured in Hounsfield units to differentiate wood from air. MRI is never

the initial study in suspected foreign body and is contraindicated if a metallic foreign body is suspected or cannot be excluded, but may be a helpful adjunct to CT (especially if a wooden foreign body is suspected) once metallic foreign bodies are ruled out.

4. Based on imaging studies, determine the location of the intraorbital foreign body and rule out optic nerve or central nervous system involvement (frontal lobe, cavernous sinus, carotid artery).

5. Perform orbital B-scan ultrasonography if a foreign body is suspected, but not detected, by CT scan. B-scan is only helpful in the anterior orbit.

6. Culture any drainage sites or foreign material as appropriate.

Treatment

1. NEVER remove an intraorbital foreign body at the slit lamp without first obtaining imaging to evaluate the depth and direction of penetration. Premature removal may result in intracranial bleeding, cerebrospinal fluid leakage, worsening of intraocular injury, etc.

2. Surgical exploration, irrigation, and extraction, based on the following indications:

   • Signs of infection or inflammation (e.g., fever, proptosis, restricted motility, severe chemosis, a palpable orbital mass, abscess on CT scan).

   • Any organic or wooden foreign body (because of the high risk for infection and sight-threatening complications). Many copper foreign bodies require removal because of a marked inflammatory reaction.

- Infectious fistula formation.
- Signs of optic nerve compression or gaze-evoked amaurosis (decreased vision in a specific gaze).
- A large or sharp-edged foreign body (independent of composition) that can be easily extracted.
- In the setting of a ruptured globe, the globe must be repaired first. The orbital foreign body may be removed as necessary thereafter.

NOTE: Posteriorly located, inorganic foreign bodies are often simply observed if inert and not causing optic nerve compression because of the risk of iatrogenic optic neuropathy or diplopia if surgical removal is attempted. Alternatively, even an inert and otherwise asymptomatic metallic foreign body that is anterior and easily accessed may be removed with relatively low morbidity.

NOTE: If the foreign body is located in the posteromedial orbit, removal may be best achieved from an endonasal approach. Consider ENT and/or neurosurgical consultation and CT protocols for image-guided surgery when appropriate.

3. Tetanus toxoid as indicated (see APPENDIX 2, TETANUS PROPHYLAXIS).
4. Consider hospitalization:
   - Administer systemic antibiotics promptly (e.g., cefazolin, 1 g i.v. q8h, for clean, inert objects). If the object is contaminated or organic, treat as orbital cellulitis (see 7.3.1, ORBITAL CELLULITIS).

- Follow vision, degree (if any) of afferent pupillary defect, extraocular motility, proptosis, and eye discomfort daily.
- Surgical exploration and removal of the foreign body when indicated (as above). Discuss with the patient and family preoperatively that successful retrieval may be impossible. Wood often splinters, and multiple procedures may be necessary to entirely remove it. Organic foreign bodies frequently cause recurrent or smoldering infection that may require months of antibiotic therapy and additional surgical exploration. This may result in progressive orbital soft tissue fibrosis and restrictive strabismus.
- If the decision is made to leave the orbital foreign body in place, discharge when stable with oral antibiotics (e.g., amoxicillin–clavulanate 250/125 to 500/125 mg p.o. q8h or 875/125 mg p.o. b.i.d.) to complete a 10- to 14-day course.

5. Patients with small inorganic foreign bodies not requiring surgical intervention may be discharged without hospitalization with oral antibiotics for a 10- to 14-day course.

Follow Up

The patient should return within 1 week of discharge (or immediately if the condition worsens). Close follow up is indicated for several weeks after the antibiotic is stopped to assure that there is no clinical evidence of infection or migration of the orbital foreign body toward a critical orbital structure (e.g., the optic nerve, EOM, globe). Reimage patient as clinically necessary. See 3.14, RUPTURED GLOBE AND PENETRATING OCULAR INJURY; 3.11, TRAUMATIC OPTIC NEUROPATHY; and 7.3.1, ORBITAL CELLULITIS.

3.13 Corneal Laceration

PARTIAL-THICKNESS LACERATION

Signs

(See Figure 3.13.1.)

The AC is not entered, and therefore, the cornea is not perforated.

Workup

1. Careful slit lamp examination should be performed to exclude ocular penetration. Carefully evaluate the conjunctiva, sclera, and cornea, checking for extension beyond the limbus in cases involving the corneal periphery. Evaluate AC depth and compare with the fellow eye. A shallow AC

3

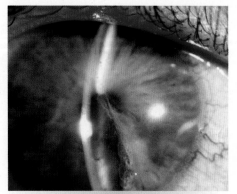

Figure 3.13.1 Corneal laceration.

indicates an actively leaking wound or a self-sealed leak (see FULL-THICKNESS CORNEAL LACERATION below). Check for iris TIDs and evaluate the lens for a cataract or a foreign body tract (must have a high level of suspicion with projectile objects). The presence of TIDs and lens abnormalities indicates a ruptured globe.

2. Seidel test (see APPENDIX 5, SEIDEL TEST TO DETECT A WOUND LEAK). If the Seidel test is positive, a full-thickness laceration is present (see FULL-THICKNESS CORNEAL LACERATION below). A negative Seidel test indicates either a partial-thickness laceration or a self-sealed full-thickness laceration.

3. Avoid IOP measurement if the Seidel test is positive. Measure IOP with caution if the Seidel test is negative to avoid opening a previously self-sealed full-thickness laceration.

Treatment

1. A cycloplegic (e.g., cyclopentolate 1% to 2%) and frequent application of an antibiotic (e.g., polymyxin B/bacitracin ointment or fluoroquinolone drops) depending on the nature of the wound.

2. When a moderate to deep corneal laceration is accompanied by wound gape, it is often best to suture the wound closed in the operating room to provide structural stability and to avoid excessive scarring with corneal irregularity, especially when in the visual axis.

3. If corneal foreign bodies are present and superficial, treat per Sections 3.3, CORNEAL AND CONJUNCTIVAL FOREIGN BODIES. If foreign bodies are in the deeper cornea, there are no signs of infection or inflammation, and are well tolerated (see 3.15, INTRAOCULAR FOREIGN BODY, for inert foreign bodies), they may be left and watched closely. If the patient is symptomatic or if signs of infection/inflammation occur, deeper corneal foreign bodies should be removed in the operating room.

4. Tetanus toxoid for dirty wounds (see APPENDIX 2, TETANUS PROPHYLAXIS).

Follow Up

Reevaluate daily until the epithelium heals.

FULL-THICKNESS CORNEAL LACERATION

(See Figure 3.13.2.)

See 3.14, RUPTURED GLOBE AND PENETRATING OCULAR INJURY. Note that small, self-sealing, or slow-leaking lacerations with formed ACs may be treated with aqueous suppressants, bandage soft contact lenses, fluoroquinolone drops q.i.d., and precautions as listed in Sections 3.14, RUPTURED GLOBE AND PENETRATING OCULAR INJURY. Avoid topical steroids. If an IOFB is present, see 3.15, INTRAOCULAR FOREIGN BODY.

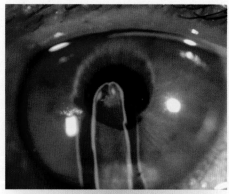

Figure 3.13.2 Full-thickness corneal laceration with positive Seidel test.

3.14 Ruptured Globe and Penetrating Ocular Injury

Symptoms

Pain, decreased vision, and loss of fluid from eye. History of trauma, fall, or sharp object entering globe.

Signs

(See Figure 3.14.1.)

Critical. Full-thickness scleral or corneal laceration, severe subconjunctival hemorrhage (especially involving 360 degrees of bulbar conjunctiva, often bullous), a deep or shallow AC compared to the fellow eye, a peaked or irregular pupil, iris TIDs, lens material or vitreous in the AC, foreign body tract or new opacity in the lens, or extraocular motility limitation (greatest in the direction of rupture). Intraocular contents may be outside of the globe.

Other. Low IOP (may also be normal or rarely increased), iridodialysis, cyclodialysis, hyphema, periorbital ecchymosis, VH, and dislocated or subluxed lens. Commotio retinae, choroidal rupture, and retinal breaks may be seen but are often obscured by VH.

Workup/Treatment

Once a ruptured globe is diagnosed, further examination should be deferred until the time of surgical repair in the operating room. This is to avoid placing any pressure on the globe and risking extrusion of intraocular contents. Diagnosis should be made by penlight, indirect ophthalmoscope, or, if possible, slit lamp examination (with minimal manipulation). Once the diagnosis is made, the following measures should be taken:

1. Protect the eye with a hard shield at all times. Do not patch the eye.

2. CT scan of the brain and orbits (axial, coronal, and parasagittal views with 1-mm sections) to rule out IOFB.

3. Gentle B-scan ultrasound may be needed to localize posterior rupture site(s) or to rule out IOFBs not visible on CT scan (nonmetallic, wood, etc.). However, B-scan should not be done in patients with an obvious anterior rupture due to the risk of extruding intraocular contents. A trained ophthalmologist should evaluate the patient before B-scan or any other manipulation is performed on a ruptured globe suspect.

4. Admit the patient to the hospital with no food or drink (NPO).

5. Place the patient on bed rest with bathroom privileges. Avoid strenuous activities, bending, and Valsalva maneuvers.

6. Systemic antibiotics should be administered within 6 hours of injury. For adults, give cefazolin 1 g i.v. q8h or vancomycin 1 g i.v. q12h, and moxifloxacin 400 mg i.v. daily (or an equivalent fluoroquinolone). For children ≤12 years, give cefazolin 25 to 50 mg/kg/d i.v. in three divided doses and gentamicin 2 mg/kg i.v. q8h. Some groups recommend 48 hours of intravenous antibiotics perioperatively. A 1-week antibiotic course is typically completed postoperatively with a broad-spectrum fluoroquinolone (e.g., levofloxacin 750 mg p.o. daily).

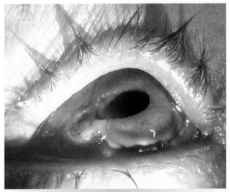

Figure 3.14.1 Ruptured globe showing flat anterior chamber (AC), iris prolapse, and peaked pupil.

NOTE: Antibiotic doses may need to be reduced if renal function is impaired. Gentamicin peak and trough levels are obtained 1/2 hour before and after the fifth dose, and blood urea nitrogen and creatinine levels are evaluated every other day.

7. Administer tetanus toxoid p.r.n. (see APPENDIX 2, TETANUS PROPHYLAXIS).
8. Administer antiemetics (e.g., ondansetron 4 or 8 mg q4–8h) p.r.n. for nausea and vomiting to prevent Valsalva and possible expulsion of intraocular contents.
9. Administer pain medicine before and after surgery p.r.n. (often intravenous).
10. Determine time of the patient's last meal. Timing of surgical repair is often influenced by this information.
11. Arrange for surgical repair to be done as soon as possible.

NOTE: In any severely traumatized eye in which there is no chance of restoring vision, potential enucleation should be discussed with the patient early on. This procedure should be performed within 7 to 14 days after the trauma to minimize the rare occurrence of sympathetic ophthalmia.

Infection is more likely to occur in eyes with dirty injuries, retained IOFBs and rupture of lens capsule and in patients with a long delay until primary surgical repair. In patients at high risk of infection, some groups recommend intravitreal antibiotics at the time of surgical closure (see 12.15, TRAUMATIC ENDOPHTHALMITIS).

NOTE: Several studies have examined prognostic factors for ocular trauma and open globe injuries. One commonly used and validated system is the Ocular Trauma Score (OTS). See **Tables 3.14.1** and **3.14.2**.

TABLE 3.14.1 Calculating the OTS

Variable	Raw Points
Initial Vision	
NLP	60
LP/HM	70
1/200 to 19/200	80
20/200 to 20/50	90
>20/40	100
Rupture	−23
Endophthalmitis	−17
Perforating injury	−14
Retinal detachment	−11
Afferent pupillary defect	−10

LP/HM, light perception/hand motion; NLP, no light perception.

REFERENCE

Kuhn F, Maisiak R, Mann L, et al. The Ocular Trauma Score (OTS). *Ophthalmol Clin North Am.* 2002;15(2):163-165.

TABLE 3.14.2 Visual Prognosis per OTS

Sum of Raw Points	OTS	No Light Perception (%)	Light Perception/ Hand Motion (%)	1/200 to 19/200 (%)	20/200 to 20/50 (%)	>20/40 (%)
0 to 44	1	74	15	7	3	1
45 to 65	2	27	26	18	15	15
66 to 80	3	2	11	15	31	41
81 to 91	4	1	2	3	22	73
92 to 100	5	0	1	1	5	94

OTS, Ocular Trauma Score.

3.15 Intraocular Foreign Body

Symptoms

Eye pain, decreased vision, or may be asymptomatic; often suggestive history (e.g., hammering metal or sharp object entering globe).

Signs

(See Figure 3.15.1.)

Critical. May have a clinically detectable corneal or scleral perforation site, hole in the iris, focal lens opacity, or an IOFB. IOFBs are often seen on CT scan (thin cuts), B-scan, and/or UBM.

Other. See 3.14, RUPTURED GLOBE AND PENETRATING OCULAR INJURY. Also, microcystic (epithelial) edema of the peripheral cornea (a clue that a foreign body may be hidden in the AC angle in the same sector of the eye). Long-standing iron-containing IOFBs may cause siderosis, manifesting as anisocoria, heterochromia, corneal endothelial and epithelial deposits, anterior subcapsular cataracts, lens dislocation, retinopathy, and optic atrophy.

Types of Foreign Bodies

1. Frequently produce severe inflammatory reactions and may encapsulate within 24 hours if on the retina.

    Magnetic: Iron, steel, and tin.

    Nonmagnetic: Copper and vegetable matter (may be severe or mild).

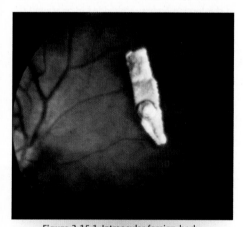

Figure 3.15.1 Intraocular foreign body.

2. Typically produce mild inflammatory reactions.

    Magnetic: Nickel.

    Nonmagnetic: Aluminum, mercury, zinc, and vegetable matter (may be severe or mild).

3. Inert foreign bodies: Carbon, gold, coal, glass, lead, gypsum plaster, platinum, porcelain, rubber, silver, and stone. Brass, an alloy of copper and zinc, is also relatively nontoxic. However, even inert foreign bodies can be toxic because of a coating or chemical additive. Most ball bearings (BBs) and gunshot pellets are made of 80% to 90% lead and 10% to 20% iron.

Workup

- History: Composition of foreign body? Time of last meal?
- Perform ocular examination, including visual acuity and careful evaluation of globe integrity. If there is an obvious perforation site, the remainder of the examination may be deferred until surgery. If there does not appear to be a risk of extrusion of intraocular contents, the globe is inspected gently to localize the perforation site and to detect the foreign body.
- Slit lamp examination; search the AC and iris for a foreign body and look for an iris TID. Examine the lens for disruption, cataract, or embedded foreign body. Check IOP.
- Consider careful gonioscopy of the AC angle if no wound leak can be detected and the globe appears intact.
- Dilated retinal examination using indirect ophthalmoscopy.
- Obtain a CT scan of the orbits and brain (coronal, axial, and parasagittal views with no larger than 1-mm sections through the orbits). MRI is contraindicated in the presence of a metallic foreign body. It may be difficult to visualize wood, glass, or plastic on a CT scan, especially acutely. Suspicion of a nonmetallic IOFB should specifically be mentioned to the reading radiologist.
- Gentle B-scan of the globe and orbit. Intraocular air can mimic a foreign body. Consider UBM to inspect the AC if IOFB is not visible on clinical examination (e.g.,

foreign body in the AC angle or sulcus). These steps should be deferred in patients with a definitive or suspected anterior rupture given the risk for extrusion of intraocular contents.

- Culture the wound site if it appears infected.
- Determine whether the foreign body is magnetic (e.g., examine material from which the foreign body came).

Treatment

1. Hospitalization with no food or drink (NPO) until repair.
2. Place a protective rigid shield over the involved eye. Do not patch the eye.
3. Tetanus prophylaxis as needed (see APPENDIX 2, TETANUS PROPHYLAXIS).
4. Broad-spectrum gram-positive and gram-negative antibiotic coverage (e.g., vancomycin 1 g i.v. q12h and ceftazidime 1 g i.v. q12h or ciprofloxacin 400 mg i.v. q12h or moxifloxacin 400 mg i.v. q.d.).

 NOTE: Fluoroquinolones are contraindicated in children and pregnant women.

5. Cycloplegia (e.g., atropine 1% b.i.d.) for posterior-segment foreign bodies.

6. Urgent surgical removal of any acute IOFB is advisable to reduce the risk of infection and development of proliferative vitreoretinopathy (PVR). For some metallic foreign bodies, a magnet may be useful during surgical extraction. Copper or contaminated foreign bodies require especially urgent removal. A chronic IOFB may require removal if associated with severe recurrent inflammation, if in the visual axis, or if causing siderosis.
7. If endophthalmitis is present, treat as per 12.15, TRAUMATIC ENDOPHTHALMITIS.

Follow Up

Observe the patient closely in the hospital for signs of inflammation or infection. If the surgeon is uncertain as to whether the foreign body was entirely removed, postoperative imaging should be considered with CT, B-scan, or UBM as above. Periodic follow up for years is required; watch for a delayed inflammatory reaction in both the traumatic and nontraumatic eye. When an IOFB is left in place, an electroretinogram (ERG) should be obtained as soon as it can be done safely. Serial ERGs should be followed to look for toxic retinopathy, which will often reverse if the foreign body is removed.

3.16 Firework or Shrapnel-/Bullet-Related Injuries

Symptoms

Ocular pain, decreased vision, foreign body sensation, tearing, redness, and photophobia; history of trauma with firework, weapons of warfare, or devices that result in high-velocity impact and shrapnel/particulate fragmentation (e.g., firecracker, sparkler, firearm, explosive, grenade).

Signs

Critical. Foreign bodies, usually irregular in shape and fragmented in nature, embedded in ocular or orbital tissues. Periocular damage secondary to associated surrounding high-energy release. Can result in open or closed globe injuries.

Other. Conjunctival injection, eyelid edema, corneal/conjunctival epithelial defects or lacerations, thermal and/or chemical burns of ocular tissues (e.g., eyelid, conjunctiva, cornea), AC reaction, hyphema, iridodialysis, angle

recession, VH, and retina or optic nerve injury. Motility deficits and globe malposition may exist if the foreign body is embedded in or around the orbit.

Workup

1. History: Mechanism of injury (e.g., detonation of an explosive, missile, or firearm; distance of patient from the instrument of injury, etc.)? Size, weight, velocity, force, shape, and composition of the object? Concurrent tinnitus or hearing loss (often associated with explosions/firearms)?
2. Document visual acuity before any procedure is performed. Topical anesthetic may be necessary to facilitate examination, but be careful not to cause expulsion of ocular tissue if open globe exists. Also evaluate optic nerve function by examining pupillary response and testing color plates.

3. Examine for orbital signs by evaluating motility, globe malposition, and sectoral chemosis/inflammation, as this might help localize the landing site of shrapnel or bullet material that has entered without exit.

4. Look for periocular tissue burns or lacerations, which may warrant evaluation by internal medicine or dermatology.

5. Check the forniceal pH if an associated chemical injury is suspected. See 3.1, CHEMICAL BURN.

6. Slit lamp examination: Locate and assess the depth of any foreign body. Examine closely for possible entry sites (rule out self-sealing lacerations), pupil irregularities, iris tears and TIDs, capsular perforations, lens opacities, hyphema, AC shallowing (or deepening in scleral perforations), and asymmetrically low IOP in the involved eye. Assess for any damage to the lacrimal apparatus.

7. Perform a dilated fundus examination to exclude possible IOFB, unless there is a risk of extrusion of intraocular contents (see 3.15, INTRAOCULAR FOREIGN BODY). Dilation should typically be deferred if there is a foreign body lodged in the iris. In cases of chemical injury, dilate with cycloplegics only and avoid alpha-agonist drops (e.g., phenylephrine), which may exacerbate limbal ischemia.

8. Consider gentle B-scan ultrasound, CT scan of the orbit (axial, coronal, and parasagittal views, 1-mm sections), or UBM to exclude an intraocular or intraorbital foreign body. Avoid MRI if history concerning for possible metallic foreign body.

Treatment and Follow Up

1. Depends on the specific injuries present. Refer to appropriate sections as needed. Depending on the number or extent of injuries, consider exploration in the OR.

2. Consider tetanus prophylaxis (see APPENDIX 2, TETANUS PROPHYLAXIS).

3. If evidence of penetrating or perforating trauma, see 3.13, CORNEAL LACERATIONS to 3.14, RUPTURED GLOBE AND PENETRATING TRAUMA INJURY.

4. If foreign bodies are present, but either inaccessible or associated with injuries that prohibit safe removal at the slit lamp, see 3.12, INTRAORBITAL FOREIGN BODY or 3.15, INTRAOCULAR FOREIGN BODY. Many inert foreign bodies are well tolerated. The risk of iatrogenic optic neuropathy or diplopia with attempted surgical removal of foreign bodies must be weighed against the risk of delayed complications if left near vital orbital structures.

5. If evidence of pH alteration, see 3.1, CHEMICAL BURN.

6. If extensive facial or skull fractures exist, comanagement with neurosurgery, otolaryngology, or oromaxillofacial surgery may be needed. Delayed reconstructive procedures are often necessary.

7. Comanage with internal medicine or dermatology if periocular or facial burns exist. The patient may require care in a burn unit.

8. Follow up depends on the extent of injuries and the conditions being treated.

3.17 Commotio Retinae

Symptoms

Decreased vision or asymptomatic; history of recent ocular trauma.

Signs

(See Figure 3.17.1.)

Critical. Confluent area of retinal whitening in the periphery or posterior pole (Berlin edema). Cherry-red spot may be present with Berlin edema. The retinal blood vessels are undisturbed in the area of retinal whitening.

Other. Additional signs of ocular trauma, such as retinal hemorrhages, may be noted.

 NOTE: Visual acuity does not always correlate with the degree of retinal whitening.

Etiology

Blunt trauma to the globe causes shock waves which disrupt the photoreceptors. Retinal whitening is the result of fragmentation of the photoreceptor outer segments and intracellular edema of the retinal pigment epithelium (RPE). The inner retinal layers may also be involved depending on the force of injury.

3

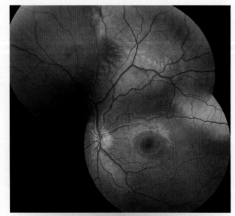

Figure 3.17.1 Commotio retinae.

Differential Diagnosis

- Retinal detachment: Retina elevated associated with retinal break or dialysis. See 11.3, RETINAL DETACHMENT.
- Retinal artery occlusion: Retinal whitening along the distribution of an artery. See 11.6, CENTRAL RETINAL ARTERY OCCLUSION and 11.7, BRANCH RETINAL ARTERY OCCLUSION.
- White without pressure: Common benign peripheral retinal finding. May be associated with a prominent vitreous base.

- Myelinated nerve fiber layer: Develops postnatally (see Figure 11.5.2).
- Chorioretinitis sclopetaria: Bare sclera visible through retinal and choroidal rupture on dilated examination. See 3.19, CHORIORETINITIS SCLOPETARIA.

Workup

Complete ophthalmic evaluation, including dilated fundus examination. Scleral depression is performed except when a ruptured globe, hyphema, microhyphema, or iritis is present. Optical coherence tomography (OCT) shows ellipsoid zone disruption.

Treatment

No treatment is required because this condition is self-limited. Some patients with foveal involvement may be left with chronic visual impairment and RPE atrophy or hyperpigmentation on fundus examination.

Follow Up

Dilated fundus examination is repeated in 1 to 2 weeks. Patients are instructed to return sooner if retinal detachment symptoms are experienced (see 11.3, RETINAL DETACHMENT).

3.18 Traumatic Choroidal Rupture

Symptoms

Decreased vision or asymptomatic. History of ocular trauma.

Signs

(See Figure 3.18.1.)

Critical. A yellow or white crescent-shaped subretinal streak, usually concentric to the optic disc. May be single or multiple. Often cannot be seen until several days or weeks after trauma because it may be obscured by overlying subretinal blood.

Other. Rarely, the rupture may be radially oriented. Choroidal neovascularization (CNV) may develop later. TON may be present.

Differential Diagnosis

- Lacquer cracks of high myopia: Often bilateral. A tilted disc, a scleral crescent adjacent to the disc, and a posterior staphyloma may also

be seen. CNV may also develop in this condition. See 11.22, HIGH MYOPIA.
- Angioid streaks: Bilateral subretinal streaks radiating from the optic disc, sometimes associated with CNV. See 11.23, ANGIOID STREAKS.

Workup

1. Complete ocular evaluation, including dilated fundus examination to rule out retinal breaks and to detect CNV.
2. Consider OCT to characterize a choroidal rupture and evaluate potential CNV.
3. Consider fluorescein angiography to confirm the presence and location of CNV if the injury is old.

Treatment

1. Observation. There are no medical or surgical treatment options in the acute setting. Consider recommending safety eyewear. An

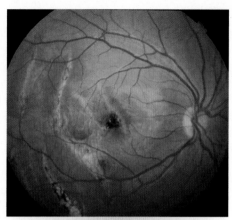

Figure 3.18.1 Choroidal rupture.

Amsler grid may be provided, and the patient is instructed to return if any change in the appearance of the grid is noted (see APPENDIX 4, AMSLER GRID).

2. Anti–vascular endothelial growth factor (VEGF) therapy may be used if CNV develops. See 11.17, NEOVASCULAR OR EXUDATIVE (WET) AGE-RELATED MACULAR DEGENERATION, for more information on CNV treatment.

Follow Up

After ocular trauma, patients with hemorrhage obscuring the underlying choroid are reevaluated every 1 to 2 weeks until the choroid can be well visualized. Although CNV is rare overall, ruptures that are particularly long or closer to the fovea are at greater risk for CNV development. Fundus examinations may be performed every 6 to 12 months depending on the severity and risk of progression to CNV. Patients treated for CNV must be followed closely after treatment to watch for persistent or new CNV (see 11.17, NEOVASCULAR OR EXUDATIVE (WET) AGE-RELATED MACULAR DEGENERATION, for further follow-up guidelines).

3.19 Chorioretinitis Sclopetaria

Symptoms

Visual loss; severity depends on the region of involvement. History of high-velocity missile injury to orbit (e.g., a BB, bullet, or shrapnel).

Signs

(See Figure 3.19.1.)

Critical. Areas of choroidal and retinal rupture leaving bare sclera visible on fundus examination, typically demonstrating a "claw-like" configuration of fundus atrophy and pigmentation.

Other. Subretinal, intraretinal, preretinal, and VH often involving the macula. Eventually blood is resorbed and the resultant defects are replaced by fibrous tissue. Intraorbital foreign body. Can have associated avulsion of vitreous base, which can cause peripheral retinal dialysis.

Etiology

Caused by a high-velocity missile passing through the orbit without perforating the globe. Resultant shock waves lead to chorioretinal rupture from the sclera.

Differential Diagnosis

• Ruptured globe: Severe subconjunctival hemorrhage and chemosis, often with deep or shallow AC; low IOP; and peaked, irregular pupil. See 3.14, RUPTURED GLOBE AND PENETRATING OCULAR INJURY.

• Choroidal rupture: White or yellow crescent-shaped subretinal streak usually concentric to the optic nerve. No retinal break is present. Initially, retinal hemorrhage in the posterior pole may obscure a choroidal rupture, which subsequently becomes apparent as the blood clears. See 3.18, TRAUMATIC CHOROIDAL RUPTURE.

• Optic nerve avulsion: Decreased vision with RAPD on examination and hemorrhagic depression or excavation of the optic disc if partial,

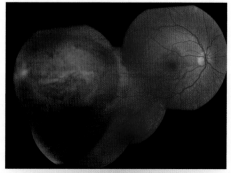

Figure 3.19.1 Chorioretinitis sclopetaria.

or retraction of entire nerve if complete. Often associated with VH. No treatment is available, and visual prognosis depends on extent of injury. See 3.11, TRAUMATIC OPTIC NEUROPATHY.

Workup

1. History: Known injury with a projectile?
2. Complete ocular evaluation including dilated fundus examination. Look for areas of retinal and choroidal rupture with underlying bare sclera. Carefully examine the conjunctiva and sclera to rule out ruptured globe. Rule out IOFB. Carefully examine the retinal periphery for retinal tears or dialysis.
3. Protect the eye with a rigid shield.
4. CT scan of the orbit (axial, coronal, and parasagittal views, 1-mm sections) to check

for intrascleral, intraocular, or intraorbital foreign bodies. Gentle B-scan or UBM may be helpful to rule out intraocular or intraorbital foreign bodies.

Treatment

Observation, as there is no effective treatment. Complications, including retinal dialysis and detachment, are treated appropriately. Surgery can be considered for nonclearing VH.

Follow Up

Sequential examinations are required every 2 to 4 weeks looking for signs of retinal detachment as blood clears. Patients should be followed until an atrophic "claw-like" scar replaces areas of hemorrhage.

3.20 Purtscher Retinopathy

Symptoms

Decreased vision, often sudden; can be severe. History of compression injury to the head, chest, or lower extremities (e.g., long bone fractures), but not a direct ocular injury.

Signs

(See Figure 3.20.1.)

Critical. Multiple cotton wool spots and/or intraretinal hemorrhages in a configuration around the optic nerve; can also have larger areas of superficial retinal whitening with perivascular clearing (Purtscher flecken). Changes are typically bilateral but may be asymmetric or unilateral.

Other. Serous macular detachment, dilated tortuous vessels, hard exudates, optic disc edema (though the disc usually appears normal), macular pseudo–cherry-red spot, RAPD, and optic atrophy when chronic.

Differential Diagnosis

1. Pseudo–Purtscher retinopathy: Several entities with the same or similar presentation but not associated with trauma (Purtscher retinopathy by definition occurs with trauma), including acute pancreatitis, malignant hypertension, thrombotic thrombocytopenic purpura (TTP), hemolytic uremic syndrome (HUS), collagen vascular diseases (e.g.,

systemic lupus erythematosus, scleroderma, dermatomyositis, Sjögren syndrome), chronic renal failure, amniotic fluid embolism, retrobulbar anesthesia, orbital steroid injection, and alcohol use.
2. Central retinal vein occlusion: Unilateral, multiple hemorrhages and cotton wool spots diffusely throughout the retina. See 11.8, CENTRAL RETINAL VEIN OCCLUSION.
3. Central retinal artery occlusion: Unilateral retinal whitening with a cherry-red spot; see 11.6, CENTRAL RETINAL ARTERY OCCLUSION.

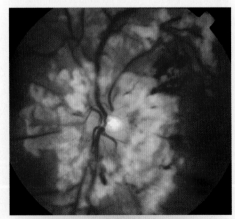

Figure 3.20.1 Purtscher retinopathy.

Etiology

Not well understood. It is felt that the findings are due to occlusion of small arterioles in the peripapillary retina by different particles depending on the associated systemic condition: complement activation, fibrin clots, platelet–leukocyte aggregates, or fat emboli.

Workup

1. History: Compression injury to the head or chest? Long bone fracture? If no trauma, any symptoms associated with causes of pseudo–Purtscher retinopathy (see above, e.g., renal failure, rheumatologic disease)?
2. Complete ocular evaluation including dilated fundus examination. Rule out direct globe injury.
3. CT of the head, chest, or long bones as indicated.
4. If characteristic findings occur in association with severe head or chest trauma, then the diagnosis is established and no further workup is required. Without trauma, the patient needs a systemic workup to investigate other causes (e.g., blood pressure measurement, basic metabolic panel [BMP], CBC, amylase, lipase, rheumatologic evaluation).
5. Fluorescein angiography: Shows patchy capillary nonperfusion in regions of retinal whitening.

Treatment

No ocular treatment available. Must treat the underlying condition if possible to prevent further damage.

Follow Up

Repeat dilated fundus examination in 2 to 4 weeks. Retinal lesions resolve over a few weeks to months. Visual acuity may remain reduced but may return to baseline in 50% of cases.

3.21 Shaken Baby Syndrome

Definition

Form of abusive head trauma characterized by intracranial hemorrhage, brain injury, multifocal fractures, and/or retinal hemorrhages due to repeated acceleration–deceleration forces with or without blunt head impact. External signs of trauma are often absent.

Symptoms

Change in mental status, new-onset seizures, poor feeding, and irritability. Child is usually <1 year of age but rarely >3 years of age. Symptoms and signs often inconsistent with history.

Signs

Critical. Retinal hemorrhages are present in ~85% of cases. Two-thirds are too numerous to count and multilayered (pre-, intra-, and subretinal), extending throughout the retina to the ora serrata. Markedly asymmetric hemorrhages in up to 20% of cases, unilateral in ~2%. Macular retinoschisis (hemorrhagic macular cysts, most often subinternal limiting membrane) may be seen with or without surrounding paramacular retinal folds. Most commonly associated brain lesions are subarachnoid and subdural hemorrhages.

Characteristic fractures include the ribs and/or long bone epiphyses. Cerebral edema and death occur in ~20% to 30% of cases.

Other. Subretinal and VH less common. Retinal detachment, papilledema, late optic atrophy, and optic nerve avulsion are infrequent. Postmortem findings include orbital, optic nerve sheath, optic nerve sheath intradural, and posterior intrascleral hemorrhage.

Differential Diagnosis

- Severe accidental injury: Accompanied by other external injuries consistent with the history. Even in the most severe accidental injuries (e.g., motor vehicle accidents [MVA]), retinal hemorrhages are uncommon. In the usual trauma of childhood, retinal hemorrhages are typically mild and do not extend to the ora serrata. Severe retinal hemorrhages similar to shaken baby syndrome have only been reported in fatal head crush, fatal MVA, and an 11-m fall onto concrete.
- Birth trauma: Retinal hemorrhages can be extensive, but nerve fiber layer hemorrhages are gone by 2 weeks, and dot/blot hemorrhages typically disappear by 4 to 6 weeks. Foveal, preretinal, and VH may persist longer.

No retinoschisis or retinal folds. Clinical history must be consistent. Most common cause of retinal hemorrhage in neonates.

- Coagulopathies, leukemia, and other blood dyscrasias. Rare, but should be ruled out. Other than leukemia, in which infiltrates are usually present, these entities do not cause extensive retinal hemorrhages.
- Hyperacute elevation of intracranial pressure (e.g., ruptured aneurysm) may cause extensive retinal hemorrhage. Easily differentiated by neuroimaging. Otherwise, increased intracranial pressure in children does NOT result in extensive retinal hemorrhage beyond the peripapillary area.
- Hypoxia, immunizations, cardiopulmonary resuscitation (CPR), meningitis, sepsis, and cortical vein thrombosis are often offered as alternate explanations in the courtroom for retinal hemorrhages, but these are not usually supported by available clinical and research evidence. Type, distribution, and number of hemorrhages is helpful in ascertaining causality.

Workup

1. History from caregiver(s) is best obtained by a child abuse pediatrician or a representative team. Be alert for history incompatible with injuries or changing versions of history.
2. Complete ophthalmic examination, including pupils (for afferent pupillary defect) and dilated fundus examination.
3. Laboratory: CBC with platelet count, PT/INR, and PTT. Consider additional evaluation based on initial screening results.
4. Imaging: CT or MRI; skeletal survey. Consider bone scan.

5. Admit patient to hospital if shaken baby syndrome is suspected. Requires coordinated care by neurosurgery, pediatrics, ophthalmology, and social services.

NOTE: Careful documentation is an integral part of the evaluation, as the medical record may be used as a legal document. Ocular photography is not the gold standard for documenting retinal hemorrhages but may be useful if available. A thorough detailed description is essential with or without a drawing, including type, number, and distribution of hemorrhages and presence/absence of retinoschisis/folds.

Treatment

Predominantly supportive. Focus is on systemic complications. Ocular manifestations are usually observed. In cases of nonabsorbing dense VH, vitrectomy may be considered due to the risk of amblyopia.

NOTE: All physicians are legally mandated to report suspected child abuse. There is legal precedence for prosecution of nonreporters.

Follow Up

Prognosis is variable and unpredictable. Survivors can suffer from significant cognitive disabilities, and severe visual loss occurs in 20% of children, usually from optic atrophy or brain injury. Even if no retinal hemorrhages exist, ophthalmologic follow up is recommended for children with brain injury.

Chapter 4

Cornea

4.1 Superficial Punctate Keratopathy

Symptoms

Pain, photophobia, red eye, foreign body sensation, and mildly decreased vision.

Signs

(See Figure 4.1.1.)

Critical. Pinpoint locations of corneal epithelial cell damage or breakdown that stain with fluorescein. May be confluent if severe. Staining pattern may allude to etiology. Pain is relieved by the instillation of anesthetic drops. Also referred to as punctate epithelial erosions.

> **NOTE:** Relief of pain with the instillation of anesthetic drops (e.g., proparacaine) strongly suggests corneal epithelial disease as the etiology of pain. Although anesthetic drop instillation is an essential part of the ocular examination, patients should NEVER be prescribed topical anesthetic drops, and the clinician should ensure the patient does not take anesthetic drops from the office. When used chronically, these drops inhibit epithelial healing and may cause corneal ulceration.

Other. Conjunctival injection and watery discharge.

Etiology

Superficial punctate keratopathy (SPK) is non-specific but is most commonly seen in the following disorders, which may be associated with a specific staining pattern:

- Superior staining
  - Contact lens–related disorder (e.g., chemical toxicity, tight lens syndrome, contact lens overwear syndrome, giant papillary conjunctivitis). See 4.20, CONTACT LENS-RELATED PROBLEMS.

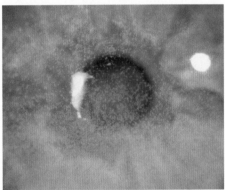

Figure 4.1.1 Superficial punctate keratopathy stained with fluorescein.

  - Foreign body under the upper eyelid: Typically linear SPK, fine epithelial defects arranged vertically.
  - Floppy eyelid syndrome: Extremely loose upper eyelids that evert easily. See 6.6, FLOPPY EYELID SYNDROME.
  - Superior limbic keratoconjunctivitis (SLK): Superior bulbar conjunctival inflammation. See 5.4, SUPERIOR LIMBIC KERATOCONJUNCTIVITIS.
  - Vernal conjunctivitis: Atopy, large conjunctival papillae under the upper eyelid and/or limbus. See 5.1, ACUTE CONJUNCTIVITIS.
- Interpalpebral staining
  - Dry eye syndrome: Poor tear lake, decreased tear break-up time, decreased Schirmer test. See 4.3, DRY EYE SYNDROME.
  - Neurotrophic keratopathy: Decreased corneal sensation. May progress to corneal ulceration. See 4.6, NEUROTROPHIC KERATOPATHY.

- Ultraviolet burn/photokeratopathy: Often in welders or from sunlamps. See 4.7, ULTRAVIOLET KERATOPATHY.
- Inferior staining
  - Blepharitis: Erythema, telangiectasias, or crusting of the eyelid margins, meibomian gland dysfunction. See 5.8, BLEPHARITIS/MEIBOMITIS.
  - Exposure keratopathy: Poor eyelid closure with failure of eyelids to cover the entire globe. See 4.5, EXPOSURE KERATOPATHY.
  - Topical drug toxicity (e.g., neomycin, gentamicin, trifluridine, atropine, as well as any drop with preservatives, including artificial tears, or any frequently used drop).
  - Conjunctivitis: Discharge, conjunctival injection, and eyelids stuck together on awakening. See 5.1, ACUTE CONJUNCTIVITIS and 5.2, CHRONIC CONJUNCTIVITIS.
  - Trichiasis/distichiasis: One or more eyelashes rubbing against the cornea (superior SPK if misdirected lashes from upper eyelid). See 6.5, TRICHIASIS.
  - Entropion or ectropion: Eyelid margin turned in or out (superior SPK if upper eyelid abnormality). See 6.3, ECTROPION and 6.4, ENTROPION.
- Other
  - Trauma: SPK can occur from relatively mild trauma, such as chronic eye rubbing.
  - Mild chemical injury: See 3.1, CHEMICAL BURN.
  - Thygeson superficial punctate keratitis: Bilateral, recurrent epithelial keratitis (raised epithelial staining lesions, not micro erosions) without conjunctival injection. See 4.8, THYGESON SUPERFICIAL PUNCTATE KERATITIS.

Workup

1. History: Trauma? Contact lens wear? Eye drops? Discharge or eyelid matting? Chemical or ultraviolet light exposure? Snoring or sleep apnea? Time of day when worse?
2. Evaluate the cornea, eyelid margin, and tear film with fluorescein. Evert the upper and lower eyelids. Check eyelid closure, position, and laxity. Look for inward-growing or misdirected lashes.

3. Inspect contact lenses for fit (if still in the eye) and for the presence of deposits, sharp edges, and cracks.

 NOTE: A soft contact lens should be removed before instillation of fluorescein.

Treatment

See the appropriate section to treat the underlying disorder. SPK is often treated nonspecifically as follows:

1. Noncontact lens wearer with a small amount of SPK
   - Artificial tears q.i.d., preferably preservative-free.
   - Can add a lubricating gel or ointment q.h.s.
2. Noncontact lens wearer with a large amount of SPK
   - Preservative-free artificial tears q2h.
   - Ophthalmic antibiotic ointment (e.g., bacitracin/polymyxin B or erythromycin q.i.d. for 3 to 5 days).
   - Consider a cycloplegic drop (e.g., cyclopentolate 1% t.i.d.) for relief of pain and photophobia.
3. Contact lens wearer with a small amount of SPK
   - Discontinue contact lens wear.
   - Artificial tears q.i.d., preferably preservative-free.
   - Can add a lubricating gel or ointment q.h.s.
4. Contact lens wearer with a large amount of SPK
   - Discontinue contact lens wear.
   - Antibiotic: Fluoroquinolone (e.g., ciprofloxacin, gatifloxacin, moxifloxacin, or besifloxacin) or aminoglycoside (e.g., tobramycin) drops four to six times per day as well as ophthalmic ointment q.h.s. (e.g., ciprofloxacin or bacitracin/polymyxin B). If confluent SPK, consider ophthalmic antibiotic ointment four to six times per day.
   - Consider a cycloplegic drop (e.g., cyclopentolate 1% t.i.d.) for relief of pain and photophobia.

NOTE: DO NOT patch contact lens–related SPK or epithelial defects because they can quickly develop into severely infected ulcers.

Follow Up

1. Noncontact lens wearers with SPK are not seen again solely for the SPK unless the patient is a child or is unreliable. Reliable patients are told to return if their symptoms worsen or do not improve within 2 to 3 days. When underlying ocular disease is responsible for the SPK, follow up is in accordance with the guidelines for the underlying problem.

2. Contact lens wearers with a large amount of SPK are seen every day or two until significant improvement is demonstrated. Contact lenses are not to be worn until the condition clears. Antibiotics may be discontinued when the SPK resolves. The patient's contact lens regimen (e.g., wearing time, cleaning routine) must be corrected or the contact lenses changed if either is thought to be responsible (see 4.20, CONTACT LENS-RELATED PROBLEMS). Contact lens wearers with a small amount of SPK are rechecked in several days to 1 week, depending on symptoms and degree of SPK.

 NOTE: Contact lens wearers should be advised not to wear contacts when their eyes feel irritated.

4.2 Recurrent Corneal Erosion

Symptoms

Recurrent attacks of acute ocular pain, photophobia, foreign body sensation, and tearing. The pain may awaken patients from sleep or occur immediately upon eye opening. There is often a history of prior corneal abrasion in the involved eye.

Signs

Critical. Localized irregularity and mobility of the corneal epithelium (fluorescein dye may outline the area with negative or positive staining) or a corneal abrasion. Epithelial changes may resolve within hours of the onset of symptoms so abnormalities may be subtle or absent when the patient is examined.

Other. Corneal epithelial dots or microcysts, a fingerprint pattern, or map-like lines may be seen in both eyes if epithelial basement membrane (map–dot–fingerprint) dystrophy is present. These findings may also be seen unilaterally and focally in any eye that has recurrent erosions.

Etiology

Damage to the corneal epithelium or epithelial basement membrane from one of the following:

- Anterior corneal dystrophy: Epithelial basement membrane (most common), Reis–Bücklers, Thiel–Behnke, and Meesmann dystrophies.
- Previous traumatic corneal abrasion: Injury may have been years before the current presentation.

- Stromal corneal dystrophy: Lattice, granular, and macular dystrophies.
- Corneal degeneration: Band keratopathy, Salzmann nodular degeneration.
- Keratorefractive, corneal transplant, cataract surgery, or any surgery in which the corneal epithelium is removed (either therapeutically or for visualization).

Workup

1. History: History of a corneal abrasion? Ocular surgery? Family history (corneal dystrophy)?

2. Slit lamp examination with fluorescein staining of both the eyes (visualization of abnormal basement membrane lines may be enhanced by instilling fluorescein and looking for areas of rapid tear break-up, referred to as "negative staining").

Treatment

1. Acute episode: Cycloplegic drop (e.g., cyclopentolate 1%) t.i.d. and ophthalmic antibiotic ointment (e.g., erythromycin, bacitracin) four to six times daily. Can use 5% sodium chloride ointment q.i.d. in addition to antibiotic ointment. If the epithelial defect is large, a bandage soft contact lens and topical antibiotic drops q.i.d. may be placed. Oral analgesics as needed.

2. Never prescribe topical anesthetic drops.

3. After epithelial healing is complete, artificial tears at least q.i.d. and artificial tear ointment q.h.s. for at least 3 to 6 months, or 5% sodium chloride drops q.i.d. and 5% sodium chloride ointment q.h.s. for at least 3 to 6 months.

4. If the corneal epithelium is loose or heaped and is not healing, consider epithelial debridement. Apply a topical anesthetic (e.g., proparacaine) and use a sterile cotton-tipped applicator or cellulose sponge (e.g., Weck-Cel surgical spear) to gently remove all of the loose epithelium.

5. For erosions not responsive to the preceding treatment, consider the following:

   • Prophylactic medical treatment with 5% sodium chloride ointment q.h.s.

   • Oral doxycycline (matrix metalloproteinase inhibitor) 50 mg b.i.d. with or without a short course of topical steroid drops (e.g., fluorometholone 0.1% b.i.d. to q.i.d. for 2 to 4 weeks).

   • Extended-wear bandage soft contact lens for 3 to 6 months with a topical antibiotic and routine changing of the lens.

   • Anterior stromal puncture can be applied to localized erosions, such as in traumatic cases, outside the visual axis in cooperative patients. It can be performed with or without an intact epithelium. Stromal puncture may be applied manually with a needle at the slit lamp or with Nd:YAG laser. This treatment may cause small permanent corneal scars that are usually of no visual significance if outside of the visual axis.

   • Epithelial debridement with diamond burr polishing of Bowman membrane or excimer laser phototherapeutic keratectomy (PTK). Both are highly effective (up to 90%) for large areas of epithelial irregularity and lesions in the visual axis. Excimer laser ablation of the superficial stroma can be particularly helpful if repeated erosions have created anterior stromal haze or scarring. It is important to keep in mind that excimer laser PTK can lead to a hyperopic refractive shift after treatment if a deep ablation is performed.

Follow Up

Every 1 to 2 days until the epithelium has healed, and then every 1 to 3 months, depending on the severity and frequency of the episodes. It is important to educate patients that persistent use of lubricating ointment (5% sodium chloride or tear ointment) for 3 to 6 months following the initial healing process reduces the chance of recurrence.

4.3 Dry Eye Syndrome

Symptoms

Burning, dryness, foreign body sensation, mildly to moderately decreased vision, and excess tearing. Often exacerbated by smoke, wind, heat, low humidity, or prolonged use of the eye (e.g., when working on a computer that results in decreased blink rate). Usually bilateral and chronic (although patients sometimes are seen with recent onset in one eye). Discomfort often out of proportion to clinical signs.

Signs

Critical
• Scanty or irregular tear meniscus seen at the inferior eyelid margin: The normal meniscus should be at least 0.5 mm in height and have a convex shape.

• Decreased tear break-up time (measured from a blink to the appearance of a tear film defect, by using fluorescein stain): Less than 10 seconds indicates tear film instability.

NOTE: Tear film defects must be randomly located, as isolated areas of repeated early tear break-up may indicate a focal corneal surface irregularity.

Other. Punctate corneal or conjunctival fluorescein, rose bengal, or lissamine green staining; usually inferiorly or in the interpalpebral area. Excess mucus or debris in the tear film and filaments on the cornea may be found in severe cases.

Differential Diagnosis

See 4.1, SUPERFICIAL PUNCTATE KERATOPATHY.

Etiology

- Idiopathic: Commonly found in menopausal and postmenopausal women.
  - Evaporative: Lipid layer tear deficiency; often associated with blepharitis or meibomian gland dysfunction. Symptoms may be worse in the morning with complaints of visual blurring upon waking.
  - Aqueous deficient: Aqueous layer tear deficiency; aqueous production decreases with age. Symptoms frequently worse later in the day or after extensive use of the eyes.
  - Combination: Evaporative and aqueous deficiency often occur together. May also include a mucin layer tear deficiency.
- Lifestyle related: Arid climate, allergen exposure, smoking, extended periods of reading/computer work/television viewing.
- Connective tissue diseases (e.g., Sjögren syndrome, rheumatoid arthritis, granulomatosis with polyangiitis [GPA, formerly Wegener granulomatosis], systemic lupus erythematosus).
- Conjunctival scarring (e.g., mucous membrane pemphigoid, Stevens–Johnson syndrome, trachoma, chemical burn).
- Drugs (e.g., oral contraceptives, anticholinergics, antihistamines, antiarrhythmics, antipsychotics, antispasmodics, tricyclic antidepressants, beta blockers, diuretics, retinoids, selective serotonin reuptake inhibitors, chemotherapy).
- Infiltration of the lacrimal glands (e.g., sarcoidosis, tumor).
- Postradiation fibrosis of the lacrimal glands.
- Vitamin A deficiency: Usually from malnutrition, intestinal malabsorption, or bariatric surgery. See 13.7, VITAMIN A DEFICIENCY.
- After cataract surgery or corneal refractive surgery such as limbal relaxing incisions, photorefractive keratectomy (PRK), laser in situ keratomileusis (LASIK), and small incision lenticule extraction (SMILE): Likely secondary to disruption of corneal nerves and interference with normal reflex tearing. The size and location of the incision or flap may be correlated to the degree of the patient's symptoms.

Workup

1. History and external examination to detect underlying etiology.

2. Slit lamp examination with fluorescein stain to evaluate the ocular surface and tear break-up time. May also use rose bengal or lissamine green stain to examine the cornea and conjunctiva. Tear meniscus is best evaluated prior to the instillation of eye drops.
3. Tear secretion testing: Technique: After drying the eyes of excess tears, Schirmer filter paper is placed at the junction of the middle and lateral one-third of the lower eyelid in each eye for 5 minutes. Eyes are to remain open with normal blinking.
   - Unanesthetized: Measures basal and reflex tearing. Normal is wetting of at least 15 mm in 5 minutes.
   - Anesthetized: Measures basal tearing only. Topical anesthetic (e.g., proparacaine) is applied before drying the eye and placing the filter paper. Abnormal is wetting of 5 mm or less in 5 minutes. Less than 10 mm may be considered borderline. We prefer the less irritating anesthetized method.
4. Other potentially helpful in-office tests include measurement of tear osmolarity and level of matrix metalloproteinase-9 (MMP-9); elevation of these factors suggests dryness and inadequate tear film. Tear lactoferrin can also be measured; low levels suggest aqueous deficient dry eye disease.
5. Consider screening for Sjögren syndrome especially if associated with dry mouth and systemic autoimmune-related symptoms.

Treatment

Mild Dry Eye

Artificial tears q.i.d., preferably preservative-free.

Moderate Dry Eye

1. Increase the frequency of artificial tear application up to q1–2h; use only preservative-free artificial tears.
2. Add a lubricating gel or ointment q.h.s.
3. Lifestyle modification (e.g., humidifiers and smoking cessation).
4. Cyclosporine 0.05% or 0.09% b.i.d. is effective for patients with chronic dry eye and decreased tears secondary to ocular inflammation. Cyclosporine often burns with application for the first several weeks and takes 1 to

3 months for significant clinical improvement. To hasten improvement and lessen side effects, consider treating patients concomitantly with a mild topical steroid drop (e.g., loteprednol 0.5%, fluorometholone 0.1%, or fluorometholone acetate 0.1%) b.i.d. to q.i.d. for 1 month while beginning cyclosporine therapy.

5. Lifitegrast 5% b.i.d. is effective for the signs and symptoms of dry eye disease. Lifitegrast may burn on instillation, may cause blurred vision for several minutes, and may leave a metallic taste in the throat. Symptomatic improvement is often noted within 2 weeks of starting lifitegrast, but can take up to 3 months.

6. If these measures are inadequate or impractical, consider punctal occlusion. Use collagen inserts (temporary) or silicone or acrylic plugs (reversible). Be sure that any inflammatory component including blepharitis is treated prior to punctal occlusion.

Severe Dry Eye

1. Cyclosporine 0.05% or 0.09% or lifitegrast 5% as described earlier.

2. Punctal occlusion, as described earlier (both lower and upper puncta if necessary), and preservative-free artificial tears up to q1–2h. Consider permanent occlusion by thermal cautery if plugs continually fall out.

3. Add lubricating gel to ointment b.i.d. to q.i.d. p.r.n.

4. Moisture chamber (plastic film sealed at orbital rim) or glasses/goggles with lubrication at night.

5. If mucus strands or filaments are present, remove with forceps and consider 10% acetylcysteine q.i.d.

6. Other therapies may include oral flaxseed oil, oral omega-3 fatty acids, autologous serum tears, topical vitamin A, bandage soft contact lens, or a scleral lens.

7. Consider a small permanent lateral tarsorrhaphy if all of the previous measures fail.

A temporary adhesive tape tarsorrhaphy (to tape the lateral one-third of the eyelid closed) can also be used, pending a surgical tarsorrhaphy.

 NOTE

1. In addition to treating the dry eye, treatment for contributing disorders (e.g., blepharitis, exposure keratopathy) should be instituted if these conditions are present.

2. Always use preservative-free artificial tears if dosing is more frequent than q.i.d. to prevent preservative toxicity.

3. If the history suggests the presence of a connective tissue disease (e.g., history of arthritic pain, dry mouth), consider blood testing for these conditions and/or referral to an internist or rheumatologist for further evaluation.

Follow Up

In days to months, depending on the severity of symptoms and degree of dryness. Anyone with severe dry eyes caused by an underlying chronic systemic disease (e.g., rheumatoid arthritis, Sjögren syndrome, sarcoidosis, ocular pemphigoid) may need to be monitored more closely.

NOTE: Patients with significant dry eye should be discouraged from contact lens wear and corneal refractive surgery such as PRK, LASIK, and SMILE. However, daily disposable soft contact lenses can be successful if fit loosely and combined with aggressive preservative-free lubrication and plugs, if needed.

Patients with Sjögren syndrome have an increased incidence of lymphoma and mucous membrane problems and may require internal medicine, rheumatologic, dental, and gynecologic follow up.

4.4 Filamentary Keratopathy

Symptoms

Moderate-to-severe pain, red eye, foreign body sensation, tearing, and photophobia.

Signs

Critical. Short fluorescein-staining strands of degenerated epithelial cells surrounding a mucus core adherent to the anterior surface of cornea.

Other. Conjunctival injection, poor tear film, and punctate epithelial defects.

Etiology

- Severe ocular dryness: Most common cause. See 4.3, DRY EYE SYNDROME.
- SLK: Filaments are located in the superior cornea, in association with superior conjunctival injection, superior punctate fluorescein staining, and superior corneal pannus. See 5.4, SUPERIOR LIMBIC KERATOCONJUNCTIVITIS.
- Recurrent corneal erosions: Recurrent spontaneous corneal abrasions often occurring upon waking. See 4.2, RECURRENT CORNEAL EROSION.
- Adjacent to irregular corneal surface (e.g., postoperative, near a surgical wound).
- Patching (e.g., postoperative, after corneal abrasions) or ptosis.
- Neurotrophic keratopathy: See 4.6, NEUROTROPHIC KERATOPATHY.

Workup

1. History, especially for the previously mentioned conditions.
2. Slit lamp examination with fluorescein staining.

Treatment

1. Treat the underlying condition.
2. Consider debridement of the filaments. After applying topical anesthetic (e.g., proparacaine), gently remove filaments at their base with fine forceps or a cotton-tipped applicator. This gives temporary relief, but the filaments will recur if the underlying etiology is not treated.
3. Treatment with one or more of the following regimens:
    - Preservative-free artificial tears six to eight times per day and lubricating gel or ointment q.h.s.
    - Punctal occlusion.
    - Acetylcysteine 10% q.i.d.

    NOTE: Acetylcysteine is not commercially available as a drop but can be made by a compounding pharmacy.

4. If the symptoms are severe or treatment fails, then consider a bandage soft contact lens (unless the patient has severe dry eyes as underlying etiology). Extended-wear bandage soft contact lenses may need to be worn for weeks to months. Concomitant prophylactic or therapeutic topical antibiotics such as fluoroquinolone drops are typically given, especially if associated with a corneal abrasion/epithelial defect. A scleral lens may be helpful in recalcitrant cases.

Follow Up

In 1 to 4 weeks. If the condition is not improved, consider repeating the filament removal or applying a bandage soft contact lens. Long-term lubrication must be maintained if the underlying condition cannot be eliminated.

4.5 Exposure Keratopathy

Symptoms

Ocular irritation, burning, foreign body sensation, tearing, and redness of one or both eyes. Usually worse in the morning.

Signs

Critical. Inadequate blinking or closure of the eyelids, leading to corneal drying. Punctate epithelial defects are found in the lower one-third of the cornea or as a horizontal band in the region of the palpebral fissure (**see Figure 4.5.1**).

Other. Conjunctival injection and chemosis, corneal erosion, infiltrate or ulcer, eyelid deformity, or abnormal eyelid closure.

Etiology

- Seventh cranial nerve palsy: Orbicularis oculi weakness (e.g., Bell palsy). See 10.9, ISOLATED SEVENTH CRANIAL NERVE PALSY.
- Sedation or altered mental status.
- Eyelid deformity (e.g., ectropion or eyelid scarring from trauma, eyelid surgery such as excisional procedure, chemical burn, or herpes zoster ophthalmicus).

4

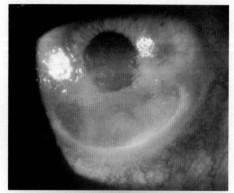

Figure 4.5.1 Exposure keratopathy with fluorescein.

- Nocturnal lagophthalmos: Failure to close the eyes during sleep.
- Proptosis (e.g., due to an orbital process such as thyroid eye disease). See 7.1, ORBITAL DISEASE.
- After ptosis repair or blepharoplasty procedures.
- Floppy eyelid syndrome. See 6.6, FLOPPY EYELID SYNDROME.
- Poor blink (e.g., Parkinson disease, neurotrophic cornea).

Workup

1. History: Previous Bell palsy or eyelid surgery? Thyroid disease?
2. Evaluate eyelid closure and corneal exposure. Ask the patient to close his or her eyes gently (as if sleeping). Assess Bell phenomenon (the patient is asked to close the eyelids forcefully against resistance; abnormal when the eyes do not rotate upward). Check for eyelid laxity.
3. Check corneal sensation before instillation of anesthetic drops. If sensation is decreased, there is greater risk for corneal complications and the patient may need further management for neurotrophic keratopathy. See 4.6, NEUROTROPHIC KERATOPATHY.
4. Slit lamp examination: Evaluate the tear film and corneal integrity with fluorescein dye. Look for signs of secondary infection (e.g., corneal infiltrate, anterior chamber reaction, severe conjunctival injection).

5. Investigate any underlying disorder (e.g., etiology of seventh cranial nerve palsy).

Treatment

Prevention is critical. All patients who are sedated or obtunded are at risk for exposure keratopathy and should receive lubrication according to the following recommendations.

In the presence of secondary corneal infection, see 4.11, BACTERIAL KERATITIS.

1. Correct any underlying disorder.
2. Preservative-free artificial tears q2–6h. Punctal occlusion with plugs may also be considered.
3. Lubricating ointment q.h.s. to q2h.
4. Consider eyelid taping or patching q.h.s. to maintain the eyelids in the closed position. If severe, consider taping the lateral one-third of the eyelids closed (leaving the visual axis open) during the day. Taping is rarely definitive but may be tried when the underlying disorder is thought to be temporary.
5. A potential in-office procedure includes placement of self-retained amniotic membrane tissue (e.g., sterilized, dehydrated amniotic membrane covered by a bandage soft contact lens or frozen, specialized plastic ring–mounted amniotic membrane such as Prokera).
6. When maximal medical therapy fails to prevent progressive corneal deterioration, one of the following surgical procedures may be beneficial:
   - Partial tarsorrhaphy (eyelids sewn or glued together).
   - Eyelid reconstruction (e.g., for ectropion).
   - Eyelid gold or platinum weight implant (e.g., for seventh cranial nerve palsy).
   - Orbital decompression (e.g., for proptosis).
   - Conjunctival flap or sutured/glued amniotic membrane graft (for severe corneal decompensation if the preceding fail).

Follow Up

Reevaluate every 1 to 2 days in the presence of corneal ulceration. Less frequent examinations (e.g., in weeks to months) are required for less severe corneal disease.

4.6 Neurotrophic Keratopathy

Symptoms

Foggy or blurry vision, red eye, and swollen eyelid. Foreign body sensation or pain is less than expected for the degree of ocular signs.

Signs

Critical. Loss of corneal sensation, interpalpebral SPK, or epithelial defects with fluorescein staining.

Other
- Early: Perilimbal injection and interpalpebral corneal punctate epithelial defects or a frank nonhealing epithelial defect with rolled edges, stromal edema, and Descemet folds. Typically located inferior to the visual axis.
- Late: Corneal ulcer usually without infectious infiltrate, although concomitant infectious keratitis may occur. The ulcer often has a gray, heaped-up epithelial border, tends to be in the lower one-half of the cornea, and is horizontally oval. Progressive thinning may occur rapidly and lead to a descemetocele (corneal stromal loss down to Descemet membrane) or corneal perforation.

Differential Diagnosis

See 4.1, SUPERFICIAL PUNCTATE KERATOPATHY.

Etiology

Occurs in eyes with diminished or absent corneal sensation. Denervation causes the corneal epithelium and tear film to become abnormal and unstable. May occur with any of the following conditions:

- Postinfection with varicella zoster virus (VZV) or herpes simplex virus (HSV).
- Following ocular surgery, particularly after corneal incisional or laser surgery (e.g., keratoplasty, LASIK, SMILE, PRK).
- Tumor (especially an acoustic neuroma, where both the fifth and seventh cranial nerves may be affected) or any neurologic insult/disease of the fifth cranial nerve (e.g., brainstem stroke, trauma, multiple sclerosis, Riley–Day syndrome).
- Chronic contact lens wear.
- Diabetic neuropathy.

- Extensive panretinal photocoagulation: May damage the long ciliary nerves (these patients often have concurrent diabetic neuropathy).
- Complication of trigeminal nerve or dental surgery.
- Complication of radiation therapy to the eye or an adnexal structure.
- Chronic topical medications (e.g., nonsteroidal anti-inflammatory agents, timolol).
- Topical anesthetic abuse.
- Crack keratopathy: Often bilateral. Take careful history for crack cocaine smoking or potential exposure. Often helpful to admit patient and remove them from their environment.
- Chemical injury or exposure to hydrogen sulfide or carbon disulfide (used in manufacturing).

Workup

1. History: Previous episodes of a red and painful eye? Prior herpes infection, cold sores, or shingles rash around the eye and/or forehead? Diabetes? History of irradiation, stroke, or hearing problem? Previous refractive procedure or other eye surgery? Chemical exposure? Smoking history? Topical medications?
2. Prior to anesthetic instillation, test corneal sensation bilaterally with a sterile cotton wisp.
3. Slit lamp examination with fluorescein staining of cornea and conjunctiva.
4. Check the skin for herpetic lesions or scars from a previous herpes zoster infection.
5. Look for signs of a corneal exposure problem (e.g., inability to close an eyelid, seventh cranial nerve palsy, absent Bell phenomenon).
6. If suspicious of a central nervous system lesion, obtain a computed tomography (CT) or magnetic resonance imaging (MRI) of the brain.

Treatment

Eyes with neurotrophic keratopathy have impaired healing ability. If not treated in a timely manner, an epithelial defect in an eye with this condition may progress to stromal lysis and possibly perforation.

1. Mild-to-moderate punctate epithelial staining: Preservative-free artificial tears q2–4h and artificial tear ointment q.h.s. Consider punctal plugs and q.h.s. patching.

2. Small corneal epithelial defect: Antibiotic ointment (e.g., erythromycin or bacitracin q.i.d. to q1–2h) until resolved. Usually requires prolonged artificial tear treatment, as described above. Consider placement of a bandage soft contact lens with prophylactic antibiotic drops (e.g., ofloxacin or moxifloxacin t.i.d. to q.i.d.) along with frequent preservative-free artificial tears (q1–2h) as an alternative to antibiotic ointment.

3. Corneal ulcer: See 4.11, BACTERIAL KERATITIS, for the workup and treatment of a secondarily infected ulceration. Treatment options for a neurotrophic ulceration include antibiotic ointment q2h, tarsorrhaphy, self-retained amniotic membrane tissue, sutured/glued amniotic membrane graft, or conjunctival flap (See TREATMENT in 4.5, EXPOSURE KERATOPATHY). Oral doxycycline (50 to 100 mg b.i.d.), a collagenase inhibitor, may slow stromal lysis. Systemic ascorbic acid (e.g., vitamin C 1 to 2 g daily) may promote collagen synthesis and reduce the level of ulceration. Autologous serum, albumin, or umbilical cord serum eye drops may also be beneficial.

4. Cenegermin-bkbj 0.002%, recombinant human nerve growth factor, is the first Food and Drug Administration–approved drug for neurotrophic keratopathy and is very effective in many eyes. It is an ophthalmic solution that is applied six times daily for an 8-week treatment course.

5. A scleral lens (e.g., prosthetic replacement of the ocular surface ecosystem [PROSE]) may be helpful long term.

6. Cornea neurotization is a complex surgical procedure whereby nerves are redirected, or more commonly grafted, to reestablish corneal sensation.

NOTE: Patients with neurotrophic keratopathy and corneal exposure often do not respond to treatment unless a tarsorrhaphy is performed. A temporary adhesive tape tarsorrhaphy (the lateral one-third of the eyelid is taped closed) may be beneficial, pending more definitive treatment.

Follow Up

1. Mild-to-moderate epithelial staining: In 3 to 14 days.

2. Corneal epithelial defect: Every 1 to 3 days until improvement demonstrated and then every 5 to 7 days until resolved.

3. Corneal ulcer: Daily until significant improvement is demonstrated. Hospitalization may be required for severe ulcers, especially if there is concern that patient may not be properly administering medication in the setting of decreased corneal sensation or the patient may be abusing anesthetic drops (see 4.11, BACTERIAL KERATITIS).

4.7 Ultraviolet Keratopathy

Symptoms

Moderate-to-severe ocular pain, foreign body sensation, red eye, tearing, photophobia, and blurred vision; often a history of welding or using a sunlamp without adequate protective eyewear. Symptoms typically worsen 6 to 12 hours after the exposure. Usually bilateral.

Signs

Critical. Dense, confluent punctate epithelial defects in an interpalpebral distribution highlighted with fluorescein staining.

Other. Conjunctival injection, mild-to-moderate eyelid edema, mild-to-no corneal edema, relatively miotic pupils that react sluggishly, and mild anterior chamber reaction.

Differential Diagnosis

• Toxic epithelial keratopathy from exposure to a chemical (e.g., solvents, alcohol) or drug (e.g., neomycin, gentamicin, antiviral agents, anesthetic drops).

• Thermal burn/keratopathy: Often from contact with curling iron, boiling fluid, fire ember, or flame. Injury usually limited to corneal epithelium; may have marked superficial corneal opacification or eschar. Treat with possible debridement of involved area and then as for corneal abrasion. See 3.2, CORNEAL ABRASION.

- See 4.1, SUPERFICIAL PUNCTATE KERATOPATHY.

Workup

1. History: Welding? Sunlamp use? Topical medications? Chemical exposure? Prior episodes? Use of protective eyewear?
2. Slit lamp examination: Use fluorescein stain. Evert the eyelids to search for a foreign body.
3. If chemical exposure suspected, check pH of tear lake in upper and lower conjunctival fornices. If not neutral (6.8 to 7.5), treat as chemical burn. See 3.1, CHEMICAL BURN.

Treatment

1. Cycloplegic drop (e.g., cyclopentolate 1%).
2. Antibiotic ointment (e.g., erythromycin or bacitracin) four to eight times per day.
3. Oral analgesics as needed.

 NOTE: A bandage soft contact lens with prophylactic topical broad-spectrum antibiotic drop may be used in place of frequent antibiotic ointment.

Follow Up

1. If a bandage soft contact lens was placed, the patient is seen in 1 to 2 days.
2. Reliable patients without a bandage soft contact lens are asked to assess their own symptoms after 24 hours.
   - If much improved, the patient continues with topical antibiotics (e.g., erythromycin or bacitracin ointment q.i.d.).
   - If still significantly symptomatic, reevaluate. If significant punctate staining is present, retreat with a cycloplegic, antibiotic as discussed previously.
3. Unreliable patients or those with an unclear etiology should not have a bandage soft contact lens placed. Such patients should be reexamined in 1 to 2 days.

4.8 Thygeson Superficial Punctate Keratitis

Symptoms

Mild-to-moderate foreign body sensation, photophobia, and tearing. No history of red eye. Usually bilateral with a chronic course of exacerbations and remissions, but may not be active in both eyes at the same time.

Signs

Critical. Coarse stellate gray-white corneal epithelial opacities that are often central, slightly elevated, and stain lightly with fluorescein. Underlying subepithelial infiltrates may be present **(see Figure 4.8.1)**.

Other. Minimal-to-no conjunctival injection, corneal edema, anterior chamber reaction, or eyelid abnormalities.

Differential Diagnosis

See 4.1, SUPERFICIAL PUNCTATE KERATOPATHY.

Treatment

Mild

1. Artificial tears, preferably preservative-free, four to eight times per day.

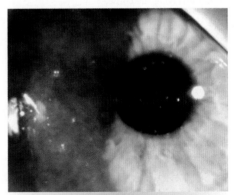

Figure 4.8.1 Thygeson superficial punctate keratitis.

2. Artificial tear ointment q.h.s.

 NOTE: Treatment is based more on patient symptoms than corneal appearance.

Moderate to Severe

1. Mild topical steroid (e.g., fluorometholone 0.1%, fluorometholone acetate 0.1%, or loteprednol 0.2% to 0.5% q.i.d.) for 1 to 4 weeks, followed by a very slow taper. May need prolonged low-dose topical steroid therapy.

2. If no improvement with topical steroids, a bandage soft contact lens can be tried.
3. Cyclosporine 0.05% or 0.09% drops daily to q.i.d. or lifitegrast 5% b.i.d. may be an alternative or adjunctive treatment, especially in patients with side effects from steroids.

Follow Up

Weekly during an exacerbation and then every 3 to 6 months. Patients receiving topical steroids require intraocular pressure (IOP) checks every 4 to 12 weeks.

4.9 Pterygium/Pinguecula

Symptoms

Irritation, redness, and decreased vision; may be asymptomatic

Signs

Critical. One of the following, almost always located at the 3-o'clock or 9-o'clock perilimbal position.

- Pterygium: Wing-shaped fold of fibrovascular tissue arising from the interpalpebral conjunctiva and extending onto the cornea. There is no associated thinning of the cornea below these lesions. Usually nasal in location **(see Figure 4.9.1)**.
- Pinguecula: Yellow-white, flat, or slightly raised conjunctival lesion, usually in the interpalpebral fissure adjacent to the limbus, but not involving the cornea.

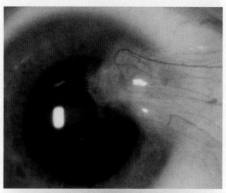
Figure 4.9.1 Pterygium.

Other. Either lesion may be highly vascularized and injected or may be associated with SPK or delle (thinning of the adjacent cornea secondary to drying). An iron line (Stocker line) may be seen in the cornea just beyond the leading edge of a pterygium.

Differential Diagnosis

- Conjunctival intraepithelial neoplasia (CIN): Unilateral papillomatous jelly-like, velvety, or leukoplakic (white) mass, often elevated and vascularized. May not be in a wing-shaped configuration and not necessarily in the typical 3-o'clock or 9-o'clock location of a pterygium or pinguecula. See 5.12, CONJUNCTIVAL TUMORS.

 NOTE: Atypical pterygia require biopsy to rule out CIN or melanoma.

- Limbal dermoid: Congenital rounded white lesion, usually at the inferotemporal limbus. See 5.12, CONJUNCTIVAL TUMORS.
- Other conjunctival tumors (e.g., papilloma, nevus, melanoma). See 5.12, CONJUNCTIVAL TUMORS.
- Pseudopterygium: Conjunctival tissue adherent to the peripheral cornea. May appear in location of previous trauma, surgery, corneal ulceration, or cicatrizing conjunctivitis. There is often associated underlying corneal thinning.
- Peripheral hypertrophic subepithelial corneal degeneration: Less common, usually bilateral, occurring mostly in Caucasian women.

Elevated peripheral subepithelial opacities with adjacent limbal vascular abnormalities.

- Pannus: Blood vessels growing into the cornea, often secondary to chronic contact lens wear, blepharitis, ocular rosacea, herpes keratitis, phlyctenular keratitis, atopic disease, trachoma, trauma, and others. Usually at the level of Bowman membrane with minimal to no elevation.
- Sclerokeratitis: See 5.7, SCLERITIS.

Etiology

Elastotic degeneration of deep conjunctival layers resulting in fibrovascular tissue proliferation. Related to sunlight exposure and chronic irritation. More common in individuals from equatorial regions.

Workup

Slit lamp examination to identify the lesion and evaluate the adjacent corneal integrity and thickness. Check for corneal astigmatism, which is often irregular but may be oriented with the rule.

Treatment

1. Protect eyes from sun, dust, and wind (e.g., ultraviolet-blocking sunglasses or goggles if appropriate).
2. Lubrication with artificial tears, preferably preservative-free, four to eight times per day to reduce ocular irritation.
3. For an inflamed pterygium or pinguecula:
   - Mild: Artificial tears q.i.d.
   - Moderate to severe: A mild topical steroid (e.g., fluorometholone 0.1%, fluorometholone acetate 0.1%, or loteprednol 0.2% to 0.5% q.i.d.), a nonsteroidal anti-inflammatory drop (e.g., ketorolac 0.4% to 0.5% q.i.d.), or a topical antihistamine ± mast cell stabilizer (e.g., bepotastine,

ketotifen, olopatadine) may be used to decrease symptoms.
4. If a delle is present, then apply artificial tear ointment q2h. See 4.23, DELLE.
5. Surgical removal is indicated when:
   - The pterygium threatens the visual axis or induces significant astigmatism.
   - The patient is experiencing excessive irritation not relieved by the aforementioned treatment.
   - The lesion is interfering with contact lens wear.
   - The lesion is visually apparent and causing cosmetic concerns.
   - Consider removal prior to cataract or refractive surgery.

NOTE: Pterygia can recur after surgical excision. Bare sclera dissection with a conjunctival autograft or amniotic membrane graft reduces the recurrence rate. Intraoperative application of an antimetabolite (e.g., mitomycin C) also reduces recurrence. Antimetabolites are more commonly reserved for excision of recurrent pterygia, as these medications are associated with an increased risk of corneoscleral thinning or necrosis.

Follow Up

1. Asymptomatic, stable patients may be checked every 1 to 2 years.
2. Pterygia should be measured periodically (every 3 to 12 months, initially) to determine the rate at which they are growing toward the visual axis.
3. If treating with a topical steroid, check after a few weeks to monitor inflammation and IOP. Taper and discontinue the steroid drop over several weeks once the inflammation has abated.

4.10 Band Keratopathy

Symptoms

Decreased vision, foreign body sensation, and corneal whitening; may be asymptomatic.

Signs

Critical. Anterior corneal plaque of calcium at the level of Bowman membrane, typically within

the interpalpebral fissure, and separated from the limbus by clear cornea. Lucid spaces may be present in the plaque, giving it a Swiss cheese appearance. The plaque usually begins at the 3-o'clock and 9-o'clock positions, adjacent to the limbus. (See Figure 4.10.1.)

Other. May have other signs of chronic eye disease.

4

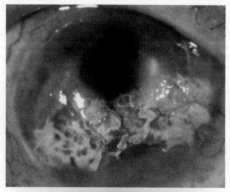

Figure 4.10.1 Band keratopathy.

Etiology

More Common. Chronic uveitis (e.g., juvenile idiopathic arthritis [JIA]), interstitial keratitis (IK), corneal edema, trauma, phthisis bulbi, long-standing glaucoma, dry eye, ocular surgery (especially retinal detachment repair with silicone oil), and idiopathic.

Less Common. Hypercalcemia (may result from hyperparathyroidism, renal failure, sarcoidosis, multiple myeloma, Paget disease of bone, vitamin D excess, etc.), hyperphosphatemia, gout, corneal dystrophy, myotonic dystrophy, long-term exposure to irritants (e.g., mercury fumes), and other causes.

Workup

1. History: Chronic eye disease? Previous ocular surgery? Chronic exposure to environmental irritants or ocular medications? Systemic disease?

2. Slit lamp examination.

3. If no signs of chronic anterior segment disease or long-standing glaucoma are present, and the band keratopathy cannot be accounted for, then consider the following workup:

   • Serum calcium, albumin, magnesium, and phosphate levels. Blood urea nitrogen and creatinine. Uric acid level if gout is suspected.

Treatment

Mild (e.g., Foreign Body Sensation)

Artificial tears, preferably preservative-free, four to six times per day and artificial tear ointment

q.h.s. to q.i.d. as needed, add antibiotic ointment (e.g., bacitracin, bacitracin-polymyxin or erythromycin) if irregular epitheium or epithelial defects over calcium deposition. Consider a bandage soft contact lens for comfort.

Severe (e.g., Obstruction of Vision, Irritation Not Relieved by Lubricants, Cosmetic Problem)

Removal of the calcium may be performed at the slit lamp or under the operating microscope by chelation using disodium ethylenediamine tetraacetic acid (EDTA):

1. Disodium EDTA 3% to 4% is obtained from a compounding pharmacy.

2. Anesthetize the eye with a topical anesthetic (e.g., proparacaine) and place an eyelid speculum.

3. Debride the corneal epithelium overlying the calcium with a sterile blade or a sterile cotton-tipped applicator.

4. Wipe a cellulose sponge or cotton swab saturated with the EDTA solution over the band keratopathy until the calcium clears (which may take 10 to 60 minutes).

5. Irrigate with normal saline, place an antibiotic ointment (e.g., erythromycin) and a cycloplegic drop (e.g., cyclopentolate 1% to 2%). Consider a bandage soft contact lens and topical antibiotic drop (e.g., moxifloxacin, gatifloxacin q.i.d.).

6. Consider giving the patient a systemic analgesic (e.g., acetaminophen with codeine).

Follow Up

1. If surgical removal has been performed, the patient should be examined every few days until the epithelial defect has healed.

2. Residual anterior stromal scarring may be amenable to excimer laser PTK to improve vision. Excimer laser PTK may also be used to try to improve the ocular surface and prevent recurrent erosions.

3. The patient should be checked every 3 to 12 months, depending on the severity of symptoms. EDTA chelation can be repeated if the band keratopathy recurs.

4.11 Bacterial Keratitis

Symptoms

Red eye, moderate-to-severe ocular pain, photophobia, decreased vision, discharge, and acute contact lens intolerance.

Signs

(See Figure 4.11.1.)

Critical. Focal white opacity (infiltrate) in the corneal stroma associated with an epithelial defect and underlying stromal thinning/tissue loss.

NOTE: An examiner using a slit beam cannot see clearly through an infiltrate or ulcer to the iris, whereas stromal edema or mild anterior stromal scars are more transparent.

Other. Epithelial defect, mucopurulent discharge, stromal edema, folds in Descemet membrane, anterior chamber reaction, endothelial fibrin/cell deposition with or without hypopyon formation (which, in the absence of globe perforation, usually represents sterile inflammation), conjunctival injection, upper eyelid edema. Posterior synechiae, hyphema, and increased IOP may occur in severe cases.

Differential Diagnosis

- Fungal: Must be considered after any traumatic corneal injury, particularly from vegetable matter (e.g., a tree branch), which may lead to filamentous fungal keratitis. Contact lens wear is another risk factor. Infiltrates commonly have feathery borders and/or may be surrounded by satellite lesions. Candida infections more frequently occur in eyes with preexisting ocular surface disease and may mimic the clinical picture of bacterial ulcers. See 4.12, FUNGAL KERATITIS.

- Acanthamoeba: This protozoan classically causes an extremely painful keratitis and/or stromal infiltrate; is associated with perineural invasion. It usually occurs in daily-wear soft contact lens wearers who may or may not practice poor lens hygiene. History of trauma or history of swimming and/or hot tubbing while wearing contact lenses may be elicited.

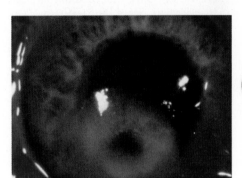

Figure 4.11.1 Bacterial keratitis.

In the early stages, the epithelial abnormality may look more like HSV keratitis than a bacterial ulcer. In the late stages (3 to 8 weeks), the infiltrate often becomes ring shaped. See 4.13, ACANTHAMOEBA KERATITIS.

- HSV: May have eyelid vesicles or corneal epithelial dendrites. A history of recurrent unilateral eye disease or known ocular herpes is common. If a staining infiltrate develops in a patient with stromal herpetic keratitis, one needs to rule out bacterial superinfection. See 4.15, HERPES SIMPLEX VIRUS.

- Atypical mycobacteria: Usually follows ocular injuries with vegetable matter or ocular surgery, such as cataract extraction, corneal grafts, and refractive surgery (especially LASIK). It has a more indolent course. Culture plates (on Lowenstein–Jensen media) must be kept for 8 weeks. An acid-fast bacillus smear may be very helpful.

- Sterile corneal thinning and ulcers: Minimal or no discharge, mild iritis, peripheral stromal infiltration with overlying staining and adjacent vascularization, and negative cultures. Corneal melting may be associated with various systemic diseases. See 4.22, PERIPHERAL CORNEAL THINNING/ULCERATION.

- Staphylococcal hypersensitivity: Peripheral corneal infiltrates, sometimes with an overlying epithelial defect; usually multiple, often bilateral, with a clear space between the infiltrate and the limbus. Conjunctival injection is localized rather than diffuse, and there is less pain. There is minimal-to-no anterior chamber reaction. Often with coexisting blepharitis/meibomitis. See 4.18, STAPHYLOCOCCAL HYPERSENSITIVITY.

- Sterile corneal infiltrates: Typically from an immune reaction to contact lens solutions or hypoxia related to contact lens wear. Usually multiple small, often peripheral, subepithelial infiltrates with little overlying staining and minimal anterior chamber reaction. Usually a diagnosis of exclusion after ruling out an infectious process. Similar lesions can occur after adenoviral conjunctivitis, but these tend to be more central and less dense with a preceding history of conjunctivitis. See 5.1, ACUTE CONJUNCTIVITIS.

- Residual corneal foreign body or rust ring: History of foreign body injury. May be accompanied by corneal stromal inflammation, edema, and sometimes, a sterile infiltrate. There may be a mild anterior chamber reaction. The infiltrate and inflammation usually clear after the foreign body and rust ring are removed, but a superinfection may occur.

- Topical anesthetic abuse: A type of neurotrophic ulcer that should be suspected when there is poor response to appropriate therapy. In the late stages of anesthetic abuse, the corneal appearance may mimic an infectious process such as Acanthamoeba or herpes simplex stromal keratitis. A large ring opacity, edema, and anterior chamber reaction are characteristic. Crack cocaine keratopathy has a similar appearance. Healing, with or without scarring, typically occurs after the exposure to anesthetic is stopped.

Etiology

Bacterial organisms are the most common cause of infectious keratitis. In general, corneal infections are assumed to be bacterial until proven otherwise by laboratory studies or until a therapeutic trial of topical antibiotics is unsuccessful. At Wills Eye, the most common causes of bacterial keratitis are Staphylococcus, Pseudomonas, Streptococcus, Moraxella, and Serratia species. Clinical findings vary widely depending on the severity of disease and on the organism involved. The following clinical characteristics may be helpful in predicting the organism involved. However, clinical impression should never take the place of broad-spectrum initial treatment and appropriate laboratory evaluation. See Appendix 8, CORNEAL CULTURE PROCEDURE.

- Staphylococcal ulcers typically have a well-defined, gray-white stromal infiltrate that may enlarge to form a dense stromal abscess.

- Streptococcal infiltrates may be either very purulent or crystalline (see 4.14, CRYSTALLINE KERATOPATHY). Acute fulminant onset with severe anterior chamber reaction and hypopyon formation are common in the former, while the latter tends to have a more indolent course and occurs in patients often on chronic topical steroids (e.g., corneal transplant patients).

- Pseudomonas typically presents as a rapidly progressive, suppurative, necrotic infiltrate associated with a hypopyon and mucopurulent discharge, commonly seen in the setting of soft contact lens wear **(see Figure 4.11.2)**.

- Moraxella may cause infectious keratitis in patients with preexisting ocular surface disease and in patients who are immunocompromised. Infiltrates are typically indolent, located in the inferior portion of the cornea, have a tendency to be full-thickness, and may rarely perforate.

Workup

1. History: Contact lens wear and care regimen should always be discussed. Sleeping in contact lenses? Daily or extended-wear lenses? Conventional, frequent replacement, or single use? Disinfecting solutions used? Recent changes in routine? Water exposure (swimming or hot tub use) with lenses? Trauma or corneal foreign body? Corneal surgery including refractive surgery? Eye care before visit (e.g., antimicrobials or topical steroids)? Previous corneal disease? Systemic illness?

2. Slit lamp examination: Stain with fluorescein to determine if there is epithelial loss overlying the infiltrate; document the size, depth, and location of the corneal infiltrate and epithelial defect. Assess the anterior chamber reaction and document the presence and size of a hypopyon. Measure the IOP, preferably with a Tono-Pen.

3. Corneal scrapings for smears and cultures if appropriate and if culture media are available. We routinely culture infiltrates if they are larger than 1 to 2 mm, in the visual axis, unresponsive to initial treatment, or if there

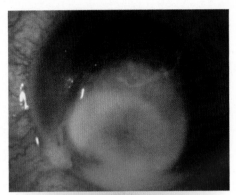

Figure 4.11.2 Pseudomonas keratitis.

is suspicion for an unusual organism based on history or examination. See Appendix 8, CORNEAL CULTURE PROCEDURE.

4. In contact lens wearers suspected of having an infectious ulcer, the contact lenses and case are cultured, if available. Explain to the patient that the cultured contact lenses will be discarded. A positive culture from a contact lens or contact lens case should be interpreted with clinical judgment. While a contaminant can be misleading, a result that supports the examination findings can be helpful.

Treatment

Ulcers and infiltrates are initially treated as bacterial unless there is a high index of suspicion of another form of infection. Initial therapy should be broad spectrum. Remember that bacterial coinfection may occasionally complicate fungal and Acanthamoeba keratitis. Mixed bacterial infections can also occur.

1. Cycloplegic drop for comfort and to prevent synechiae formation (e.g., cyclopentolate 1% t.i.d.; atropine 1% b.i.d. to t.i.d. recommended if a hypopyon in present). The specific medication depends on severity of anterior chamber inflammation.

2. Topical antibiotics according to the following algorithm:

Low Risk of Visual Loss

Small, nonstaining peripheral infiltrate with at most minimal anterior chamber reaction and no discharge:

- Noncontact lens wearer: Broad-spectrum topical antibiotics (e.g., fluoroquinolone [moxifloxacin, gatifloxacin, besifloxacin, levofloxacin] or polymyxin B/trimethoprim drops q1–2h while awake).

- Contact lens wearer: Fluoroquinolone (e.g., moxifloxacin, gatifloxacin, ciprofloxacin, besifloxacin, levofloxacin) drops q1–2h while awake ± polymyxin B/trimethoprim drops q1–2h while awake; can add tobramycin or ciprofloxacin ointment one to four times a day.

Borderline Risk of Visual Loss

Medium size (1 to 1.5 mm diameter) peripheral infiltrate, or any smaller infiltrate with an associated epithelial defect, mild anterior chamber reaction, or moderate discharge:

- Fluoroquinolone (e.g., moxifloxacin, gatifloxacin, ciprofloxacin, besifloxacin, levofloxacin) q1h around the clock ± polymyxin B/trimethoprim q1h around the clock. Consider starting with a loading dose of q5min for five doses and then q30min until midnight then q1h.

NOTE: Moxifloxacin and besifloxacin have slightly better gram-positive coverage. Gatifloxacin and ciprofloxacin have slightly better Pseudomonas and Serratia coverage.

Vision Threatening

Our current practice at Wills Eye is to start fortified antibiotics for most ulcers larger than 1.5 to 2 mm, in the visual axis, or unresponsive to initial treatment. See Appendix 9, FORTIFIED TOPICAL ANTIBIOTICS/ANTIFUNGALS, for directions on making fortified antibiotics. If fortified antibiotics are not immediately available, start with a fluoroquinolone and polymyxin B/trimethoprim until fortified antibiotics can be obtained from a formulating pharmacy.

- Fortified tobramycin or gentamicin (15 mg/mL) q1h, alternating with fortified cefazolin (50 mg/mL) or vancomycin (25 mg/mL) q1h. This means that the patient will be placing a drop in the eye every one-half hour around the clock. Vancomycin drops should be reserved for resistant organisms, patients at risk for resistant organisms (e.g., due to hospital or antibiotic exposure, unresponsive to initial treatment), and for patients who are allergic to penicillin or cephalosporins. An increasing number of methicillin-resistant

Staphylococcus aureus (MRSA) infections are now community acquired. If the ulcer is severe and Pseudomonas is suspected, consider starting fortified tobramycin every 30 minutes and fortified cefazolin q1h around the clock; in addition, consider fortified ceftazidime q1h or a fluoroquinolone q1h around the clock.

4

NOTE: All patients with borderline risk of visual loss or severe vision-threatening ulcers are initially treated with loading doses of antibiotics using the following regimen: One drop every 5 minutes for five doses, then every 30 to 60 minutes around the clock.

1. In some cases, topical steroids are added after the bacterial organism and sensitivities are known, the infection is under control, and severe inflammation persists. Infectious keratitis may worsen significantly with topical steroids, especially when caused by fungus, atypical mycobacteria, Nocardia or Pseudomonas.

2. Eyes with corneal thinning should be protected by a shield without a pressure patch (a patch is never placed over an eye thought to have an infection). The use of a matrix metalloproteinase inhibitor (e.g., doxycycline 100 mg p.o. b.i.d.) and a collagen synthesis promoter such as systemic ascorbic acid (e.g., vitamin C 1 to 2 g daily) may help to suppress connective tissue breakdown and prevent the perforation of the cornea.

3. No contact lens wear.

4. Oral pain medication as needed.

5. Oral fluoroquinolones (e.g., ciprofloxacin 500 mg p.o. b.i.d.; moxifloxacin 400 mg p.o. daily) penetrate the eye well. These may have added benefit for patients with scleral extension or for those with frank or impending perforation. Ciprofloxacin is preferred for Pseudomonas and Serratia.

6. Systemic antibiotics are also necessary for Neisseria infections (e.g., ceftriaxone 1 g intravenously [i.v.] q12–24h if corneal involvement, or a single 1 g intramuscular [i.m.] dose if there is only conjunctival involvement) and for Haemophilus infections (e.g., oral amoxicillin/clavulanate [20 to 40 mg/kg/d in three divided doses]) because of occasional extraocular involvement such as otitis media, pneumonia, and meningitis.

NOTE: Systemic fluoroquinolones were historically used for *Neisseria gonorrhoeae,* but are no longer recommended to treat gonococcal infections (especially in men who have sex with men, in areas of high endemic resistance, and in patients with a recent foreign travel history) due to increased resistance. Additionally, they are contraindicated in pregnant women and children.

7. Admission to the hospital may be necessary if:
   - Infection is sight threatening and/or impending perforation.
   - Patient has difficulty administering the antibiotics at the prescribed frequency.
   - High likelihood of noncompliance with drops or daily follow up.
   - Suspected topical anesthetic abuse.
   - Intravenous antibiotics are needed (e.g., gonococcal conjunctivitis with corneal involvement). Often employed in the presence of corneal perforation and/or scleral extension of infection.

8. For atypical mycobacteria, consider prolonged treatment (q1h for 1 week, then gradually tapering) with one or more of the following topical agents: fluoroquinolone (e.g., moxifloxacin or gatifloxacin), fortified amikacin (15 mg/mL), clarithromycin (1% to 4%), or fortified tobramycin (15 mg/mL). Consider oral treatment with clarithromycin 500 mg b.i.d. Previous LASIK has been implicated as a risk factor for atypical mycobacteria infections.

Follow Up

1. Daily evaluation at first, including repeat measurements of the size of the infiltrate, epithelial defect and hypopyon. The most important criteria in evaluating treatment response are the amount of pain, the epithelial defect size (which may initially increase because of scraping for cultures and smears), the size and depth of the infiltrate, and the anterior chamber reaction. The IOP must be checked and treated if elevated (see 9.7, Inflammatory Open Angle Glaucoma). Reduced pain is often the first sign of a positive response to treatment.

2. If improving, the antibiotic regimen is gradually tapered but is never tapered past the minimum dose to inhibit the emergence of resistance (usually t.i.d. to q.i.d. depending on the agent). Otherwise, the antibiotic regimen is adjusted according to the culture and sensitivity results.

3. Consider new or repeat cultures and stains (without stopping treatment) in the setting of non-responsive or worsening infiltrate/ulcer. Treat with fortified antibiotics and modify based on culture results and the clinical course. Hospitalization may be recommended. See Appendix 8, CORNEAL CULTURE PROCEDURE.

4. A corneal biopsy may be required if the condition is worsening and infection is still suspected despite negative cultures.

5. For an impending or a complete corneal perforation, a corneal transplant or patch graft is considered. Cyanoacrylate tissue glue may also work in a treated corneal ulcer that has perforated despite infection control. Frequent antibiotics are continued after application of glue to treat the infection.

 NOTE: Outpatients are told to return immediately if the pain increases, vision decreases, or they notice an increase in the size of the ulcer when they look in the mirror.

4.12 Fungal Keratitis

Symptoms

Pain, photophobia, redness, tearing, discharge, foreign body sensation. Often history of minor trauma particularly with vegetable matter (e.g., a tree branch), contact lens wear, chronic eye disease, and/or a history of poor response to conventional antibacterial therapy. Usually more indolent than bacterial keratitis.

Signs

Critical

- Filamentous fungi: Corneal stromal gray-white opacity (infiltrate) with a feathery border. The epithelium over the infiltrate may be elevated above the remainder of the corneal surface, or there may be an epithelial defect with stromal thinning (ulcer).
- Nonfilamentous fungi: A gray-white stromal infiltrate similar to a bacterial ulcer.

Other. Satellite lesions surrounding the primary infiltrate, conjunctival injection, mucopurulent discharge, anterior chamber reaction, hypopyon. The infiltrate is more likely to extend beyond the epithelial defect than in bacterial ulcers.

Differential Diagnosis

See 4.11, BACTERIAL KERATITIS.

Etiology

- Filamentous fungi (e.g., Fusarium or Aspergillus species most commonly): Usually from trauma with vegetable matter in previously healthy eyes or associated with contact lens wear.
- Nonfilamentous fungi (e.g., Candida species): Usually in previously diseased eyes (e.g., dry eyes, herpes simplex or varicella zoster keratitis, exposure keratopathy, and chronic use of steroid drops), see **Figure 4.12.1**.

Workup

See 4.11, BACTERIAL KERATITIS for complete workup and culture procedure.

1. Whenever smears and cultures are done, include a Gram, Giemsa, calcofluor white, or KOH stain for organisms; periodic acid-Schiff, Gomori methenamine silver, and hematoxylin and eosin (H&E) stains can also be used. Scrape

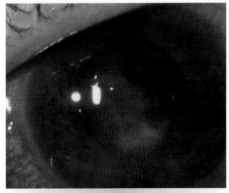
Figure 4.12.1 Candida fungal keratitis.

deep into the edge of the ulcer for material. See Appendix 8, CORNEAL CULTURE PROCEDURE.

2. If an infectious etiology is still suspected despite negative cultures, consider a corneal biopsy to obtain further diagnostic information.

3. Consider cultures and smears of contact lens case and solution.

4. Sometimes all tests are negative, yet the disease continues to progress and therapeutic penetrating keratoplasty (PK) is necessary for diagnosis and treatment.

Treatment

Corneal infiltrates and ulcers of unknown etiology are treated as bacterial until proven otherwise (see 4.11, BACTERIAL KERATITIS). If the stains or cultures indicate a fungal keratitis, institute the following measures:

1. Natamycin 5% drops (especially for filamentous fungi), amphotericin B 0.15% drops (especially for Candida), and/or topical fortified voriconazole 1% initially q1–2h around the clock, then taper over the next several weeks based on response to therapy, (see Appendix 9, FORTIFIED TOPICAL ANTIBIOTICS/ANTIFUNGALS).

> **NOTE:** Natamycin is the only commercially available topical antifungal agent; all others must be compounded.

2. Cycloplegic drop (e.g., cyclopentolate 1% t.i.d.; atropine 1% b.i.d. to t.i.d. is recommended if hypopyon, fibrin or significant anterior chamber reaction is present).

3. No topical steroids. If the patient is currently taking steroids, they should be tapered rapidly and discontinued.

4. Consider adding oral antifungal agents (e.g., fluconazole or itraconazole 200 to 400 mg p.o. loading dose, then 100 to 200 mg p.o. daily, posaconazole 300 mg p.o. b.i.d. for 1 day then 300 mg p.o. q.d., or voriconazole 200 mg p.o.

b.i.d.). Oral antifungal agents are often used for deep corneal ulcers or suspected fungal endophthalmitis.

5. Consider epithelial debridement to facilitate the penetration of antifungal medications. Topical antifungals do not penetrate the cornea well, especially through an intact epithelium. When culture results and sensitivities are known, intrastromal depot injections of amphotericin (10 mcg/0.1 mL) or voriconazole (voriconazole 50 mcg/0.1 mL) can also be considered.

6. Measure IOP (preferably with Tono-Pen). Treat elevated IOP if present (see 9.7, INFLAMMATORY OPEN ANGLE GLAUCOMA).

7. Eye shield, without patch, in the presence of corneal thinning.

8. Admission to the hospital may be necessary if patient compliance is an issue. It may take weeks to achieve complete healing.

9. If unable to adequately control the infection despite prolonged treatment, a therapeutic penetrating keratoplasty can be considered, ideally before the infection reaches the limbus. Intracameral antifungal medications (e.g., voriconazole 50 mcg/0.1 mL or amphotericin 10 mcg in 0.1 mL) at the time of therapeutic keratoplasty should be considered. Anterior lamellar keratoplasty is relatively contraindicated because there is a high risk of recurrence of infection.

Follow Up

Patients are reexamined daily at first. However, the initial clinical response to treatment in fungal keratitis is much slower compared to bacterial keratitis. Stability of infection after initiation of treatment is often a favorable sign. Unlike bacterial ulcers, epithelial healing in fungal keratitis is not always a sign of positive response. Fungal infections in deep corneal stroma may be recalcitrant to therapy. These ulcers may require weeks to months of treatment, and therapeutic corneal transplantation may be necessary for infections that progress despite maximal medical therapy or corneal perforation.

4.13 Acanthamoeba Keratitis

Symptoms

Can vary from foreign body sensation to severe ocular pain (often out of proportion to the early clinical findings), redness, and photophobia over a period of several weeks.

Signs

(See Figures 4.13.1 and 4.13.2.)

Critical. Early: Epitheliitis with pseudodendrites, whorls, epithelial ridges, and/or diffuse

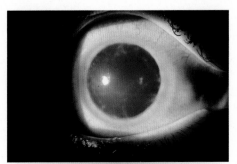

Figure 4.13.1 Acanthamoeba keratitis with radial keratoneuritis.

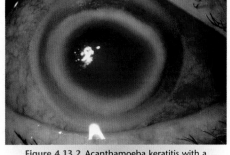

Figure 4.13.2 Acanthamoeba keratitis with a dense ring infiltrate.

4

subepithelial microcysts. Subepithelial infiltrates (sometimes along corneal nerves, producing a radial keratoneuritis).

Late (3 to 8 weeks): Ring-shaped corneal stromal infiltrate.

NOTE: Acanthamoeba keratitis should be considered in any patient with a history of soft contact lens wear, poor contact lens hygiene (e.g., using tap water to clean lenses, infrequent disinfection), and/or history of trauma or exposure to water (swimming, fishing, hot tub use) while wearing contact lenses. Although most patients with Acanthamoeba have a history of contact lens use, some patients do not and these patients often have a delayed diagnosis. Cultures for bacteria are negative (unless superinfection present). The condition usually does not improve with antibiotic or antiviral medications and commonly follows a chronic, progressive, downhill course. Acanthamoeba is important to consider in patients with seemingly unresponsive HSV keratitis, as HSV keratitis usually responds well to appropriate treatment. The diagnosis of HSV keratitis in a contact lens wearer should always include consideration of Acanthamoeba, as the clinical appearance of these two entities can be similar in the early stages of disease.

Other. Eyelid swelling, conjunctival injection (especially circumcorneal), cells and flare in the anterior chamber. Minimal discharge or corneal vascularization. Coinfection with bacteria or fungi may occur later in the course.

Differential Diagnosis

HSV keratitis is first in the differential. See 4.11, BACTERIAL KERATITIS and 4.15, HERPES SIMPLEX VIRUS.

Workup

See 4.11, BACTERIAL KERATITIS for a general workup. One or more of the following are obtained when Acanthamoeba is suspected:

1. Corneal scrapings for Gram, Giemsa, calcofluor white, and periodic acid-Schiff stains (Giemsa and periodic acid-Schiff stains may show typical cysts). See Appendix 8, CORNEAL CULTURE PROCEDURE.

2. Consider a culture on nonnutrient agar with *Escherichia coli* overlay.

3. Consider a corneal biopsy if the stains and cultures are negative and the condition is not improving on the current regimen.

4. Consider cultures and smears of contact lens and case.

5. Confocal biomicroscopy may be helpful if available.

Treatment

One or more of the following are usually used in combination, sometimes in the hospital initially:

1. Polyhexamethylene biguanide 0.02% (PHMB) drops q1h or chlorhexidine 0.02% drops q1h.

2. Propamidine isethionate 0.1% drops q1h are typically added in addition to PHMB or chlorhexidine. Dibromopropamidine isethionate 0.15% ointment is also available.

3. Consider an oral antifungal agent (e.g., itraconazole 400 mg p.o. for one loading dose, then 100 to 200 mg p.o. daily, ketoconazole 200 mg p.o. daily, or voriconazole 200 mg p.o. daily to b.i.d.).

All patients:

4. Miltefosine is designated by the FDA as an orphan drug for the treatment of acanthamoeba keratitis and can be considered as an adjunctive treatment to the topical therapy. At Wills, we typically begin this medication upon pathologic identification of acanthamoeba cysts and prescribe 50 mg b.i.d. to t.i.d. for a 4 week course. Basic metabolic panel, liver function tests, and pregnancy test (if applicable) should be obtained prior to starting miltefosine, which is known to cause serious risks in pregnancy. Note that there may be rebound inflammation after the miltefosine is stopped, which can respond to topical steroids.

 NOTE: Alternative therapy includes hexamidine 0.1%, clotrimazole 1% drops, miconazole 1% drops, or paromomycin drops q2h. Low-dose steroid drops may be helpful in reducing inflammation after the infection is controlled, but steroid use is controversial.

5. Discontinue contact lens wear in both eyes.
6. Cycloplegic drop (e.g., cyclopentolate 1% t.i.d. or atropine 1% b.i.d.).

7. In presence of inflammation, pain, and/or scleritis, oral nonsteroidal anti-inflammatory agents (e.g., naproxen 250 to 500 mg p.o. b.i.d.) may be used. Additional narcotic oral analgesics are often needed.

NOTE: Corneal transplantation may be indicated for medical failures, but this procedure can be complicated by recurrent infection. It is best delayed for 6 to 12 months after medical treatment is completed.

Follow Up

Every 1 to 4 days until the condition is consistently improving, and then every 1 to 4 weeks. Medication may then be tapered judiciously. Treatment is usually continued for 3 months after resolution of inflammation, which may take up to 6 to 12 months.

NOTE

1. Propamidine isethionate 0.1% drops are available in the United Kingdom and other countries; it may be compounded in the United States.
2. PHMB is available in the United Kingdom as Cosmocil. It can be prepared by a compounding pharmacy in the United States from Baquacil, a swimming pool disinfectant.

4.14 Crystalline Keratopathy

Symptoms

Decreased vision, photophobia, decreased corneal sensation may occur. May be asymptomatic.

Signs

Crystals seen in subepithelial and/or stromal regions of the cornea. May or may not have an overlying epithelial defect. In the presence of a corneal transplant, the crystalline opacities frequently are localized along an existing suture track.

Etiology

- Infectious crystalline keratopathy: Seen in corneal grafts and chronically inflamed

corneas. *Streptococcus viridans* is the most common organism; other organisms include *Staphylococcus epidermidis*, Corynebacterium species, *Pseudomonas aeruginosa*, and fungi. Patients with history of refractive surgery are at a higher risk for atypical mycobacteria and Alternaria species.

- Schnyder corneal dystrophy: Slowly progressive, autosomal dominant. Subepithelial corneal crystals in 50% of patients (cholesterol and phospholipids), central and midperipheral corneal haze, dense arcus, decreased corneal sensation. Local disorder of corneal lipid metabolism but can be associated with hyperlipidemia and hypercholesterolemia. Higher prevalence in patients with Swede–Finn descent. See 4.25, CORNEAL DYSTROPHIES.

- Bietti crystalline corneoretinal dystrophy: Rare, autosomal recessive. Retinal crystals (decrease with time) and sparkling, yellow-white spots at the corneal limbus in the superficial stroma and subepithelial layers of the cornea.
- Cystinosis: Rare, autosomal recessive, systemic metabolic defect. Infantile form (nephropathic): dwarfism, progressive renal dysfunction, and polychromatic cystine crystals in conjunctiva, corneal stroma (densest in peripheral cornea but present throughout anterior stroma), trabecular meshwork. Intermediate/ adolescent form: less severe renal involvement. Adult form: normal life expectancy.
- Lymphoproliferative disorders (e.g., monoclonal gammopathy of undetermined significance, essential cryoglobulinemia, or multiple myeloma): Fine crystalline opacities are diffusely distributed throughout the cornea more commonly in the anterior stroma and peripheral cornea than the posterior stroma and central cornea.

Workup

1. Infectious crystalline keratopathy: Culture as outlined in Appendix 8, CORNEAL CULTURE PROCEDURE. Obtain mycobacterial cultures/ acid-fast bacillus stain (especially in patients with history of refractive surgery).
2. Fasting lipid profile in patients with Schnyder corneal dystrophy.
3. Electroretinogram may be decreased in later stages of Bietti crystalline dystrophy.
4. Cystinosis: Very high level of suspicion required, especially for infantile form, which

can be fatal in the first decade of life without a renal transplant. Conjunctival biopsy, blood or bone marrow smear.

5. If a lymphoproliferative disorder is suspected, consult hematology and consider complete blood count with differential, serum chemistries (including calcium), creatinine, albumin, lactate dehydrogenase, beta-2 microglobulin, C-reactive protein (CRP), serum protein electrophoresis (SPEP), urine protein electrophoresis (UPEP), and peripheral/bone marrow smear.

Treatment

1. Infectious crystalline keratopathy: Treat as outlined in see 4.11, BACTERIAL KERATITIS, and 4.29, CORNEAL REFRACTIVE SURGERY COMPLICATIONS. If patient is on topical steroid therapy, decrease frequency or steroid strength rather than stopping the steroid abruptly.
2. Schnyder corneal dystrophy: Excimer laser PTK may be effective for subepithelial crystals. Corneal transplantation for severe cases. Diet and/or medications if associated systemic dyslipidemia.
3. No specific treatment for Bietti crystalline dystrophy.
4. Cystinosis: Topical cysteamine drops reduce the density of crystalline deposits and corneal pain. PK for severe cases (although corneal deposits may recur). Patients must get systemic evaluation by primary care physician and/or geneticist.
5. Lymphoproliferative disorder: Consult a hematologist and/or oncologist.

4.15 Herpes Simplex Virus

Symptoms

Red eye, pain, foreign body sensation, photophobia, tearing, decreased vision, skin (e.g., eyelid) vesicular rash, history of previous episodes; usually unilateral.

Signs

Primary HSV infection is usually not apparent clinically. However, neonatal primary herpes infection

is a rare, potentially devastating disease associated with localized skin, eye, or oral infection and severe central nervous system and multiorgan system infection (see 8.9, OPHTHALMIA NEONATORUM [NEWBORN CONJUNCTIVITIS]). Compared to adults, children tend to exhibit more severe disease that may be bilateral, recurrent, and associated with extensive eyelid involvement, multiple corneal/ conjunctival dendrites, and a greater degree of secondary corneal scarring and astigmatism. Possible triggers for recurrence include ocular surgery, certain topical medications, fever, stress, menstruation, and upper respiratory tract infection. Infection may be characterized by any or all of the following:

Eyelid/Skin Involvement

Clear vesicles on an erythematous base that progress to crusting, heal without scarring, cross dermatomes, but are typically unilateral (only 10% of primary HSV dermatitis is bilateral).

Conjunctivitis

Conjunctival injection with acute unilateral follicular conjunctivitis, with or without conjunctival dendrites or geographic ulceration.

Epithelial Keratitis

(See Figure 4.15.1.)

May be seen as macropunctate keratitis, dendritic keratitis (a thin, linear, branching epithelial ulceration with club-shaped terminal bulbs at the end of each branch), or a geographic ulcer (a large, amoeba-shaped corneal ulcer with a dendritic edge). The edges of herpetic lesions are heaped up with swollen epithelial cells that stain well with rose bengal or lissamine green; the central ulceration stains well with fluorescein. Corneal sensitivity may be decreased. Subepithelial scars and haze (ghost dendrites) may develop as epithelial dendrites resolve. Epithelial keratitis is considered to be live, replicating viral disease, and treatment is directed accordingly.

Differential Diagnosis of Corneal Dendrites

A "true" dendrite (branching epithelial ulceration with terminal end-bulbs) is pathognomonic for HSV however there are many similar appearing lesions that should be distinguished:

- VZV: Pseudodendrites in VZV are slightly elevated and are without central ulceration. They do not have true terminal bulbs and do not typically stain well with fluorescein. See 4.16, HERPES ZOSTER OPHTHALMICUS/VARICELLA ZOSTER VIRUS.
- Recurrent corneal erosion or any recent corneal abrasion: A healing epithelial defect often has a dendritiform appearance. Recurrent erosions in patients with lattice dystrophy can have a geographic shape. See 4.2, RECURRENT CORNEAL EROSION.

- Acanthamoeba keratitis pseudodendrites: History of soft contact lens wear, pain often out of proportion to inflammation, chronic course. These are raised epithelial lesions, not epithelial ulcerations. See 4.13, ACANTHAMOEBA KERATITIS.
- Others: Cornea verticillata from medications or Fabry disease, and rarely tyrosinemia.

Stromal Keratitis

- Stromal keratitis without ulceration (alternate terms: nonnecrotizing keratitis, immune stromal keratitis, interstitial keratitis): Unifocal or multifocal stromal haze or whitening, often with stromal edema, in the absence of epithelial ulceration. Accompanying stromal vascularization indicates chronicity or prior episodes. The differential of stromal keratitis without ulceration includes any cause of IK (see below). HSV stromal keratitis is considered an immune reaction rather than active infectious process and therefore treatment is directed accordingly.
- Stromal keratitis with ulceration (necrotizing keratitis): Suppurative stromal inflammation, thinning, with an adjacent or overlying epithelial defect. Appearance may be indistinguishable from infectious keratitis (fungal, bacterial, parasitic) and therefore infection should be ruled out. Stromal keratitis may lead to thinning or scarring and therefore must be treated diligently.
- Endothelial keratitis (disciform keratitis): Corneal stromal and epithelial edema in a round or discrete pattern, associated with an area of keratic precipitates often out of proportion to the amount of anterior chamber inflammation.

Neurotrophic Ulcer

- A chronic presentation in a relatively neurotrophic cornea due to fifth cranial nerve sensory damage following prior keratitis. A sterile ulcer with smooth epithelial margins over an area of interpalpebral stromal disease that persists or worsens despite antiviral therapy. May be associated with stromal melting and perforation. Without a known history or HSV keratitis, other causes of neurotrophic keratitis should be considered, including: VZV, diabetes, cranial surgery, or radiation.

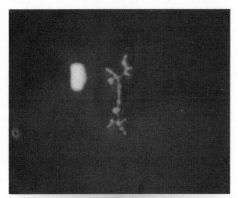

Figure 4.15.1 Herpes simplex dendritic keratitis.

Uveitis

- An anterior chamber inflammatory reaction may develop during corneal stromal disease or independently from keratitis. Elevated IOP secondary to trabeculitis is often suggestive of herpetic uveitis. Patchy iris transillumination defects are also characteristic.

Retinitis

Rare. See 12.8, ACUTE RETINAL NECROSIS.

Workup

1. History: Previous episodes? History of corneal abrasion; contact lens wear; or previous nasal or oral sores? Recent topical or systemic steroids? Immune deficiency state? Recent fever or sun/UV exposure? History of shingles?
2. External examination: Note the distribution of skin vesicles if present. The lesions are more suggestive of HSV than VZV if concentrated around the eye without extension onto forehead, scalp, and tip of nose. HSV often involves both the upper and lower eyelids.
3. Check corneal sensation (before instillation of topical anesthetic), which may be decreased in HSV and VZV.
4. Slit lamp examination with IOP measurement.
5. DFE: Viral retinitis must be ruled out in all new presentations.
6. Herpes simplex is usually diagnosed clinically and requires no confirmatory laboratory tests. If the diagnosis is in doubt, any of the following tests may be helpful:

- Viral PCR (or culture): A sterile, cotton-tipped applicator is used to swab the cornea, conjunctiva, or skin (after unroofing vesicles with a sterile needle) and is placed in the viral transport medium. Readily available in most laboratory settings with a relatively good sensitivity.
- Scrapings of a corneal or skin lesion (scrape the edge of a corneal ulcer or the base of a skin lesion) for Giemsa stain, which shows multinucleated giant cells (this will not help differentiate HSV from other herpes family viruses). Enzyme-linked immunosorbent assay testing specific to HSV also is available.
- HSV antibody titers are frequently present in patients. They rise after primary but not recurrent infection. The absence of HSV1 antibodies helps rule out HSV as a cause of stromal keratitis. Positive titer is nonspecific as HSV is ubiquitous and exposure rates in the general population are extremely high.

Treatment

Blepharoconjunctivitis: Skin/Eyelid/Conjunctivitis

1. Self-limited, however treatment may shorten course and reduce corneal exposure to live virus. Systemic (acyclovir 400 mg five times daily or valacyclovir 500 mg twice daily or famciclovir 250 mg twice daily for 7 to 10 days) or topical (ganciclovir 0.15% ophthalmic gel five times daily or trifluridine 1% nine times daily for 7 to 10 days) therapy may be helpful.

Epithelial Keratitis

1. Either systemic or topical antiviral therapy may be used. Many cornea specialists now prefer systemic treatment for greater intraocular concentration, ease of use, and reduction of corneal medication toxicity.

- Dendritic: Oral treatment (acyclovir 400 mg five times daily or valacyclovir 500 mg twice to three times daily or famciclovir 250 mg twice to three times daily) for 7 to 10 days or topical ganciclovir 0.15% ophthalmic gel or 3% acyclovir ophthalmic ointment five times per day until healed, then three times per day for 7 days

4

or trifluridine 1% drops nine times per day until healed then five times daily for 7 days (but not exceeding 21 days). Topical ganciclovir gel and acyclovir ointment appear to have a lower incidence of corneal toxicity than trifluridine drops.

- Geographic: Oral treatment (acyclovir 400 to 800 mg five times daily or valacyclovir 500 to 1,000 mg twice to three times daily or famciclovir 250 to 500 mg twice to three times daily) for 14 to 21 days or topical therapy as described above.

2. Consider cycloplegic drop (e.g., cyclopentolate 1% t.i.d.) if an anterior chamber reaction or photophobia is present.

3. Topical antibiotic (drop or ointment) may be given at a prophylaxis dose to prevent bacterial superinfection until epithelium is healed.

4. Patients taking topical steroids should have them tapered rapidly.

5. Limited debridement of infected epithelium can be used as an adjunct to antiviral agents.

- Technique: After topical anesthetic instillation, a sterile, moistened cotton-tipped applicator or semisharp instrument is used carefully to peel off the lesions at the slit lamp. After debridement, antiviral treatment should be instituted or continued as described earlier.

6. For epithelial defects that do not resolve after 1 to 2 weeks, bacterial coinfection or Acanthamoeba keratitis should be suspected. Noncompliance and topical antiviral toxicity should also be considered. At that point, the topical antiviral agent should be discontinued, and a nonpreserved artificial tear ointment or an antibiotic ointment (e.g., erythromycin) should be used four to eight times per day for several days with careful follow up. Smears for Acanthamoeba should be performed whenever the diagnosis is suspected.

Stromal Keratitis Without Epithelial Ulceration

- Therapeutic dose topical steroid: Prednisolone acetate 1% six to eight times daily tapered slowly. Patients may require low dose/potency maintenance therapy indefinitely.

- Prophylactic oral antiviral: Acyclovir 400 mg twice daily or valacyclovir 500 mg once or twice daily or famciclovir 250 mg once or twice daily.

- Microbial superinfections must be ruled out and treated. Tissue adhesive or corneal transplantation may be required if the cornea perforates.

Stromal Keratitis With Epithelial Ulceration

- Limited dose of topical steroid: Prednisolone acetate 1% twice daily.

- Therapeutic dose of oral antiviral for 7 to 10 days: Acyclovir 800 mg three to five times daily or valacyclovir 1 g two to three times daily or famciclovir 500 mg two to three times daily. The oral antiviral agent is reduced to prophylactic dose as long as topical steroids are continued.

Endothelial Keratitis

Therapeutic dose of topical steroid and therapeutic dose of oral antiviral (see dosing above).

Neurotrophic Ulcer

See 4.6, NEUROTROPHIC KERATOPATHY.

 NOTE: Chronic use of prophylactic oral antivirals may help prevent subsequent episodes of HSV keratouveitis.

- Adjunctive medications which may be used include:
  - Topical antibiotic (e.g., erythromycin ointment) in the presence of epithelial defects.
  - Aqueous suppressants for increased IOP. Avoid prostaglandin analogues due to association with recurrent HSV infections and uveitis.

NOTE

1. Topical steroids are contraindicated in those with infectious epithelial disease.

2. Rarely, a systemic steroid (e.g., prednisone 40 to 60 mg p.o. daily tapered rapidly) is given to patients with severe stromal disease accompanied by an epithelial defect and hypopyon. Cultures should be done to rule out a superinfection.

3. While oral antivirals (e.g., acyclovir, valacyclovir, and famciclovir) have not been shown to be beneficial in the treatment of stromal disease, they are typically employed, and

may be beneficial in the treatment of herpetic uveitis (see 12.1, ANTERIOR UVEITIS [IRITIS/IRIDOCYCLITIS]).

4. Valacyclovir has greater bioavailability than acyclovir. Little has been published on famciclovir for HSV, but it may be better tolerated in patients who have side effects to acyclovir such as headache, fatigue, or gastrointestinal upset.

5. Dosing of antivirals discussed above (e.g., acyclovir, valacyclovir, and famciclovir) needs to be adjusted in patients with renal insufficiency. Checking BUN and creatinine is recommended in patients at risk for renal disease before starting high doses of these medications.

6. Valacyclovir should be used with caution in patients with human immunodeficiency virus due to reports of thrombocytopenic purpura and hemolytic uremic syndrome in this population.

7. The persistence of an ulcer with stromal keratitis is commonly due to the underlying inflammation (requiring cautious steroid therapy); however, it may be due to antiviral toxicity or active HSV epithelial infection. When an ulcer deepens, a new infiltrate develops, or the anterior chamber reaction increases, smears and cultures should be considered for bacteria and fungi. See Appendix 8, CORNEAL CULTURE PROCEDURE.

Follow Up

1. Patients are reexamined in 2 to 7 days to evaluate the response to treatment and then every 1 to 2 weeks, depending on the clinical findings. The following clinical parameters are evaluated: the size of the epithelial defect and ulcer, the corneal thickness and the depth of corneal involvement, the anterior chamber reaction, and the IOP (see 9.7, INFLAMMATORY OPEN ANGLE GLAUCOMA, for glaucoma management). Patients with necrotizing keratitis need to be followed daily or admitted if there is threat of perforation.

2. Topical antiviral medications for corneal dendrites and geographic ulcers should not be continued for greater than 14 to 21 days (see dosing above).

3. Topical steroids used for corneal stromal disease are tapered slowly (often over months to years). The initial concentration of the steroid (e.g., prednisolone acetate 1%) is eventually reduced (e.g., loteprednol 0.5% or prednisolone acetate 0.125%). Extended taper includes dosing q.o.d., twice weekly, once weekly, etc., especially with a history of flareups when steroids are stopped. Prophylactic systemic antiviral agents (see dosing above) are used until steroids are used once daily or less, at which point they can be continued or stopped.

4. Corneal transplantation may eventually be necessary if inactive postherpetic scars significantly affect vision, though a rigid gas permeable (RGP) contact lens and maximization of the ocular surface with aggressive lubrication should be tried first. The eye should be quiet for at least 3 to 6 months prior to surgery. Systemic antiviral prophylaxis is typically continued for at least 1 year (often indefinitely) following surgery.

5. Recommend long-term oral antiviral prophylaxis (e.g., acyclovir 400 mg b.i.d.) if a patient has had multiple episodes of epithelial disease or stromal disease.

4.16 Herpes Zoster Ophthalmicus/Varicella Zoster Virus

Symptoms

Dermatomal pain, paresthesias, and skin rash or discomfort. May be preceded by headache, fever, or malaise, and accompanied or followed by blurred vision, eye pain, and red eye.

Signs

Critical. Acute vesicular dermatomal skin rash along the first division of the fifth cranial nerve. Characteristically, the rash is unilateral and typically spares the lower eyelid. Hutchinson sign (tip of the nose involved in the distribution of the nasociliary branch of V1) predicts higher risk of ocular involvement. While the associated edema of the vesicular rash may extend bilaterally, the lesions always respect the midline.

Other. Less commonly, the lower eyelid and cheek on one side (V2), and, rarely, one side of the jaw (V3) are involved. Conjunctivitis, corneal involvement (e.g., multiple small epithelial dendritiform lesions early, followed by larger pseudodendrites [raised mucous plaques which may be present on cornea or conjunctiva, see **Figure 4.16.1**], SPK, immune stromal keratitis, neurotrophic keratitis), uveitis, sectoral iris atrophy, scleritis, retinitis, choroiditis, optic neuritis, cranial nerve palsies, and elevated IOP can occur. Late postherpetic neuralgia also may occur.

> **NOTE:** Corneal disease may follow the acute skin rash by several days, weeks, or months and can last for years. Occasionally, the diagnosis can be more difficult to determine in cases where a clinical rash never develops or cases where corneal disease precedes the skin rash. There is a rise in VZV titers after zoster.

Differential Diagnosis

- HSV: Patients are often younger; rash is not dermatomal. See 4.15, HERPES SIMPLEX VIRUS.

Workup

1. History: Duration of rash and pain? Immunocompromised or risk factors for HIV/AIDS? Hearing changes, facial pain or weakness, vertigo (cranial nerve VII involvement [Ramsay Hunt syndrome])? Rashes elsewhere?
2. Complete ocular examination, including a slit lamp evaluation with fluorescein or rose bengal staining, IOP check, and dilated fundus examination with careful evaluation for acute retinal necrosis (ARN) in immunocompetent patients and progressive outer retinal necrosis (PORN) in patients with immunodeficiency. See 12.8, ACUTE RETINAL NECROSIS (ARN).
3. Consider medical evaluation for immuno-compromised status if immunodeficiency is suspected from the history.
4. If patient is >60 years old (especially if systemic steroid therapy is to be initiated), or if any other organ systems or nonophthalmic sites are involved, evaluation by the patient's primary medical doctor or other subspecialist(s) is warranted.

Treatment

See **Table 4.16.1**.

> **NOTE:** Immunocompromised patients should not receive systemic steroids.

Skin Involvement

1. In adults with a moderate-to-severe skin rash for <4 days in which active skin lesions are present and consider if the patient presents later in the first week with active lesions:
   - Oral antiviral agent (e.g., acyclovir 800 mg p.o. five times per day, valacyclovir 1,000 mg p.o. t.i.d., or famciclovir 500 mg p.o. t.i.d.) for 7 to 10 days. If the condition is severe, as manifested by orbital, optic nerve, or cranial nerve involvement, or the patient is systemically ill, hospitalize and prescribe acyclovir 5 to 10 mg/kg i.v. q8h for 5 to 10 days.
   - Ophthalmic antibiotic ointment (e.g., bacitracin or erythromycin) to skin lesions b.i.d.
   - Warm compresses to periocular skin t.i.d.
2. Adults with a skin rash of more than 1-week duration or without active skin lesions:
   - Ophthalmic antibiotic ointment (e.g., bacitracin or erythromycin) to skin lesions b.i.d.
   - Warm compresses to periocular skin t.i.d.
3. Children: Discuss with a pediatrician and consider weight-based acyclovir dosing (20 mg/kg q8h) for children <12 years of age or under 40 kg, otherwise use adult dosage above. For systemic spread, hospitalize and prescribe intravenous acyclovir in conjunction with pediatric and infectious disease comanagement.

Ocular Involvement

> **NOTE:** It is common clinical practice at Wills Eye for all patients with VZV ocular findings to receive 7 to 10 days of systemic oral antivirals (e.g., acyclovir 800 mg p.o. five times per day, valacyclovir 1,000 mg p.o. t.i.d., or famciclovir 500 mg p.o. t.i.d.) usually in conjunction with the following therapies.

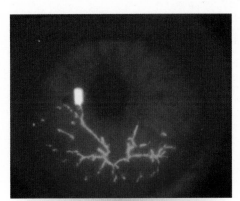

Figure 4.16.1 Herpes zoster keratitis with pseudodendrites.

1. Conjunctival involvement: Cool compresses and ophthalmic ointment (e.g., bacitracin or erythromycin) to the eye b.i.d.
2. SPK: Lubrication with preservative-free artificial tears q1–2h and ointment q.h.s.
3. Corneal or conjunctival mucous plaque pseudodendrites: Lubrication with preservative-free artificial tears q1–2h and ointment q.h.s. Consider antibiotic ointment to prevent bacterial superinfection. Topical antivirals (e.g., ganiciclovir gel four to five times daily) may be helpful for recalcitrant corneal mucous plaque pseudodendrites.
4. Immune stromal keratitis: Topical steroid (e.g., prednisolone acetate 1%) started at a frequency of four to eight times per day and adjusted according to clinical response. Topical steroids are tapered over months to years using weaker steroids with a goal of less than daily dosing (e.g., q.o.d., twice weekly, once weekly, etc.).
5. Uveitis (with or without immune stromal keratitis): Topical steroid (e.g., prednisolone acetate 1%) four to eight times per day and cycloplegic drop (e.g., cyclopentolate 1% t.i.d.). See 12.1, ANTERIOR UVEITIS (IRITIS/IRIDOCYCLITIS). Treat increased IOP with aggressive aqueous suppression; avoid prostaglandin analogues.
6. Neurotrophic keratitis: Treat mild epithelial defects with ophthalmic antibiotic ointment (e.g., erythromycin) four to eight times per day. If a corneal infiltrate occurs, obtain appropriate smears and cultures to rule out infection (see 4.11, BACTERIAL KERATITIS). If the infiltrate is sterile, and there is no response to ointment, consider punctal plugs, bandage soft contact lens, tarsorrhaphy, amniotic membrane tissue, autologous serum tears, recombinant nerve growth factor, or conjunctival flap along with prophylactic topical antibiotics (see 4.6, NEUROTROPHIC KERATOPATHY).
7. Scleritis: See 5.7, SCLERITIS.
8. Retinitis, choroiditis, optic neuritis, or cranial nerve palsy: Acyclovir 10 mg/kg i.v. q8h for 1 week and prednisone 60 mg p.o. for 3 days, then taper over 1 week. Management of ARN or PORN may require intraocular antivirals (see 12.8, ACUTE RETINAL NECROSIS). Infectious disease and neurologic consultation to rule out central nervous system involvement should be considered. Patients with severe disease can develop a large vessel cranial arteritis resulting in a massive cerebrovascular accident.
9. Increased IOP: May be steroid response or secondary to inflammation. If uveitis is present, increase the frequency of the steroid administration for a few days and use topical aqueous suppressants (e.g., timolol 0.5% daily or b.i.d., brimonidine 0.2% t.i.d., or dorzolamide 2% t.i.d.; see 9.7, INFLAMMATORY OPEN ANGLE GLAUCOMA, and 9.9, STEROID-RESPONSE GLAUCOMA). Oral carbonic anhydrase inhibitors may be necessary if the IOP is >30 mm Hg. If IOP remains increased and the inflammation is controlled, substitute fluorometholone 0.1% or loteprednol 0.5% drops for prednisolone acetate and attempt to taper the dose.

NOTE: Pain may be severe during the first 2 weeks, and narcotic analgesics may be required. An antidepressant (e.g., amitriptyline 25 mg p.o. t.i.d.) may be beneficial for both postherpetic neuralgia and depression that can develop in VZV. Capsaicin 0.025% or doxepin ointment may be applied to the skin t.i.d. to q.i.d. after the rash heals (not around the eyes) for postherpetic neuralgia. Oral gabapentin or pregabalin can be helpful for acute pain and for postherpetic neuralgia. Management of postherpetic neuralgia should involve the patient's primary medical doctor or a pain management specialist.

TABLE 4.16.1   Antiviral Therapy Guidelines for Varicella Zoster Virus

Drug	Dosing Information	Toxicities	Contraindications
Acyclovir	If immunocompetent, 800 mg p.o. five times per day; if immunocompromised, start 10/mg/kg i.v. q8h (q12h if creatinine >2.0) for 7 to 10 d, followed by 800 mg p.o. five times per day to prevent reactivation.	Intravenous: reversible renal and neurologic toxicity	Use with caution in patients with a history of renal impairment.
Famciclovir	500 mg p.o. q8h. Adjust dosage for creatinine clearance <60 mL/min.	Headache, nausea, diarrhea, dizziness, fatigue	Use with caution in patients with a history of renal impairment.
Valacyclovir	1 g p.o. q8h. Adjust dosage for creatinine clearance <60 mL/min.	Headache, nausea, vomiting, diarrhea	TTP/HUS has been reported in patients with advanced HIV/AIDS.

Follow Up

If ocular involvement is present, examine the patient every 1 to 7 days, depending on the severity. Patients without ocular involvement can be followed every 1 to 4 weeks. After the acute episode resolves, check the patient every 3 to 6 months (3 if on steroids) because relapses may occur months to years later, particularly as steroids are tapered. Systemic steroid use is controversial.

NOTE: VZV is contagious for children and adults who have not had chickenpox or the chickenpox vaccine and is spread by inhalation. Varicella-naïve pregnant women must be especially careful to avoid contact with a VZV-infected patient. A vaccine for shingles is recommended for people aged 50 years or older.

VARICELLA ZOSTER VIRUS (CHICKENPOX)

Symptoms

Facial rash, red eye, foreign body sensation.

Signs

Early: Acute conjunctivitis with vesicles or papules at the limbus, on the eyelid, or on the conjunctiva. Pseudodendritic corneal epithelial lesions, stromal keratitis, anterior uveitis, optic neuritis, retinitis, and ophthalmoplegia occur rarely.

Late: Immune stromal or neurotrophic keratitis.

Treatment

1. Conjunctival involvement and/or corneal epithelial lesions: Cool compresses and ophthalmic antibiotic ointment (e.g., erythromycin t.i.d.) to the eye and periorbital lesions.
2. Stromal keratitis with uveitis: Topical steroid (e.g., prednisolone acetate 1% q.i.d.), cycloplegic drop (e.g., cyclopentolate 1% t.i.d.)
3. Neurotrophic keratitis: Uncommon; see 4.6, NEUROTROPHIC KERATOPATHY.
4. Canalicular obstruction: Uncommon. Managed by intubation of puncta.

 NOTE

1. Aspirin is contraindicated in children because of the risk of Reye syndrome.
2. Immunocompromised children with chickenpox may require i.v. acyclovir.

Follow Up

1. Follow up in 1 to 7 days, depending on the severity of ocular disease. Taper the topical steroids slowly.
2. Watch for stromal or neurotrophic keratitis approximately 4 to 6 weeks after the chickenpox infection resolves.

4.17 Interstitial Keratitis

IK is broadly defined as any non-ulcerating inflammation of the corneal stroma without epithelial or endothelial involvement, but often with neovascularization. IK is the common end-point of many corneal diseases.

Signs

Acute Phase

Critical. Marked corneal stromal blood vessels and edema.

Other. Anterior chamber cells and flare, fine keratic precipitates on the corneal endothelium, conjunctival injection.

Chronic Phase

(See Figure 4.17.1.)

Deep corneal haze or scarring, corneal stromal blood vessels containing minimal or no blood (ghost vessels), stromal thinning.

Etiology

Most Common. HSV is the most common cause of IK (see 4.15, HERPES SIMPLEX VIRUS). Other common causes include: VZV, congenital syphilis (bilateral in 80% of cases, often occurs in the first or second decade of life, rare in first years of life. Affects both eyes within 1 year of each other, more commonly occurs as late inactive/immune-mediated disease and less often as acute/infectious disease), acquired syphilis, and tuberculosis (TB, unilateral and often sectoral).

Less Common. Epstein-Barr virus (EBV) Lyme disease, leprosy, and Cogan syndrome (autoimmune disorder characterized by bilateral IK, vertigo, tinnitus, hearing loss, and negative syphilis serologies; also associated with systemic vasculitis [e.g., polyarteritis nodosa] and typically occurs in young adults).

Workup

For active IK or old, previously untreated IK:

1. History: Venereal disease in the mother during pregnancy or in the patient? Hearing loss or tinnitus? Prior HSV or shingles infections?

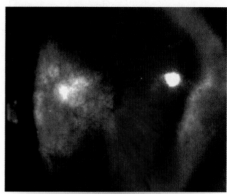

Figure 4.17.1 Interstitial keratitis.

2. External examination: Look for saddle-nose deformity, Hutchinson teeth, frontal bossing, or other signs of congenital syphilis. Look for hypopigmented or anesthetic skin lesions and thickened skin folds, loss of the temporal eyebrow, and loss of eyelashes, as in leprosy.

3. Slit lamp examination: Examine corneal nerves for segmental thickening, like beads on a string (leprosy). Examine the iris for nodules (leprosy) and hyperemia with fleshy, pink nodules (syphilis). Check IOP.

4. Dilated fundus examination: Look for classic salt-and-pepper chorioretinitis or optic atrophy of syphilis.

5. Laboratory evaluation: Fluorescent treponemal antibody absorption (FTA-ABS) or treponemal-specific assay (e.g., microhemagglutination-*Treponema pallidum* [MHA-TP]) for prior exposure; Venereal Disease Research Laboratory test (VDRL) or rapid plasma reagin (RPR) for disease activity. See 12.12, SYPHILIS.

6. Purified protein derivative (PPD) or interferon-gamma release assay (IGRA) (e.g., QuantiFERON-TB Gold),

7. Lyme serology if in endemic region.

8. Chest radiograph or chest CT if negative FTA-ABS (or MHA-TP) or positive PPD or IGRA.

9. Consider erythrocyte sedimentation rate, rheumatoid factor, complete blood count, and EBV antibody.

Treatment

1. Acute disease:
   - Topical cycloplegic drop (e.g., cyclopentolate 1% t.i.d. or atropine 1% b.i.d.).
   - Topical steroid (e.g., prednisolone acetate 1% q2–6h depending on the degree of inflammation).
   - Treat any underlying disease.
2. Old inactive disease with central scarring:
   - RGP or scleral contact lens if vision decreased from irregular astigmatism
   - Corneal transplantation may improve vision if minimal amblyopia is present.
3. Recently inactive or old inactive disease:
   - If the treponemal-specific assay or FTA-ABS is positive and the patient has active or untreated syphilis, or if the VDRL or RPR titer is positive and has not declined the expected amount after treatment, then treatment for syphilis is indicated. See 12.12, SYPHILIS.
   - If PPD or IGRA is positive and the patient is <35 years and has not been treated for TB in the past, or there is evidence of active systemic TB (e.g., positive finding on chest radiograph), then refer the patient to an internist and infectious disease specialist for TB treatment.
   - If Cogan syndrome is present, refer the patient to an otolaryngologist and rheumatologist.
   - If Lyme antibody and titers are positive, treat per 13.4, LYME DISEASE.

Follow Up

1. Acute disease: Every 3 to 7 days initially, and then every 2 to 4 weeks. The frequency of steroid administration is slowly reduced as the inflammation subsides over the course of months (may take years). IOP is monitored closely and reduced with medications based on the degree of IOP elevation and overall health of the optic nerve (see 9.7, INFLAMMATORY OPEN ANGLE GLAUCOMA).
2. Old inactive disease: Yearly follow up, unless treatment is required for underlying etiology.

4.18 Staphylococcal Hypersensitivity

Symptoms

Mild photophobia, mild pain, localized red eye, chronic eyelid crusting, foreign body sensation or dryness. History of recurrent acute episodes, chalazia, or styes.

Signs

(See Figure 4.18.1.)

Critical. Singular or multiple, unilateral or bilateral, peripheral corneal stromal infiltrates often with a clear space between the infiltrates and the limbus. Variable staining with fluorescein. Minimal anterior chamber inflammation. Sectoral conjunctival injection typically occurs.

Other. Blepharitis, inferior SPK, phlyctenule (a wedge-shaped, raised, vascularized sterile infiltrate near the limbus, usually in children). Peripheral scarring and corneal neovascularization. Findings often present in the contralateral eye or elsewhere in the affected eye.

Differential Diagnosis

- Infectious corneal infiltrates: Often round, painful, and associated with an anterior chamber reaction. Not usually multiple and recurrent. See 4.11, BACTERIAL KERATITIS.
- Other causes of marginal thinning/infiltrates: See 4.22, PERIPHERAL CORNEAL THINNING/ULCERATION.

Etiology

Infiltrates are believed to be a cell-mediated, or delayed, type IV hypersensitivity reaction to bacterial antigens in the setting of staphylococcal blepharitis.

NOTE: Patients with ocular rosacea (e.g., meibomian gland inflammation and telangiectasias of the eyelids) are especially susceptible to this condition.

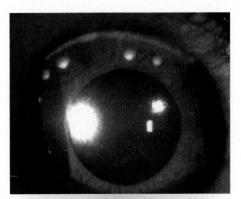

Figure 4.18.1 Staphylococcal hypersensitivity.

Workup

1. History: Recurrent episodes? Contact lens wearer (a risk factor for infection)?
2. Slit lamp examination with fluorescein staining and IOP measurement.
3. If an infectious infiltrate is suspected, then corneal scrapings for cultures and smears should be obtained. See Appendix 8, CORNEAL CULTURE PROCEDURE.

Treatment

Mild

Warm compresses, eyelid hygiene, and an antibiotic drop q.i.d. (e.g., fluoroquinolone or trimethoprim/polymyxin B) and antibiotic ophthalmic ointment q.h.s. (e.g., bacitracin, erythromycin, bacitracin/polymyxin B). See 5.8, BLEPHARITIS/MEIBOMITIS.

Moderate to Severe

- Treat as described for mild, but add a low-dose topical steroid (e.g., loteprednol 0.5%,

fluorometholone 0.1%, fluorometholone acetate 0.1% or prednisolone acetate 0.125% q.i.d.) with an antibiotic (e.g., fluoroquinolone or trimethoprim/polymyxin B q.i.d.). A combination antibiotic/steroid can also be used q.i.d. (e.g., loteprednol 0.5%/tobramycin 0.3%, dexamethasone 0.1%/tobramycin 0.3% or dexamethasone 0.05%/tobramycin 0.3%). Steroid use without antibiotic coverage is not recommended. Maintain until the symptoms improve and then slowly taper.

- If episodes recur despite eyelid hygiene, add systemic doxycycline (100 mg p.o. b.i.d., for 2 weeks, and then daily for 1 month, and then 50 to 100 mg daily titrated as necessary) until the ocular disease is controlled for several months. This medication has an anti-inflammatory effect on the sebaceous glands in addition to its antimicrobial action. Topical azithromycin q.h.s., erythromycin q.h.s. or cyclosporine b.i.d. may be helpful in controlling eyelid inflammation.

- Low-dose antibiotics (e.g., bacitracin or erythromycin ointment q.h.s.) may have to be maintained indefinitely.

> **NOTE:** Tetracyclines such as doxycycline are contraindicated in children <8 years old, pregnant women, and breast feeding mothers. Erythromycin 200 mg p.o. one to two times per day can be used in children to decrease recurrent disease.

Follow Up

In 2 to 7 days, depending on the clinical picture. IOP is monitored while patients are taking topical steroids.

4.19 Phlyctenulosis

Symptoms

Tearing, irritation, pain, mild-to-severe photophobia. History of similar episodes or chalazia. Corneal phlyctenules are more symptomatic than conjunctival phlyctenules.

Signs

Critical

- Conjunctival phlyctenule: A small, rounded, white inflammatory nodule on the bulbar

conjunctiva, often at or near the limbus, in the center of a hyperemic area.

- Corneal phlyctenule: A small, white nodule, initially at the limbus, with dilated conjunctival blood vessels approaching it. Often associated with epithelial ulceration and central corneal migration, producing wedge-shaped corneal neovascularization and scarring behind the leading edge of the lesion. Can be bilateral and recurrent **(see Figure 4.19.1)**.

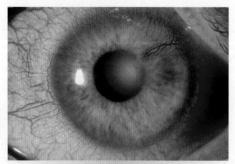

Figure 4.19.1 Corneal phlyctenule.

Other. Conjunctival injection, blepharitis, corneal scarring.

Differential Diagnosis

- Inflamed pinguecula: Uncommon in children. Located in the palpebral fissure. Connective tissue often seen from lesion to the limbus. Often bilateral. See 4.9, PTERYGIUM/PINGUECULA.
- Infectious corneal ulcer: With migration, corneal phlyctenules produce a sterile ulcer surrounded by a white infiltrate. When an infectious ulcer is suspected (e.g., increased pain, anterior chamber reaction), appropriate antibiotic treatment and diagnostic smears and cultures are necessary. See Appendix 8, CORNEAL CULTURE PROCEDURE.
- Staphylococcal hypersensitivity: Peripheral corneal infiltrates, sometimes with an overlying epithelial defect; usually multiple, often bilateral, with a clear space between the infiltrate and the limbus. Minimal anterior chamber reaction. See 4.18, STAPHYLOCOCCAL HYPERSENSITIVITY.
- Ocular rosacea: Corneal neovascularization with thinning and subepithelial infiltration may develop in an eye with rosacea. See 5.9, OCULAR ROSACEA.
- Herpes simplex keratitis: May produce corneal neovascularization associated with a stromal infiltrate. Usually unilateral. See 4.15, HERPES SIMPLEX VIRUS.

Etiology

Delayed hypersensitivity reaction usually as a result of one of the following:

- Staphylococcus: Usually related to blepharitis. See 4.18, STAPHYLOCOCCAL HYPERSENSITIVITY.

- Rarely TB or another infectious agent (e.g., Coccidiomycosis, Candidiasis, lymphogranuloma venereum).

Workup

1. History: TB or recent infection?
2. Slit lamp examination: Inspect the eyelid margin for signs of Staphylococcal anterior blepharitis and rosacea.
3. PPD and/or IGRA in patients without blepharitis and those at high risk for TB.
4. Chest radiograph or chest CT if high suspicion for TB or positive PPD or IGRA.

Treatment

Indicated for symptomatic patients.

1. Topical steroid (e.g., loteprednol 0.5% or prednisolone acetate 1% q.i.d., depending on the severity of symptoms). A combination antibiotic/steroid can also be used q.i.d. (e.g., loteprednol 0.5%/tobramycin 0.3% or dexamethasone 0.1%/tobramycin 0.3%).
2. Topical ophthalmic antibiotic regimen in the presence of corneal ulcer. See 4.11, BACTERIAL KERATITIS. Otherwise antibiotic ointment (e.g., erythromycin, bacitracin) q.h.s.
3. Eyelid hygiene b.i.d. to t.i.d. for blepharitis. See 5.8, BLEPHARITIS/MEIBOMITIS.
4. Preservative-free artificial tears four to six times per day.
5. In severe cases of blepharitis or acne rosacea, use doxycycline 100 mg p.o. daily. to b.i.d., or erythromycin 200 mg p.o. daily to b.i.d. See 5.8, BLEPHARITIS/MEIBOMITIS.
6. If the PPD, IGRA, or chest radiograph is positive for TB, refer the patient to an internist or infectious disease specialist for management.

Follow Up

Recheck in several days. Healing usually occurs over a 10- to 14-day period, with a residual stromal scar. When the symptoms have significantly improved, slowly taper the steroid. Maintain the antibiotic ointment and eyelid hygiene indefinitely. Continue oral antibiotics for 3 to 6 months. Topical cyclosporine may be a beneficial steroid-sparing agent in patients with recurrent inflammation.

4.20 Contact Lens–Related Problems

Symptoms

Pain, photophobia, foreign body sensation, decreased vision, red eye, itching, discharge, burning, and contact lens intolerance.

> **NOTE:** Any contact lens wearer with pain or redness should remove the lens immediately and have a thorough ophthalmic examination as soon as possible if symptoms persist or worsen.

Signs

See the distinguishing characteristics of each etiology.

Etiology

- Infectious corneal infiltrate/ulcer (bacterial, fungal, Acanthamoeba): White corneal lesion that may stain with fluorescein. Must always be ruled out in contact lens patients with eye pain. See 4.11, BACTERIAL KERATITIS, 4.12, FUNGAL KERATITIS, and 4.13, ACANTHAMOEBA KERATITIS.

- Giant papillary conjunctivitis: Itching, mucous discharge, and lens intolerance in a patient with large superior tarsal conjunctival papillae. See 4.21, CONTACT LENS–INDUCED GIANT PAPILLARY CONJUNCTIVITIS.

- Hypersensitivity/toxicity reactions to preservatives in solutions: Conjunctival injection and ocular irritation typically develop shortly after lens cleaning and insertion, but can be present chronically. A recent change from one type or brand of solution is common. It not only occurs more often in patients using older preserved solutions (e.g., thimerosal or chlorhexidine as a component) but also is seen with newer "all-purpose" solutions. May be due to inadequate rinsing of lenses after enzyme use. Signs include SPK, conjunctival injection, bulbar conjunctival follicles, subepithelial or stromal corneal infiltrates, superior epithelial irregularities, and superficial scarring.

- Contact lens deposits: Multiple small deposits on the contact lens, leading to corneal and conjunctival irritation. The contact lens is often old and may not have been cleaned or enzyme-treated properly in the past.

- Tight lens syndrome: Symptoms may be severe and often develop within 1 or 2 days of contact lens fitting (usually a soft lens), especially if patient sleeps overnight with daily-wear lenses. No lens movement with blinking and lens appears "sucked-on" to the cornea (this can occur after rewearing a soft lens that has dried out and then been rehydrated). An imprint in the conjunctiva is often observed after the lens is removed. Central corneal edema, SPK, anterior chamber reaction, and sometimes a sterile hypopyon may develop.

- Contact lens–associated red eye (CLARE): Red eye, corneal edema, iritis with or without hypopyon, hypoxic subepithelial, or stromal infiltrates (often multiple) may be present.

- Corneal warpage: Seen predominantly in long-term polymethylmethacrylate hard contact lens wearers. Initially, the vision becomes blurred with glasses ("spectacle blur") but remains good with contact lenses. Keratometry reveals distorted mires and corneal topography shows irregular astigmatism that usually eventually resolves after lens discontinuation.

- Corneal neovascularization: Patients are often asymptomatic until the visual axis is involved. Superficial corneal neovascularization for 1 mm is common and usually not a concern in aphakic contact lens wearers. With any sign of chronic hypoxia, the goal is to increase oxygen permeability, increase movement, and discontinue extended-wear lenses.

- Limbal stem cell deficiency: Early signs include punctate staining in a whorl-like pattern of the epithelium near the limbus, often superiorly. If untreated, the epitheliopathy can extend to involve the entire cornea. Neovascularization and haze can develop.

- Contact lens keratopathy (pseudo-SLK): Hyperemia and fluorescein staining of the superior bulbar conjunctiva, particularly at the limbus. SPK, subepithelial infiltrates, stromal haze, and irregularity may be found on the superior cornea. This may represent a hypersensitivity or toxicity reaction to preservatives in contact lens solutions (classically thimerosal, but newer preservatives as well). No corneal filaments, papillary reaction, or association with thyroid disease.

4

- Displaced contact lens: Most commonly the lens has actually fallen out of the eye and been lost. If retained, the lens is usually found in the superior fornix and may require double eversion of the upper eyelid to remove. Fluorescein will stain a soft lens to aid in finding it.
- Others: Contact lens inside out, corneal abrasion (see 3.2, CORNEAL ABRASION), poor lens fit, damaged contact lens, and change in refractive error.

Workup

1. History: Main complaint (mild-to-severe pain, discomfort, itching)? Type of contact lens (soft, hard, gas-permeable, extended wear, frequent replacement, or single-use daily disposable)? Age of lens? When lens last worn? Continuous time lens are worn? Sleeping in lenses? How are the lenses cleaned and disinfected? Are enzyme tablets used? Preservative-free products? Recent changes in contact lens habits or solutions? How is the pain related to wearing time? Is pain relieved by removal of the lens?
2. In noninfectious conditions, while the contact lens is still in the eye, evaluate its fit and examine its surface for deposits, irregularities, and defects at the slit lamp.
3. Remove lens and examine the eye with fluorescein. Evert the upper eyelids of both eyes and inspect the superior tarsal conjunctiva for papillae.
4. Smears and cultures are taken when an infectious corneal ulcer is suspected with infiltrate >1 mm, involvement of visual axis, or when an unusual organism is suspected (e.g., Acanthamoeba or fungus). See 4.11, BACTERIAL KERATITIS, 4.12, FUNGAL KERATITIS, 4.13, ACANTHAMOEBA KERATITIS, and Appendix 8, CORNEAL CULTURE PROCEDURE.
5. The contact lenses and lens case are also cultured occasionally.

Treatment

When the diagnosis of infection is suspected:

1. Discontinue contact lens wear.
2. Antibiotic treatment regimen varies with diagnosis as follows:

Possible Corneal Ulcer (Corneal Infiltrate, Epithelial Defect, Anterior Chamber Reaction, Pain)

a. Obtain appropriate smears and cultures. See Appendix 8, CORNEAL CULTURE PROCEDURE.
b. Start intensive topical antibiotics, See 4.11, BACTERIAL KERATITIS.

Small Subepithelial Infiltrates, Corneal Abrasion, or Diffuse SPK

a. Topical antibiotic (e.g., fluoroquinolone) drops four to eight times per day and a cycloplegic drop.
b. Can also add fluoroquinolone or bacitracin/polymyxin B ointment q.h.s. Beware of toxicity with long-term use.
c. See 3.2, CORNEAL ABRASION or 4.1, SUPERFICIAL PUNCTATE KERATOPATHY for specific details.

NOTE: Never pressure patch a contact lens wearer because of the risk of rapid development of infection.

When a specific contact lens problem is suspected, it may be treated as follows:

Giant Papillary Conjunctivitis

(See 4.21, CONTACT LENS–INDUCED GIANT PAPILLARY CONJUNCTIVITIS)

Hypersensitivity/Toxicity Reaction

a. Discontinue contact lens wear.
b. Preservative-free artificial tears four to six times per day.
c. On resolution of the condition, the patient may return to new contact lenses, preferably daily disposable lenses. If the patient desires frequent-replacement or conventional lenses, hydrogen peroxide-based systems are recommended, and appropriate lens hygiene is reviewed.

Contact Lens Deposits

a. Discontinue contact lens wear.
b. Replace with a new contact lens once the symptoms resolve. Consider changing the

brand of contact lens, or change to daily disposable or frequent replacement lens.

c. Teach proper contact lens care, stressing weekly enzyme treatments for lenses replaced less frequently than every 2 weeks.

Tight Lens Syndrome and CLARE

a. Discontinue contact lens wear.

b. Consider a topical cycloplegic drop (e.g., cyclopentolate 1% t.i.d.) in the presence of an anterior chamber reaction.

c. Once resolved, refit patients with a flatter and more oxygen-permeable contact lens. Discontinue extended-wear contact lenses.

d. If a soft lens has dried out, discard and refit.

> **NOTE:** Patients with small hypopyon do not need to be cultured when tight lens syndrome is highly suspected (i.e., if epithelium intact, with edema but no infiltrate).

Corneal Warpage

a. Discontinue contact lens wear. Explain to patients that vision may be poor for the following 2 to 6 weeks, and they may require a change in spectacle prescription. May need to discontinue lenses one eye at a time so patient can function.

b. A gas-permeable hard contact lens should be refitted when the refraction and keratometric readings have stabilized.

Corneal Neovascularization

a. Discontinue contact lens wear.

b. Consider a topical steroid (e.g., prednisolone 1% q.i.d. or loteprednol 0.5% q.i.d.) for extensive deep neovascularization (rarely necessary).

c. Refit carefully with a highly oxygen-transmissible, daily-wear disposable contact lens that moves adequately over the cornea.

Limbal Stem Cell Deficiency

a. Discontinue contact lens wear.

b. Use preservative-free artificial tears and lubricating ointment.

c. Consider punctal occlusion.

d. Consider a short course of topical steroids (e.g., loteprednol 0.5%, fluorometholone 0.1% or fluorometholone acetate 0.1%).

e. Consider autologous serum drops (e.g. 20% q.i.d.).

f. In more advanced cases surgical considerations including selective epithelial debridement for partial limbal stem cell deficiency or limbal stem cell grafting in complete limbal stem cell deficiency may be indicated.

Pseudo-Superior Limbic Keratoconjunctivitis

a. Treat as described for hypersensitivity/toxicity reactions. Use preservative-free artificial tears. When a large subepithelial opacity extends toward the visual axis, topical steroids may be added cautiously (e.g., loteprednol 0.5% q.i.d.), but they are often ineffective. Steroid use in contact lens–related problems should have concomitant antibiotic coverage.

Displaced Lens

a. Inspect lens carefully for damage. If lens is undamaged, clean and disinfect it; if damaged, discard and replace. Recheck fit when symptoms have resolved.

Follow Up

1. Next day if infection cannot be ruled out. Treatment is maintained until the condition clears.

2. In noninfectious conditions, reevaluate in 1 to 4 weeks, depending on the clinical situation. Contact lens wear is resumed when the condition resolves. Patients using topical steroids should be followed more closely with attention to IOP monitoring.

3. The following regimen for contact lens care is one we recommend if single-use daily disposable lenses are not possible:

a. Daily cleaning and disinfection with removal of lenses while sleeping for all lens types, including those approved for "extended wear" and "overnight wear." We prefer standard rather than hyperoxygen-transmissible lenses for frequent replacement, as the latter may allow greater adherence for organisms.

b. Daily cleaning regimen for soft contact lenses:
- Preservative-free daily cleaner.
- Preservative-free saline.
- Disinfectant, preferably hydrogen peroxide type.
- Disinfection solutions must be used for recommended time (hours) prior to lens reinsertion.

- Weekly treatment with enzyme tablets (not necessary in disposable lenses replaced every 2 to 4 weeks or less).

c. RGP lenses: Cleaning/soaking/rinsing all in one solution. Lenses can be reinserted soon after the removal from disinfecting solution.

4.21 Contact Lens–Induced Giant Papillary Conjunctivitis

Symptoms

Itching, mucous discharge, contact lens intolerance, increased contact lens awareness, and excessive lens movement.

Signs

Critical. Giant papillae on the superior tarsal conjunctiva **(see Figure 4.21.1).**

> **NOTE:** The upper eyelid must be everted to make the diagnosis. Upper eyelid eversion should be part of the routine eye examination in any patient who wears contact lenses.

Other. Contact lens coatings, high-riding lens, mild conjunctival injection, ptosis (usually a late sign).

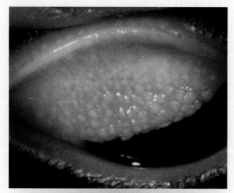

Figure 4.21.1 Giant papillary conjunctivitis.

Differential Diagnosis

- Vernal keratoconjunctivitis: Bilateral allergic conjunctivitis more commonly seen in younger patients. Seasonal variation (spring and summer tend to be the worst). Gelatinous limbal papillae (Horner–Trantas Dots) and shield ulcer may be present.
- Atopic keratoconjunctivitis: History of atopy, dermatitis, and/or asthma. Giant papillae occasionally seen in both superior and inferior conjunctiva.

> **NOTE:** Consider alternative etiology if no improvement of papillae with discontinuation of contact lens wear or if systemic symptoms present.

Workup

1. History: Details of contact lens use, including the age of lenses, daily or extended wear, the frequency of replacement, and the cleaning and enzyme treatment regimen.
2. Slit lamp examination: Evert the upper eyelids and examine for large papillae (≥1 mm).

Treatment

1. Modify contact lens regimen as follows:

Mild-to-Moderate Giant Papillary Conjunctivitis

a. Replace and refit the contact lens. Consider planned replacement or daily disposable lenses (daily disposable lenses preferred).

b. Reduce contact lens wearing time (switch from extended-wear contact lens to daily-wear).

c. Have the patient clean the lenses more thoroughly, preferably by using preservative-free solutions, preservative-free saline, and a hydrogen peroxide–based disinfection system.

d. Increase enzyme use (use at least every week).

Severe Giant Papillary Conjunctivitis

a. Suspend contact lens wear.

b. Restart with a new contact lens when the symptoms and signs clear (usually 1 to 4 months), preferably with daily disposable soft contact lenses.

c. Careful lens hygiene as described earlier.

d. Start a topical mast cell stabilizer or combination antihistamine/mast cell stabilizer (e.g., pemirolast, nedocromil, lodoxamide, cromolyn, alcaftadine, olopatadine, bepotastine, or epinastine).

e. In unusually severe cases, short-term use of a low-dose topical steroid may be considered (e.g., loteprednol 0.5%, fluorometholone 0.1% or fluorometholone acetate 0.1% q.i.d.). Contact lenses should not be worn while using a topical steroid.

f. Steroid sparring topical anti-inflammatory agents such as cyclosporine 0.05% or 0.09% or lifitegrast 5% may be beneficial if long-term treatment is needed.

Follow Up

In 2 to 4 weeks. The patient may resume contact lens wear once the symptoms are resolved. Symptoms may improve before papillae resolve. Mast cell stabilizers are continued while the signs remain, and they may need to be used chronically to maintain contact lens tolerance. If topical steroids are used, they are usually slowly tapered and patients need to be monitored for steroid side effects.

NOTE: Giant papillary conjunctivitis can result not only from contact lens wear and atopic/vernal conjunctivitis, but also an exposed suture or an ocular prosthesis. Exposed sutures are removed. Prostheses should undergo routine cleaning and polishing. A coating can be placed on the prosthesis to reduce giant papillary conjunctivitis. Otherwise, these entities are treated as described earlier.

4.22 Peripheral Corneal Thinning/Ulceration

Symptoms

Pain, photophobia, red eye; may be asymptomatic.

Signs

Peripheral corneal thinning (best seen with a narrow slit beam); may be associated with sterile infiltrate or ulcer.

Differential Diagnosis

Infectious infiltrate or ulcer. Lesions are often treated as infectious until cultures come back negative. See 4.11, BACTERIAL KERATITIS.

Etiology

• Peripheral ulcerative keratitis (PUK), idiopathic or related to systemic connective tissue disease: Rheumatoid arthritis, GPA, relapsing polychondritis, polyarteritis nodosa, systemic lupus erythematosus, others. Peripheral (unilateral or bilateral) corneal thinning/ulcers may be associated with sterile inflammatory infiltrates. The sclera may be involved. May progress circumferentially to involve the entire peripheral cornea. Perforation may occur. This may be the first manifestation of systemic disease (see Figure 4.22.1).

• Terrien marginal degeneration: Usually bilateral, often asymptomatic. Slowly progressive thinning of the peripheral cornea; typically superior; more often in men. The anterior chamber is quiet, and the eye is typically not injected although may be associated with inflammatory signs and symptoms secondary to epithelial breakdown and inflammatory or infectious infiltrates. A yellow line (lipid) may appear, with a fine pannus along the central edge of the thinning. The thinning may slowly spread circumferentially. Refractive changes,

4

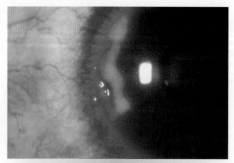

Figure 4.22.1 Peripheral ulcerative keratitis.

including irregular and against-the-rule astigmatism are often present. The epithelium usually remains intact, but perforation may occur with minor trauma.

- Mooren ulcer: Unilateral or bilateral. Painful corneal thinning and ulceration with inflammation. Initially starts as a focal area in the peripheral cornea, nasally or temporally with involvement of the limbus; later extends circumferentially or centrally. Unlike PUK, Mooren ulcer usually does not involve the sclera. An epithelial defect, stromal infiltrate/thinning, and an undermined leading edge are typically present. Limbal blood vessels may grow into the ulcer, and perforation can occur. Idiopathic (autoimmunity may play a key role); diagnosis of exclusion after ruling out the aforementioned systemic causes of PUK. Mooren-like ulcer has been associated with systemic hepatitis C virus infection. Bilateral cases are more resistant to treatment than unilateral cases.

- Pellucid marginal degeneration: Painless, noninflammatory bilateral asymmetric corneal thinning of the inferior peripheral cornea (usually from the 4- to 8-o'clock portions). There is no anterior chamber reaction, conjunctival injection, lipid deposition, or vascularization. The epithelium is intact. Corneal protrusion may be seen above the area of thinning. The thinning may slowly progress.

- Furrow degeneration: Painless corneal thinning just peripheral to an arcus senilis, typically in the elderly. Noninflammatory without vascularization. Perforation is rare. Usually nonprogressive and does not require treatment.

- Delle: Painless oval corneal thinning resulting from corneal drying and stromal dehydration

adjacent to an abnormal conjunctival or corneal elevation. The overlying epithelium may be compromised but is often intact. See 4.23, DELLE.

- Staphylococcal hypersensitivity/marginal keratitis: Peripheral, white corneal infiltrate(s) with limbal clearing that may have an epithelial defect and mild thinning. See 4.18, STAPHYLOCOCCAL HYPERSENSITIVITY.

- Dry eye syndrome: Peripheral (or central) sterile corneal melts may result from severe cases of dry eye. See 4.3, DRY EYE SYNDROME.

- Exposure/neurotrophic keratopathy: In severe cases, a sterile oval ulcer may develop in the inferior interpalpebral portion of the cornea without signs of significant inflammation. May be associated with an eyelid abnormality, a fifth or seventh cranial nerve defect, or proptosis. The ulcer may become superinfected. See 4.5, EXPOSURE KERATOPATHY and 4.6, NEUROTROPHIC KERATOPATHY.

- Sclerokeratitis: Corneal ulceration may be associated with scleritis. Scleral edema with or without nodules develops, scleral vessels become engorged, and the sclera may develop a blue hue. An underlying connective tissue disease, especially GPA, must be ruled out. See 5.7, SCLERITIS.

- Ocular rosacea: Typically affects the inferior cornea in middle-aged patients. Erythema and telangiectasia of the eyelid margins, corneal neovascularization. See 5.9, OCULAR ROSACEA.

- Others: Cataract surgery, inflammatory bowel disease, previous HSV or VZV infections, and leukemia can rarely cause peripheral corneal thinning/ulceration.

Workup

1. History: Contact lens wearer or previous HSV or VZV keratitis? Connective tissue disease or inflammatory bowel disease? Other systemic symptoms? Seasonal conjunctivitis with itching (vernal)? Prior ocular surgery?

2. External examination: Old facial scars of VZV? Lagophthalmos or other eyelid closure problem causing exposure? Blue tinge to the sclera? Rosacea facies?

3. Slit lamp examination: Look for infiltrate, corneal ulcer, hypopyon, uveitis, scleritis, old

herpetic corneal scarring, poor tear lake, SPK, blepharitis. Check corneal sensation prior to instilling anesthetic. Look for giant papillae on the superior tarsal conjunctiva or limbal papillae. Measure IOP.

4. Schirmer test (see 4.3, DRY EYE SYNDROME).

5. Dilated fundus examination: Look for cotton–wool spots consistent with connective tissue disease or evidence of posterior scleritis (e.g., vitritis, subretinal fluid, chorioretinal folds, exudative retinal detachment).

6. Corneal scrapings and cultures when infection is suspected. See Appendix 8, CORNEAL CULTURE PROCEDURE.

7. Consider systemic workup including serum erythrocyte sedimentation rate, complete blood count with differential, rheumatoid factor, antinuclear antibody, antineutrophilic cytoplasmic antibody levels, angiotensin-converting enzyme, and chest x-ray or CT to rule out connective tissue disease and leukemia.

8. Scleritis workup, when present (see 5.7, SCLERITIS).

9. Refer to an internist (and/or rheumatologist) when connective tissue disease is suspected.

Treatment

See sections on delle, staphylococcal hypersensitivity, dry eye syndrome, exposure and neurotrophic keratopathies, scleritis, vernal conjunctivitis, and ocular rosacea.

1. PUK associated systemic immune-mediated disease: Management is usually coordinated with an internist or rheumatologist.
   - Ophthalmic antibiotic ointment (e.g., erythromycin ointment) or preservative-free artificial tear ointment q2h.
   - Cycloplegic drop (e.g., cylopentolate 1% or atropine 1% b.i.d. to t.i.d.) when an anterior chamber reaction or pain is present.
   - Consider doxycycline 100 mg p.o. b.i.d. for its metalloproteinase inhibition properties and ascorbic acid (vitamin C 1 to 2 g daily) as a collagen synthesis promoter.
   - Systemic steroids (e.g., prednisone 60 to 100 mg p.o. daily; dosage is adjusted according to the response) and antiulcer prophylaxis (e.g., ranitidine 150 mg p.o. b.i.d. or pantoprazole 40 mg daily) are used for significant and progressive corneal thinning, but not for perforation.
   - An immunosuppressive agent (e.g., methotrexate, mycophenolate mofetil, infliximab, azathioprine, cyclophosphamide) is often required, especially for GPA. This should be done in coordination with the patient's internist or rheumatologist.
   - Excision or recession of adjacent inflamed conjunctiva is occasionally helpful when the condition progresses despite treatment.
   - Punctal occlusion if dry eye syndrome is present. Topical cyclosporine 0.05% to 2% b.i.d. to q.i.d. or lifitegrast 5% b.i.d. may also be helpful. See 4.3, DRY EYE SYNDROME.
   - Consider cyanoacrylate tissue adhesive or corneal transplantation surgery for an impending or actual corneal perforation. A conjunctival flap or amniotic membrane graft can also be used for an impending corneal perforation.
   - Patients with significant corneal thinning should wear their glasses (or protective glasses [e.g., polycarbonate lens]) during the day and an eye shield at night.

NOTE: Topical steroids should be used with caution in the presence of significant corneal thinning because of the risk of perforation. Gradually taper topical steroids if the patient is already taking them. Notably, corneal thinning due to relapsing polychondritis may improve with topical steroids (e.g., prednisolone acetate 1% q1–2h).

2. Terrien marginal degeneration: Correct astigmatism with glasses or contact lenses if possible. Protective eyewear should be worn if significant thinning is present. Lamellar grafts can be performed if thinning is extreme.

3. Mooren ulcer: Underlying systemic diseases must be ruled out before this diagnosis can be made. Topical steroids, topical cyclosporine 0.05% to 2%, limbal conjunctival excision, corneal gluing, and lamellar or penetrating keratoplasty may be beneficial. Systemic immunosuppression (e.g., oral steroids, methotrexate, cyclophosphamide, and cyclosporine) has been described.

4. Pellucid marginal degeneration: See 4.24, KERATOCONUS.

5. Furrow degeneration: No treatment is required.

Follow Up

Patients with severe disease are examined daily; those with milder conditions are checked less frequently. Watch carefully for signs of superinfection (e.g., increased pain, stromal infiltration, anterior chamber cells and flare, conjunctival injection), increased IOP, and progressive corneal thinning. Treatment is maintained until the epithelial defect over the ulcer heals and is then gradually tapered. As long as an epithelial defect is present, there is risk of progressive thinning and perforation.

4.23 Delle

Symptoms

Irritation and foreign body sensation or may be asymptomatic.

Signs

Critical. Corneal thinning, usually at the limbus, often in the shape of an ellipse, accompanied by an adjacent focal conjunctival or corneal elevation.

Other. Fluorescein pooling in the area but can stain. No infiltrate, no anterior chamber reaction, mild-to-moderate hyperemia.

Differential Diagnosis

See 4.22, Peripheral Corneal Thinning/Ulceration.

Etiology

Poor spread of the tear film over a focal area of cornea (with resultant stromal dehydration) due to an adjacent surface elevation (e.g., chemosis, conjunctival hemorrhage, filtering bleb, pterygium, tumor, and poststrabismus surgery).

Workup

1. History: Previous eye surgery?

2. Slit lamp examination with fluorescein staining: Look for an adjacent area of elevation.

Treatment

1. Lubricating or antibiotic ophthalmic ointment every 2 to 4 hours and q.h.s. Temporary patching can be helpful in promoting corneal stromal rehydration in presence of excessive thinning.

2. Treat the causative elevated lesion according to etiology. Surgical excision may be necessary.

3. If the cause cannot be removed (e.g., filtering bleb), lubricating ointment should be applied nightly, and viscous artificial tear drops should be used four to eight times per day. If drops are needed more than four times per day, a preservative-free drop should be used.

Follow Up

Unless there is severe thinning, reexamination can be performed in 1 to 7 days, at which time the cornea can be expected to be of normal thickness. If it is not, continue aggressive lubrication.

4.24 Keratoconus

Symptoms

Progressive decrease in vision, starbursts and halos, usually beginning in adolescence and continuing into middle age. Acute corneal hydrops can cause a sudden decrease in acuity, pain, red eye, photophobia, and profuse tearing.

Signs

(See Figure 4.24.1.)

Critical. Non-inflammatory ectasia of corneal stroma seen as slowly progressive irregular astigmatism resulting from paracentral (usually inferior) thinning and bulging of the cornea (maximal thinning near the apex of the protrusion), vertical tension lines in the posterior cornea (Vogt striae), an irregular corneal retinoscopic reflex (scissor reflex), and egg-shaped mires on keratometry. Inferior steepening is seen on corneal topographic evaluation, and inferocentral posterior elevation and thinning are seen on tomographic evaluation. Almost always bilateral but often asymmetric.

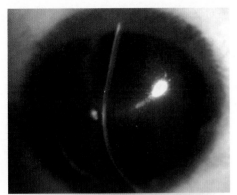

Figure 4.24.1 Keratoconus.

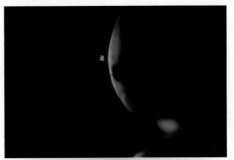

Figure 4.24.2 Acute corneal hydrops.

4

Other. Fleischer ring (epithelial iron deposits at the base of the cone), bulging of the lower eyelid when looking downward (Munson sign), superficial apical scarring. Corneal hydrops (sudden development of corneal edema) results from a rupture in Descemet membrane **(see Figure 4.24.2)**.

Associations

Keratoconus is associated with sleep apnea, floppy eyelid syndrome, Down syndrome, atopic disease, Turner syndrome, Leber congenital amaurosis, mitral valve prolapse, retinitis pigmentosa, and Marfan syndrome. It frequently is related to chronic eye rubbing. Family history of keratoconus is also a risk factor.

Differential Diagnosis

- Pellucid marginal degeneration: Uncommon, nonhereditary. Corneal thinning in the inferior periphery from 4 to 8 o'clock, 1 to 2 mm from the limbus. Absence of inflammation. The cornea protrudes superior to the band of thinning manifesting in high irregular against the rule astigmatism.

NOTE: Treatment for pellucid marginal degeneration is the same as for keratoconus, except corneal transplantation (penetrating or lamellar) is technically more difficult due to peripheral thinning and has a higher failure rate because larger grafts are necessary.

- Keratoglobus: Rare, congenital, nonhereditary, nonprogressive. Uniform globular-shaped cornea with thinning from limbus to limbus. Associated with Ehlers–Danlos syndrome and blue sclera.
- Post-refractive surgery ectasia: After lamellar refractive surgery such as LASIK and SMILE, and rarely surface ablation, a condition very similar to keratoconus can develop. It is treated in the same manner as keratoconus.

Workup

1. History: Duration and rate of decreased vision? Frequent change in eyeglass prescriptions? History of eye rubbing? Allergies? Medical problems? Family history? Previous refractive surgery?
2. Slit lamp examination with close attention to location and characteristics of corneal thinning, Vogt striae, and a Fleischer ring (may be best appreciated with cobalt blue light).
3. Retinoscopy and refraction. Look for irregular astigmatism and a waterdrop or scissors red reflex.
4. Corneal topography (can show central and inferior steepening), tomography (can show posterior corneal elevation, thinning, and inferior displacement of the thinnest location), and keratometry (irregular mires and steepening).

Treatment

1. Patients are instructed not to rub their eyes.
2. Correct refractive errors with glasses or soft contact lenses (for mild cases) or RGP or scleral contact lenses (successful in most cases). Hybrid or piggyback contact lenses are other options.

3. Partial-thickness (deep anterior lamellar keratoplasty) or full-thickness corneal transplantation surgery is usually indicated when contact lenses cannot be tolerated or no longer produce satisfactory vision.

4. Intracorneal ring segments have been successful in getting some patients back into contact lenses, especially in mild-to-moderate keratoconus.

5. Corneal cross-linking (CXL) is a procedure performed to slow or arrest actively progressive disease by strengthening molecular bonds between collagen fibrils. The currently FDA approved protocol involves creation of a 9 mm corneal epithelial defect after which riboflavin drops are placed on the cornea for at least 30 minutes and then ultraviolet light is applied to the cornea for another 30 minutes. While FDA approved for ages 14 years and older, it can be performed off-label for younger children.

Acute corneal hydrops:

- Descemet membrane usually heals and edema resolves by 3 months. However, treatment may be helpful.
- Cycloplegic agent (e.g., cyclopentolate 1% t.i.d) may be beneficial for relief of pain if there is an associated anterior chamber reaction. In some patients, dilating the pupil can exacerbate photosensitivity,
- Consider an aqueous suppressant such as brimonidine 0.1% b.i.d. to t.i.d.

- Start sodium chloride 5% ointment b.i.d. to q.i.d. until resolved (usually several weeks to months).
- Consider topical steroids to suppress corneal neovascularization and/or enhance ocular comfort.
- Glasses or a shield should be worn by patients at risk for trauma or by those who rub their eyes.
- Intracameral air, SF_6, or C_3F_8 may help edema resolve more quickly, but may be equivalent to conservative management in final BCVA. Such intervention can cause cataract and pupillary block glaucoma. Rarely, full thickness corneal suturing of the cleft may speed resolution but may also cause aqueous leakage.

> **NOTE:** Acute hydrops is not an indication for emergency corneal transplantation, except in the extremely rare case of corneal perforation (which is first treated medically and sometimes with tissue adhesives). Slow aqueous leakage through the stromal fluid cleft and edematous epithelium can occur and usually resolves on its own.

Follow Up

Every 3 to 12 months, depending on the progression of symptoms. After an episode of hydrops, examine the patient every 1 to 4 weeks until resolved (which can take several months).

4.25 Corneal Dystrophies

Typically bilateral, progressive corneal disorders without inflammation or corneal neovascularization. No relationship to environmental or systemic factors. Most are autosomal dominant disorders except for macular dystrophy, type 3 lattice dystrophy, and congenital hereditary endothelial dystrophy (autosomal recessive).

> **NOTE:** The IC3D (International Committee for Classification of Corneal Dystrophies) system of corneal dystrophy classification has described dystrophies according to the layer chiefly affected; epithelial and subepithelial, epithelial-stromal, stromal, and those affecting Descemet membrane and the endothelium. Dystrophies with a known common genetic basis (TGFBI) are also grouped together.

EPITHELIAL AND SUBEPITHELIAL DYSTROPHIES

Epithelial Basement Membrane Dystrophy (Map–Dot–Fingerprint Dystrophy)

Most common anterior dystrophy. Diffuse gray patches (maps), creamy white cysts (dots), or fine refractile lines (fingerprints) in the corneal epithelium, best seen with retroillumination or a broad slit lamp beam angled from the side **(see Figures 4.25.1** and **4.25.2)**. Spontaneous painful corneal erosions may develop, particularly on opening the eyes after sleep. May cause decreased vision, monocular diplopia, and shadow images. See 4.2, RECURRENT CORNEAL EROSION, for treatment.

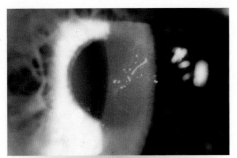

Figure 4.25.1 Epithelial basement membrane dystrophy with multiple "maps and dots" centrally.

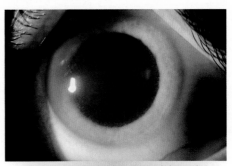

Figure 4.25.3 Meesmann corneal dystrophy demonstrating multiple tiny discrete vesicles in direct illumination.

Meesmann Dystrophy

Rare, epithelial dystrophy that is seen in the first years of life, but is usually asymptomatic until middle age. Retroillumination shows discrete, tiny epithelial vesicles involving the whole cornea but can be segmental **(see Figures 4.25.3 and 4.25.4)**. Although treatment is usually not required, bandage soft contact lenses or superficial keratectomy may be beneficial if significant photophobia is present or if visual acuity is severely affected.

Epithelial-Stromal TGFBI Dystrophies: Reis–Bücklers and Thiel–Behnke

Appears early in life. Subepithelial, gray reticular opacities are seen primarily in the central cornea **(see Figure 4.25.5)**. Painful episodes from recurrent erosions are relatively common and require treatment. Corneal transplantation surgery may be necessary to improve vision, but the dystrophy often recurs in the graft. Excimer laser PTK or superficial lamellar keratectomy may be adequate treatment in many cases.

CORNEAL STROMAL DYSTROPHIES

When these conditions cause reduced vision, patients usually benefit from a corneal transplant (lamellar or penetrating) or excimer laser PTK.

Lattice Dystrophy

Four clinical forms:

- Type 1 (most common): Refractile branching lines, white subepithelial dots, and scarring of the corneal stroma centrally, best seen with retroillumination. Recurrent erosions are common (see 4.2, RECURRENT CORNEAL EROSION). The corneal periphery is typically clear **(see Figure 4.25.6)**. Tends to recur within 5 years after excimer laser PTK or corneal transplantation.

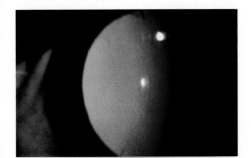

Figure 4.25.2 Epithelial basement membrane dystrophy depicting multiple "fingerprint" lines.

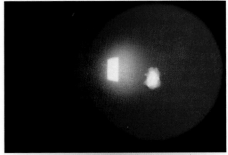

Figure 4.25.4 Meesmann corneal dystrophy demonstrating multiple tiny discrete vesicles in retroillumination.

4

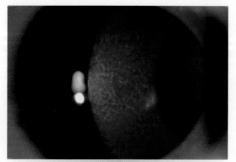

Figure 4.25.5 Reis–Bücklers corneal dystrophy.

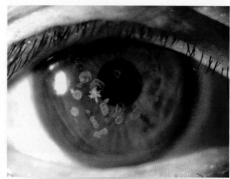

Figure 4.25.7 Granular dystrophy with discrete opacities.

- Type 2 (Meretoja syndrome): Associated with systemic amyloidosis, mask-like facies, ear abnormalities, cranial and peripheral nerve palsies, dry and lax skin.
- Types 3 and 4: Symptoms delayed until fifth to seventh decades.

Granular Dystrophy, Type I

Classic granular dystrophy. White anterior stromal deposits in the central cornea, separated by discrete clear intervening spaces ("bread-crumb-like" opacities) **(see Figure 4.25.7)**. The corneal periphery is spared. Appears in the first decade of life but rarely becomes symptomatic before adulthood. Recurrent erosions can occur. Also may recur after excimer laser PTK or corneal transplantation within 5 years.

Granular Dystrophy, Type II

Also known as combined granular-lattice dystrophy or Avellino dystrophy. Similar to granular dystrophy type I but with significant amyloid deposition consistent with lattice dystrophy.

Macular Dystrophy

Gray-white stromal opacities with ill-defined edges extending from limbus to limbus with cloudy intervening spaces **(see Figure 4.25.8)**. Can involve the full thickness of the stroma, more superficial centrally and deeper peripherally. Corneas tend to be flatter and thinner than normal. Causes late decreased vision more commonly than recurrent erosions. May recur many years after corneal transplantation. Autosomal recessive.

Schnyder Corneal Dystrophy

Fine, yellow-white anterior stromal crystals located in the central cornea are seen in half of the patients **(see Figure 4.25.9)**. Later develop full-thickness central haze and a dense arcus

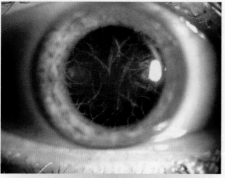

Figure 4.25.6 Lattice dystrophy with branching lines.

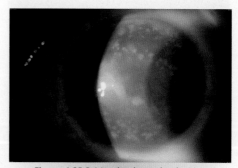

Figure 4.25.8 Macular dystrophy showing opacities with ill-defined borders.

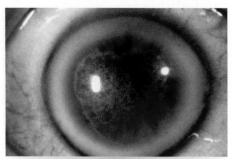

Figure 4.25.9 Anterior stromal crystals in Schnyder corneal dystrophy.

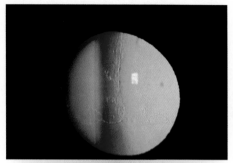

Figure 4.25.10 Posterior polymorphous corneal dystrophy with linear bands.

senilis. Workup includes fasting serum cholesterol and triglyceride levels due to association with systemic lipid abnormalities. Can compromise vision enough to require excimer laser PTK or corneal transplantation. See 4.14, CRYSTALLINE KERATOPATHY.

DESCEMET MEMBRANE AND ENDOTHELIAL DYSTROPHIES

Fuchs Dystrophy

See 4.26, FUCHS ENDOTHELIAL DYSTROPHY.

Posterior Polymorphous Corneal Dystrophy

Changes at the level of Descemet membrane, including vesicles arranged in a linear or grouped pattern, diffuse blotchy gray haze, or broad bands with irregular, scalloped edges (see Figure 4.25.10). Iris abnormalities, including iridocorneal adhesions and corectopia (a decentered pupil), may be present and are occasionally associated with corneal edema. Glaucoma may occur. See 8.12, DEVELOPMENTAL ANTERIOR SEGMENT AND LENS ANOMALIES/DYSGENESIS, FOR DIFFERENTIAL DIAGNOSIS. Treatment includes management of corneal edema and corneal transplantation for severe cases.

Congenital Hereditary Endothelial Dystrophy

Bilateral corneal edema (often asymmetric), normal corneal diameter, normal IOP, and no cornea guttae. Present at birth, nonprogressive, associated with nystagmus. Pain or photophobia uncommon. Rare. Autosomal recessive. (See 8.11, CONGENITAL/INFANTILE GLAUCOMA, for differential diagnosis.)

Treatment

Some patients may benefit from a corneal transplant (endothelial or penetrating keratoplasty).

4.26 Fuchs Endothelial Dystrophy

Symptoms

Glare and blurred vision, worse on awakening. May progress to severe pain due to ruptured bullae. Symptoms usually develop in the fifth and sixth decades.

Signs

Critical. Cornea guttae with stromal +/- epithelial edema (see Figure 4.26.1). Bilateral, but may be asymmetric.

NOTE: Central cornea guttae without stromal edema is called endothelial dystrophy (see Figure 4.26.2). This condition may progress to Fuchs dystrophy over years.

Other. Fine pigment dusting on the endothelium, central epithelial edema and bullae, folds in Descemet membrane, stromal edema, subepithelial haze, or scarring.

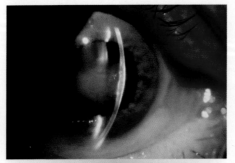

Figure 4.26.1 Corneal edema secondary to Fuchs endothelial dystrophy.

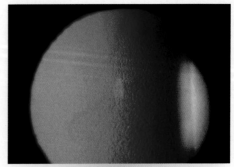

Figure 4.26.2 Corneal guttae in endothelial dystrophy.

Differential Diagnosis

- Postsurgical corneal edema (also known as aphakic or pseudophakic bullous keratopathy): History of cataract surgery or other anterior segment surgery (e.g., tube shunt). See 4.27, APHAKIC BULLOUS KERATOPATHY/PSEUDOPHAKIC BULLOUS KERATOPATHY.
- Congenital hereditary endothelial dystrophy: Bilateral corneal edema at birth. See 4.25, CORNEAL DYSTROPHIES.
- Posterior polymorphous corneal dystrophy: Seen early in life. Corneal endothelium shows grouped vesicles, geographic gray lesions, or broad bands. Occasionally corneal edema. See 4.25, CORNEAL DYSTROPHIES.
- Iridocorneal endothelial syndrome: "Beaten metal" corneal endothelial appearance, with corneal edema, peripheral anterior synechiae, increased IOP, variable iris thinning, corectopia, and polycoria. Typically unilateral, in young to middle-aged adults. See 9.15, IRIDOCORNEAL ENDOTHELIAL SYNDROME.

Workup

1. History: Previous surgery?
2. Slit lamp examination: Cornea guttae are best seen with retroillumination. Fluorescein staining may demonstrate intact or ruptured bullae.
3. Measure IOP.
4. Corneal pachymetry to determine the central corneal thickness.
5. Consider specular microscopy to evaluate the endothelial cells although may be difficult to image the endothelial layer through an edematous cornea and in between guttate changes.
6. Consider corneal tomography to help monitor progression of disease.

Treatment

1. Topical sodium chloride 5% drops q.i.d. and ointment q.h.s.
2. May gently blow warm air from a hair dryer at arm's length toward the eyes for a few minutes every morning to dehydrate the cornea.
3. IOP reduction if indicated; also may help with corneal edema.
4. Ruptured corneal bullae are painful and should be treated as recurrent erosions (see 4.2, RECURRENT CORNEAL EROSION).
5. Surgery: Endothelial keratoplasty (Descemet membrane endothelial keratoplasty [DMEK] or Descemet stripping endothelial keratoplasty [DSEK]) is usually indicated when visual acuity decreases due to corneal edema; PK is indicated if significant anterior stromal scarring is present. Descemet stripping only (DSO) may be an option for milder forms of Fuchs endothelial dystrophy.

Follow Up

Every 3 to 12 months to check IOP and assess corneal edema. The condition progresses very slowly, and visual acuity typically remains good until stromal edema, epithelial edema, and/or corneal scarring develop.

4.27 Aphakic Bullous Keratopathy/Pseudophakic Bullous Keratopathy

Symptoms

Decreased vision, pain, tearing, foreign body sensation, photophobia, and redness. History of cataract surgery in the involved eye.

Signs

(See Figure 4.27.1.)

Critical. Corneal edema in an eye in which the native lens has been removed.

Other. Corneal bullae, Descemet folds, subepithelial haze or scarring, corneal neovascularization, with or without preexisting guttae. Cystoid macular edema (CME) may be present.

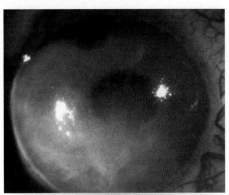

Figure 4.27.1 Pseudophakic bullous keratopathy.

Etiology

Multifactorial: Corneal endothelial damage, intraocular inflammation, vitreous or subluxed intraocular lens or tube shunt touching (or intermittently touching) the cornea, preexisting endothelial dysfunction, and glaucoma.

Workup

1. Slit lamp examination: Stain the cornea with fluorescein to check for denuded epithelium. Check the position of the intraocular lens if present, determine whether vitreous is touching the corneal endothelium, and evaluate the eye for inflammation. Check for subepithelial haze or scarring. Evaluate the fellow eye for endothelial dystrophy.
2. Check IOP.
3. Dilated fundus examination: Look for CME.
4. Consider a fluorescein angiogram or optical coherence tomography to help detect CME, although evaluation may be limited by corneal opacification.

Treatment

1. Topical sodium chloride 5% drops q.i.d. and ointment q.h.s., if epithelial edema is present.
2. Reduce IOP with medications if needed. Avoid epinephrine derivatives and prostaglandin analogs, if possible, because of the risk of CME (see 9.1, PRIMARY OPEN ANGLE GLAUCOMA).
3. Ruptured epithelial bullae (producing corneal epithelial defects) may be treated with the following:
   - An ophthalmic antibiotic drops or ointment (e.g., erythromycin or bacitracin) and a cycloplegic (e.g., cyclopentolate 1% t.i.d.). The topical antibiotic can be used frequently (e.g., q2h) without patching.
   - Alternatively, sodium chloride 5% drops or ointment q.i.d., a bandage soft contact lens, or, in patients with limited visual potential, anterior stromal micropuncture or excimer laser PTK can be used for recurrent ruptured epithelial bullae (see 4.2, RECURRENT CORNEAL EROSION).
4. Full-thickness corneal transplant or endothelial keratoplasty (DMEK or DSEK) combined with possible intraocular lens repositioning, replacement, or removal and/or vitrectomy may be indicated when vision fails or when the disease becomes advanced and painful. Anterior stromal micropuncture, excimer laser PTK, conjunctival flap, or amniotic membrane graft surgery may be considered for a painful eye with poor visual potential.
5. See 11.14, CYSTOID MACULAR EDEMA, for treatment of CME.

NOTE: Although both CME and corneal disease may contribute to decreased vision, the precise role of each is often difficult to determine preoperatively. CME is less likely with posterior chamber or open-loop anterior chamber intraocular lenses than closed-loop anterior chamber intraocular lenses, which are no longer used.

Follow Up

If ruptured bullae, every 1 to 3 days until improvement demonstrated, and then every 5 to 7 days until the epithelial defect heals. Otherwise, every 1 to 6 months, depending on symptoms.

4.28 Corneal Graft Rejection

Symptoms

Decreased vision, mild pain, redness, and photophobia with history of prior corneal transplantation, usually months to years beforehand. Often asymptomatic and diagnosed on routine follow-up examination.

Signs

(See Figure 4.28.1.)

Critical. New keratic precipitates are localized to the donor endothelium. May be associated with stromal and/or epithelial edema, a line of keratic precipitates on the corneal endothelium (endothelial rejection line or Khodadoust line), subepithelial infiltrates (Krachmer spots), an irregularly elevated epithelial line (epithelial rejection line), or localized stromal neovascularization.

Other. Conjunctival injection (particularly circumcorneal), anterior chamber inflammation, neovascularization growing up to or extending onto the graft, and broken graft suture. Tearing may occur, but a mucoid discharge is not present.

Differential Diagnosis

- Suture abscess or corneal infection: May have a corneal infiltrate, hypopyon, or a purulent discharge. Remove the suture (by pulling the contaminated portion through the shortest track possible) and obtain smears and cultures, including a culture of the suture. Steroid frequency is usually reduced. Treat with intensive topical fluoroquinolone or fortified antibiotics and monitor closely, sometimes in the hospital. See 4.11, BACTERIAL KERATITIS.
- Uveitis: Anterior chamber cells and flare with keratic precipitates that are not limited to the graft endothelium. Often, a previous history of uveitis is obtained, but it is best to treat as

if it were a graft rejection. If known history of HSV, add suppressive antiviral therapy if not on it already. HSV iritis is frequently associated with elevated IOP. SEE Chapter 12, UVEITIS.

- Epithelial downgrowth: May present as an advancing line with smooth or scalloped borders on the endothelial surface. Can be present on the donor and/or the recipient endothelium. Will not respond to steroids and is associated with less corneal edema.
- Increased IOP: A markedly increased IOP may produce epithelial corneal edema without other graft rejection signs. Edema clears after the IOP is reduced.
- Other causes of graft failure: Non–immune-mediated late corneal graft endothelial decompensation or recurrent disease in the graft (e.g., herpes keratitis, corneal dystrophy).

Workup

1. History: Time since corneal transplantation? Current eye medications? Compliance with eye medications and postoperative follow up. Recent change in topical steroid regimen? Indication for corneal transplantation (e.g., HSV)?
2. Slit lamp examination, with careful inspection for endothelial rejection line, keratic precipitates, subepithelial infiltrates, and other signs listed above.

Treatment

Endothelial Rejection (Endothelial Rejection Line, Corneal Edema, and/or Keratic Precipitates)

1. Topical steroids (e.g., prednisolone acetate 1% q1h or difluprednate 0.05% q2h while awake; can add dexamethasone 0.1% ointment q.h.s.).

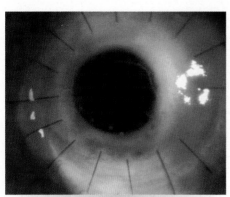

Figure 4.28.1 Corneal graft rejection with endothelial rejection line and keratic precipitates.

2. If rejection is severe, recurrent, or recalcitrant, consider systemic steroids (e.g., prednisone 40 to 80 mg p.o. daily) or, rarely, subconjunctival steroids (e.g., betamethasone 3 mg per 0.5 mL). In high-risk patients with severe rejection, consider hospitalization and methylprednisolone 500 mg i.v. for a total of one to three doses.

3. In select cases, other systemic immunosuppressives may be considered including cyclosporine and tacrolimus.

4. Cycloplegic agent (e.g., cyclopentolate 1% t.i.d.).

5. Control IOP if increased. See 9.7, INFLAMMATORY OPEN ANGLE GLAUCOMA.

6. Topical cyclosporine 0.05% to 2% b.i.d. to q.i.d. may be helpful in the treatment and prevention of graft rejection.

Epithelial and Stromal Rejection (Subepithelial Infiltrates or Epithelial Rejection Line)

1. Double the current level of topical steroids or use prednisolone acetate 1% q.i.d. (whichever is more).

2. Cycloplegic agent, topical cyclosporine, and IOP control as above.

Follow Up

Institute treatment immediately to maximize the likelihood of graft survival. Examine the patient every 3 to 7 days. Once improvement is noted, the steroids are tapered very slowly and may need to be maintained at low doses for months to years. IOP must be checked regularly in patients taking topical steroids.

4.29 Corneal Refractive Surgery Complications

The basic principle of corneal refractive surgery is to induce a change in the curvature of the cornea to correct a preexisting refractive error.

COMPLICATIONS OF SURFACE ABLATION PROCEDURES (PHOTOREFRACTIVE KERATECTOMY, LASER SUBEPITHELIAL KERATECTOMY, AND EPITHELIAL LASER IN SITU KERATOMILEUSIS)

In PRK, the corneal epithelium is removed and the corneal stroma is ablated using an argon-fluoride excimer laser (193 nm, ultraviolet) to correct a refractive error. In laser subepithelial keratomileusis (LASEK), the epithelium is *chemically* separated from the Bowman layer, moved to the side before laser ablation of the stroma, and then repositioned centrally. In epithelial laser in situ keratomileusis (epi-LASIK), the epithelium is *mechanically* separated from the Bowman layer,

moved to the side before laser ablation of the stroma, and then repositioned centrally or discarded (see **Table 4.29.1**).

Symptoms

Early (1 to 14 Days). Decreasing visual acuity and increased pain.

> **NOTE:** The induced epithelial defect at surgery, which usually takes a few days to heal, normally will cause postoperative pain. A bandage soft contact lens is used to minimize this discomfort.

Later (2 Weeks to Several Months). Decreasing visual acuity, severe glare, and monocular diplopia.

Signs

Corneal infiltrate and central corneal scar.

TABLE 4.29.1   Refractive Surgery Characteristics

	PRK	LASEK	Epi-LASIK	LASIK	SMILE
Epithelial flap or method of stromal exposure	No flap. Epithelium removed by blade, spatula, brush, excimer laser, or dilute absolute alcohol.	Epithelial flap created by 20% absolute alcohol concentrated on epithelium by marker well.	Epithelial flap created by a blunt blade epi-keratome. Epithelial flap may be replaced (epi-on) or discarded (epi-off).	Epithelial and stromal flap created by sharp microkeratome or femtosecond laser.	No flap. Thin disc of stroma created by femtosecond laser and then mechanically extracted through small incision.
Depth of exposure	Bowman membrane	Bowman membrane	Bowman membrane	Anterior stroma (sub-Bowman keratomileusis provides more superficial stromal exposure)	Anterior stroma
Typical refractive limitations	Spherical range: −8.0D to +3.0D, cylinder range up to 3.0D	Spherical range: −8.0D to +3.0D, cylinder range up to 3.0D	Spherical range: −8.0D to +3.0D, cylinder range up to 3.0D	Spherical range: −10.0D to +3.0D, cylinder range up to 3.0D	Spherical range: −10.0D to −1.0D, cylinder range up to 3.0D
Advantages	Useful in thin corneas, epithelial pathology. No stromal flap healing issues.	Useful in thin corneas, epithelial pathology. No stromal flap healing issues.	Useful in thin corneas, epithelial pathology. No stromal flap healing issues.	Minimal pain, rapid visual recovery, minimal stromal haze.	Minimal pain, rapid visual recovery. No flap complications. Possibly less dry eye than LASIK.
Disadvantages	Postoperative pain, slower visual recovery, higher risk of subepithelial haze.	Postoperative pain, slower visual recovery, higher risk of subepithelial haze.	Postoperative pain, slower visual recovery, higher risk of subepithelial haze. Not ideal with significant glaucoma or anterior corneal scarring.	Not ideal for thin corneas, epithelial dystrophies, severe dry eyes, significant glaucoma. Presence of flap with possible complications (see text).	Currently only for myopia or myopic astigmatism in the US. Not ideal for thin corneas or in corneas with epithelial pathology. Removal of stromal lenticule can be technically difficult. SMILE enhancements complex; reoperations often done with PRK.

Etiology

Early

- Dislocated or poorly fit bandage soft contact lens (see 4.20, CONTACT LENS-RELATED PROBLEMS).
- Nonhealing epithelial defect (see 3.2, CORNEAL ABRASION). Must also consider HSV keratitis.
- Corneal ulcer (see 4.11, BACTERIAL KERATITIS).
- Medication allergy (see 5.1, ACUTE CONJUNCTIVITIS).

Later

- Undercorrection or overcorrection.
- Corneal haze (scarring) noted in anterior corneal stroma.
- Irregular astigmatism (e.g., central island, decentered ablation).
- Regression or progression of refractive error.
- Steroid-induced glaucoma or ocular hypertension (see 9.9, STEROID-RESPONSE GLAUCOMA).

Workup

1. Complete ophthalmic examination, including IOP measurement by Tonopen and applanation. IOP may be underestimated given decreased corneal thickness.
2. Refraction if change in refractive error suspected. Hard contact lens overrefraction corrects irregular astigmatism.
3. Corneal topography and/or tomography if irregular astigmatism is suspected.

Treatment and Follow Up

1. Epithelial defect (see 3.2, CORNEAL ABRASION).
2. Infectious keratitis (see 4.15, HERPES SIMPLEX KERATITIS and 4.11, BACTERIAL KERATITIS).
3. Corneal haze: Increase steroid drop frequency. Follow up in 1 to 2 weeks. Cases of severe haze may respond to excimer laser PTK with mitomycin C.
4. Refractive error or irregular astigmatism: Consider surface ablation enhancement. If irregular astigmatism present, topography-guided surface ablation, excimer laser PTK, or hard contact lens may be needed.
5. Steroid-induced glaucoma. See 9.9, STEROID-RESPONSE GLAUCOMA.

COMPLICATIONS OF LASER IN SITU KERATOMILEUSIS

In LASIK, a hinged, partial-thickness corneal flap is created using a microkeratome or femtosecond laser, and then the underlying stroma is ablated with an excimer laser to correct refractive error. The corneal flap is repositioned over the stromal bed without sutures.

Symptoms

Early (1 to 14 Days). Decreasing visual acuity and increased pain.

Later (2 Weeks to Several Months). Decreasing visual acuity, severe glare, monocular diplopia, and dry eye symptoms.

Signs

Severe conjunctival injection, corneal infiltrate, large fluorescein-staining epithelial defect, dislocated corneal flap, interface inflammation, epithelial ingrowth under the flap, central corneal scar, SPK, scissoring of the light reflex or retinoscopy, and irregular corneal thinning or steepening

Etiology

Early

- Dry eye/neurotrophic keratopathy. By far the most common early complication.
- Folding, dislocation, or loss of corneal flap.
- Large epithelial defect.
- Diffuse lamellar keratitis (DLK). Also known as "sands of the Sahara" because of its appearance (multiple fine inflammatory infiltrates in the flap interface). Usually occurs within 5 days of surgery **(see Figure 4.29.1)**.
- Corneal ulcer and/or infection in flap interface. See 4.11, BACTERIAL KERATITIS.
- Central toxic keratopathy (CTK). Central corneal stromal opacification and consolidation of unknown etiology, causing corneal thinning and flattening. It tends to improve over 6 to 12 months.
- Medication allergy. See 5.1, ACUTE CONJUNCTIVITIS.

NOTE: Patients after LASIK have reduced corneal sensation in the area of the flap for at least 3 months (returns to essentially normal in 6 to 12 months).

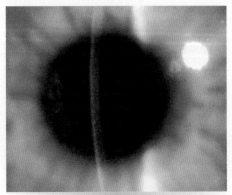

Figure 4.29.1 Diffuse lamellar keratitis.

Later

- Epithelial ingrowth into flap interface.
- Corneal haze (scarring): Less common than after surface ablation procedures.
- Irregular astigmatism (e.g., decentered ablation, central island, flap irregularity, ectasia).
- Regression or progression of refractive error.
- Dry eye syndrome/neurotrophic keratopathy.
- DLK can occur weeks to years after LASIK in response to a corneal insult such as corneal abrasion, recurrent erosion, or viral keratitis.
- Pressure-induced stromal keratitis (PISK). High IOP (often secondary to steroid response) can cause the development of fluid in the interface with a clinical appearance similar to DLK. IOP measurements are falsely low due to the fluid cleft, and pressure should be measured with a Tonopen or other handheld tonometer both on the central cornea and peripheral to the LASIK flap.

Workup

1. Complete slit lamp examination, including fluorescein staining and IOP measurement by Tono-Pen and applanation. IOP may be underestimated given flap creation and decreased corneal thickness. Check IOP peripheral to the flap edge if suspect PISK.
2. Schirmer test, as needed.
3. Refraction on all patients who do not have uncorrected vision of 20/20. Refraction with hard contact lens for irregular astigmatism.
4. Corneal topography and/or tomography for suspected irregular astigmatism.

Treatment and Follow Up

1. Flap abnormalities:
   - Visually significant stromal folds: Lift flap and refloat within 24 hours.
   - Flap dislocation: Requires urgent surgical repositioning.
   - Persistent symptomatic flap striae may require flap lifting and suturing.
2. Lost corneal flap: Treat as epithelial defect. See 3.2, CORNEAL ABRASION.
3. Epithelial defect. See 3.2, CORNEAL ABRASION.
4. SPK and dry eye. See 4.1, SUPERFICIAL PUNCTATE KERATOPATHY and 4.3, DRY EYE SYNDROME.
5. DLK: Aggressive treatment with frequent topical steroids (e.g., prednisolone acetate 1% q1h). If severe, may also require lifting of flap and irrigation of interface. Treat any underlying cause, such as an epithelial defect.
6. CTK: No proven treatment. Lubrication and observation.
7. PISK: Ocular hypotensive medications and rapid tapering of steroids.
8. Corneal infiltrate. See 4.11, BACTERIAL KERATITIS and Appendix 8, CORNEAL CULTURE PROCEDURE. The flap may need to be lifted to obtain the best culture results.
9. Epithelial ingrowth: Observation if very peripheral and not affecting vision. Surgical debridement if dense, affecting the health of flap, approaching visual axis, or affecting vision. Small pockets may also be treated with a YAG laser.
10. Corneal haze: Increase steroid drop frequency. Follow up in 1 to 2 weeks.
11. Refractive error or irregular astigmatism: Appropriate refraction. Consider PRK or LASIK enhancement. If irregular astigmatism, consider flap repositioning, custom or topography guided enhancement, or contact lens fitting.
12. Consider CXL for ectasia.

COMPLICATIONS OF SMALL INCISION LENTICULE EXTRACTION

In SMILE, a femtosecond laser is used to create a thin disc of tissue (lenticule) inside the corneal stroma, which is then mechanically dissected and extracted through a small peripheral incision.

Symptoms

Early (1 to 14 days). Decreasing visual acuity and increased pain.

Later (2 weeks to Several Months). Decreasing visual acuity, severe glare, monocular diplopia, and dry eye symptoms.

Signs

Severe conjunctival injection, corneal infiltrate, large epithelial defect, interface inflammation, epithelial ingrowth into interface, central corneal scar, scissoring of the light reflex or retinoscopy, and irregular corneal thinning or steepening.

Etiology

Early

- Cap microstriae.
- Large epithelial defect.
- DLK: Also known as "sands of the Sahara" because of its appearance (multiple fine inflammatory infiltrates in the interface). Usually occurs within 5 days of surgery.
- Corneal ulcer and/or infection in interface. See 4.11, BACTERIAL KERATITIS.
- Dry eye/neurotrophic keratopathy.
- Medication allergy. See 5.1, ACUTE CONJUNCTIVITIS.

> 📝 **NOTE:** Early postoperative dry eye symptoms of SMILE are comparable to LASIK but often with faster recovery.

Later

- Epithelial ingrowth into stromal pocket (interface).
- Corneal haze (scarring): Less common than after surface ablation procedures.
- Irregular astigmatism (e.g., retained lenticule fragments, decentered treatment, ectasia).
- Regression or progression of refractive error.
- Dry eye syndrome/neurotrophic keratopathy.
- DLK can occur weeks to years after SMILE in response to a corneal insult such as corneal abrasion, recurrent erosion, or viral keratitis.
- PISK: High IOP (often secondary to steroid response) can cause the development of fluid in the interface with a clinical appearance similar to DLK. IOP measurements are falsely low by the fluid cleft, and pressure should be measured with a Tono-Pen or other handheld tonometer both on the central cornea and peripheral to the SMILE cap.

Workup

1. Complete slit lamp examination, including fluorescein staining and IOP measurement by Tono-Pen and applanation. IOP may be underestimated given lenticule extraction and decreased corneal thickness. Check IOP peripheral to the cap edge if suspect PISK.
2. Schirmer test, as needed.
3. Refraction on all patients who do not have uncorrected vision of 20/20. Refraction with hard contact lens for irregular astigmatism.
4. Corneal topography and/or tomography for suspected irregular astigmatism.

Treatment and Follow Up

1. Cap microstriae: Gentle cap massage, frequent topical steroids.
2. Epithelial defect. See 3.2, CORNEAL ABRASION.
3. SPK and dry eye. See 4.1, SUPERFICIAL PUNCTATE KERATOPATHY and 4.3, DRY EYE SYNDROME.
4. DLK: Aggressive treatment with frequent topical steroids (e.g., prednisolone acetate 1% q1h). If severe, may also require lifting of flap and irrigation of interface. Treat any underlying cause, such as an epithelial defect.
5. PISK: Ocular hypotensive medications and rapid tapering of steroids.
6. Corneal infiltrate. See 4.11, BACTERIAL KERATITIS and Appendix 8, CORNEAL CULTURE PROCEDURE.
7. Epithelial ingrowth: Observation if very peripheral and not affecting vision. Conversion of cap into a flap and surgical debridement if dense, affecting the health of cap, approaching visual axis, or affecting vision. Small pockets can also be treated with a YAG laser.
8. Corneal haze: Increase steroid drop frequency. Follow up in 1 to 2 weeks.
9. Refractive error or irregular astigmatism: Appropriate refraction. Consider PRK enhancement. If irregular astigmatism, consider custom or topography guided enhancement or contact lens fitting.
10. Consider CXL for ectasia.

COMPLICATIONS OF RADIAL KERATOTOMY

In radial keratotomy (RK), partial-thickness, spoke-like cuts are made in the peripheral cornea using a diamond blade (often 90% to 95% depth), which results in a flattening of the central cornea and correction of myopia. Astigmatic keratotomy (AK) is a similar procedure in which arcuate or tangential relaxing incisions are made to correct astigmatism. Now rarely used given complication rate and advancement of technology.

Symptoms

Early (1 to 14 Days). Decreasing visual acuity and increased pain.

Later (2 Weeks to Years). Decreasing visual acuity, severe glare, and monocular diplopia.

> **NOTE:** RK weakens the corneal integrity placing patients at higher risk for rupture after trauma.

Signs

Corneal infiltrate, large fluorescein-staining epithelial defect, rupture at RK incision site after trauma, and anterior chamber reaction.

Etiology

Early

- Large epithelial defect. See 3.2, CORNEAL ABRASION.
- Corneal ulcer/infection in RK incision. See 4.11, BACTERIAL KERATITIS.
- Medication allergy. See 5.1, ACUTE CONJUNCTIVITIS.
- Very rarely, endophthalmitis. See 12.13, POSTOPERATIVE ENDOPHTHALMITIS.

Later

- RK incisions approaching the visual axis causing glare and starbursts.
- Irregular astigmatism.
- Regression of refractive error; common in first few months after surgery.
- Progression of refractive effect (consecutive hyperopia); common after first few years after surgery.
- Ruptured globe at RK incision site after trauma. See 3.14, RUPTURED GLOBE AND PENETRATING OCULAR INJURY.

Workup

1. Complete slit lamp examination, including IOP measurement and fluorescein staining.
2. Refraction on all patients who do not have uncorrected vision of 20/20. Refraction with hard contact lens for irregular astigmatism.
3. Corneal topography and/or tomography if irregular astigmatism suspected.

Treatment and Follow Up

1. Corneal infiltrate: See 4.11, BACTERIAL KERATITIS and Appendix 8, CORNEAL CULTURE PROCEDURE.
2. Epithelial defect: See 3.2, CORNEAL ABRASION.
3. Endophthalmitis: See 12.13, POSTOPERATIVE ENDOPHTHALMITIS.
4. Refractive error or irregular astigmatism: Appropriate refraction. Consider enhancement of RK incisions or AK. Rarely, surface laser ablation with mitomycin C can be used. Irregular astigmatism may require a hard contact lens.
5. Ruptured globe at RK incision: Requires surgical repair. See 3.14, RUPTURED GLOBE AND PENETRATING OCULAR INJURY.

Chapter 5

Conjunctiva/Sclera/Iris/ External Disease

5.1 Acute Conjunctivitis

Symptoms

"Red eye" (conjunctival hyperemia), discharge, eyelids sticking or crusting (worse upon awakening from sleep), and foreign body sensation, with <4-week duration of symptoms (otherwise, see 5.2, CHRONIC CONJUNCTIVITIS) **(see Figure 5.1.1).**

VIRAL CONJUNCTIVITIS/EPIDEMIC KERATOCONJUNCTIVITIS

Symptoms

Itching, burning, tearing, and gritty or foreign body sensation; history of recent upper respiratory tract infection or contact with someone with viral conjunctivitis. Often starts in one eye and involves the fellow eye a few days later.

Signs

(See Figure 5.1.2.)

Critical. Inferior palpebral conjunctival follicles **(see Figure 5.1.3)** and tender palpable preauricular lymph node.

Other. Watery discharge, red and edematous eyelids, pinpoint subconjunctival hemorrhages, punctate keratopathy (epithelial erosion in severe cases), and membrane/pseudomembrane **(see Figure 5.1.4)**. Fine intraepithelial microcysts are an early corneal finding, which, if present, can be helpful in diagnosis. Subepithelial (anterior stromal) infiltrates (SEIs) can develop 1 to 2 weeks after the onset of the conjunctivitis.

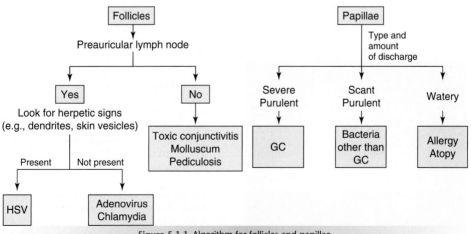

Figure 5.1.1 Algorithm for follicles and papillae.

5

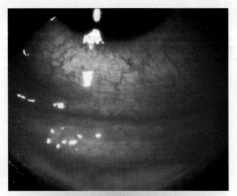

Figure 5.1.2 Viral conjunctivitis.

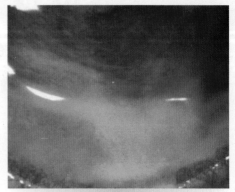

Figure 5.1.4 Viral conjunctivitis with pseudomembranes.

Etiology and Variants of Viral Conjunctivitis

- Most commonly adenovirus: Epidemic keratoconjunctivitis is most commonly caused by subgroup D of serotypes 8, 19, and 37. Pharyngoconjunctival fever is associated with pharyngitis and fever, usually in children, and is most commonly caused by serotypes 3 and 7.
- Acute hemorrhagic conjunctivitis: Associated with prominent subconjunctival hemorrhages, usually 1 to 2 weeks in duration, and tends to occur in tropical regions. Caused by enterovirus 70 (rarely followed by polio-like paralysis), coxsackievirus A24, and adenovirus serotype 11.

NOTE: Many systemic viral syndromes (e.g., measles, mumps, influenza, and coronavirus) can cause a nonspecific conjunctivitis. The underlying condition should be managed appropriately; the eyes are treated with artificial tears four to eight times per day. If tears are used more than four times daily, preservative-free tears are recommended.

Workup

No conjunctival cultures/swabs are indicated unless the discharge is excessive or the condition becomes chronic (see 5.2, CHRONIC CONJUNCTIVITIS).

Treatment

1. Counsel the patient that viral conjunctivitis is a self-limited condition that typically gets worse for the first 4 to 7 days after the onset and may not resolve for 2 to 3 weeks (potentially longer with corneal involvement).
2. Viral conjunctivitis is highly contagious (usually for 10 to 12 days from the onset) when the eyes are red (when not on steroids) or have active discharge/tearing. Patients should avoid touching their eyes, shaking hands, sharing towels or pillows, etc. Restrict work and school for patients with significant exposure to others while the eyes are red and weeping.
3. Frequent hand washing.

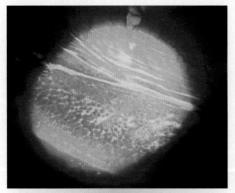

Figure 5.1.3 Follicles on the inferior palpebral conjunctiva.

4. Application of preservative-free artificial tears or tear ointment four to eight times per day for 1 to 3 weeks. Advise single-use vials to limit tip contamination and spread of the condition.

5. Cool compresses several times per day.

6. Application of antihistamine drops (e.g., epinastine 0.05% b.i.d.) if itching is severe.

7. If a membrane/pseudomembrane is present, it should be gently peeled with a cotton-tip applicator or smooth forceps to enhance comfort, minimize corneal defects, and help prevent symblepharon formation.

8. If a membrane/pseudomembrane is present or if SEIs reduce vision and/or cause significant photophobia, topical steroids should be initiated. For membranes/pseudomembranes, use a more frequent steroid dose or stronger steroid (e.g., loteprednol 0.5% or prednisolone acetate 1% q.i.d.). Consider a steroid ointment (e.g., fluorometholone 0.1% ointment q.i.d. or dexamethasone/tobramycin 0.1%/0.3% ointment q.i.d.) in the presence of significant tearing to maintain longer medication exposure. For SEIs alone, a weaker steroid with less frequent dosing is usually sufficient (e.g., loteprednol 0.2% or 0.5% b.i.d.). Given the possible side effects, prescription of topical steroids is cautionary in the emergency room setting or in patients with questionable follow up. Steroids may hasten the resolution of the symptoms but prolong the infectious period. Additionally, steroids often necessitate a long-term taper, and delayed SEIs can recur during or after such a taper. Steroids should not be prescribed if the patient has not been examined by an eye care professional using a slit lamp.

NOTE: Routine use of topical antibiotics for viral conjunctivitis is discouraged unless corneal erosions are present or there is mucopurulent discharge suggestive of bacterial conjunctivitis (see BACTERIAL CONJUNCTIVITIS).

Follow Up

In 2 to 3 weeks, but sooner if the condition worsens significantly or if topical steroids are prescribed.

HERPES SIMPLEX VIRUS CONJUNCTIVITIS

See 4.15, HERPES SIMPLEX VIRUS, for a detailed discussion. Patients may have a history of perioral cold sores. Manifests with a unilateral (sometimes recurrent) follicular conjunctival reaction, palpable preauricular node, and, occasionally, concurrent herpetic skin vesicles along the eyelid margin or periocular skin. Systemic (7 to 10 days of acyclovir 400 mg five times daily or valacyclovir 500 mg two to three times a day or famciclovir 250 mg two to three times a day) or topical (ganciclovir 0.15% ophthalmic gel five times daily, acyclovir ointment five times daily or trifluridine 1% nine times daily for 7 to 10 days) antiviral therapy and warm compresses. Steroids are contraindicated.

ALLERGIC CONJUNCTIVITIS

Symptoms

Itching, watery discharge, and a history of allergies are typical. Usually bilateral.

Signs

Chemosis, red and edematous eyelids, conjunctival papillae, periocular hyperpigmentation, and no preauricular node **(see Figure 5.1.5)**.

Treatment

1. Eliminate the inciting agent. Frequent washing of hair and clothes may be helpful.

2. Cool compresses several times per day.

3. Topical drops, depending on the severity:

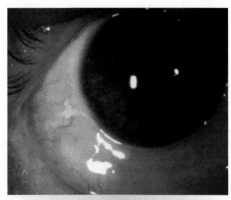

Figure 5.1.5 Allergic conjunctivitis.

- Mild: Artificial tears four to eight times per day.
- Moderate: Use antihistamine and/or mast-cell stabilizer drops. Convenient medications with daily dosing include olopatadine 0.2% (over-the-counter) or 0.7% and alcaftadine 0.25% drops. Common medications with b.i.d. dosing include cetirizine 0.24%, azelastine 0.05%, olopatadine 0.1% (over-the-counter), epinastine 0.05%, nedocromil 2%, bepotastine 1.5%, or ketotifen 0.025% (over-the-counter) drops. Pemirolast 0.1% and lodoxamide 0.1% drops can also reduce symptoms but are recommended at q.i.d. dosing.

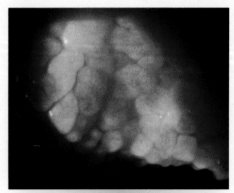

Figure 5.1.6 Vernal/atopic conjunctivitis with large superior tarsal papillae.

> **NOTE:** An ophthalmic nonsteroidal anti-inflammatory drug (NSAID) such as ketorolac 0.5% q.i.d. can also be effective in reducing ocular inflammation, but its use should be monitored given the known risk of corneal toxicity with chronic instillation.

- Severe: Mild topical steroid (e.g., loteprednol 0.2% q.i.d., fluorometholone 0.1% q.i.d. or fluorometholone acetate 0.1% q.i.d. for 1 to 2 weeks) in addition to the preceding medications.

4. Oral antihistamine (e.g., diphenhydramine 25 mg p.o. t.i.d. to q.i.d. or loratadine 10 mg p.o. daily) in moderate-to-severe cases can be very helpful.

> **NOTE:** Routine use of topical antibiotics or steroids for allergic conjunctivitis is discouraged.

Follow Up

Two weeks. If topical steroids are used, tapering is required and patients should be monitored for side effects.

VERNAL/ATOPIC CONJUNCTIVITIS

Symptoms

Usually bilateral but frequently asymmetric itching with thick, ropy discharge. More common in boys. Seasonal (spring/summer) recurrences in vernal conjunctivitis; history of atopy, dermatitis, and/or asthma without seasonal correlation in atopic conjunctivitis. Vernal conjunctivitis is usually seen in younger patients.

Signs

Critical. Large conjunctival papillae seen under the upper eyelid or along the limbus (limbal vernal) **(see Figure 5.1.6)**.

Other. Superior corneal "shield" ulcer (a well-delineated, sterile, gray-white infiltrate with overlying epithelial defect), limbal raised white dots (Horner–Trantas dots) of degenerated eosinophils **(see Figure 5.1.7)**, and superficial punctate keratopathy (SPK).

Treatment

1. Treat as for allergic conjunctivitis except for ensuring prophylactic use of a mast-cell stabilizer or a combination of antihistamine/mast-cell stabilizer (e.g., olopatadine 0.2% or

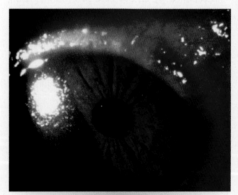

Figure 5.1.7 Vernal/atopic conjunctivitis with raised white dots of eosinophils along limbus.

0.7% daily, alcaftadine 0.25% daily, olopatadine 0.1% b.i.d., ketotifen 0.1% b.i.d., lodoxamide 0.1% q.i.d., and pemirolast 0.1% q.i.d.) for 2 to 3 weeks before the allergy season starts.
2. If a shield ulcer is present, add:
  • Topical steroid (e.g., loteprednol 0.5% or prednisolone acetate 1% drops, dexamethasone 0.1% ointment) four to six times per day.
  • Topical antibiotic drop (trimethoprim/polymyxin B q.i.d) or ointment (e.g., erythromycin q.i.d., bacitracin/polymyxin B q.i.d.).
  • Cycloplegic agent (e.g., cyclopentolate 1% t.i.d.).

NOTE: Shield ulcers may need to be scraped to remove the superficial plaque-like material before re-epithelialization can occur.

3. Cool compresses q.i.d.
4. Consider cyclosporine 0.05% to 2% b.i.d. to q.i.d. if not responding to the preceding treatment. Inform the patient that the maximal effect of this drop is not seen for several weeks.
5. If associated with atopic dermatitis of eyelids, consider applying tacrolimus 0.03% to 0.1% ointment q.h.s. or b.i.d. (preferred), pimecrolimus 1% cream b.i.d., or topical steroid ophthalmic ointment (e.g., fluorometholone 0.1% q.i.d.) to the affected skin for 1 to 2 weeks.

Follow Up

Every 1 to 3 days in the presence of a shield ulcer; otherwise, every few weeks. Topical medications are tapered slowly as improvement is noted. Antiallergy drops are maintained for the duration of the season and are often reinitiated a few weeks before the next spring. Patients on topical steroids should be monitored regularly with attention to IOP, even if used only on the skin.

BACTERIAL CONJUNCTIVITIS (NONGONOCOCCAL)

Symptoms

Redness, foreign body sensation, and discharge; itching is much less prominent.

Signs

Critical. Purulent white-yellow discharge of mild-to-moderate degree.

Other. Conjunctival papillae, chemosis, preauricular node typically absent (unlike gonococcal in which a preauricular node is often palpable).

Etiology

Commonly *Staphylococcus aureus* (associated with blepharitis, phlyctenules, and marginal sterile infiltrates), *Staphylococcus epidermidis*, *Haemophilus influenzae* (especially in children and commonly associated with otitis media), *Streptococcus pneumoniae*, and *Moraxella catarrhalis*.

NOTE: Suspect gonococcal infections if onset is hyperacute with significant discharge, see GONOCOCCAL CONJUNCTIVITIS in this section.

Workup

If severe, recurrent, or recalcitrant, send conjunctival scrapings for immediate Gram stain (to evaluate for gonococcus) and for routine culture and sensitivity tests (e.g., blood and chocolate agar).

Treatment

1. Use topical antibiotic therapy (e.g., trimethoprim/polymyxin B or fluoroquinolone drops or ointment q.i.d.) for 5 to 7 days.
2. *H. influenzae* conjunctivitis should be treated with oral amoxicillin/clavulanate (20 to 40 mg/kg/d in three divided doses) because of occasional extraocular involvement (e.g., otitis media, pneumonia, and meningitis).
3. If associated with dacryocystitis, systemic antibiotics are necessary. See 6.9, DACRYOCYSTITIS/INFLAMMATION OF THE LACRIMAL SAC.

Follow Up

Every 2 to 3 days initially, then every 5 to 7 days when stable until resolved. Antibiotic therapy is adjusted according to culture and sensitivity test results.

GONOCOCCAL CONJUNCTIVITIS

Signs

Critical. Severe purulent discharge, hyperacute onset (classically within 12 to 24 hours).

Other. Conjunctival papillae, marked chemosis, preauricular adenopathy, and eyelid swelling. See 8.9, OPHTHALMIA NEONATORUM (NEWBORN CONJUNCTIVITIS), for a detailed discussion of gonococcal conjunctivitis in the newborn.

Workup

1. Examine the entire cornea for peripheral ulcers (especially superiorly) because of the risk for rapid progression to perforation (see Figure 5.1.8).
2. Send conjunctival scrapings for immediate Gram stain and for culture and sensitivity tests (e.g., chocolate agar or Thayer–Martin agar).

Treatment

Initiated if the Gram stain shows Gram-negative intracellular diplococci or there is a high clinical suspicion of gonococcal conjunctivitis.

1. A dual treatment regimen of ceftriaxone 1 g intramuscularly (i.m.) PLUS azithromycin 1 g p.o. both in a single dose is recommended. If corneal involvement exists, or cannot be excluded because of chemosis and eyelid swelling, hospitalize the patient and treat with ceftriaxone 1 g intravenously (i.v.) every 12 to 24 hours in place of i.m. ceftriaxone. The duration of treatment may depend on the clinical response. Consider an infectious disease consultation in all cases of gonococcal conjunctivitis.
2. If ceftriaxone is not available or unable to be tolerated (e.g., cephalosporin-allergic patients), consider the following treatment regimens:
   - Gemifloxacin 320 mg p.o. in a single dose PLUS azithromycin 2 g p.o. in a single dose
   - Gentamicin 240 mg i.m. in a single dose PLUS azithromycin 2 g p.o. in a single dose

NOTE: Not only are oral fluoroquinolones contraindicated in pregnant women and children, but also due to increased resistance, they are no longer recommended monotherapy for the treatment of gonococcal infections. Note that topical fluoroquinolones, such as moxifloxacin, are used safely in children >4 months old.

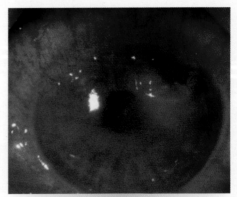

Figure 5.1.8 Gonococcal conjunctivitis with corneal involvement.

3. Topical fluoroquinolone ointment q.i.d. or fluoroquinolone drop q2h. If the cornea is involved, use a fluoroquinolone drop q1h (e.g., gatifloxacin, moxifloxacin, besifloxacin, levofloxacin, or ciprofloxacin).
4. Saline irrigation q.i.d. until the discharge resolves.
5. Treat for possible chlamydial coinfection (e.g., azithromycin 1 g p.o. single dose or doxycycline 100 mg p.o. b.i.d. for 7 days).
6. Treat sexual partners with oral antibiotics for both gonorrhea and chlamydia as described.

Follow Up

Daily until consistent improvement is noted and then every 2 to 3 days until the condition resolves. The patient and sexual partners should be evaluated by their medical doctors for other sexually transmitted diseases.

PEDICULOSIS (LICE, CRABS)

Typically develops from contact with pubic lice (usually sexually transmitted). Can be unilateral or bilateral.

Symptoms

Itching and mild conjunctival injection.

Signs

Critical. Adult lice, nits, and blood-tinged debris on the eyelids and eyelashes (see Figure 5.1.9).

Other. Follicular conjunctivitis.

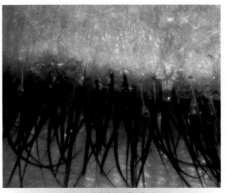

Figure 5.1.9 Pediculosis.

Treatment

1. Mechanical removal of lice and eggs with jeweler's forceps.

2. Any bland ophthalmic ointment (e.g., erythromycin) to the eyelids t.i.d. for 10 days to smother the lice and nits.
3. Anti-lice lotion and shampoo as directed to nonocular areas for patient and close contacts.
4. Thoroughly wash and dry all clothes, towels, and linens.

> **NOTE:** In children, pediculosis is suspicious for possible sexual abuse, and the involvement of social services and/or child protection agencies is recommended.

For chlamydial, toxic, and molluscum contagiosum-related conjunctivitis, see 5.2, CHRONIC CONJUNCTIVITIS.

Also see related sections: 5.10, OCULAR CICATRICIAL PEMPHIGOID; 8.9, OPHTHALMIA NEONATORUM (NEWBORN CONJUNCTIVITIS); and 13.6, STEVENS–JOHNSON SYNDROME (ERYTHEMA MULTIFORME MAJOR).

5.2 Chronic Conjunctivitis

Symptoms

"Red eye" (conjunctival hyperemia), conjunctival discharge, eyelids sticking (worse on awakening from sleep), and foreign body sensation, duration >4 weeks (otherwise see 5.1, ACUTE CONJUNCTIVITIS).

Differential Diagnosis

- Parinaud oculoglandular conjunctivitis (see 5.3, PARINAUD OCULOGLANDULAR CONJUNCTIVITIS).
- Silent dacryocystitis (see 6.9, DACRYOCYSTITIS/INFLAMMATION OF THE LACRIMAL SAC).
- Contact lens-related (see 4.20, CONTACT LENS-RELATED PROBLEMS).
- Conjunctival tumors (see 5.12, CONJUNCTIVAL TUMORS).
- Autoimmune disease (e.g., reactive arthritis, sarcoidosis, discoid lupus, and others).

CHLAMYDIAL INCLUSION CONJUNCTIVITIS

Sexually transmitted, due to *Chlamydia trachomatis* serotypes D–K, and typically found in young adults. A history of vaginitis, cervicitis, or urethritis may be present.

Signs

Inferior tarsal or bulbar conjunctival follicles, superior corneal pannus, palpable preauricular node, or peripheral SEIs. A stringy, mucous discharge may be present.

Workup

1. History: Determine the duration of red eye, any prior treatment, concomitant vaginitis, cervicitis, or urethritis. Sexually active?
2. Slit lamp examination.
3. In adults, direct chlamydial immunofluorescence test, DNA probe, chlamydial culture, or polymerase chain reaction of the conjunctival sample.

> **NOTE:** Topical fluorescein can interfere with immunofluorescence test results.

4. Consider conjunctival scraping for Giemsa stain: Shows basophilic intracytoplasmic inclusion

bodies in epithelial cells, polymorphonuclear leukocytes, and lymphocytes in newborns.

Treatment

1. Azithromycin 1 g p.o. single dose, doxycycline 100 mg p.o. b.i.d., or erythromycin 500 mg p.o. q.i.d. for 7 days is given to the patient and his or her sexual partners.
2. Topical erythromycin or tetracycline ointment b.i.d. to t.i.d. for 2 to 3 weeks.

Follow Up

In 2 to 3 weeks, depending on the severity. The patient and sexual partners should be evaluated by their medical doctors for other sexually transmitted diseases. Occasionally a 6-week course of doxycycline may be required.

TRACHOMA

Principally occurs in developing countries in areas of poor sanitation and crowded conditions. Due to *C. trachomatis* serotypes A–C.

Signs

(See Figure 5.2.1.)

Macallan Classification

- Stage 1: Superior tarsal follicles, mild superior SPK, and pannus, often preceded by purulent discharge and tender preauricular node.
- Stage 2: Florid superior tarsal follicular reaction (2a) or papillary hypertrophy (2b) associated with superior corneal SEIs, pannus, and limbal follicles.
- Stage 3: Follicles and scarring of superior tarsal conjunctiva.
- Stage 4: No follicles, extensive conjunctival scarring.
- Late complications: Severe dry eyes, trichiasis, entropion, keratitis, corneal scarring, superficial fibrovascular pannus, Herbert pits (scarred limbal follicles), corneal bacterial superinfection, and ulceration.

World Health Organization Classification

- TF (trachomatous inflammation: follicular): More than five follicles on the upper tarsus.

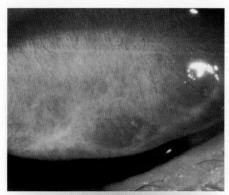

Figure 5.2.1 Trachoma showing Arlt line, or scarring, of the surgery tarsal conjunctiva.

- TI (trachomatous inflammation: intense): Inflammation with thickening obscuring >50% of the tarsal vessels.
- TS (trachomatous scarring): Cicatrization of tarsal conjunctiva with fibrous white bands.
- TT (trachomatous trichiasis): Trichiasis of at least one eyelash.
- CO (corneal opacity): Corneal opacity involving at least part of the pupillary margin.

Workup

1. History of exposure to endemic areas (e.g., North Africa, Middle East, India, Southeast Asia).
2. Examination and diagnostic studies as above (e.g., chlamydial inclusion conjunctivitis).

Treatment

1. Azithromycin 20 mg/kg p.o. single dose, doxycycline 100 mg p.o. b.i.d., or erythromycin 500 mg p.o. q.i.d. for 2 weeks.
2. Tetracycline, erythromycin, or sulfacetamide ointment b.i.d. to q.i.d. for 3 to 4 weeks.

NOTE: Tetracycline derivatives are contraindicated in children younger than 8 years, pregnant women, and nursing mothers.

Follow Up

Every 2 to 3 weeks initially, and then as needed. Although treatment is usually curative, reinfection is common if hygienic conditions do not improve.

NOTE: Currently, the World Health Organization is conducting a large-scale program to eradicate trachoma through intermittent widespread distribution of azithromycin as well as improving facial cleanliness and water sanitation in endemic areas. The aim is the global elimination of trachoma by the year 2030.

MOLLUSCUM CONTAGIOSUM

Signs

Critical. Dome-shaped, single or multiple, and umbilicated shiny nodule(s) on the eyelid or eyelid margin.

Other. Follicular conjunctival response from toxic viral products, corneal pannus, and SPK. Immunocompromised patients may have larger (up to 5 mm) and more numerous lesions along with less conjunctival reaction. An increased incidence associated with pediatric atopic dermatitis has been observed.

Treatment

When associated with chronic conjunctivitis, lesions should be removed by simple excision, incision, and curettage, or cryosurgery.

Follow Up

Every 2 to 4 weeks until the conjunctivitis resolves, which often takes 4 to 6 weeks. If many lesions are present, consider human immunodeficiency virus (HIV) testing.

MICROSPORIDIAL KERATOCONJUNCTIVITIS

Signs

Diffuse, coarse, raised punctate keratitis, and nonpurulent papillary or follicular conjunctivitis not responsive to conservative treatment. In immunocompromised patients, a corneal stromal keratitis resembling HSV or fungal keratitis can

occur. Diagnosis is based on scrapings or biopsy of the conjunctiva or cornea; obligate intracellular parasites can be identified with Gram stain, Giemsa stain, electron microscopy, and confocal microscopy in vivo.

Treatment

Regimens of antiparasitic and/or antibiotic agents are recommended. Topical fumagillin, polyhexamethylene biguanide (PHMB), and/or oral antiparasitic medications (e.g., itraconazole 200 mg p.o. daily or albendazole 400 mg p.o. b.i.d.) have been used. Epithelial debridement followed by antibiotic ointment (e.g., erythromycin, ciprofloxacin, or bacitracin/polymyxin B t.i.d.) may be useful. Treat any systemic infestation. Consider HIV testing and infectious disease consultation.

TOXIC CONJUNCTIVITIS/ MEDICAMENTOSA

Signs

Inferior papillary reaction and/or inferior conjunctival staining with fluorescein from topical eye drops. Most notably from IOP-lowering medications, aminoglycosides, antivirals, and preserved drops (especially those containing benzalkonium chloride). With long-term use, usually more than 1 month, a follicular response can be seen with other medications including atropine, miotics, epinephrine agents, and nonaminoglycoside antibiotics. Inferior SPK and scant discharge may be noted.

Treatment

Usually sufficient to discontinue the offending eye drop. Can add preservative-free artificial tears four to eight times per day. In severe cases, topical steroids can help quiet the conjunctival inflammation and render the eye more comfortable.

Follow Up

In 1 to 4 weeks, as needed.

5.3 Parinaud Oculoglandular Conjunctivitis

Symptoms

Red eye, mucopurulent discharge, and foreign body sensation.

Signs

Critical. Granulomatous nodule(s) on the palpebral and bulbar conjunctiva; visibly swollen ipsilateral preauricular or submandibular lymph nodes.

Other. Fever, rash, and follicular conjunctivitis.

Etiology

- Cat-scratch disease from *Bartonella henselae* (most common cause): Often a history of being scratched or licked by a kitten within 2 weeks of symptoms.
- Tularemia: History of contact with rabbits, other small wild animals, or ticks. Patients have severe headache, fever, and other systemic manifestations.
- Tuberculosis and other mycobacteria.
- Rare causes: Syphilis, leukemia, lymphoma, mumps, Epstein–Barr virus, HSV, fungi, sarcoidosis, listeria, typhus, and others.

Workup

Initiated when etiology is unknown (e.g., no recent cat scratch). Consider:

1. Conjunctival biopsy with scrapings for Gram, Giemsa, and acid-fast stains.
2. Conjunctival cultures on blood, Löwenstein–Jensen, Sabouraud, and thioglycolate media.
3. Complete blood count, rapid plasma reagin (RPR) or VDRL, fluorescent treponemal antibody absorption (FTA-ABS) or treponemal-specific assay (e.g., MHA-TP), angiotensin-converting enzyme (ACE), and, if the patient is febrile, blood cultures.
4. Chest radiograph, purified protein derivative (PPD) of tuberculin, and/or interferon-gamma release assay (IGRA) (e.g., QuantiFERON-TB Gold).
5. If tularemia is suspected, serologic titers are necessary.

6. If diagnosis of cat-scratch disease is uncertain, then cat-scratch serology and cat-scratch skin test (Hanger–Rose) can be performed.

Treatment

1. Warm compresses for tender lymph nodes.
2. Antipyretics as needed.
3. Disease specific:

   - Cat-scratch disease: Generally resolves spontaneously in 6 weeks. Consider azithromycin 500 mg p.o. q.i.d., then 250 mg daily for four doses (for children, 10 mg/kg q.i.d., then 5 mg/kg daily for four doses); alternatives include trimethoprim/sulfamethoxazole (160/800 mg b.i.d.) or ciprofloxacin 500 mg p.o. b.i.d. Duration should be individualized. Use a topical antibiotic (e.g., bacitracin/polymyxin B ointment or gentamicin drops q.i.d.). The cat does not need to be removed.
   - Tularemia: Recommended therapy is gentamicin 5 mg/kg once daily i.m. or i.v. for 10 days. For mild illness, alternative therapies include ciprofloxacin 500 mg p.o. b.i.d. for 10 to 14 days or doxycycline 100 mg p.o. b.i.d. for 14 to 21 days. Systemic medication should coincide with gentamicin 0.3% drops q2h for 1 week and then five times per day until resolved. Often patients are systemically ill and under the care of a medical internist for tularemia; if not, refer to a medical internist for systemic management.
   - Tuberculosis: Refer to an internist for antituberculosis medication.
   - Syphilis: Systemic penicillin (dose depends on the stage of syphilis) and topical tetracycline ointment (see 12.12, SYPHILIS).

Follow Up

Repeat the ocular examination in 1 to 2 weeks. Conjunctival granulomas and lymphadenopathy can take 4 to 6 weeks to resolve for the cat-scratch disease.

5.4 Superior Limbic Keratoconjunctivitis

Symptoms

Red eye, burning, foreign body sensation, pain, tearing, itching mild photophobia, and frequent blinking. The course can be chronic with exacerbations and remissions.

Signs

Critical. Sectoral thickening, inflammation, and radial injection of the superior bulbar conjunctiva, especially at the limbus. Superior bulbar conjunctivochalasis often present **(see Figure 5.4.1).**

Other. Fine papillae on the superior tarsal conjunctiva; fine punctate fluorescein staining on the superior cornea, limbus, and conjunctiva; superior corneal micropannus and filaments. Usually bilateral, frequently asymmetric.

Workup

1. History: Recurrent episodes? Thyroid disease?
2. Slit lamp examination with fluorescein, lissamine green, or rose bengal staining, particularly of the superior cornea and adjacent conjunctiva. Lift the upper eyelid to see the superior limbal area and then evert to visualize the tarsus. Sometimes the localized hyperemia is best appreciated by direct inspection with room light rather than at the slit lamp, by raising the eyelids of the patient on downgaze.

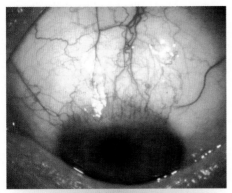

Figure 5.4.1 Superior limbic keratoconjunctivitis.

3. Thyroid function tests (there is a 50% prevalence of current or remote thyroid disease in patients with superior limbic keratoconjunctivitis).

Treatment

Mild

1. Aggressive lubrication with preservative-free artificial tears four to eight times per day and artificial tear ointment q.h.s.
2. Consider punctal occlusion with plugs or cautery because of association with dry eyes.
3. Treat any concurrent blepharitis.
4. Consider treatment with cyclosporine 0.05%, cyclosporine 0.09%, or lifitegrast 5% b.i.d. if not responding to lubrication.
5. In the absence of dry eyes, a therapeutic bandage disposable soft contact lens can be placed to help relieve symptoms and facilitate healing.

Moderate to Severe (in Addition to Preceding)

1. Autologous serum drops may be tried with intermittent dosing throughout the day.
2. Consider treatment with topical tacrolimus 0.03% ointment b.i.d. if there is no improvement with aggressive lubrication (off-label in the eye).
3. If a significant amount of mucus or filaments are present, add acetylcysteine 10% drops four to six times per day. Low potency topical steroids such as loteprednol, rimexolone, or fluorometholone can be used for short courses to treat exacerbations.
4. Application of silver nitrate 0.5% solution on a cotton-tipped applicator for 10 to 20 seconds to the superior tarsal and superior bulbar conjunctiva after topical anesthesia (e.g., proparacaine). This is followed by irrigation with saline and use of antibiotic ointment (e.g., erythromycin) q.h.s. for 1 week.

NOTE: Do not use silver nitrate (75% to 95%) cautery sticks, which cause severe ocular burns.

5. A low dose of doxycycline can be a helpful adjuvant to counteract matrix metalloproteinase upregulation caused by superior limbic keratoconjunctivitis.

6. Botulinum toxin can be injected into the muscle of Riolan for temporary relief of symptoms.

7. Surgical considerations include conjunctival cautery, cryotherapy, conjunctival resection (with or without amniotic membrane graft), recession of the superior bulbar conjunctiva, or high-frequency radiowave electrosurgery.

Follow Up

Every 2 to 4 weeks during an exacerbation. If signs and symptoms persist despite multiple medical treatment strategies, surgical options should be considered.

5.5 Subconjunctival Hemorrhage

Symptoms

Red eye, foreign body sensation, but usually asymptomatic unless there is associated chemosis.

Signs

Blood underneath the conjunctiva, often in one sector of the eye. The entire view of the sclera can be obstructed by blood **(see Figure 5.5.1)**.

Differential Diagnosis

• Kaposi sarcoma: Red or purple lesion beneath the conjunctiva, usually elevated slightly. HIV/AIDS testing should be performed.

• Other conjunctival lesions (e.g., lymphoma or amyloid) with secondary hemorrhage.

Etiology

• Valsalva (e.g., coughing, sneezing, vomiting, bearing down with constipation, or other forms of straining).

• Traumatic: Can be isolated or associated with a retrobulbar hemorrhage or ruptured globe.

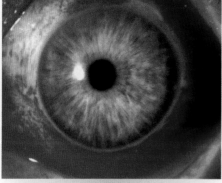

Figure 5.5.1 Subconjunctival hemorrhage.

• Hypertension and diabetes.

• Bleeding disorder.

• Antiplatelet or anticoagulant medications (e.g., aspirin, clopidogrel, warfarin, ticagrelor, dabigatran, rivaroxaban, apixaban, and edoxaban).

• Topical steroid therapy.

• Hemorrhage due to orbital mass (rare).

• Idiopathic.

Workup

1. History: Bleeding or clotting problems? Medications? Eye rubbing, trauma, heavy lifting, or Valsalva? Recurrent subconjunctival hemorrhage? Acute or chronic cough?

2. Check blood pressure.

3. Ocular examination: If recurrent, rule out a conjunctival lesion when resolved. If severe, check extraocular motility, resistance to retropulsion, and IOP. In traumatic cases, rule out other ocular injuries (e.g., a ruptured globe [signs may include reduced visual acuity, abnormally deep or shallow anterior chamber, severe bullous subconjunctival hemorrhage, hyphema, vitreous hemorrhage, or uveal prolapse], retrobulbar hemorrhage [associated with proptosis and increased IOP], or orbital fracture). See 3.14, RUPTURED GLOBE AND PENETRATING OCULAR INJURY, 3.10, TRAUMATIC RETROBULBAR HEMORRHAGE, and 3.9, ORBITAL BLOWOUT FRACTURE.

4. If the patient has recurrent subconjunctival hemorrhages or a history of bleeding problems, prothrombin time, activated partial thromboplastin time, complete blood count with differential and peripheral blood smear

(to evaluate for thrombocytopenia or leukemia), liver function tests, and protein C and S should be obtained.

5. If orbital signs are present (proptosis, decreased extraocular motility, elevated IOP) in atraumatic cases, perform axial, coronal, and parasagittal imaging (computed tomography [CT], or magnetic resonance imaging [MRI]) of the orbits with and without contrast to evaluate for an orbital mass (e.g., neuroblastoma in children or lymphangioma in adults). In traumatic cases, image as appropriate based on clinical findings, mechanism of injury, etc. (see Chapter 3, Trauma).

Treatment

None required. Artificial tear drops q.i.d. can be given if mild ocular irritation is present. In addition, *elective* use of aspirin products and NSAIDs should be discouraged unless in the context of coexisting medical conditions. Blood thinners should not be stopped unless a patient is cleared by their primary medical physician.

Follow Up

Usually resolves spontaneously within 2 to 4 weeks. Patients are told to return if the blood does not fully resolve or if they experience a recurrence. Referral to an internist or family physician should be made as indicated for hypertension or a bleeding diathesis.

5.6 Episcleritis

Symptoms

Acute or rapid onset of redness and mild pain in one or both eyes, typically in young-to middle-aged adults, more common in women; a history of recurrent episodes is common. No discharge or photophobia.

Signs

Critical. Sectoral (and, less commonly, diffuse) redness of one or both eyes, mostly due to engorgement of the episcleral vessels. These vessels are large, run in a radial direction beneath the conjunctiva, and can be moved slightly with a cotton-tip applicator **(see Figure 5.6.1)**.

Other. Mild-to-moderate tenderness over the area of episcleral injection or a nodule that can be moved slightly over the underlying sclera may be seen. Fluorescein staining can sometimes be seen over the nodule. Associated anterior uveitis and corneal involvement are rare. Vision is normal.

Differential Diagnosis

- Scleritis: Typically older patient. May have known underlying immune-mediated disease (e.g., collagen vascular disease). Pain is deep, severe, and often radiates to the ipsilateral side of the head or face. The sclera may have a violaceous hue when observed in natural light. Scleral (and deep episcleral) vessels, as well as conjunctival and superficial episcleral vessels, are injected. The scleral vessels do not blanch on application of topical phenylephrine 2.5%. Possible corneal involvement with adjacent peripheral stromal keratitis. See 5.7, Scleritis.

- Iritis: Cells and flare in the anterior chamber. May be present with scleritis. See 3.5, Traumatic Iritis and 12.1, Anterior Uveitis (Iritis/Iridocyclitis).

- Conjunctivitis: Diffuse redness and discharge with follicles or papillae. See 5.1, Acute Conjunctivitis and 5.2, Chronic Conjunctivitis.

- Contact lens-related: Overwear, tight contact lens syndrome, or reaction to contact lens solution. Must be considered in all contact lens wearers. See 4.20, Contact Lens-Related Problems.

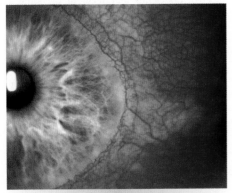

Figure 5.6.1 Episcleritis.

Etiology

- Idiopathic: Most common; 60% of patients have no underlying systemic disease.
- Infectious: Herpes zoster virus (scars from an old facial rash may be present, may cause episcleritis or scleritis), sexually transmitted infections, protozoa, and others.
- Medications (e.g., topiramate and pamidronate).
- Others: Rosacea, atopy, collagen vascular diseases (e.g., rheumatoid arthritis, inflammatory bowel disease, ankylosing spondylitis, psoriatic arthritis, systemic lupus erythematosus), vasculitides, and gout.

Workup

1. History: Assess for a history of rash, arthritis, venereal disease, recent viral illness, and other medical problems.
2. External examination in natural light: Look for the violaceous hue of scleritis.
3. Slit lamp examination: Anesthetize (e.g., topical proparacaine) and move the conjunctiva with a cotton-tipped applicator to determine the depth of the injected blood vessels. Evaluate for any corneal or anterior chamber involvement. Check IOP.
4. Place a drop of phenylephrine 2.5% in the affected eye and re-examine the vascular pattern 10 to 15 minutes later. Episcleral vessels should blanch, highlighting any underlying scleral vascular engorgement.
5. If the history suggests an underlying etiology (systemic disease usually precedes ocular involvement), or in cases with multiple recurrences, the appropriate laboratory tests should be obtained (e.g., complete blood count, comprehensive metabolic panel, antinuclear antibody [ANA], rheumatoid factor, anticyclic citrullinated peptide [anti-CCP], erythrocyte sedimentation rate [ESR], serum uric acid level, RPR or VDRL, FTA-ABS or treponemal-specific assay, antineutrophil cytoplasmic antibody [ANCA]).

Treatment

1. If mild, treat with artificial tears q.i.d.
2. If moderate to severe, a topical NSAID (e.g., diclofenac 0.1% q.i.d., bromfenac 0.07% or 0.09% daily) or a mild topical steroid (e.g., fluorometholone 0.1% or 0.25%, fluorometholone acetate 0.1% or loteprednol 0.5% q.i.d.) often relieves the discomfort. Occasionally, more potent or frequent topical steroid application is necessary.
3. Oral NSAIDs may be used as an alternate steroid-sparing initial therapy and should be given with food or antacids (e.g., ibuprofen 200 to 600 mg p.o. t.i.d. to q.i.d., naproxen 250 to 500 mg p.o. b.i.d., or flurbiprofen 50 to 100 mg p.o. b.i.d. to t.i.d.) for at least 10 to 14 days.

 NOTE: Many physicians prefer oral NSAIDs to topical NSAIDs or steroids as initial therapy.

Follow Up

Patients treated with artificial tears need not be seen for several weeks unless discomfort worsens or persists. If topical steroids are used, recheck every 2 to 3 weeks until symptoms resolve. The frequency of steroid administration is then tapered. Episcleritis may recur in the same or contralateral eye.

5.7 Scleritis

Symptoms

Severe and boring eye pain (most prominent feature), which may radiate to the forehead, brow, jaw, or sinuses and classically awakens the patient at night. Pain worsens with eye movement and with touch. Gradual or acute onset with red eye. May have tearing, photophobia, or a decrease in vision. Recurrent episodes are common. Scleromalacia perforans (necrotizing scleritis without inflammation) may have minimal symptoms.

Signs

Critical. Inflammation of scleral, episcleral, and conjunctival vessels (scleral vessels are large, deep vessels that cannot be moved with a cotton swab and do not blanch with topical 2.5% or 10% phenylephrine). Can be sectoral, nodular, or diffuse with associated scleral edema. Characteristic violaceous scleral hue (best seen in natural light by gross inspection). Areas of scleral thinning or remodeling may appear with recurrent episodes, allowing the underlying uvea to become visible or even bulge outward.

Other. Scleral nodules, corneal changes (peripheral keratitis, limbal guttering, or keratolysis), glaucoma, uveitis, or cataract.

Signs of Posterior Scleritis. Subretinal granuloma, circumscribed fundus mass, choroidal folds, retinal striae, exudative retinal detachment, optic disc swelling, macular edema, proptosis, or rapid-onset hyperopia.

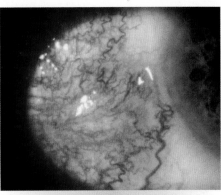

Figure 5.7.1 Nodular scleritis.

Differential Diagnosis

- Episcleritis: Sclera not involved. Blood vessels blanch with topical phenylephrine. Usually more acute onset than scleritis. Patients tend to be younger and have mild symptoms, if any. See 5.6, EPISCLERITIS.
- Vogt–Koyanagi–Harada (VKH) disease, choroidal melanoma, metastatic choroidal tumor, and choroidal hemangioma can mimic posterior scleritis.
- Scleritis associated with other orbital inflammatory foci (myositis, dacryoadenitis, etc.) may be part of idiopathic orbital inflammatory syndrome (IOIS) commonly known as orbital pseudotumor.
- Orbital cellulitis.

Etiology

Up to 50% of patients with scleritis have an associated systemic disease, typically connective tissue or vasculitic in nature. Workup indicated if no known underlying disease is present.

More Common. Connective tissue disease (e.g., rheumatoid arthritis, granulomatosis with polyangiitis, relapsing polychondritis, systemic lupus erythematosus, reactive arthritis, polyarteritis nodosa, ankylosing spondylitis, inflammatory bowel disease), infectious (e.g., *Pseudomonas*, atypical mycobacteria, fungi, *Nocardia*, herpes zoster, syphilis), trauma including status-post surgery (especially scleral buckle or pterygium surgery with mitomycin-C or beta irradiation), and gout.

Less Common. Varicella zoster, tuberculosis, Lyme disease, other bacteria (e.g., *Pseudomonas* species with scleral ulceration, *Proteus* species

associated with scleral buckle), sarcoidosis, foreign body, or parasite.

Classification

1. Diffuse anterior scleritis: Widespread inflammation of the anterior segment.
2. Nodular anterior scleritis: Immovable inflamed nodule(s) **(see Figure 5.7.1)**.
3. Necrotizing anterior scleritis with inflammation **(see Figure 5.7.2)**: Extreme pain. The sclera becomes transparent (choroidal pigment visible) because of necrosis. High association with systemic inflammatory diseases.
4. Necrotizing anterior scleritis without inflammation (scleromalacia perforans): Typically asymptomatic. Seen most often in older women with long-standing rheumatoid arthritis.
5. Posterior scleritis: May start posteriorly, or rarely be an extension of anterior scleritis,

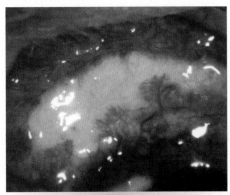

Figure 5.7.2 Necrotizing scleritis with thin, bluish sclera.

or simulate an amelanotic choroidal mass. Associated with exudative retinal detachment, disc swelling, retinal hemorrhage, choroidal folds, choroidal detachment, restricted motility, proptosis, pain, or tenderness.

Workup

1. History: Previous episodes? History of ocular trauma or surgery? Medical problems? An associated systemic disease is more common in patients >50 years old.
2. Examine the sclera in all directions of gaze by gross inspection in natural light or adequate room light.
3. Slit lamp examination with a red-free filter (green light) to determine whether avascular areas of the sclera exist. Check for corneal or anterior chamber involvement.
4. Dilated fundus examination to rule out posterior involvement.
5. B-scan ultrasonography to detect posterior scleritis (e.g., T-sign).
6. Fluorescein angiography in eyes with posterior scleritis may show multiple areas of pinpoint leakage, choroidal folds, and subretinal fluid.
7. Complete physical examination (especially joints, skin, and cardiovascular and respiratory systems) by an internist or a rheumatologist.
8. Complete blood count, creatinine, ESR, CRP, uric acid, RPR or VDRL, FTA-ABS or treponemal-specific assay (e.g., MHA-TP), ANCA, rheumatoid factor, anti-CCP, ANA, ACE, CH50 (total complement activity assay), C3, C4, and urinalysis.
9. Other tests if clinical suspicion warrants additional workup: PPD or IGRA, Lyme antibody, chest radiograph, HLA B27, radiograph of sacroiliac joints, and MRI or CT scan if indicated. Cultures should be taken if infection is suspected.

Treatment

1. Diffuse and nodular scleritis: One or more of the following may be required. Concurrent antiulcer medication (e.g., proton-pump inhibitor [e.g., omeprazole 20 mg p.o. daily] or histamine type 2 receptor blocker [e.g., ranitidine 150 mg p.o. b.i.d.]) may be helpful.
   - Oral NSAIDs (e.g., flurbiprofen 100 mg t.i.d., naproxen 250 to 500 mg p.o.

b.i.d., or indomethacin 25 to 50 mg p.o. t.i.d.): Several different NSAIDs may be tried before therapy is considered a failure. If there is still no improvement, consider systemic steroids.

   - Oral steroids: Prednisone 60 to 80 mg p.o. daily for 1 week, followed by a taper to 20 mg daily over the next 2 to 6 weeks, followed by a slower taper. Once daily calcium with vitamin D (e.g., 600 mg with 400 iU) supplements should be given to reduce the risk of osteoporosis. An oral NSAID often facilitates the tapering of the steroid but significantly increases the risk of gastric ulceration. If unsuccessful or disease requires >7.5 to 10 mg prednisone/day for long-term control, immunosuppressive therapy is indicated.
   - Intravenous steroids: Methylprednisolone succinate 1,000 mg daily for 3 days (followed by oral steroids as above) is preferable to prednisone >80 mg/d because of reduced risk of ischemic necrosis of bone.
   - Immunosuppressive therapy (e.g., cyclophosphamide, methotrexate, cyclosporine, azathioprine, mycophenolate mofetil, anti-TNFα agents, and other biologics): If one drug is ineffective or not tolerated, additional agents should be tried. Systemic steroids may be used in conjunction. Immunosuppressive therapy should be coordinated with an internist, rheumatologist, or uveitis specialist. Topical cyclosporine is rarely effective.
   - Conventional teaching is that topical therapy is of little benefit. However, difluprednate 0.05% drops are sometimes helpful (with or without a topical NSAID) and thus, in mild cases, may spare the need for systemic immunosuppressive agents.
   - Subconjunctival steroid injections (e.g., 0.1 to 0.3 mL of triamcinolone acetonide 40 mg/mL or dexamethasone sodium phosphate 4 mg/mL): May be very helpful in patients unable to tolerate systemic therapy. Side effects may include subconjunctival hemorrhage, cataract, glaucoma, and (rarely) catastrophic scleral melting. Do not use in cases of necrotizing scleritis.

2. Necrotizing scleritis:
   - Necrotizing scleritis associated with rheumatoid arthritis is associated with increased mortality due to coronary arteritis or cerebral angiitis and requires urgent, aggressive immunosuppressive therapy.
   - Systemic steroids and immunosuppressive therapies are used as above during the first month; the former is tapered slowly.
   - Scleral patch grafting may be necessary if there is a significant risk of perforation, ideally once the inflammation is better controlled.
3. Posterior scleritis: Therapy may include systemic aspirin, NSAIDs, steroids, or immunosuppressive therapy as described previously. Consult a retina or uveitis specialist.
4. Infectious etiologies: Debridement and cultures/stains are essential. Treat with appropriate topical and systemic antimicrobials.

Oral fluoroquinolones have good ocular tissue penetration. If a foreign body (e.g., scleral buckle [associated with *Proteus* or *Pseudomonas*]) is present, surgical removal is indicated.

5. Glasses or eye shield should be worn at all times if there is significant thinning and risk of perforation.

> **NOTE:** Remember that periocular steroids are contraindicated in necrotizing scleritis where they can lead to further scleral thinning and possible perforation.

Follow Up

Depends on the severity of the symptoms and the degree of scleral thinning. Decreased pain is the first sign of response to treatment, even if inflammation appears unchanged.

5.8 Blepharitis/Meibomitis

Symptoms

Itching, burning, mild pain, foreign body sensation, tearing, erythema of the eyelids, and crusting around the eyes upon awakening. This is in contrast to dry eye syndrome in which symptoms are usually worse later in the day.

Signs

Critical. Crusty, red, thickened eyelid margins with prominent blood vessels **(see Figure 5.8.1)** or inspissated oil glands at the eyelid margins **(see Figure 5.8.2)**. Crusting, collarettes, and/or cylindrical sleeves around lashes.

Other. Conjunctival injection, swollen eyelids, mild mucous discharge, and SPK. Rosacea may be present. Corneal infiltrates, pannus, and phlyctenules may be present.

Differential Diagnosis

- Pediculosis. See 5.1, ACUTE CONJUNCTIVITIS.
- Demodicosis. *Demodex* mites may play a role in patients with chronic blepharitis. Look for cylindrical sleeves on lashes. Microscopic evaluation of epilated eyelash is diagnostic.

Treatment

See 5.9, OCULAR ROSACEA, for treatment options in the presence of acne rosacea.

1. Scrub the eyelid margins twice a day with a commercial eyelid scrub or mild shampoo on a washcloth.
2. Warm compresses for 5 to 10 minutes b.i.d. to q.i.d.

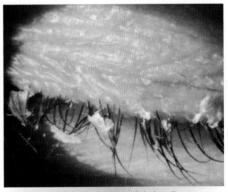

Figure 5.8.1 Blepharitis with lash collarettes.

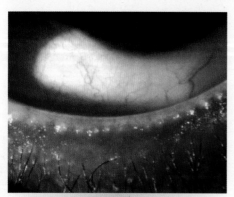

Figure 5.8.2 Meibomitis with inspissated meibomian glands.

3. If associated with dry eyes, use preservative-free artificial tears four to eight times per day.

4. If moderately severe, add erythromycin ointment or azithromycin gel-drop to the eyelids q.h.s.

5. Consider omega-3 fatty acid oral supplementation as well as cyclosporine 0.05%, cyclosporine 0.09%, or lifitegrast 5% drops b.i.d.

6. Unresponsive meibomitis can be treated with topical ophthalmic antibiotic/steroid ointments (e.g., tobramycin 0.3%/dexamethasone 0.1% or tobramycin 0.3%/dexamethasone 0.05% b.i.d. to t.i.d.). Also consider an oral agent such as doxycycline 100 mg p.o. daily for 1 to 2 weeks; slowly taper to one-fourth full dose and maintain for 3 to 6 months. Oral azithromycin

500 mg/d × 3 days for 3 cycles with 7-day intervals may also be used.

7. If *Demodex* mite infestation is suspected, due to the presence of collarettes, and patients have failed the above regimen, consider tea-tree oil eyelid scrubs or an eyelid cleansing agent with hypochlorous acid once or twice daily for a minimum of 6 weeks.

8. If little improvement has been made, consider thermal treatment to the meibomian glands with expression, intense pulsed light laser therapy, microblepharoexfoliation, and probing of meibomian glands.

NOTE: Tetracycline derivatives such as doxycycline should not be used in pregnant women, nursing mothers, or children ≤8 years. Erythromycin 200 mg p.o. b.i.d. is an alternative in these cases.

Follow Up

Two to four weeks depending on the severity of presenting symptoms. Eyelid scrubs and warm compresses may be reduced to once daily as the condition improves but may need to be maintained indefinitely.

NOTE: Intractable, unilateral, or asymmetric (not only of eye laterality but also upper versus lower eyelid) blepharitis is rarely a manifestation of sebaceous carcinoma of the eyelid and warrants appropriate clinical workup. See 6.11, MALIGNANT TUMORS OF THE EYELID.

5.9 Ocular Rosacea

Symptoms

Bilateral chronic ocular irritation, dry eyes, redness, burning, photophobia, and foreign body sensation. Typically middle-aged adults, but it can be found in children. More common in women. Associated facial symptoms include recurrent facial flushing episodes, persistent midfacial erythema, and papular skin lesions.

Signs

Critical. Telangiectasias, pustules, papules, or erythema of the cheeks, forehead, and nose. Findings may be subtle especially in heavily pigmented individuals, often best seen under natural light. Superficial or deep corneal vascularization, particularly in the inferior cornea, is sometimes seen and may extend into a stromal infiltrate.

Other. Rhinophyma of the nose occurs in the late stages of the disease, especially in men. Blepharitis (telangiectasias of the eyelid margin with inflammation) and a history of recurrent chalazia are common. Conjunctival injection, SPK, phlyctenules, perilimbal infiltrates of staphylococcal hypersensitivity, iritis, or even corneal perforation (rare) may occur.

Differential Diagnosis

• Herpes simplex keratitis: Usually unilateral. Stromal keratitis with neovascularization may appear similar. See 4.15, HERPES SIMPLEX VIRUS.
• See 4.1, SUPERFICIAL PUNCTATE KERATOPATHY, for additional differential diagnoses.
• See 4.22, PERIPHERAL CORNEAL THINNING/ ULCERATION for peripheral ulcerative keratitis associated with systemic disease.

Etiology

Unknown, but signs and symptoms are often induced by certain environmental/local factors, including hot beverages (e.g., coffee or tea), tobacco, vasodilating medications, alcohol, and emotional stress.

Workup

1. External examination: Look at the face for the characteristic skin findings.
2. Slit lamp examination: Look for telangiectasias and meibomitis on the eyelids, conjunctival injection, and corneal scarring and vascularization.

Treatment

1. Warm compresses and eyelid hygiene for blepharitis or meibomitis (see 5.8, BLEPHARITIS/MEIBOMITIS). Treat dry eyes if present (see 4.3, DRY EYE SYNDROME).
2. Avoidance of exacerbating foods, beverages, and environmental factors.
3. Doxycycline 100 mg p.o. b.i.d. for 1 to 2 weeks and then daily; taper the dose slowly once relief from symptoms is obtained. Some patients are maintained on low-dose doxycycline (e.g., 20 to 100 mg p.o. daily or less than daily) indefinitely if the active disease

recurs when the patient is off medication. Erythromycin 250 mg q.i.d. or oral azithromycin 500 mg/d × 3 days for 3 cycles with 7-day intervals is an alternative if doxycycline is contraindicated.

 NOTE: Tetracycline derivatives such as doxycycline should not be given to pregnant women, nursing women, or children ≤8 years. Patients should be warned of increased sunburn susceptibility with the use of this medication.

 NOTE: Asymptomatic ocular rosacea without progressively worsening eye disease does not require oral antibiotics.

4. Consider oral omega-3 fatty acid supplements, cyclosporine 0.05%, cyclosporine 0.09%, or lifitegrast 5% drops b.i.d., and topical steroids for chronic rosacea-related ocular and eyelid inflammation (see 5.8, BLEPHARITIS/ MEIBOMITIS).
5. Facial lesions can be treated with metronidazole gel (0.75%) application b.i.d.
6. Treat chalazia as needed (see 6.2, CHALAZION/ HORDEOLUM).
7. Corneal perforations may be treated with cyanoacrylate tissue adhesive if small (<1-2 mm), whereas larger perforations may require surgical correction. Doxycycline is indicated if there is a concern for corneal melting due to its anticollagenase properties.
8. If infiltrates stain with fluorescein, an infectious corneal ulcer may be present. Smears, cultures, and antibiotic treatment may be necessary. See 4.11, BACTERIAL KERATITIS and Appendix 8, CORNEAL CULTURE PROCEDURE.

Follow Up

Variable; depends on the severity of the disease. Patients without corneal involvement are seen weeks to months later. Those with corneal involvement are examined more often. Patients with moderate-to-severe facial disease should also seek dermatologic consultation.

5.10 Mucous Membrane Pemphigoid (Ocular Cicatricial Pemphigoid)

Systemic autoimmune disease leading to mucocutaneous inflammation and eventual scarring.

Symptoms

Insidious onset of dryness, redness, blepharospasm, itching, foreign body sensation, tearing, burning, decreased vision, and photophobia. Bilateral involvement. The course is characterized by remissions and exacerbations. Usually occurs in patients older than 55 years.

Signs

Critical. Inferior symblepharon (linear folds of conjunctiva connecting the palpebral conjunctiva of the lower eyelid to the inferior bulbar conjunctiva), foreshortening and tightness of the lower fornix, and scarring of palpebral conjunctiva on eyelid eversion **(see Figure 5.10.1)**.

Other. Secondary bacterial conjunctivitis, SPK, and corneal ulcer. Potential later findings include poor tear film, resulting in severe dry eye syndrome; entropion; trichiasis or distichiasis (if present, carefully examine fornices for symblepharon); corneal opacification with pannus, neovascularization, and keratinization; obliteration of the fornices, with eventual limitation of ocular motility; and ankyloblepharon.

Systemic. Mucous membrane (e.g., oropharynx, esophagus, anus, vagina, and urethra) vesicles; scarring or strictures; ruptured or formed bullae; denuded epithelium. Desquamative gingivitis is

common. Cutaneous vesicles and bullae may occur, sometimes with erythematous plaques or scars near affected mucous membranes.

Based on clinical findings, the disease can be divided into four stages:

1. Stage I—Chronic conjunctivitis with mild corneal involvement.

2. Stage II—Cicatrization with conjunctival shrinkage and foreshortening of fornices.

3. Stage III—Above with the additional presence of symblepharon. Subepithelial scarring leads to distortion of lashes.

4. Stage IV—End stage, with ankyloblepharon and severe corneal involvement (persistent epithelial defects, stromal ulcers, scarring, neovascularization, and diffuse keratinization).

Differential Diagnosis

- Stevens–Johnson syndrome (erythema multiforme major) and toxic epidermal necrolysis (TEN): Acute onset, but similar ocular involvement as ocular pemphigoid. Often precipitated by drugs (e.g., sulfa, penicillin, other antibiotics, phenytoin) or infections (e.g., herpes and mycoplasma). See 13.6, STEVENS–JOHNSON SYNDROME (ERYTHEMA MULTIFORME MAJOR).

- History of membranous conjunctivitis with scarring: Usually adenovirus or beta-hemolytic *Streptococcus*. See 5.1, ACUTE CONJUNCTIVITIS and 5.2, CHRONIC CONJUNCTIVITIS.

- Severe chemical burns. See 3.1, CHEMICAL BURN.

- Chronic topical medicine: Examples include glaucoma medications (especially pilocarpine or phospholine iodide) and antiviral agents.

- Others: Atopic keratoconjunctivitis, radiation treatment, and squamous cell carcinoma.

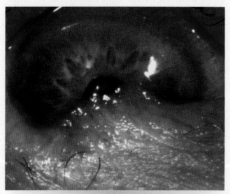

Figure 5.10.1 Mucous membrane pemphigoid with symblepharon.

NOTE: Symblepharon is a nonspecific finding and can follow severe conjunctivitis, chemical injury, trauma, radiation exposure, etc. However, symblepharon associated with mucous membrane pemphigoid (MMP)/ocular cicatricial pemphigoid (OCP) is usually progressive.

Workup

1. History: Long-term topical medications? Acute onset of severe systemic illness in the past? Recent systemic medications?
2. Skin and mucous membrane examination.
3. Slit lamp examination: Especially for forniceal foreshortening or inferior symblepharon (most easily achieved by pulling down the lower eyelid during upgaze) and for palpebral conjunctival scarring on eyelid eversion. Check IOP.
4. Gram stain and culture of the cornea or conjunctiva if a secondary bacterial infection is suspected. See Appendix 8, CORNEAL CULTURE PROCEDURE.
5. Consider a biopsy of the conjunctiva or other involved mucous membranes for direct immunofluorescence studies, or indirect immunofluorescence for the presence of antibodies.
6. Obtain appropriate consults, as below.

Treatment

A multidisciplinary approach is often needed, including dermatology, oculoplastics, cornea, otolaryngology, gastroenterology, and pulmonology. Early diagnosis of the ocular involvement is critical for optimal management.

1. Preservative-free artificial tears 4 to 10 times per day. Can add an artificial tear ointment b.i.d. to q.i.d. and q.h.s. Autologous serum drops 20% to 50% four times a day may also be added.
2. Treat blepharitis vigorously with eyelid hygiene, warm compresses, and antibiotic ointment (e.g., erythromycin t.i.d.). Oral doxycycline can be used if blepharitis is present (for its anti-inflammatory properties). See 5.8, BLEPHARITIS/MEIBOMITIS.
3. Goggles or glasses with sides to provide a moist environment for the eyes.
4. Fitting of scleral lenses to maintain ocular surface integrity.
5. Punctal occlusion if puncta are not already closed by scarring.

6. Topical steroids may rarely help in suppressing acute exacerbations, but be cautious of corneal melting.
7. Systemic steroids (e.g., prednisone 60 mg p.o. daily) may also help in suppressing acute exacerbations but are most effective when used with other immune modulators.
8. Immunosuppressive agents (e.g., mycophenolate mofetil, methotrexate, cyclophosphamide, rituximab, and intravenous immunoglobulin) are typically used for progressive disease.
9. Dapsone is occasionally used for progressive disease. The starting dose is 25 mg p.o. for 3 to 7 days; increase by 25 mg every 4 to 7 days until the desired result is achieved (usually 100 to 150 mg p.o. daily). Dapsone is maintained for several months and tapered slowly.

NOTE: Dapsone can cause a dose-related hemolysis. A complete blood count and glucose-6-phosphate dehydrogenase (G-6-PD) level must be checked before administration. Dapsone should be avoided in patients with G-6-PD deficiency. A complete blood count with reticulocyte count is obtained weekly as the dose is increased every 3 to 4 weeks until blood counts are stable and then every few months.

10. Consider surgical correction of entropion and cryotherapy or electrolysis for trichiasis. Surgery carries the risk of further scarring and is best performed when inflammation is absent.
11. Mucous membrane grafts (e.g., buccal or amniotic membrane graft) can be used to reconstruct the fornices if needed.
12. Consider a keratoprosthesis in an end-stage eye with good macular and optic nerve function if the inflammation and IOP are controlled. The surgical prognosis for the long-term survival of the keratoprosthesis is guarded.

Follow Up

Every 1 to 2 weeks during acute exacerbations and every 1 to 6 months during remissions.

5.11 Contact Dermatitis

Symptoms

Sudden onset of a periorbital rash, usually pruritic, and/or eyelid swelling.

Signs

Critical. Periorbital edema, erythema, vesicles, and lichenification of the skin. Conjunctival chemosis out of proportion to injection and papillary response **(see Figure 5.11.1)**.

Other. Watery discharge; crusting of the skin may develop.

Differential Diagnosis

• Varicella zoster virus (shingles): Dermatomal pattern with severe pain. See 4.16, HERPES ZOSTER OPHTHALMICUS/VARICELLA ZOSTER VIRUS.
• Eczema: Recurrent in nature and is markedly pruritic.
• Impetigo: Pruritic with honey-colored crusts.
• Orbital cellulitis or preseptal cellulitis: See 7.3.1, ORBITAL CELLULITIS and 6.10, PRESEPTAL CELLULITIS.

Etiology

Most commonly eye drops and cosmetics.

Treatment

1. Avoid the offending agent(s).
2. Cool compresses four to six times per day.
3. Preservative-free artificial tears four to eight times per day and topical antihistamines (e.g., levocabastine 0.05% q.i.d.).

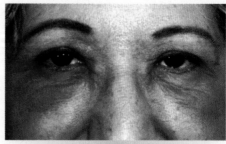

Figure 5.11.1 Contact dermatitis.

4. Consider tacrolimus 0.03% to 0.1% q.h.s. or b.i.d. (preferred).
5. Consider a mild steroid ointment (e.g., fluorometholone 0.1%, or loteprednol 0.5%) applied to the periocular area b.i.d. to t.i.d. for 4 to 5 days for skin involvement.
6. Consider an oral antihistamine (e.g., diphenhydramine 25 to 50 mg p.o. t.i.d. to q.i.d.) for several days.

Follow Up

Re-examine within 1 week.

5.12 Conjunctival Tumors

The following are the most common and important conjunctival tumors. Pterygium/pinguecula and phlyctenulosis are discussed in Sections 4.9 and 4.19, respectively.

AMELANOTIC LESIONS

Limbal Dermoid

A congenital benign tumor, usually located in the inferotemporal quadrant of the limbus, can involve the more central cornea. Lesions are white, solid, fairly well circumscribed, elevated, and can have hair arising from their surface. May enlarge, particularly at puberty. With time, intracorneal lipid deposition can occur at the leading edge of the dermoid. Associated with eyelid coloboma, preauricular skin tags, and vertebral abnormalities (Goldenhar syndrome). Surgical removal may be performed for cosmetic purposes or if they are

affecting the visual axis, although a white corneal scar may persist postoperatively and cause astigmatism. Penetrating keratoplasty may be needed.

> **NOTE:** The cornea or sclera underlying a dermoid can be very thin or even absent. Penetration of the eye can occur with surgical resection. Ultrasound biomicroscopy or anterior segment optical coherence tomography may be helpful to determine the depth.

Dermolipoma

A congenital benign tumor, usually occurring under the bulbar conjunctiva temporally, often superotemporally. Yellow-white, solid tumor. Can have hair arising from its surface and fat within the stroma. High association with Goldenhar syndrome. Surgical removal is avoided because of the frequent posterior extension of this tumor into the orbit. If necessary, partial resection of the anterior portion can usually be done.

Pyogenic Granuloma

Benign, deep-red, and pedunculated mass. Typically develops at a site of prior surgery, trauma, or chalazion. This lesion consists of exuberant granulation tissue. May respond to topical steroids. A topical steroid–antibiotic combination (e.g., dexamethasone/tobramycin 0.1%/0.3% q.i.d. for 1 to 2 weeks) can be helpful because infection can be present. Excision is required if it persists.

Lymphangioma

Probably congenital but often not detected until years after birth. A slowly progressive benign lesion that appears as a diffuse, multiloculated, and cystic mass. Seen most commonly between birth and young adulthood, often before 6 years of age. Hemorrhage into the cystic spaces can produce a "chocolate cyst." Can enlarge, sometimes due to an upper respiratory tract infection. Concomitant eyelid, orbital, facial, nasal, or oropharyngeal lymphangiomas can be present. Surgical excision may be performed for cosmetic or functional purposes, but it often must be repeated because it is difficult to remove the entire tumor with one surgical procedure. Sclerotherapy, in which intralesional injections of 2 to 4 mg of 1 mg/mL bleomycin are administered every 4 weeks depending on clinical response, can lead to involution and fibrosis of the lesion. This technique is typically employed for more advanced or chronically recurrent tumors. Lesions often stabilize in early adulthood. These lesions do not regress like capillary hemangiomas.

Granuloma

Can occur at any age, predominantly on the tarsal conjunctiva. No distinct clinical appearance, but patients can have an associated embedded foreign body, sarcoidosis, tuberculosis, or another granulomatous disease. For systemic granulomatous diseases (e.g., sarcoidosis), conjunctival granulomas can be an excellent source of diagnostic tissue. Management often includes a course of topical steroids or excisional biopsy.

Papilloma

1. Viral: Frequently multiple pedunculated or sessile lesions in children and young adults.

May occur on the palpebral or bulbar conjunctiva. They are benign and are usually left untreated because of their high recurrence rate (which is often multiple) and their tendency for spontaneous resolution. They can also be treated with oral cimetidine (30 mg/kg/d in children or 150 mg p.o. b.i.d. in adults) because of the drug's immune-stimulating properties or they can respond to topical or lesional injection of interferon alfa 2b.

2. Nonviral: Typically, a single sessile or pedunculated lesion is found in older patients. These are located more commonly near the limbus and can represent precancerous lesions with malignant potential. Complete wide excisional biopsy with cryotherapy at the conjunctival margin is the preferred treatment since it may be difficult to differentiate from squamous cell carcinoma.

NOTE: In dark-skinned individuals, papillomas can appear pigmented and can be mistaken for malignant melanoma.

Kaposi Sarcoma

Malignant, nontender vascular subconjunctival nodule. Usually red and may simulate a conjunctival hemorrhage. Perform HIV/AIDS testing. Kaposi sarcoma lesions may resolve when patients are placed on highly active antiretroviral therapy. Other treatments include vinblastine, vincristine, excision, cryotherapy, interferon alfa 2b, or irradiation.

Conjunctival Intraepithelial Neoplasia (Dysplasia and Carcinoma In Situ)

Typically occurs in middle-aged to elderly people. Leukoplakic or gray-white, gelatinous lesion that usually begins at the limbus. Occasionally, a papillomatous, fern-like vascular appearance develops. Usually unilateral and unifocal. Can evolve into invasive squamous cell carcinoma **(see Figure 5.12.1)** if not treated early and successfully. Can spread over the cornea or, less commonly, invade the eye or metastasize. The preferred treatment is a complete excisional biopsy followed by supplemental cryotherapy to the remaining adjacent conjunctiva. Excision may require lamellar dissection into the corneal stroma and sclera in recurrent or long-standing lesions. Topical forms of mitomycin C, 5-fluorouracil, and interferon

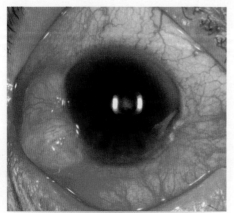

Figure 5.12.1 Conjunctival squamous cell carcinoma.

have also been used. Periodic follow-up examinations are required to detect recurrences.

Lymphoid Tumors (Range from Benign Reactive Lymphoid Hyperplasia to Lymphoma)

Can occur in young to middle-aged adults, but the mean age of diagnosis is 61 years. Usually appears as a light pink, salmon-colored lesion. Can appear in the bulbar conjunctiva, where it is typically oval, or in the fornix, where it is usually horizontal, conforming to the contour of the fornix **(see Figure 5.12.2)**. An excisional or incisional biopsy is performed for immunohistochemical studies (require fresh nonfixed tissue). Symptomatic benign reactive lymphoid hyperplasia can be treated by excisional biopsy or topical steroid drops. Lymphomas should be completely excised

when possible, without damage to the extraocular muscles or excessive sacrifice of the conjunctiva. If not possible, an incisional biopsy is justified and subsequent treatment with rituximab, chemotherapy, or low dose radiotherapy is advised. Refer to an internist or oncologist for systemic evaluation. Systemic lymphoma may develop, if it is not already present.

Epibulbar Osseous Choristoma

Congenital, benign, hard, bony mass, usually on the superotemporal bulbar conjunctiva. Surgical removal can be performed for cosmetic purposes.

Amyloid

Smooth, waxy, and yellow-pink masses are seen especially in the lower fornix when the conjunctiva is involved. Often there are associated small hemorrhages. A definitive diagnosis is made with a biopsy. Consider workup for systemic amyloidosis, although most cases in the conjunctiva are localized and solitary **(see Figure 5.12.3)**.

Amelanotic Melanoma

Pigmentation of conjunctival melanoma is variable. Look for bulbar or limbal lesions with significant vascularity to help make this difficult diagnosis. Look carefully for primary acquired melanosis.

Sebaceous Carcinoma

Although usually involving the palpebral conjunctiva, this tumor can involve the bulbar conjunctiva (when there is a pagetoid invasion of the conjunctiva). This diagnosis should always be considered in older patients with refractory unilateral blepharoconjunctivitis.

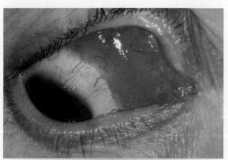

Figure 5.12.2 Conjunctival lymphoma (salmon patch).

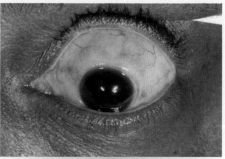

Figure 5.12.3 Conjunctival amyloid.

(See 6.11, MALIGNANT TUMORS OF THE EYELID, for a detailed discussion of sebaceous carcinoma.)

MELANOTIC LESIONS

Nevus

Commonly develops during puberty, most often within the palpebral fissure on the bulbar conjunctiva. Usually well demarcated with variable pigmentation. The degree of pigmentation can also change with time. A key sign in the diagnosis is the presence of small cysts in the lesion. Benign nevi can enlarge; however, a melanoma can occasionally develop from a nevus, and enlargement can be an early sign of malignant transformation. Nevi of the palpebral conjunctiva are rare, and primary acquired melanosis and malignant melanoma must be considered in such lesions. A baseline photograph of the nevus should be taken, and the patient should be observed every 6 to 12 months. Surgical excision is elective. Nevi may be amelanotic **(see Figure 5.12.4)**.

Ocular or Oculodermal Melanocytosis

A congenital episcleral (not conjunctival) lesion, as demonstrated (after topical anesthesia) by moving the conjunctiva back and forth over the area of pigmentation with a cotton-tipped swab (conjunctival pigmentation will move with the conjunctiva). Typically, the lesion is unilateral, blue-gray, and often accompanied by a darker ipsilateral iris and choroid. In oculodermal melanocytosis, also called nevus of Ota, the periocular skin is also pigmented. These lesions are slightly pigmented at birth but can become more pigmented at puberty. Both conditions predispose to melanoma of the uveal tract, orbit, and brain (most commonly in whites) and glaucoma. It is estimated that 1/400 affected patients develop uveal melanoma.

Primary Acquired Melanosis

Flat, brown patches of pigmentation, without cysts, in the conjunctiva. Usually arise during or after middle age and almost always occur in whites. Classically, approximately 10% to 30% of these lesions develop into melanoma. Malignant transformation should be suspected when an elevation or increase in vascularity in one of these areas develops. Management options depend on the lesion size. If 1 to 2 clock hour size, then careful observation with photographic comparison is

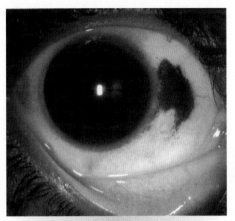

Figure 5.12.4 Conjunctival nevus.

advised. If 2 to 4 clock hour size, then excisional biopsy followed by cryotherapy is advised. If >4 clock hour size, then incisional biopsy plus cryotherapy is performed.

Malignant Melanoma

Typically occurs in middle-aged to elderly patients. The lesion is a nodular brown mass. Well vascularized. Often a large conjunctival feeding vessel is present. May develop *de novo*, from a nevus, or from primary acquired melanosis. Check for an underlying ciliary body melanoma (dilated fundus examination, transillumination, and ultrasonographic biomicroscopy). Intraocular and orbital extension can occur. Excisional biopsy using a "no-touch technique" (with supplemental cryotherapy) is performed unless intraocular or orbital involvement is present. In advanced cases, orbital exenteration is necessary. Sentinel lymph node biopsy is advised to detect early metastatic disease **(see Figure 5.12.5)**.

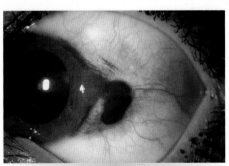

Figure 5.12.5 Conjunctival melanoma.

Less Common Causes of Conjunctival Pigmentation

1. Ochronosis with alkaptonuria: Autosomal recessive enzyme deficiency. Occurs in young adults with arthritis and dark urine. The pigment is at the level of the sclera, which can cause a "pigmented pinguecula." Blue-black discoloration of the ear cartilage.
2. Argyrosis: Silver deposition causes black discoloration. Patients may have a history of long-term use of silver nitrate drops.
3. Hemochromatosis: Can cause darkening of the skin, termed bronze diabetes.
4. Ciliary staphyloma: Scleral thinning with uveal show.
5. Adrenochrome deposits: Long-term epinephrine or dipivefrin use.
6. Mascara deposits: Usually occurs in the inferior fornix and becomes entrapped in epithelium or cysts.

5.13 Malignant Melanoma of the Iris

Malignant melanoma of the iris can occur as a localized or diffuse pigmented (melanotic) or nonpigmented (amelanotic) lesion.

Signs

Critical. Unilateral brown or translucent iris mass lesion exhibiting slow growth. It is more common in the inferior half of the iris and in light-skinned individuals. Rare in blacks **(see Figure 5.13.1)**.

Other. A localized melanoma is usually >3 mm in diameter at the base and >1 mm in depth with a variable prominent feeder vessel. Can produce a sector cortical cataract, ectropion iridis, spontaneous hyphema, seeding of tumor cells into the anterior chamber, or direct invasion of tumor into the trabecular meshwork and secondary glaucoma. A diffuse melanoma causes progressive darkening of the involved iris, loss of iris crypts, and increased IOP. Focal iris nodules can be present.

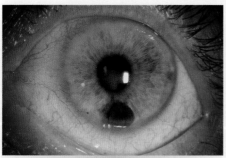
Figure 5.13.1 Iris melanoma.

Differential Diagnosis

Melanotic Masses

- Nevi: Typically become clinically apparent at puberty, usually flat or minimally elevated (i.e., <1 mm) and uncommonly exceed 3 mm in diameter. Can cause ectropion iridis, sector cortical cataract, or secondary glaucoma. Usually not vascular. More common in the inferior half of the iris. Nevi do not usually grow.
- Tumors of the iris pigment epithelium: Usually black in contrast to melanomas, which are often brown or amelanotic. Found on the posterior aspect of the iris.

Amelanotic Masses

- Metastasis: Grows rapidly. More likely to be multiple or bilateral than melanoma. Frequently liberates cells and produces a pseudohypopyon. Involves the superior and inferior halves of the iris equally.
- Leiomyoma: Transparent and vascular. Difficult to distinguish from an amelanotic melanoma.
- Iris cyst: Unlike melanoma, most transmit light with transillumination. Can arise from the iris pigment epithelium or within the iris stroma. Each with very different clinical features.
- Inflammatory granuloma: Sarcoidosis, tuberculosis, juvenile xanthogranuloma, and others. Often have other signs of inflammation such as keratic precipitates, synechiae, and posterior subcapsular cataracts. A history of iritis or a systemic inflammatory disease may be elicited. See Chapter 12, UVEITIS.

Diffuse Lesions

- Congenital iris heterochromia: The darker iris is present at birth or in early childhood. It is nonprogressive and usually is not associated with glaucoma. The iris has a smooth appearance.
- Fuchs heterochromic iridocyclitis: Asymmetry of iris color, mild iritis in the eye with the lighter-colored iris, usually unilateral. Often associated with a cataract or glaucoma. See 12.1, ANTERIOR UVEITIS (IRITIS/IRIDOCYCLITIS).
- Iris nevus syndrome: Corneal edema, peripheral anterior synechiae, iris atrophy, or an irregular pupil can be present along with multiple iris nodules and glaucoma.
- Pigment dispersion: Usually bilateral. The iris is rarely heavily pigmented (although the trabecular meshwork can be), and iris transillumination defects are often present. See 9.10, PIGMENT DISPERSION SYNDROME/PIGMENTARY GLAUCOMA.
- Hemosiderosis: A dark iris can result after iron breakdown products from old blood deposits on the iris surface. Patients have a history of a traumatic hyphema or vitreous hemorrhage.
- Siderosis from a retained metallic foreign body.

Workup

1. History: Previous cancer, ocular surgery, or trauma? Weight loss? Anorexia?

2. Slit lamp examination: Carefully evaluate the irides. Check IOP.
3. Gonioscopy.
4. Dilated fundus examination using indirect ophthalmoscopy.
5. Transillumination of iris mass (helps differentiate epithelial cysts that transmit light from pigmented lesions that do not).
6. Photograph the lesion and accurately draw it in the chart, including dimensions. Ultrasonographic biomicroscopy and anterior segment optical coherence tomography can be helpful.

Treatment/Follow Up

1. Observe the patient with periodic examinations and photographs every 3 to 12 months, depending on the suspicion of malignancy.
2. Surgical resection is indicated if growth is documented, the tumor interferes with vision, or it produces intractable glaucoma.
3. Diffuse iris melanoma with secondary glaucoma may require enucleation.

NOTE: Avoid filtering surgery for glaucoma associated with possible iris melanoma because of the high risk of tumor dissemination.

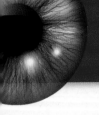

Chapter 6

Eyelid

6.1 Ptosis

Symptoms

Drooping upper eyelid, superior visual field compromise. Occasional visual compromise often gets worse with reading and at night. Concerning associated symptoms include diplopia, headache, and neck pain.

Signs

(See Figure 6.1.1.)

Critical. Drooping upper eyelid.

Other. Concerning associated signs include anisocoria, proptosis, and ocular motility deficits. See individual entities.

Etiology

NOTE: Although the majority of ptosis is aponeurotic and of benign etiology, certain entities must be ruled out by careful examination.

1. Horner syndrome.
2. Third cranial nerve (CN) palsy (complete, partial, or aberrant CN III regeneration).
3. Myasthenia gravis.
4. Orbital tumor.
5. Eyelid/conjunctival tumor.
6. Chronic progressive external ophthalmoplegia (CPEO) (particularly Kearns–Sayre syndrome, see 10.12, CHRONIC PROGRESSIVE EXTERNAL OPHTHALMOPLEGIA).

Categories:
- Myogenic: While this term is often used to describe aponeurotic ptosis, true myogenic ptosis is nearly always congenital. It is present at birth and is caused by localized dysgenesis of the levator palpebrae superioris. It results in poor levator function (0 to 5 mm) and poor or

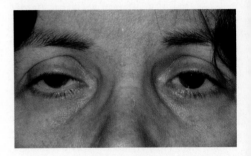

Figure 6.1.1 Ptosis.

absent eyelid crease. A poor Bell phenomenon (palpebral oculogyric reflex), lagophthalmos in downgaze, and upgaze limitation may indicate a double elevator palsy. Acquired myogenic ptosis is uncommon and may be seen with muscular dystrophy and CPEO.
- Aponeurotic: Common cause of ptosis. Occurs secondary to levator dehiscence and is characterized by a high or absent eyelid crease, moderate degree of ptosis, and preserved levator function (10 to 15 mm). Often gets worse in downgaze. Levator stretching or dehiscence can result from normal aging, repetitive eye rubbing, use of rigid contact lenses (pulling on the eyelids to put in or take out), trauma, or previous intraocular surgery (speculum-related muscle damage).
- Neurogenic: Third CN palsy (often complete ptosis, never an isolated abnormality; congenital, compressive, or vasculopathic, see 10.5, ISOLATED THIRD CRANIAL NERVE PALSY); Horner syndrome (mild, ~2 mm upper and lower eyelid ptosis, see 10.2, HORNER SYNDROME); myasthenia gravis (variable degree, duration, and laterality, worsens with fatigue, see 10.11, MYASTHENIA GRAVIS); Marcus Gunn jaw-winking syndrome (ptotic

eyelid elevates with jaw movement); ophthalmoplegic migraine; and multiple sclerosis.

- Mechanical: Foreign-body or retained contact lens in upper fornix; upper eyelid or forniceal inflammation (chalazion, giant papillary conjunctivitis, posttraumatic or postsurgical edema); and neoplasm.
- Traumatic: Eyelid laceration with levator involvement, levator contusion, tethering or ischemia within an orbital roof fracture, late dehiscence, or cicatricial changes.
- Pseudoptosis: Contralateral eyelid retraction or proptosis, ipsilateral enophthalmos or hypertropia, microphthalmia, phthisis bulbi, dermatochalasis, brow ptosis, eyelid tumor, edema, blepharospasm, or Duane syndrome.

Workup

1. History: Onset and duration? Present since birth? Old photographs (e.g., driver's license) and family members' opinions are useful adjuncts to the history. Prior surgery in either eye? Trauma? Fluctuation throughout the day? Associated diplopia, headache, or neck pain? Trouble breathing or swallowing, associated drooling? History of autoimmune disease?

2. Mandatory documentation: Must carefully check and document pupillary size and extraocular motility, even if normal. If anisocoria is present, measurements should be documented under light and dark conditions. Additional pharmacologic testing may be indicated (see 10.1, ANISOCORIA). If extraocular muscle dysfunction is noted, additional testing with prism bars may be indicated.

3. Complete orbital examination: Measure and compare globe position with Hertel exophthalmometry, margin reflex distance, levator function (full upper eyelid excursion with frontalis muscle held inactive at the brow), and upper eyelid crease position of both eyes. Is there lagophthalmos? Associated lower eyelid "ptosis" (elevation of ipsilateral lower eyelid retractors) is often seen in Horner syndrome. Proptosis or eyelid lag may masquerade as contralateral ptosis. Signs of aberrant eyelid movements like jaw-winking, variability and/or fatigue, orbicularis weakness, and eyelid retraction with adduction and/or infraduction? Resistance to retropulsion? Palpate superior orbit to rule out a mass or superior orbital rim deformity.

4. Complete ocular examination: Flip upper eyelid to examine conjunctival surface and superior fornix. Dilated fundus examination to look for pigmentary changes in adolescents and young adults who present with ptosis, poor levator function, and external ophthalmoplegia (possible CPEO and Kearns–Sayre syndrome).

5. Corneal protective mechanisms: Document presence or absence of lagophthalmos, orbicularis function, Bell phenomenon, and tear production. Check the cornea carefully for any abnormalities or dystrophies, which may predispose the patient to keratopathy.

6. Other tests
   - Ice test: Apply ice pack to ptotic eye(s) for 2 minutes, measuring eyelid position before and after. Improvement in eyelid position is highly suggestive of myasthenia gravis.
   - Phenylephrine test: Instill one drop of 2.5% phenylephrine in the ptotic eye(s). Patients with an improvement of ptosis after 5 to 7 minutes may be good candidates for ptosis correction by Müller muscle-conjunctival resection.
   - Apraclonidine, cocaine, and hydroxyamphetamine tests. See 10.2, HORNER SYNDROME.

NOTE: In recent years, limited access to ophthalmic cocaine and hydroxyamphetamine has reduced their utility in the clinical setting.

7. Imaging studies: In cases where a systemic or neurologic cause is suspected:
   - Computed tomography (CT) or magnetic resonance imaging (MRI) of orbit if a superior orbital mass is suspected.
   - CT/computed tomography angiogram (CTA) or MRI/magnetic resonance angiogram (MRA) of the head and neck if Horner syndrome is present. This should be performed emergently if there is clinical suspicion for carotid artery dissection (neck pain, acute onset, and a history of trauma). Imaging of the head alone is inadequate. See 10.2, HORNER SYNDROME.

- Emergent CT/CTA, MRI/MRA, or conventional angiography to rule out posterior communicating artery aneurysm is indicated for all third CN palsies whether pupil-involving or pupil-sparing. See 10.5, ISOLATED THIRD CRANIAL NERVE PALSY.
- Chest CT if either Horner syndrome (to rule out apical lung mass compressing sympathetic ganglion) or myasthenia gravis (to rule out thymoma) is suspected. See 10.2, HORNER SYNDROME and 10.11, MYASTHENIA GRAVIS.

8. Ancillary studies:
- If myasthenia gravis is suspected, acetylcholine receptor antibody (binding, blocking, and modulating) testing, single-fiber electromyography (including the orbicularis muscle), and/or edrophonium chloride testing under monitored conditions may be indicated. See 10.11, MYASTHENIA GRAVIS.
- Urgent ECG and cardiology consult if Kearns–Sayre syndrome is suspected. These patients can have heart block, resulting in sudden death.

Treatment

1. Depends on the underlying etiology (see 10.2, HORNER SYNDROME; 10.5, ISOLATED THIRD CRANIAL NERVE PALSY; 10.11, MYASTHENIA GRAVIS).
2. Nonsurgical options: Observation. Taping upper eyelids open and eyelid crutches attached to glasses in neurogenic and myogenic ptosis. Management of chalazion with warm compresses and/or topical or intralesional steroid/antibiotic.
3. Surgical options: Excision of eyelid and/or orbital lesions, transcutaneous levator advancement, transconjunctival levator advancement, frontalis muscle suspension, Fasanella–Servat procedure, or Müller muscle-conjunctival resection (Müllerectomy). The surgical approach depends on preoperative evaluation and the underlying etiology of ptosis.

Follow Up

1. Congenital: Close follow up is required to monitor for possible amblyopia (deprivation versus refractive secondary to induced corneal astigmatism), abnormal head positioning, and exposure keratopathy.
2. Traumatic: Observation for 6 months before considering surgical intervention. Many improve or completely resolve.
3. Neurologic: Reevaluate based on particular entity.
4. Postoperative (after ptosis repair):
- *Acute:* Monitor for infection and hemorrhage.
- *Subacute:* Monitor for exposure keratopathy and asymmetry that may require postoperative readjustment. Mild lagophthalmos is common for 2 to 3 weeks after surgical repair and usually resolves.
- *Chronic:* Monitor for ptosis recurrence and exposure keratopathy.

6.2 Chalazion/Hordeolum

Symptoms

Acute or chronic eyelid lump, swelling, and tenderness.

Signs

(See Figure 6.2.1.)

Critical. Visible or palpable, well-defined, subcutaneous nodule in the eyelid. In some cases, a nodule cannot be identified.

Other. Blocked meibomian gland orifice, eyelid swelling and erythema, focal tenderness, associated blepharitis, or acne rosacea. May also note lesion coming to a head or draining mucopurulent material.

Definitions

Chalazion: Focal, tender, or nontender inflammation within the eyelid secondary to obstruction of a meibomian gland or gland of Zeis.

Hordeolum: Acute, tender infection; can be external (abscess of a glands of Zeis on eyelid margin) or internal (abscess of the meibomian gland). Usually involves *Staphylococcus* species and occasionally evolves into preseptal cellulitis.

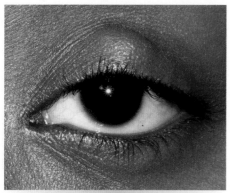

Figure 6.2.1 Chalazion.

Differential Diagnosis

- Preseptal cellulitis: Eyelid and periorbital erythema, edema, and warmth. See 6.10, PRESEPTAL CELLULITIS.
- Forniceal foreign body: eyelid swelling, particularly in soft contact lens wearers or those with a history of trauma. See 3.3, CORNEAL AND CONJUNCTIVAL FOREIGN BODIES.
- Sebaceous carcinoma: Suspect in older patients with recurrent chalazia, eyelid thickening, madarosis, or chronic unilateral blepharitis. See 6.11, MALIGNANT TUMORS OF THE EYELID.
- Pyogenic granuloma: Benign, deep-red, pedunculated conjunctival lesion often associated with chalazia, hordeola, trauma, or surgery. May be excised or treated with a topical antibiotic–steroid combination such as neomycin/polymyxin B/dexamethasone q.i.d. for no more than 1 to 2 weeks. Intraocular pressure must be monitored if topical steroids are used.

Workup

1. History: Previous ocular surgery or trauma? Previous chalazia or eyelid lesions?
2. External examination: Palpate involved eyelid for a nodule. Look for rosacea.
3. Slit lamp examination: Evaluate meibomian glands for inspissation and evert the eyelid. Assess for madarosis, poliosis, and ulceration to rule out other etiologies.

Treatment

1. Warm compresses for at least 10 minutes q.i.d. with gentle massage over the lesion.

2. Consider a short course of a topical antibiotic for hordeolum (e.g., bacitracin, tobramycin, or erythromycin ointment b.i.d. for 1 to 2 weeks) or a short course of topical antibiotic/steroid for chalazion (e.g., neomycin/polymyxin B/dexamethasone ointment b.i.d. for 1 to 2 weeks). Consider chronic low-dose doxycycline 20 to 50 mg p.o. daily to b.i.d. for its antibacterial and anti-inflammatory properties (e.g., for multiple or recurrent chalazia and/or ocular rosacea).

3. If a hordeolum worsens, consider incision and drainage and management as per preseptal cellulitis (see 6.10, PRESEPTAL CELLULITIS).

4. If the chalazion fails to resolve after 3 to 4 weeks of medical therapy and the patient desires surgical intervention, incision and curettage may be performed. Alternatively, an intralesional steroid injection may be performed (e.g., 0.2 to 1.0 mL of triamcinolone 40 mg/mL mixed 1:1 with 2% lidocaine with epinephrine). Alternate steroid formulations include various combinations of betamethasone sodium phosphate and betamethasone acetate 6 mg/mL or dexamethasone sodium phosphate 4 mg/mL. Total dosage depends on the lesion size. It is recommended that all chalazia, especially recurrent or atypical chalazia, be sent for pathology upon removal.

NOTE: A steroid injection can lead to permanent depigmentation or atrophy of the skin at the injection site, especially in dark-skinned individuals. Similarly, a vigorous injection can rarely result in retrograde intra-arterial infiltration with resultant central retinal artery occlusion. Because of these risks, some manufacturers of injectable steroids (e.g., triamcinolone and betamethasone) have historically recommended against their use intraocularly and in the periocular region. Off-label use of the medications should include a detailed discussion between physician and patient.

Follow Up

Patients are not routinely seen after instituting medical therapy unless the lesion persists beyond 3 to 4 weeks. Patients who have a procedure such as incision and curettage are usually reexamined as needed.

6.3 Ectropion

Symptoms

Tearing, irritation, redness, and mucous discharge. May be asymptomatic.

Signs

(See Figure 6.3.1.)

Critical. Outward turning of the eyelid margin.

Other. Superficial punctate keratopathy (SPK) from corneal exposure; conjunctival injection and thickening and eventual keratinization from chronic dryness. Eyelid scarring may be seen in cicatricial cases. Facial hemiparesis and lagophthalmos may be seen in paralytic cases.

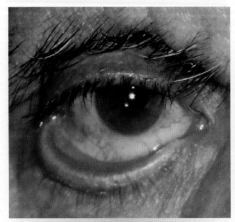

Figure 6.3.1 Ectropion.

Etiology

- Involutional: Horizontal eyelid laxity related to aging. Most common.
- Paralytic: CN VII palsy.
- Cicatricial: Anterior lamellar shortening from burn injury, prior surgery or trauma, actinic damage, chronic inflammation, skin diseases (e.g., eczema and ichthyosis), and others.
- Mechanical: Due to herniated orbital fat, eyelid tumor, and others.
- Allergic: Contact dermatitis.
- Congenital: Facial dysmorphic syndromes (e.g., Treacher Collins syndrome), Down syndrome, or isolated abnormality.

Workup

1. History: Previous surgery, trauma, chemical burn, or CN VII palsy?
2. External examination: Check orbicularis oculi function and assess horizontal eyelid laxity and punctal location. Look for an eyelid tumor, scarring, herniated orbital fat, and so on. If there is concomitant CN VII palsy and CN VIII deficit (hearing loss), consider CT or MRI brain to rule out acoustic neuroma.
3. Slit lamp examination: Evaluate for exposure keratopathy and conjunctival inflammation.

Treatment

1. Treat exposure keratopathy with lubricating agents. See 4.5, EXPOSURE KERATOPATHY.
2. Treat an inflamed, exposed eyelid margin with warm compresses and antibiotic ointment (e.g., bacitracin or erythromycin q.i.d.). A short course of combination antibiotic–steroid ointment (e.g., neomycin/polymyxin B/dexamethasone) may be helpful if close follow up is ensured.
3. Taping the eyelids into position may be a temporizing measure.
4. Definitive treatment usually requires surgery. Surgery is delayed for 3 to 6 months in patients with CN VII palsy because the ectropion may resolve spontaneously (see 10.9, ISOLATED SEVENTH CRANIAL NERVE PALSY). Corneal exposure may make the repair more urgent.

Follow Up

Patients with corneal or conjunctival exposure are examined as needed based on the severity of signs and symptoms. If the tissues are relatively healthy, follow up is not urgent. Patients using topical steroids need to be followed up routinely for steroid-induced side effects.

6

6.4 Entropion

Symptoms

Irritation, foreign-body sensation, tearing, and redness.

Signs

(See Figure 6.4.1.)

Critical. Inward turning of the eyelid margin that pushes otherwise normal lashes onto the globe.

Other. SPK from eyelashes contacting the cornea, conjunctival injection. Corneal epithelial defect, thinning, and/or ulceration in severe cases.

Etiology

- Involutional: Age-induced horizontal eyelid laxity, retractor disinsertion, and orbicularis override.
- Cicatricial: Due to conjunctival scarring in mucous membrane pemphigoid, Stevens–Johnson syndrome, chemical burns, trauma, trachoma, and others.
- Spastic: Sustained orbicularis contraction due to surgical trauma, ocular irritation, or blepharospasm.
- Congenital.

Workup

1. History: Previous surgery, trauma, chemical burn, or infection (trachoma, herpes simplex, varicella zoster)?
2. Slit lamp examination: Check for corneal involvement and conjunctival or eyelid scarring.

Treatment

If blepharospasm is present, see 6.7, BLEPHAROSPASM.

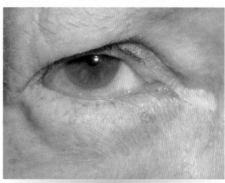

Figure 6.4.1 Entropion.

1. Aggressive lubrication and antibiotic ointment (e.g., erythromycin or bacitracin q.i.d.).
2. Everting the eyelid margin away from the globe and taping it in place with lateral traction may be a temporizing measure.
3. For spastic entropion, a Quickert suture placed at the bedside or in the office can temporarily resolve the eyelid malposition by tightening the lower eyelid retractors and rotating the eyelid margin anteriorly.
4. Surgery is often required for permanent correction.

Follow Up

If the cornea is uninvolved, the condition does not require urgent attention or follow up. If the cornea is significantly damaged, aggressive treatment is indicated (see 4.1, SUPERFICIAL PUNCTATE KERATOPATHY). Follow up is determined by the severity of corneal involvement.

6.5 Trichiasis

Symptoms

Irritation, foreign-body sensation, tearing, redness, and photophobia.

Signs

Critical. Misdirected eyelashes rubbing against the globe.

Other. Conjunctival injection; SPK; corneal epithelial defect, infiltrate, or scarring.

Etiology

- Entropion: Inward turning of eyelid pushing normal lashes onto the cornea. See 6.4, ENTROPION.

- Epiblepharon: Congenital or familial condition in which redundant lower eyelid anterior lamella redirects lashes into a vertical position, where they may contact the globe. Most common in Asian individuals, especially children.
- Distichiasis: An aberrant second row of lashes arising from meibomian gland orifices. Most commonly acquired in the setting of trauma or chronic inflammation (e.g., blepharitis, mucous membrane pemphigoid). Congenital distichiasis is a rare, sometimes hereditary, condition in which the meibomian glands are replaced by an extra row of eyelashes.
- Idiopathic.
- Chronic blepharitis: Inflamed eyelid margin. See 5.8, BLEPHARITIS/MEIBOMITIS.
- Cicatricial: Eyelid scarring from trauma, surgery, mucous membrane pemphigoid (see 5.10, MUCOUS MEMBRANE PEMPHIGOID), trachoma, Stevens–Johnson syndrome, chemical and thermal burns, medications, and others.
- Medication-induced: systemic and topical (e.g., prostaglandin analogs).

Workup

1. History: Recurrent episodes? Prior severe systemic illness or allergic reaction? Prior trauma?

2. Slit lamp examination: Evert the eyelids and inspect the palpebral conjunctiva for scarring and symblepharon. Assess eyelid position for inward rotation statically and dynamically. Check the cornea for epithelial defects, infiltrates, and scarring.

Treatment

1. Remove the misdirected lashes.
   - A few misdirected lashes: Perform epilation/removal at the slit lamp with fine forceps. Recurrence is common without follicular destruction.
   - Diffuse, severe, or recurrent trichiasis: Definitive therapy usually requires electrolysis, cryotherapy, radiofrequency epilation, argon laser, or eyelid surgery.
2. Treat SPK with antibiotic ointment (e.g., erythromycin or bacitracin b.i.d. to q.i.d.).
3. Treat any underlying blepharitis. See 5.8, BLEPHARITIS/MEIBOMITIS.
4. Address eyelid malposition if present. See 6.4, ENTROPION.

Follow Up

As needed based on symptom severity and corneal integrity. Closer follow up is needed if there is evidence of SPK or corneal epithelial defect.

6.6 Floppy Eyelid Syndrome

Symptoms

Chronically red, irritated eye(s) with mild mucous discharge, often worse upon awakening due to eyelid eversion during sleep. Usually bilateral, but often asymmetric. Typically seen in obese patients due to the strong association with sleep apnea, with a slight male predilection.

Signs

Critical. Upper eyelids are easily everted without an accessory finger or cotton-tipped applicator exerting counterpressure.

Other. Rubbery, atrophic superior tarsal plate with conjunctival injection and chronic papillary conjunctivitis, SPK, ptosis with lash ptosis, and/or lower eyelid laxity. Associations include obstructive sleep apnea, obesity, keratoconus, and Down syndrome.

Differential Diagnosis

The key differentiating factor is increased horizontal laxity and spontaneous eversion of the upper eyelids.

- Vernal conjunctivitis: Seasonal, itching, and giant papillary reaction. See 5.2, CHRONIC CONJUNCTIVITIS.
- Giant papillary conjunctivitis: Often related to contact lens wear or an exposed suture. See 4.21, CONTACT LENS–INDUCED GIANT PAPILLARY CONJUNCTIVITIS.
- Superior limbic keratoconjunctivitis: Hyperemia, thickening, and inflammation of the superior bulbar conjunctiva, limbus, and cornea. Often associated with thyroid dysfunction, keratoconjunctivitis sicca, and rheumatoid arthritis. See 5.4, SUPERIOR LIMBIC KERATOCONJUNCTIVITIS.

- Toxic keratoconjunctivitis: Papillae or follicles are typically more pronounced inferiorly in patients using eye drops. See 5.2, CHRONIC CONJUNCTIVITIS.
- Ectropion: Outward turning of the eyelid margin, often leading to tearing, irritation, and eyelid thickening. See 6.3, ECTROPION.

Etiology

The underlying etiology is not definitively known. Studies have suggested locally elevated matrix metalloproteinase (MMP) levels and elastin loss. Symptoms are thought to result from spontaneous eversion of the upper eyelid during sleep, allowing the superior palpebral conjunctiva to rub against pillows or sheets. Unilateral or asymmetric symptoms occur in those who tend to sleep prone on the affected side.

Workup

1. Pull the upper eyelid toward the patient's forehead to determine if it spontaneously everts or is abnormally lax.
2. Conduct slit lamp examination of the cornea and conjunctiva with fluorescein staining, looking for superior palpebral conjunctival papillae and SPK.
3. Ask about history of snoring and obstructive sleep apnea.

Treatment

1. Topical antibiotic ointment for any mild corneal or conjunctival abnormality (e.g., erythromycin ointment b.i.d. to q.i.d.). May change to artificial tear ointment when lesions resolve.
2. The eyelids may be taped closed during sleep, or a shield may be worn to protect the eyelid from rubbing against the pillow or bed. Patients are asked to refrain from sleeping face down. Asking patients to sleep on their contralateral side may be therapeutic as well as diagnostic.
3. Surgical horizontal tightening of the eyelid with lateral tarsal strip or wedge resection is often required for definitive treatment.

Follow Up

1. Every few days to weeks initially, followed by weeks to months as the condition stabilizes.
2. Refer to an internist, otolaryngologist, or pulmonologist for evaluation and management of possible obstructive sleep apnea. Evaluation is important because of the systemic sequelae of untreated sleep apnea and for anesthesia risk assessment before eyelid surgery.

6.7 Blepharospasm

Symptoms

Uncontrolled blinking, twitching, or closure of the eyelids. Always bilateral, but may briefly be unilateral at the first onset. Occasionally may have mid to lower face and/or neck spasms. Can also be associated with oromandibular dystonia that results in spasms in the jaw and tongue, as well as laryngeal and cervical dystonia, a condition referred to as Meige syndrome.

Signs

Critical. Bilateral, episodic, and involuntary contractions of the orbicularis oculi muscles.

Other. Disappears during sleep.

Differential Diagnosis

- Hemifacial spasm: Unilateral contractures of the entire side of the face that do not disappear during sleep. Usually idiopathic but may be related to prior CN VII palsy, injury at the level of the brainstem, or compression of CN VII by a blood vessel or tumor. MRI of the cerebellopontine angle should be obtained in all patients to rule out tumors. Treatment options include observation, botulinum toxin injections, or neurosurgical decompression of CN VII.
- Ocular irritation induced blepharospasm (e.g., corneal or conjunctival foreign body, trichiasis, blepharitis, iritis, and dry eye).
- Eyelid myokymia: Subtle eyelid twitch felt by the patient but difficult to observe, commonly brought on by stress, caffeine, alcohol, or ocular irritation. Usually unilateral lower eyelid involvement. Typically self-limited. Treat by avoiding precipitating factors and/or administering small doses of botulinum toxin.

- Tourette syndrome: Multiple compulsive muscle spasms associated with utterances of bizarre sounds or obscenities.
- Tic douloureux (trigeminal neuralgia): Acute episodes of pain in the CN V distribution, often causing a wince or tic.
- Tardive dyskinesia: Orofacial dyskinesia, often with dystonic movements of the trunk and limbs, typically from long-term use of antipsychotic medications.
- Apraxia of eyelid opening. Usually associated with Parkinson disease. Unlike blepharospasm, apraxia of eyelid opening does not feature orbicularis spasm. Instead, apraxic patients simply cannot open their eyelids voluntarily.

Etiology

- Idiopathic and likely multifactorial, possibly involving dopaminergic pathways within the basal ganglia.

Workup

1. History: Unilateral or bilateral? Does the episode involve the eyelids alone or is the lower face also involved? Are limb muscles involved? Medications?
2. Slit lamp examination: Examination for dry eye, blepharitis, or foreign body.
3. Neuroophthalmic examination to rule out other accompanying abnormalities.

4. Typical blepharospasm does not require central nervous system imaging as part of the workup. MRI of the brain with attention to the posterior fossa and path of CN VII is reserved for atypical cases or other diagnoses (e.g., hemifacial spasm).

Treatment

1. Treat any underlying eye disorder causing ocular irritation. See 4.3, DRY EYE SYNDROME and 5.8, BLEPHARITIS/MEIBOMITIS.
2. Consider botulinum toxin (onabotulinumtoxinA, incobotulinumtoxinA, and abobotulinumtoxinA) injections into the orbicularis muscles around the eyelids if the blepharospasm is severe. Can also be used to treat orofacial dyskinesia.
3. If the spasm is not relieved with botulinum toxin injections, consider surgical excision of the orbicularis muscle (myectomy) from the upper and lower eyelids and brow.
4. Muscle relaxants and sedatives are rarely of value but can be helpful in some patients. Oral medications such as lorazepam can help, but their use is often limited by their sedative qualities. Oral methylphenidate may be helpful in patients with severe spasm.

Follow Up

Not an urgent condition, but patients with severe blepharospasm can be functionally blind.

6.8 Canaliculitis

Symptoms

Tearing or discharge, red eye, and mild tenderness over the nasal aspect of the lower or upper eyelid.

Signs

(See Figure 6.8.1.)

Critical. Erythematous "pouting" of the punctum and erythema of the surrounding skin. Expression of mucopurulent discharge or concretions from the punctum is diagnostic.

Other. Recurrent conjunctivitis confined to the nasal aspect of the eye, gritty sensation on probing of the canaliculus, and focal injection of the nasal conjunctiva.

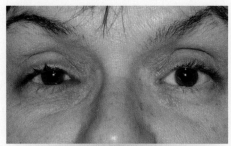

Figure 6.8.1 Canaliculitis.

Differential Diagnosis

- Dacryocystitis: Infection of the lacrimal sac with more lacrimal sac swelling, tenderness, and pain than canaliculitis. See 6.9, DACRYOCYSTITIS/INFLAMMATION OF THE LACRIMAL SAC.

- Chalazion: Focal inflammatory eyelid nodule without discharge from punctum. See 6.2, CHALAZION/HORDEOLUM.
- Nasolacrimal duct obstruction: Tearing, minimal-to-no erythema or tenderness around the punctum. See 8.10, CONGENITAL NASOLACRIMAL DUCT OBSTRUCTION.

Etiology

- *Actinomyces israelii* (streptothrix): Most common. Gram-positive rod with fine, branching filaments. Produces sulfur-rich stones.
- Other bacteria (e.g., *Fusobacterium* and *Nocardia* species).
- Fungal (e.g., *Candida*, *Fusarium*, and *Aspergillus* species).
- Viral (e.g., herpes simplex and varicella zoster).
- Retained punctal plug or foreign body.

Workup

1. Apply gentle pressure over the lacrimal sac with a cotton-tipped swab and roll it toward the punctum while observing for mucopurulent discharge or concretions.
2. Smears and cultures of the material expressed from the punctum, including slides for Gram stain and Giemsa stain. Consider thioglycolate and Sabouraud cultures.
3. Ask about a history of punctal plug placement in the past.

Treatment

1. Remove obstructing concretions or retained plug. Concretions may be expressed through the punctum at the slit lamp. A canaliculotomy is usually required for complete removal or in the setting of a retained punctal plug. If necessary, marsupialize the horizontal canaliculus from a conjunctival approach and allow the incision to heal by secondary intention.
2. If concretions are removed, consider irrigating the canaliculus with an antibiotic solution (e.g., trimethoprim sulfate/polymyxin B, moxifloxacin, penicillin G solution 100,000 units/mL, iodine 1% solution). The patient is irrigated while in the upright position, so the solution drains out of the nose and not into the nasopharynx.
3. Treat the patient with antibiotic drops (e.g., trimethoprim sulfate/polymyxin B or moxifloxacin q.i.d.) and oral antibiotics for 1 to 2 weeks (e.g., doxycycline 100 mg b.i.d.).
4. If a fungus is found on smears and cultures, nystatin 1:20,000 drops t.i.d. and nystatin 1:20,000 solution irrigation several times per week may be effective.
5. Apply warm compresses to the punctal area for 5 to 10 minutes q.i.d.

Follow Up

Five to seven days depending on severity. This is usually not an urgent condition.

6.9 Dacryocystitis/Inflammation of the Lacrimal Sac

Symptoms

Pain, redness, and swelling over the lacrimal sac in the innermost aspect of the lower eyelid. Tearing, discharge, fever, or chills may also be present. Symptoms may be recurrent.

Signs

(See Figure 6.9.1.)

Critical. Erythematous, tender, tense swelling over the nasal aspect of the lower eyelid and extending around the periorbital area. Mucoid or purulent discharge can be expressed from the punctum when pressure is applied over the lacrimal sac.

NOTE: Swelling in dacryocystitis is below the medial canthal tendon. Suspect lacrimal sac tumor (rare) if the mass is above the medial canthal tendon.

Other. Fistula formation from the skin below the medial canthal tendon. A lacrimal sac cyst or mucocele can occur in chronic cases. Progression to a lacrimal sac abscess, and rarely, orbital or facial cellulitis may occur.

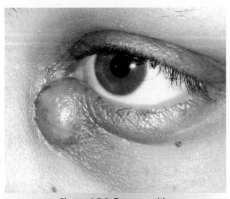

Figure 6.9.1 Dacryocystitis.

6

Differential Diagnosis

- Facial cellulitis involving the medial canthal area: No discharge from punctum with pressure over the lacrimal sac. The lacrimal drainage system is patent on irrigation. See 6.10, PRESEPTAL CELLULITIS.

- Dacryocystocele: Mild enlargement of non-inflamed lacrimal sac in an infant. Present at birth, but may not be detected until later. Caused by nasolacrimal duct obstruction or entrapment of mucus or amniotic fluid in the lacrimal sac and usually unilateral. If bilateral, assess breathing to rule out nasal obstruction. Conservative therapy with digital massage, antibiotic ointment, and warm compresses is usually sufficient for nonobstructive cases.

- Acute ethmoid sinusitis: Pain, tenderness, nasal obstruction, and erythema over the nasal bone, just medial to the inner canthus. Patients may be febrile. Imaging is diagnostic.

- Frontal sinus mucocele/mucopyocele: Swelling typically occurs well above the medial canthal tendon. Proptosis, downward and lateral displacement of the globe, and external ophthalmoplegia are often present. Imaging is diagnostic.

Etiology

- Almost always related to nasolacrimal duct obstruction.

- Uncommon causes include lacrimal sac diverticula, dacryoliths, nasal or sinus surgery, trauma, and rarely lacrimal sac tumors.

- Gram-positive bacteria are the most common pathogens; gram-negative and atypical organisms are seen more commonly in diabetics, immunocompromised, and nursing home patients.

Workup

1. History: Distinguish reflex tearing from epiphora. Previous episodes? Concomitant ear, nose, or throat infection? Underlying sinus disease? Prior trauma or surgery?

2. External examination: Apply gentle pressure to the lacrimal sac in the nasal corner of the lower eyelid with a cotton-tipped swab in an attempt to express discharge from the punctum. Perform bilaterally to uncover subtle contralateral dacryocystitis.

3. Evaluation for orbital signs: Assess pupillary response, extraocular motility, globe position for proptosis, and other evidence of potentially concurrent orbital cellulitis.

4. Obtain Gram stain and blood agar culture (consider chocolate agar culture in children given the higher incidence of *Haemophilus influenzae*) of any discharge expressed from the punctum.

5. Consider a CT scan of the orbits and paranasal sinuses in atypical cases, severe cases, and those that do not respond to appropriate antibiotics.

> **NOTE:** Do not attempt to probe or irrigate the lacrimal system during the acute infection. If a large abscess is present superficially, incision and drainage will alleviate pain and hasten healing.

Treatment

1. Systemic antibiotics in the following regimen: *Children older than 5 years and <40 kg:*
   - Afebrile, systemically well, mild case, and reliable parent: Amoxicillin/clavulanate: 25 to 45 mg/kg/d p.o. in two divided doses for children, with a maximum daily dose of 90 mg/kg/d.
   - Alternative treatment: Cefpodoxime: 10 mg/kg/d p.o. in two divided doses for children, with a maximum daily dose of 400 mg.
   - Febrile, acutely ill, moderate-to-severe case, or unreliable parent: Hospitalize and treat

with cefuroxime, 50 to 100 mg/kg/d i.v. in three divided doses in consultation with an infectious disease specialist.

Adults:

- Afebrile, systemically well, mild case, and reliable patient: Cephalexin 500 mg p.o. q6h or amoxicillin/clavulanate 500/125 mg t.i.d. or 875/125 mg p.o. b.i.d.

- If exposure to methicillin-resistant *Staphylococcus aureus* (MRSA) is suspected, then start one to two tablets double-strength trimethoprim–sulfamethoxazole 160/800 mg p.o. q12h for adults. Alternatively, start clindamycin 300 mg p.o. t.i.d. In addition to covering MRSA, this antibiotic also gives good coverage for anaerobes, streptococci, and methicillin-sensitive *S. aureus.*

- Febrile, acutely ill, or unreliable: Hospitalize and treat with cefazolin 1 g i.v. q8h. See 7.3.1, ORBITAL CELLULITIS.

    The antibiotic regimen is adjusted according to the clinical response and culture/sensitivity test results. I.V. antibiotics can be changed to comparable p.o. antibiotics depending on the rate of improvement, but systemic antibiotic therapy should be continued for at least a full 10- to 14-day course.

2. Topical antibiotic drops (e.g., trimethoprim/polymyxin B q.i.d.) may be used in addition to systemic therapy. Topical therapy alone is not adequate.

3. Apply warm compresses and gentle massage to the inner canthal region for 5 to 10 minutes q.i.d.

4. Administer pain medication (e.g., acetaminophen with or without codeine) p.r.n.

5. Consider incision and drainage of a pointing abscess.

6. Once infection has resolved, evaluate patency of the nasolacrimal duct system with probing and irrigation. If an obstruction is present, consider surgical correction (e.g., dacryocystorhinostomy with silicone intubation). In cases of recurrent or chronic dacryocystitis, surgical correction is recommended.

Follow Up

Daily, until improvement is confirmed. If outpatient condition worsens, hospitalization and i.v. antibiotics are recommended. Upon resolution of acute infection, probing and irrigation are required at the follow up to assess the patency of the nasolacrimal drainage system.

6.10 Preseptal Cellulitis

Symptoms

Tenderness, redness, warmth, and swelling of the eyelid and periorbital area. Often there is a history of local skin abrasions, penetrating injury/trauma, hordeolum, or insect bites. Can be associated with sinusitis, although this is more common with postseptal infections. May complain of fever or chills.

Signs

(See Figures 6.10.1 and 6.10.2.)

Critical. Eyelid erythema, tense edema, warmth, and tenderness. No proptosis, no optic neuropathy, no extraocular motility restriction, usually little to no conjunctival injection, and no pain with eye movement (unlike orbital cellulitis). The patient may not be able to open the eye because of eyelid edema. Visual changes such as blurred vision or monocular diplopia attributed to swollen eyelids.

Other. Tightness of eyelid skin or fluctuant eyelid edema. The eye itself may be slightly injected but is relatively uninvolved.

Differential Diagnosis

- Orbital cellulitis: Proptosis, pain with eye movement, restricted motility, and possible visual compromise. See 7.3.1, ORBITAL CELLULITIS.

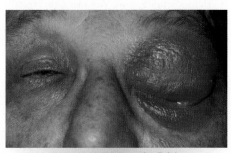
Figure 6.10.1 Preseptal cellulitis.

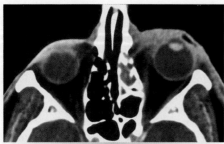

Figure 6.10.2 CT of preseptal cellulitis.

- Chalazion: Focal inflammatory eyelid nodule. See 6.2, CHALAZION/HORDEOLUM.
- Allergic: Sudden onset, nontender, itchy, and swollen eyelids. See 5.11, CONTACT DERMATITIS.
- Erysipelas: Rapidly advancing streptococcal cellulitis, often with a clear demarcation line, high fever, and chills.
- Necrotizing fasciitis: Severe bacterial infection involving subcutaneous soft tissue and deep fascia. Typically due to group A beta-hemolytic streptococci and *S. aureus*. Gray to purple skin discoloration with local hypesthesia is characteristic. Patients are often septic and may rapidly deteriorate. This potentially fatal condition requires emergent surgical debridement with i.v. antibiotic treatment.
- Viral conjunctivitis with secondary eyelid swelling: Follicular conjunctivitis is present. See 5.1, ACUTE CONJUNCTIVITIS.
- Cavernous sinus thrombosis: Proptosis with multiple cranial neuropathies. See 10.10, CAVERNOUS SINUS AND ASSOCIATED SYNDROMES (MULTIPLE OCULAR MOTOR NERVE PALSIES).
- Varicella zoster virus: Vesicular rash that respects midline. See 4.16, HERPES ZOSTER OPHTHALMICUS/VARICELLA ZOSTER VIRUS.
- Herpes simplex virus: Vesicular rash, typically unilateral, but does not respect midline/dermatomes. May be associated with ipsilateral follicular conjunctivitis. See 4.15, HERPES SIMPLEX VIRUS.
- Other orbital disorders: Proptosis, globe displacement, or restricted ocular motility. See 7.1, ORBITAL DISEASE.
- Others: Insect bite, angioedema, trauma, maxillary osteomyelitis, and others.

Etiology

- Adjacent infection (e.g., hordeolum or dacryocystitis).
- Trauma (e.g., puncture wound, laceration, insect bite).

Organisms

S. aureus and *Streptococcus* are most common, but *H. influenzae* should be considered in nonimmunized children. Suspect anaerobes if foul-smelling discharge or necrosis is present or if there is a history of an animal or human bite. Consider a viral cause if preseptal cellulitis is associated with a vesicular skin rash (e.g., herpes simplex or varicella zoster).

Workup

1. History: Pain with eye movements? Double vision? Prior trauma, sinus surgery or disease, cancer, chalazia, insect bites, or hair epilation? Sinus congestion or purulent nasal discharge? Recent vaccination? Prior antibiotic-resistant infections?
2. Complete ocular examination: Evaluate for ocular motility restriction, proptosis, afferent pupillary defect, dyschromatopsia, and disc edema. An eyelid speculum or Desmarres eyelid retractor may facilitate ocular examination if the eyelids are excessively swollen.
3. Check facial sensation in the distribution of first and second divisions of the trigeminal nerve.
4. Palpate the periorbital area and the head and neck lymph nodes for a mass.
5. Check vital signs.
6. Obtain Gram stain and culture of any open wound or drainage.
7. Perform CT scan of the orbits and sinuses (axial and coronal views) with contrast if there is a history of significant trauma or a concern for orbital or intraocular foreign body, orbital cellulitis, subperiosteal abscess, paranasal sinusitis, cavernous sinus thrombosis, or malignancy. Consider CT scan of the brain if any relevant history, signs, or symptoms necessitate this. Consider MRI or angiographic imaging if cavernous sinus or intracranial pathology is suspected, or if radiology recommends based on CT findings.

8. Consider obtaining a complete blood count with differential to identify a leukocytosis and blood cultures in severe cases or when fever is present.

Treatment

1. Antibiotic therapy

   a. Mild preseptal cellulitis, older than 5 years (<40 kg), afebrile, reliable patient/parent:

   - Amoxicillin/clavulanate: 25 to 45 mg/kg/d p.o. in two divided doses for children, a maximum daily dose of 90 mg/kg/d; 875/125 mg p.o. q12h for adults.

     or

   - Cefpodoxime: 10 mg/kg/d p.o. in two divided doses for children, a maximum daily dose of 400 mg; 200 mg p.o. q12h for adults.

     or

   - Cefdinir: 14 mg/mg/d p.o. in two divided doses for children with a maximum daily dose of 600 mg; 600 mg p.o. once daily for adults.

     If the patient is allergic to penicillin, then:

   - Trimethoprim/sulfamethoxazole: 8 to 12 mg/kg/d trimethoprim with 40 to 60 mg/kg/d sulfamethoxazole p.o. in two divided doses for children; 160 to 320 mg trimethoprim with 800 to 1600 mg sulfamethoxazole (one to two double-strength tablets) p.o. b.i.d. for adults.

     or

   - Moxifloxacin 400 mg p.o. daily (contraindicated in children).

     If exposure to MRSA is suspected, then:

   - Trimethoprim/sulfamethoxazole: 8 to 12 mg/kg/d trimethoprim with 40 to 60 mg/kg/d sulfamethoxazole p.o. in two divided doses for children; one to two tablets double-strength trimethoprim-sulfamethoxazole 160/800 mg p.o. q12h for adults.

     or

   - Doxycycline: 100 mg p.o. b.i.d. (contraindicated in children, pregnant women, and nursing mothers).

     or

   - Clindamycin: 10 to 30 mg/kg/d p.o. in three to four divided doses for children;

450 mg p.o. t.i.d. for adults. In addition to covering MRSA, this antibiotic also gives good coverage for streptococci and methicillin-sensitive *S. aureus*.

 NOTE: Patients with the following risk factors should be covered for MRSA: history of MRSA infection or colonization, recurrent skin infections, contact with someone known to have MRSA, admission to a healthcare or long-term care facility within the past year, placement of a permanent indwelling catheter, on hemodialysis, i.v. drug use, incarceration within the past 12 months, participation in sports that include skin-to-skin contact or sharing of equipment and clothing, and poor personal hygiene.

 NOTE: Oral antibiotics are maintained for 10 to 14 days.

   b. Moderate-to-severe preseptal cellulitis or any one of the following:

   - Patient appears toxic.
   - Patient may be noncompliant with outpatient treatment and follow up.
   - Child 5 years or younger.
   - No noticeable improvement or worsening after 24 to 48 hours of oral antibiotics.

     Admit to the hospital for i.v. antibiotics as follows:

   - Vancomycin: 10 to 15 mg/kg i.v. every 6 hours in children; 0.5 to 1 g i.v. q12h for adults. (Dose adjustment is needed in cases of impaired renal function.)

     Plus one of the following:

   - Ampicillin/sulbactam: 300 mg/kg/d i.v. in four divided doses for children; 3.0 g i.v. q6h for adults.
   - Piperacillin–tazobactam: 240 mg/kg/d i.v. in three divided doses for children; 4.5 g i.v. q6h adults.
   - Ceftriaxone: 80 to 100 mg/kg/d i.v. in two divided doses for children with a maximum of 4 g/d; 2 g i.v. q12h for adults.
   - Cefepime: 50 mg/kg q12h (max 2 g/dose) in children; 1 to 2 g i.v. q12h in adults.

6

- Ceftazidime: 90 to 150 mg/kg/day i.v. in three divided doses for children; 1 g i.v. q8–12h in adults.

  If the patient is allergic to penicillin, see 7.3.1, ORBITAL CELLULITIS, for alternatives.

> **NOTE:** Intravenous antibiotics can be changed to comparable oral antibiotics after significant improvement is observed. Systemic antibiotics are maintained for a complete 10- to 14-day course. See 7.3.1, ORBITAL CELLULITIS, for alternative treatment. In complicated cases or patients with multiple allergies, consider consultation with an infectious disease specialist for antibiotic management.

2. Warm compresses to the inflamed area t.i.d. p.r.n.
3. Polymyxin B/bacitracin ointment to the eye q.i.d. if secondary conjunctivitis is present.
4. Tetanus toxoid if needed. (See Appendix 2, TETANUS PROPHYLAXIS).
5. Nasal decongestants if sinusitis is present.
6. Orbital exploration and debridement are warranted if a fluctuant mass or abscess is present, or if a retained foreign body is suspected. Obtain Gram stain and culture of any drainage to guide antibiotic coverage. Avoid the orbital septum if possible. A drain may need to be placed.
7. Consider an infectious disease consult for patients who have failed oral antibiotics and require i.v. treatment.
8. Consider systemic steroids. As with orbital cellulitis, preseptal cellulitis will improve with proper antibiotic treatment of bacteria and surgical treatment of any nidus. In some cases, the inflammatory cascade caused by the infection is significant and may be slow to resolve. This may improve more quickly with a short course of steroids during or after antibiotic treatment for the infection. Steroid dosing and timing of initiation vary among clinicians. Physicians may start steroids simultaneously with antibiotics, after 24 to 48 hours of antibiotic coverage, or not at all.

Follow Up

Daily until clear and consistent improvement is demonstrated, then every 2 to 7 days until the condition has totally resolved. If preseptal cellulitis progresses despite antibiotic therapy, the patient is admitted to the hospital and a repeat (or initial) orbital CT scan is obtained. For patients already on p.o. antibiotics, switch to i.v. antibiotics (see 7.3.1, ORBITAL CELLULITIS).

6.11 Malignant Tumors of the Eyelid

Symptoms

Asymptomatic or mildly irritating eyelid lump.

Signs

Skin ulceration and inflammation with distortion of normal eyelid anatomy. Abnormal color, texture, or persistent bleeding. Loss of eyelashes (madarosis) or whitening of eyelashes (poliosis) over the lesion. Sentinel vessels may be seen. Diplopia or external ophthalmoplegia are ominous signs of a possible orbital invasion.

Differential Diagnosis of Benign Eyelid Tumors

- Seborrheic keratosis: Middle-aged or elderly patients. Brown-black, well-circumscribed, crust-like lesion, usually slightly elevated, with or without surrounding inflammation. May be removed by shave biopsy.
- Chalazion/hordeolum: Acute, erythematous, tender, well-circumscribed lesion. See 6.2, CHALAZION/HORDEOLUM.
- Cysts: Well-circumscribed white, yellow, or clear/skin-colored lesions on the eyelid margin or underneath the skin. Epidermal inclusion cysts, sebaceous cysts, and eccrine or apocrine hidrocystomas may be excised.
- Molluscum contagiosum: A viral infection of the epidermis, typically seen in children. Multiple small papules characterized by central umbilication. Can be severe in HIV-positive patients. May produce a chronic follicular conjunctivitis. Treatment is by unroofing and curettage. While some recommend curettage until bleeding occurs, there is no clear evidence that this is more effective. A variety of other therapies (e.g., cryotherapy, cautery, chemical peel, and laser) are used for lesions found elsewhere on the body but are typically

not necessary for periocular regions and may cause injury to the ocular surface. See 5.2, CHRONIC CONJUNCTIVITIS.

- Nevus: Benign melanocytic neoplasm, which may involve the dermis, the dermis–epidermis junction, or both. Congenital nevi may be present at, or shortly after, birth; however, most nevi appear during childhood and may enlarge during puberty. Nevi are well-circumscribed lesions, usually round or oval, with uniform pigmentation. Melanomas may develop within preexisting nevi and may manifest as a changing pigmented lesion and/or as a pigmented lesion with asymmetry of shape, irregular borders, color variegation, and possibly pruritus or bleeding. Suspicious lesions should be biopsied, preferably with the removal of the entire lesion to the subcutaneous fat.

- Xanthelasma: Multiple, often bilateral, soft yellow plaques of lipid-laden macrophages in the medial upper and sometimes lower eyelids. Patients 40 years and younger should have a serum cholesterol and lipid profile evaluation to rule out hypercholesterolemia. Surgical excision can be performed for cosmesis; however, recurrence is possible.

- Squamous papilloma: Soft, skin-colored lesions that may be smooth, rounded, or pedunculated. May enlarge or multiply over time. Often spontaneously regress. Occasionally squamous carcinomas can appear papillomatous. Therefore, excisional biopsy should be performed for suspicious lesions.

- Actinic keratosis: Round, erythematous, premalignant lesion with a scaly surface. Found in sun-exposed areas of skin. Treated by excisional biopsy.

- Inflammatory conditions: Blepharitis and blepharoconjunctivitis.

- Allergic conditions: Chronic contact dermatitis can appear unilateral, cause cilia loss, and simulate malignancy.

- Others: Verrucae from human papillomavirus, benign tumors of hair follicles, or sweat glands (e.g., syringoma), inverted follicular keratosis, neurofibroma, neurilemmoma, capillary hemangioma, cavernous hemangioma, and pseudoepitheliomatous hyperplasia. Necrobiotic xanthogranuloma nodules of multiple myeloma appear as yellow plaques or nodules that are often mistaken for xanthelasma.

Etiology

- Basal cell carcinoma: Most common malignant eyelid tumor, usually on the lower eyelid or medial canthus of middle-aged or elderly patients. Rarely metastasizes, but may be locally invasive, particularly when present in the medial canthal region. There are two major forms:
  - Nodular: Indurated, firm mass, commonly with telangiectasias over tumor margins. Sometimes the lesion center is ulcerated **(see Figure 6.11.1)**. On rare occasions, a cystic variant is seen.
  - Infiltrative: The classic variant of this form is the morpheaform lesion. A firm, flat, subcutaneous lesion with indistinct borders. More difficult to excise and may result in a large eyelid defect.

- Squamous cell carcinoma: Variable presentation, often appearing similar to basal cell carcinoma. Regional metastasis may occur and can be extensive with the propensity for perineural invasion. A premalignant lesion, actinic keratosis, may appear either as a scaly, erythematous flat lesion or as a cutaneous horn.

- Keratoacanthoma: This lesion was previously considered to be benign and self-limiting; however, it is now regarded as a low-grade squamous cell carcinoma. Clinically may resemble basal and squamous cell carcinomas. Typically, the lesion is elevated with rolled margins and a large central ulcer filled with keratin. Rapid growth with slow regression and even spontaneous resolution has been observed. Lesions usually involve the lower eyelid and can be destructive. Complete excision is recommended.

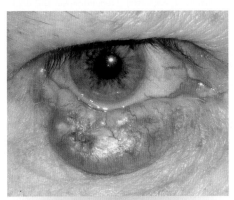
Figure 6.11.1 Basal cell carcinoma.

- Sebaceous carcinoma: More common in middle-aged or elderly patients, usually elderly women. Most common on the upper eyelid but may be multifocal, involving both the upper and the lower eyelids. Often confused with recurrent chalazia or intractable blepharitis. Loss of eyelashes and destruction of the meibomian gland orifices in the region of the tumor may occur. Regional and systemic metastasis or orbital extension is possible. Can occur many decades after prior radiation exposure to the eyelids **(see Figure 6.11.2)**.

- Others: Malignant melanoma, lymphoma, sweat gland carcinoma, metastasis (usually breast or lung), Merkel cell tumor, Kaposi sarcoma, and others.

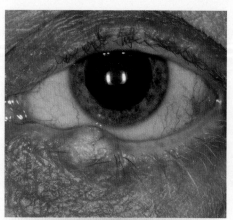

Figure 6.11.2 Sebaceous carcinoma.

Workup

1. History: Duration? Rapid or slow growth? Previous malignant skin lesion or other malignancies? Previous treatment of inflammatory or allergic condition? Previous radiation therapy? Associated pain?

2. External examination: Check the skin for additional lesions, palpate the preauricular, submaxillary, and cervical nodes to evaluate for metastasis.

3. Slit lamp examination: Look for telangiectasias on nodular tumors, loss of eyelashes in the region of the tumor, and meibomian orifice destruction. Evert eyelids of all patients with eyelid complaints.

4. Photograph or draw the lesion and its location for documentation.

5. Perform a biopsy of the lesion. An incisional biopsy is commonly performed when a malignancy is suspected. Depending on the depth of invasion, sentinel node biopsy may be indicated with melanoma and sebaceous carcinoma. Histopathologic confirmation must precede any extensive procedures.

6. Sebaceous carcinoma may be difficult to diagnose histopathologically. In the past, fresh tissue with oil red-O staining was recommended. This is no longer necessary if the pathologist is experienced with this malignancy.

7. For lymphoma, the pathologist would prefer the tissue to be sent fresh for flow cytometry. Contact the pathologist first. If confirmed, a systemic workup is indicated. See 7.4.2, ORBITAL TUMORS IN ADULTS.

Treatment

1. Basal cell carcinoma: Surgical excision with histologic evaluation of tumor margins either by frozen sections or by Mohs techniques. The entire tumor should be excised with clean margins. Cryotherapy and radiation are used rarely. Topical imiquimod, an immune modulator, might be beneficial but could be toxic to the ocular surface. Unresectable tumors can be treated by the oral Hedgehog pathway inhibitor vismodegib, although it is expensive and can cause systemic side effects. Patients are informed about the etiologic role of the sun and are advised to avoid unnecessary sunlight exposure and to use protective sunscreens.

2. Squamous cell carcinoma: Surgical excision is considered as first-line treatment. Radiation therapy is the second-best treatment after surgical excision. Topical imiquimod and topical or injectable interferon can be beneficial for elderly patients who are not surgical candidates. Patients are informed about the etiologic role of the sun. Referral to an oncologist or internist for regional and/or systemic workup and surveillance is important.

3. Sebaceous carcinoma: The approach is two-staged with stage 1 using map biopsies on the entire surface of the eye to ascertain the extent of Pagetoid spread or deep tumor. Stage 2 is performed after all biopsies are reviewed; Pagetoid spread is treated with cryotherapy whereas deep tumor requires

excision. Reconstruction is then provided. Close follow up of regional nodes is indicated. Exenteration is often required when orbital invasion is present. Referral to an oncologist or internist for systemic workup and surveillance is important with attention to the lymph nodes, lungs, brain, liver, and bone.

4. Malignant melanoma: Treatment requires wide surgical excision. The margins must be free of tumor and require permanent sections. Sentinel lymph node biopsy may be required depending on tumor depth. Referral to an oncologist or internist for regional and/or systemic workup and surveillance is imperative.

NOTE: Because both melanoma and sebaceous carcinoma are difficult to diagnose by frozen section, multiple excisions utilizing permanent sectioning may be necessary until all surgical margins are free of tumor. The cornea and globe must be protected during this interim time with lubrication or temporary tarsorrhaphy.

Follow Up

Initial follow up is every 1 to 4 weeks to ensure proper healing of the surgical site. Patients are then reevaluated every 6 to 12 months, or more frequently, for more aggressive lesions. Patients who have had one skin malignancy are at greater risk for additional malignancies.

6

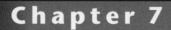

Chapter 7

Orbit

7.1 Orbital Disease

This section provides a framework to evaluate a variety of orbital disorders.

Symptoms

Eyelid swelling, bulging eye(s), and double vision are common. Pain, decreased visual acuity, decreased color vision, and changes in facial sensation can occur.

Signs

Critical. Globe dystopia (e.g., proptosis/exophthalmos, hypoglobus, and hyperglobus) and restriction of ocular motility, which can be confirmed by forced duction testing (see Appendix 6, FORCED DUCTION TEST AND FORCE GENERATION TEST). Resistance to retropulsion of the globe is common.

Differential Diagnosis of Proptosis

- Mass effect (e.g., infiltration or displacement of soft tissues by inflammatory, neoplastic, vascular, or infectious etiologies).
- Enlarged globe (e.g., myopia). Large, myopic eyes frequently have tilted discs and peripapillary crescents, and ultrasonography (US) reveals a long axial length. Asymmetric myopia may be present as a unilateral pseudoproptosis.
- Enophthalmos of the fellow eye (e.g., after an orbital floor fracture).
- Asymmetric eyelid position: Unilateral upper and/or lower eyelid retraction, or contralateral upper eyelid ptosis.
- Physiologically shallow orbits.

Etiology

Specific signs of orbital disease are rarely diagnostic. Orbital disease can be grouped into six broad categories to help tailor the necessary workup:

1. Inflammatory: Thyroid eye disease (TED), idiopathic orbital inflammatory syndrome (IOIS), sarcoidosis, granulomatosis with polyangiitis (GPA, formerly Wegener granulomatosis), reactive inflammation from paranasal sinusitis, IgG4-related disease, etc.
2. Infectious: Orbital cellulitis, subperiosteal abscess (SPA), mucormycosis, etc.
3. Neoplastic (discrete, infiltrative, or hematologic): Typically categorized as primary (e.g., solitary fibrous tumor), secondary (e.g., extension of sinus mucocele or intracranial meningioma, etc.), or metastatic. May be benign or malignant.

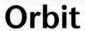 **NOTE:** As a general rule, any patient with a history of cancer and a new orbital process should be assumed to have metastatic disease unless proven otherwise.

4. Trauma: Orbital fracture, retrobulbar hemorrhage, orbital foreign body with or without secondary infection, carotid–cavernous fistula, etc.
5. Malformation: Skeletal abnormalities, congenital/genetic syndromes, etc.
6. Vascular: Usually either congenital or acquired and categorized as primary arterial (e.g., carotid–cavernous fistula) or venous (e.g., varix). Lymphangioma may also cause proptosis from intralesional hemorrhage.

Workup

1. History: Rapid or slow onset? Pain? Ocular bruit and/or pulsation? Fever, chills, systemic symptoms, skin rash, weight change? History of malignancy, diabetes, pulmonary disease, or renal disease? Trauma? History of sinonasal congestion, epistaxis? Smoking? Up to date

with health maintenance and age-appropriate screenings (e.g., mammography, prostate examination/screening)? Presence of systemic symptoms—weight loss/gain, fever, chills, night sweats, change in bowel habits, heat/cold intolerance?

2. Examination:

- Review vital signs, particularly temperature.
- Check visual acuity, size and reactivity of pupils, visual fields, color vision, and intra-ocular pressure. Check for pulsatility of semicircles on Goldmann tonometry.
- Check extraocular movements. Measure any ocular misalignment ([prisms or Maddox rod], see Appendix 3, COVER/UNCOVER AND ALTERNATE COVER TESTS and 10.7, ISOLATED FOURTH CRANIAL NERVE PALSY). Consider forced duction and force generation testing in select cases (see Appendix 6, FORCED DUCTION TEST AND FORCE GENERATION TEST).
- Check for globe dystopia. Tilt the patient's head back and look from below ("ant's-eye view"). Measure with a Hertel exophthalmometer. Position the exophthalmometer against the lateral orbital rims, not the lateral canthi. The average value is 17 mm with the upper limit of normal about 22 to 24 mm. A difference between the two eyes of more than 2 mm is considered abnormal. Can be used in conjunction with a Valsalva maneuver if a venous malformation is suspected. In addition to classic axial exophthalmos, also look for nonaxial displacement of the globe (e.g., hypoglobus and hyperglobus).
- Test resistance to retropulsion by gently pushing each globe into the orbit with your thumbs. Feel along the orbital rim for a mass. Check the conjunctival cul-de-sacs carefully and evert the upper eyelid.
- Check trigeminal and facial nerve function. Check for preauricular and cervical adenopathy.
- Perform a dilated examination to evaluate the optic nerves (pallor and swelling), posterior pole (especially for chorioretinal folds), and peripheral retina.

3. Consider automated perimetry if compressive optic neuropathy is suspected.

4. Imaging studies: Orbital computed tomography (CT, axial, coronal, and parasagittal views) or magnetic resonance imaging (MRI) with gadolinium and fat suppression, depending on suspected etiology. Orbital B-scan US with or without color Doppler imaging is useful if the diagnosis is uncertain or when a cystic or vascular lesion is suspected. Consider optical coherence tomography (OCT) to assess optic nerve contour. See Chapter 14, IMAGING MODALITIES IN OPHTHALMOLOGY.

5. Laboratory tests when appropriate: Triiodothyronine (T3), thyroxine (T4), thyroid-stimulating hormone (TSH), anti-thyroid autoantibodies (thyroid-stimulating immunoglobulin [TSI] and antithyroid peroxidase antibody [TPO]), angiotensin-converting enzyme (ACE), cytoplasmic staining, and perinuclear staining antineutrophil cytoplasmic antibody (cANCA and pANCA), lactate dehydrogenase (LDH), IgG/IgG4 levels, antinuclear antibody (ANA), serum protein electrophoresis (SPEP), complete blood count (CBC) with differential, blood urea nitrogen (BUN)/creatinine (especially if CT contrast or gadolinium is indicated), fasting blood sugar/hemoglobin A1c, blood cultures, etc.

6. Consider further systemic workup and additional imaging, depending on clinical suspicion and radiologic findings (e.g., metastasis, lymphoma, etc.).

7. Consider an excisional or incisional biopsy, as dictated by the working diagnosis. Fine-needle aspiration biopsy has a limited role in orbital diagnosis.

Additional workup, treatment, and follow-up vary according to the suspected diagnosis. See individual sections.

REFERENCES

Srinivasan A, Kleinberg T, Murchison AP, Bilyk JR. Serologic investigations in inflammatory orbital disease: part I. *Ophthalmic Plast Reconstr Surg.* 2016;32:321-328.

Srinivasan A, Kleinberg T, Murchison AP, Bilyk JR. Serologic investigations in inflammatory orbital disease: part II. *Ophthalmic Plast Reconstr Surg.* 2017;33:1-8.

7.2 Inflammatory Orbital Disease

7.2.1 THYROID EYE DISEASE

SYNONYMS: THYROID-RELATED ORBITOPATHY, GRAVES' DISEASE

Ocular Symptoms

Early: Nonspecific complaints including foreign-body sensation, redness, tearing, photophobia, and morning puffiness of the eyelids. Early symptoms are often nonspecific and may mimic allergy, blepharoconjunctivitis, chronic conjunctivitis, etc. Upper eyelid retraction tends to develop early.

Late: Additional eyelid and orbital symptoms including lateral flare, prominent eyes, persistent eyelid swelling, chemosis, double vision, "pressure" behind the eyes, and decreased vision.

Signs

(See Figure 7.2.1.1.)

Critical. Retraction of the upper eyelids with lateral flare (highly specific) and eyelid lag on downward gaze (von Graefe sign), lagophthalmos. Lower eyelid retraction is a very nonspecific sign and often presents as a normal finding. Unilateral or bilateral axial proptosis with variable resistance to retropulsion. When extraocular muscles are involved, elevation and abduction are commonly restricted and there is resistance on forced duction testing. Although often bilateral, unilateral or asymmetric TED is also frequently seen. Thickening of the extraocular muscles (inferior, medial, superior, and lateral, in order of frequency) without the involvement of the associated tendons may be noted on orbital imaging. Isolated enlargement of lateral rectus muscles is highly atypical of TED and requires further workup and possibly a biopsy. Isolated enlargement of the superior rectus/levator complex can occur in TED, but should be followed carefully for alternative causes, especially when upper eyelid retraction is not present.

Other. Reduced blink rate, significantly elevated IOP (especially in upgaze), injection of the blood vessels over the insertion sites of horizontal rectus muscles, superior limbic keratoconjunctivitis, superficial punctate keratopathy, or infiltrate or

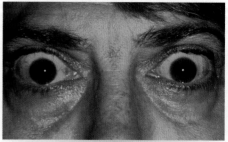

Figure 7.2.1.1 Thyroid-related orbitopathy with eyelid retraction and proptosis of the right eye.

ulceration from exposure keratopathy, afferent pupillary defect, dyschromatopsia, optic nerve swelling/pallor, and rarely choroidal folds.

> **NOTE:** Thickening of the extraocular muscles (EOMs) at the orbital apex can result in optic nerve compression and manifest in afferent pupillary defect, reduced color vision, visual field and visual acuity loss. Compressive optic neuropathy occurs in a minority of patients (5% to 7%) with TED, but must be ruled out in every patient at every visit. The optic neuropathy of TED almost invariably occurs in the setting of restrictive strabismus and increased resistance to retropulsion. Of note, in typical cases of compressive optic neuropathy from TED, axial proptosis is usually either absent or mild.

Systemic Signs

Hyperthyroidism is common (at least 80% of patients with TED). Symptoms include a rapid pulse, hot and dry skin, diffusely enlarged thyroid gland (goiter), weight loss, muscle wasting with proximal muscle weakness, hand tremor, pretibial dermopathy or myxedema, cardiac arrhythmias, and change in bowel habits. Some patients are hypothyroid (5% to 10%) or euthyroid (5% to 10%). Euthyroid patients should undergo thyroid function testing every 6 to 12 months; a significant proportion will develop thyroid abnormalities within 2 years. TED does not necessarily follow the associated thyroid dysfunction and may occur months to years before or after the thyroid dysfunction. The clinical progression of TED also has only a minor correlation with control of the thyroid dysfunction. A family history of thyroid dysfunction is common.

Concomitant myasthenia gravis with fluctuating double vision and ptosis may occur in a minority of patients. Always ask about bulbar symptoms (e.g., dysphagia, dysphonia, difficulty with breathing, weakness in proximal muscles, etc.) and fatigue in patients with suspected myasthenia gravis. The presence of ptosis (rather than upper eyelid retraction) or an adduction deficit in a patient with thyroid dysfunction and diplopia/external ophthalmoplegia should raise the possibility of myasthenia gravis (See 10.11, MYASTHENIA GRAVIS).

Differential Diagnosis of Upper Eyelid Retraction

- Previous eyelid surgery or trauma may produce eyelid retraction or eyelid lag.
- Severe contralateral ptosis may produce eyelid retraction because of Hering law, especially if the nonptotic eye is amblyopic.
- Oculomotor nerve palsy with aberrant regeneration: The upper eyelid may elevate with downward gaze, simulating eyelid lag (pseudo-von Graefe sign). Ocular motility may be limited, but the results of forced duction testing and orbital imaging are normal. Eyelid retraction is typically accentuated in adduction or in downgaze. See 10.6, ABERRANT REGENERATION OF THE THIRD CRANIAL NERVE.
- Parinaud syndrome: Eyelid retraction and limitation of upward gaze may accompany convergence-retraction nystagmus and mildly dilated pupils that react poorly to light with an intact near response (light-near dissociation).

Workup

1. History: Duration of symptoms? Pain? Change in vision? Known history of cancer or thyroid dysfunction? Smoker? Last mammogram, chest X-ray (especially in smokers), prostate examination/prostate-specific antigen (PSA) level?

2. Complete ocular examination to evaluate for exposure keratopathy (slit-lamp examination with fluorescein staining) and optic nerve compression (afferent pupillary defect, dyschromatopsia, optic nerve edema, automated perimetry, OCT). Extraocular motility (versions and ductions). Diplopia is measured with prisms or Maddox rod (see Appendix 3, COVER/UNCOVER AND ALTERNATE COVER TESTS and 10.7, ISOLATED FOURTH CRANIAL NERVE PALSY). Proptosis is measured with a Hertel exophthalmometer. Check for resistance to retropulsion. Check IOP in both primary and upgaze (increase in upgaze correlates with severity of inferior rectus muscle enlargement in TED). Dilated fundus examination with optic nerve assessment.

3. Imaging: CT of the orbit (axial and coronal views without contrast) is performed when the presentation is atypical (e.g., most cases of unilateral proptosis or any bilateral proptosis without upper eyelid retraction), or in the presence of severe congestive orbitopathy or optic neuropathy. CT in TED varies from patient to patient. In patients with restrictive strabismus and minimal proptosis ("myogenic variant"), imaging will show thickened EOMs without the involvement of the associated tendons and "apical crowding"—the loss of fat signal in the orbital apex because of enlarged EOMs. In patients with full or nearly full extraocular motility, severe proptosis, and exposure keratopathy ("lipogenic variant"), increased fat volume with minimal muscle involvement is typical.

4. Thyroid function tests (TFTs) (T3, T4, and TSH). These may be normal. TSI and TPO may sometimes be ordered and can be followed over time, and recent evidence suggests a correlation with disease activity. An elevated TSI and TPO may help guide the clinician toward a diagnosis of TED in atypical cases and guide treatment (see below).

5. Serum vitamin D level. Recent studies have shown that a subnormal result increases the risk of progressive orbitopathy.

6. Workup for suspected myasthenia gravis is necessary in selected cases. See 10.11, MYASTHENIA GRAVIS.

Treatment

1. Smoking cessation: All patients with TED who smoke must be explicitly told that continued tobacco use increases the risk of progression and the severity of orbitopathy. This conversation should be clearly documented in the medical record.

7

2. Consider teprotumumab (i.v. infusion of 10 mg/kg for the initial dose followed by an i.v. infusion of 20 mg/kg every 3 weeks for 7 additional infusions).

3. Refer the patient to a medical internist or endocrinologist for management of systemic thyroid disease, if present. If TFTs are normal, the patient's TFTs should be checked every 6 to 12 months. Not infrequently, a euthyroid patient with TED will have an elevated TSI and/or TPO.

4. Treat exposure keratopathy with artificial tears and lubrication or by taping eyelids closed at night (see 4.5, EXPOSURE KERATOPATHY). Wearing swim goggles at night may be helpful. The use of topical cyclosporine or lifitegrast drops for the treatment of ocular surface inflammation in TED is still under investigation, but is a reasonable long-term treatment option if dry eye syndrome is present.

5. Treat eyelid edema with cold compresses in the morning and head elevation at night. This management may not be very effective. Avoid diuretics.

6. Indications for orbital decompression surgery include optic neuropathy, worsening or severe exposure keratopathy despite adequate treatment, globe luxation, uncontrollably high IOP, and morbid proptosis.

7. A stepwise approach is used for surgical treatment, starting with orbital decompression (if needed), followed by strabismus surgery (for significant strabismus, if present), followed by eyelid surgery. Alteration of this sequence may lead to unpredictable results. Note that only a minority of patients with TED will need to undergo the entire surgical algorithm.

Other Treatment Modalities

• Corticosteroids: During the acute inflammatory phase, prednisone 1 mg/kg p.o. daily, tapered over 4 to 6 weeks, is a reasonable temporizing measure to improve proptosis and diplopia in preparation for orbital decompression surgery. There is evidence that the use of a 12-week course of pulsed intravenous corticosteroids (methylprednisolone 500 mg i.v. weekly for 6 weeks, followed by 250 mg i.v. weekly for 6 weeks) followed by a course of oral corticosteroids may result in better long-term control of TED with fewer systemic side effects than oral corticosteroids

and is a reasonable option to offer patients in the acute phase of TED. Other experts question the long-term efficacy of this regimen. Periorbital corticosteroid injections are also used by some experts, but may be suboptimal to oral corticosteroids. Chronic systemic corticosteroids for long-term management should be avoided because of the systemic side effects. If systemic corticosteroids are used, a detailed discussion of the potential short- and long-term risks should be documented. The patient should undergo a baseline dual-energy X-ray absorptiometry bone density scan and be started on vitamin D/calcium supplements and gastric prophylaxis with a proton pump inhibitor. Close follow up with a primary care provider is also important for the management of blood sugar elevations and other side effects.

• Orbital radiation: The use and efficacy of low-dose orbital radiation in the management of TED remain controversial. It may be used as a modality in the acute inflammatory phase of TED or as a means to limit progression and provide long-term control. Radiation therapy appears to decrease the severity and progression of restrictive strabismus in patients with active TED; efficacy in managing other aspects of TED (including optic neuropathy) has not been proved definitively, but is advocated by some experts. Radiation therapy should be used with caution in patients with diabetes, as it may worsen diabetic retinopathy, and in vasculopaths, as it may increase the risk of radiation retinopathy or optic neuropathy, although neither of these risks have been proven definitively. All patients offered radiation therapy should be informed of the potential risks. If used, radiation is best performed according to strict protocols with carefully controlled dosage and shielding under the supervision of a radiation oncologist familiar with the technique. Typically, a total dose of 20 Gy is administered in 10 to 14 fractions over 2 weeks. Treatment may transiently exacerbate inflammatory changes and an oral prednisone taper may mitigate these symptoms. Improvement is often seen within a few weeks of treatment, but may take several months to attain the maximal effect.

• Selenium supplementation: Data from Europe confirm that the use of selenium supplementation (an antioxidant) reduces the severity and progression of mild-to-moderate

TED. It remains unclear whether this finding is applicable in the United States, where no dietary selenium deficiency (as is present in certain European countries) exists. It is reasonable to offer this therapy to women with mild-to-moderate, active TED at a dose of 100 μg p.o. b.i.d for 6 months. Caution should be used in the use of selenium supplementation in men, especially with a family history of prostate cancer; some studies have suggested an increased risk of prostate cancer in males with high selenium levels, although this issue does not appear to have been settled conclusively.

- Vitamin D supplementation: Recent evidence suggests that vitamin D deficiency may be a risk factor for TED. Vitamin D supplementation has been recommended with the hope of decreasing the risk of TED progression.
- Biologics: Limited data are available on the use of biologic agents (e.g., rituximab, infliximab, adalimumab, etc.), with some studies showing efficacy and others finding none. Their use as primary therapy *in lieu* of more conventional modalities is, at present, off-label and controversial. Furthermore, there appears to be little consensus as to the most effective, specific biologic target in TED. Recently, the use of teprotumumab, a monoclonal antibody inhibitor of the insulin-like growth factor I receptor (IGF-IR) has shown promise in the management of TED. It is the only FDA-approved targeted therapy for patients with moderate to severe TED; the drug is effective in decreasing exophthalmos and diplopia.
- Visual loss from optic neuropathy: Treat immediately with prednisone 1 mg/kg/d with close monitoring. In cases of severe visual loss, admission for pulsed intravenous therapy may be indicated. Radiation therapy may be offered for mild-to-moderate optic neuropathy, with the understanding that there is typically a lag in the treatment effect. Posterior orbital decompression surgery (for mild-to-severe optic neuropathy), either medial or lateral, is essential and usually effective in rapidly reversing or stabilizing the optic neuropathy. Anterior orbital decompression is usually ineffective in treating TED optic neuropathy. Teprotumumab has also been shown to effectively manage optic neuropathy in TED based on small series of patients.

Follow Up

1. Optic nerve compression requires immediate attention and close follow up.
2. Patients with advanced exposure keratopathy and severe proptosis also require prompt attention and close follow up.
3. Patients with minimal-to-no exposure problems and mild-to-moderate proptosis are re-evaluated every 3 to 6 months. Because of the potential risk of optic neuropathy, patients with restrictive strabismus may be followed more frequently.
4. Patients with fluctuating diplopia or ptosis should be evaluated for myasthenia gravis (see 10.11, MYASTHENIA GRAVIS).
5. All patients with TED are instructed to return immediately with any new visual problems, worsening diplopia, or significant ocular irritation. All smokers with TED must be reminded to discontinue smoking at every office visit, and appropriate referral to their primary physician for a smoking cessation program is indicated.

REFERENCES

Marcocci C, Kahaly GJ, Krassas GE, et al. Selenium and the course of mild Graves' orbitopathy. *N Engl J Med.* 2011;364:1920-1931.

Heisel CJ, Riddering AL, Andrews CA, Kahana A. Serum vitamin D deficiency is an independent risk factor for thyroid eye disease. Ophthalmic Plast Reconstr Surg. 2020;36(1):17-20.

Bradley EA, Gower EW, Bradley DJ, et al. Orbital radiation for graves ophthalmopathy: a report by the American Academy of Ophthalmology. *Ophthalmology.* 2008;115(2):398-409.

Smith TJ, Kahaly GJ, Ezra DG, et al. Teprotumumab for thyroid-associated ophthalmopathy. *N Engl J Med.* 2017;376:1748-1761.

7.2.2 IDIOPATHIC ORBITAL INFLAMMATORY SYNDROME

SYNONYM: INFLAMMATORY ORBITAL PSEUDOTUMOR

Symptoms

May be acute, recurrent, or chronic. An explosive, painful onset is the hallmark of IOIS, but is present in only 65% of patients; the remainder may have a more insidious and relatively painless presentation. Pain, prominent red eye, "boggy" pink eyelid edema, double vision, or decreased vision. Children may have concomitant constitutional symptoms (fever, headache, vomiting, abdominal pain, and lethargy) and bilateral or sequential presentation, neither of which is typical in adults.

Signs

Critical. Proptosis and/or ocular motility restriction, usually unilateral, typically of explosive onset. On imaging studies, soft tissue anatomy is involved in varying degrees. The EOMs are thickened in cases of myositis; involvement of the tendon may occur, but is by no means essential or pathognomonic. The sclera (in posterior scleritis), Tenon capsule (in tenonitis), orbital fat, or lacrimal gland (in dacryoadenitis) may be involved. The paranasal sinuses are usually clear.

Other. Boggy, pink eyelid erythema and edema, conjunctival injection and chemosis, lacrimal gland enlargement or a palpable orbital mass, decreased vision, uveitis, increased IOP, hyperopic shift (typically in posterior scleritis), optic nerve swelling or atrophy (uncommon), and chorioretinal folds.

> **NOTE:** Bilateral IOIS in adults can occur, but should prompt a careful evaluation to rule out a systemic cause (e.g., sarcoidosis, GPA, IgG4-related orbitopathy, metastases [especially breast cancer], and lymphoma). Children may have bilateral disease in one-third of cases and may have associated systemic disorders.

Differential Diagnosis

- Orbital cellulitis and/or abscess.
- TED.
- Other noninfectious orbital inflammatory conditions: sarcoidosis, GPA, IgG4-related orbitopathy, amyloidosis, eosinophilic GPA, Sjögren syndrome, rheumatoid arthritis, systemic lupus erythematosus, histiocytosis, etc.
- Lymphoproliferative disease (including lymphoma).

- Primary orbital malignancy (e.g., rhabdomyosarcoma).
- Metastasis.
- Leaking dermoid cyst.
- Lymphangioma with acute hemorrhage.
- Vascular malformation, including carotid-cavernous fistula (CCF).
- Spontaneous orbital hemorrhage.
- Necrotic uveal melanoma.

Workup

See 7.1, ORBITAL DISEASE, for general orbital workup.

1. History: Previous episodes? Any other systemic symptoms or diseases? History of cancer? Smoking? Last mammogram, chest X-ray, colonoscopy, prostate examination? History of breathing problems? A careful review of systems is warranted. Fever, night sweats, and weight loss?

2. Complete ocular examination, including color vision, extraocular motility, exophthalmometry, IOP, and dilated funduscopic evaluation.

3. Vital signs, particularly temperature.

4. Imaging: Orbital CT (axial, coronal, and parasagittal views) with contrast: may show a thickened posterior sclera (the "ring sign" of 360 degrees of scleral thickening), orbital fat or lacrimal gland involvement, or thickening of the extraocular muscles (± their tendons). Bony erosion is very rare in IOIS and warrants further workup. Orbital MRI with contrast and fat suppression: May show EOM enlargement, infiltration of orbital fat, enlargement of the lacrimal gland, thickening of posterior Tenon/sclera, and enhancement along the optic nerve (perineuritis). In IOIS, the enhancement tends to "spill over" from an anatomic nidus into adjacent tissue (e.g., from EOM into surrounding orbital fat).

5. Blood tests as needed (e.g., bilateral or atypical cases): Westergren ESR, CBC with differential, ANA, ACE, cANCA, pANCA, LDH, IgG4/IgG levels, SPEP, BUN/creatinine, and fasting blood sugar/hemoglobin A1c (before instituting systemic corticosteroids). If sarcoidosis is suspected, consider chest CT which is

significantly more sensitive than chest X-ray (CXR). Mammography and prostate evaluation are warranted in specific or atypical cases. Consider QuantiFERON-TB Gold testing before instituting corticosteroids in at-risk patients.

6. If possible, perform an incisional biopsy of involved orbital tissue if easily accessible with minimal morbidity *before* instituting corticosteroid therapy (corticosteroid therapy may mask the true diagnosis). The lacrimal gland is often involved in IOIS and is relatively easy to access surgically; strong consideration should be given to biopsy all cases of suspected inflammatory dacryoadenitis. However, a biopsy of other orbital structures (extraocular muscle and orbital apex) is typically avoided in cases of classic IOIS because of the potential surgical risks; biopsy of these structures is reserved for atypical or recurrent cases. Always be suspicious of metastatic disease in any patient with a history of cancer.

Treatment

1. Prednisone 1 to 1.2 mg/kg/d as an initial dose in adults and children, along with gastric prophylaxis (e.g., omeprazole 40 mg p.o. daily). All patients are warned about potential systemic side effects and are instructed to follow up with their primary physicians to monitor blood sugar and electrolytes.

2. Low-dose radiation therapy may be used when the patient does not respond to systemic corticosteroids, when the disease recurs as corticosteroids are tapered, or when corticosteroids pose a significant risk to the patient. Radiation therapy should only be used once orbital biopsy, if anatomically and medically feasible, has excluded other etiologies.

3. Steroid-sparing agents (e.g., methotrexate, cyclophosphamide, etc.) in cases that do not respond to or recur with corticosteroid therapy. Biopsy of affected tissue, when feasible, is indicated to rule out malignancy.

4. Biologic therapy may be considered in cases that fail other modalities. The efficacy of specific biologic agents (e.g., CD20 antibody, tumor necrosis factor-α (TNF-α) antibody, etc.) in IOIS is not known. There is evidence

that IOIS is a T-cell driven process with elevated cytokines (including TNF-α); infliximab and adalimumab may be reasonable biologics to consider in recalcitrant or recurrent IOIS.

Follow Up

Re-evaluate in 1 to 2 days. Patients who respond dramatically to corticosteroids are maintained at the initial dose for 3 to 5 days, followed by a slow taper to 40 mg/d over 2 weeks, and an even slower taper below 20 mg/d, usually over several weeks. If the patient does not respond dramatically to appropriate corticosteroid doses, biopsy should be strongly considered. Recurrences of IOIS are not uncommon, especially at lower corticosteroid doses.

NOTE: IgG4-related disease is a recently described fibroinflammatory condition typified by lymphoplasmacytic infiltration of soft tissues by IgG4+ plasma cells, often with systemic involvement. Elevated serum levels of IgG4 may be present. Clinical management follows the typical algorithm of other orbital inflammations: systemic corticosteroids followed by steroid-sparing agents in chronic or recalcitrant cases. IgG4-related orbitopathy may involve any of the orbital soft tissues, but does not usually present in the explosive fashion of classic IOIS; enlargement and infiltration of sensory nerves on orbital imaging studies is a classic feature of IgG4-related orbitopathy. Definitive diagnosis requires histopathologic confirmation and IgG4 immunostaining. There is evidence from East Asia that IgG4-related disease may increase the risk of eventual lymphoma.

REFERENCES

Mombaerts I, Rose GE, Garrity JA. Orbital inflammation: biopsy first. *Surv Ophthalmol.* 2016;61:664-669.

Mombaerts I, Bilyk JR, Rose GE, et al. Consensus on diagnostic criteria of idiopathic orbital inflammation using a modified Delphi approach. *JAMA Ophthalmol.* 2017;135:769-776.

McNab AA, McKelvie P. IgG4-related ophthalmic disease. Part I: background and pathology. *Ophthalmic Plast Reconstr Surg.* 2015;31:83-88.

McNab AA, McKelvie P. IgG4-related ophthalmic disease. Part II: clinical aspects. *Ophthalmic Plast Reconstr Surg.* 2015;31:167-178.

7.3 Infectious Orbital Disease

7.3.1 ORBITAL CELLULITIS

Symptoms

Red eye, pain, blurred vision, double vision, eyelid and/or periorbital swelling, nasal congestion/discharge, sinus headache/pressure/congestion, tooth pain, infra- and/or supraorbital pain, or hypesthesia.

Signs

(See Figures 7.3.1.1 and 7.3.1.2.)

Critical. Eyelid edema, erythema, warmth, and tenderness. Conjunctival chemosis and injection, proptosis, and restricted extraocular motility with pain on attempted eye movement are usually present. Signs of optic neuropathy (e.g., afferent pupillary defect and dyschromatopsia) may be present in severe cases.

Other. Decreased vision, retinal venous congestion, optic disc edema, purulent discharge, decreased periorbital sensation, and fever. CT scan usually shows adjacent sinusitis (typically at least an ethmoid sinusitis) and possibly a subperiosteal orbital collection.

Differential Diagnosis

See 7.1, ORBITAL DISEASE.

Etiology

- Direct extension from a paranasal sinus infection (especially ethmoiditis), focal periorbital infection (e.g., infected hordeolum, dacryoadenitis, dacryocystitis, and panophthalmitis), or dental infection.
- Sequela of orbital trauma (e.g., orbital fracture, penetrating trauma, and retained intraorbital foreign body).
- Sequela of eyelid, orbital, or paranasal sinus surgery.
- Sequela of other ocular surgery or intraocular infection (e.g., panophthalmitis) (less common).
- Vascular extension (e.g., seeding from a systemic bacteremia or locally from facial cellulitis via venous anastomoses).
- Extension from a septic cavernous sinus thrombosis.

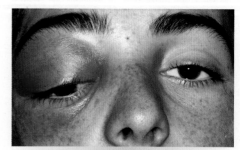

Figure 7.3.1.1 Orbital cellulitis.

NOTE: In cases of unsuspected retained foreign body, cellulitis may develop months after injury (see 3.12, INTRAORBITAL FOREIGN BODY).

Organisms

- Adult: *Staphylococcus* species, *Streptococcus* species, and *Bacteroides* species.
- Children: *Haemophilus influenzae* (rare in vaccinated children).
- Following trauma: Gram-negative rods.
- Dental abscess: Mixed, aggressive aerobes and anaerobes.
- Immunocompromised patients (diabetes, chemotherapy, and HIV infection): Fungi

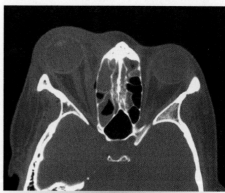

Figure 7.3.1.2 CT of right orbital cellulitis showing fat stranding and right ethmoiditis.

including those that produce zygomycosis infections (e.g., *Mucor*) and *Aspergillus*.

Workup

See 7.1, ORBITAL DISEASE, for a nonspecific orbital workup.

1. History: Trauma or surgery? Ear, nose, throat, or systemic infection? Tooth pain or recent dental abscess? Stiff neck or mental status changes? Diabetes or an immunosuppressive illness? Use of immunosuppressive agents?

2. Complete ophthalmic examination to evaluate for orbital signs including afferent pupillary defect, restriction or pain with ocular motility, proptosis, increased resistance to retropulsion, elevated IOP, decreased color vision, decreased skin sensation, or an optic nerve or fundus abnormality.

3. Check vital signs, mental status, and neck flexibility. Check for preauricular or cervical lymphadenopathy. Evaluate nasal passages for signs of eschar/fungal involvement in diabetic, acidotic, or immunocompromised patients.

4. Imaging: CT scan of the orbits and paranasal sinuses (axial, coronal, and parasagittal views, with contrast if possible) to confirm the diagnosis and to rule out a retained foreign body, orbital or SPA, paranasal sinus disease, cavernous sinus thrombosis, or intracranial extension.

5. Laboratory studies: CBC with differential and blood cultures.

6. Explore and debride any penetrating wound, if present, and obtain a Gram stain and culture of any drainage (e.g., blood and chocolate agars, Sabouraud dextrose agar, and thioglycolate broth). Obtain CT before wound exploration to rule out skull base foreign body.

7. Consult neurosurgery for suspected meningitis for management and possible lumbar puncture. If paranasal sinusitis is present, consider a consultation with otorhinolaryngology for possible surgical drainage. Consider an infectious disease consultation in atypical, severe, or unresponsive cases. If a dental source is suspected, oral maxillofacial surgery should be consulted urgently for assessment, since infections from this area tend to be aggressive, potentially vision threatening, and may spread into the cavernous sinus.

NOTE: Zygomycosis is an orbital, nasal, and sinus disease occurring in diabetic or otherwise immunocompromised patients. Typically associated with severe pain and external ophthalmoplegia. Profound visual loss may rapidly occur. Metabolic acidosis may be present. Sino-orbital zygomycosis is rapidly progressive and life threatening. See 10.10, CAVERNOUS SINUS AND ASSOCIATED SYNDROMES (MULTIPLE OCULAR MOTOR NERVE PALSIES).

Treatment

1. Admit the patient to the hospital and consider consult with an infectious disease specialist and otorhinolaryngologist.

2. Broad-spectrum intravenous antibiotics to cover Gram-positive, Gram-negative, and anaerobic organisms are recommended for 48 to 72 hours, followed by oral medication for at least 1 week. The specific antibiotic agents vary.

   - In patients from the community with no recent history of hospitalization, nursing home stay, or institutional stay, we currently recommend ampicillin–sulbactam 3 g i.v. q6h for adults; 300 mg/kg per day in four divided doses for children, a maximum daily dose of 12 g ampicillin–sulbactam (8 g ampicillin component);

     or

   - piperacillin–tazobactam 4.5 g i.v. q8h or 3.375 g q6h for adults; 240 mg of piperacillin component/kg/day in three divided doses for children, and a maximum daily dose of 18 g piperacillin.

   - In patients suspected of harboring hospital-associated methicillin-resistant *Staphylococcus aureus* (HA-MRSA) or in those with suspected meningitis, add concurrent intravenous vancomycin at 15 to 20 mg/kg q8–12h for adults with normal renal function and 40 to 60 mg/kg/d in three or four divided doses for children, with a maximum daily dose of 2 g. *For adults who are allergic to penicillin but can tolerate cephalosporins, use vancomycin as dosed above plus:* Ceftriaxone 2 g i.v. daily and metronidazole 500 mg i.v. q8h (not to exceed 4 g/d).

   - For adults who are allergic to penicillin/cephalosporin, treat with a combination of

7

a fluoroquinolone (for patients >17 years of age, moxifloxacin 400 mg i.v. daily or ciprofloxacin 400 mg i.v. q12h or levofloxacin 750 mg i.v. daily) and metronidazole 500 mg i.v. q8h.

> **NOTE:** Antibiotic dosages may need to be reduced in the presence of renal insufficiency or failure. Peak and trough levels of vancomycin are usually monitored, and dosages are adjusted as needed. BUN and creatinine levels are monitored closely. Also, be aware that many antibiotics (especially tetracycline derivatives) may change the efficacy of warfarin and other anticoagulants. It is prudent to obtain internal medicine consultation for the management of anticoagulants while the patient is using antibiotics.

> **NOTE:** The incidence of community-acquired methicillin-resistant *S. aureus* (CA-MRSA) is increasing in the United States, especially in urban areas. It is extremely difficult to clinically distinguish CA-MRSA from more conventional microbial pathogens. CA-MRSA may progress more rapidly and present with greater clinical severity than typical bacterial pathogens, but these are subjective criteria. It is prudent to cover CA-MRSA in severe cases of orbital cellulitis, in cases with a suspected skin source, in cases that have failed conventional therapy, or in areas of high CA-MRSA incidence. CA-MRSA is typically treated with tetracycline or a tetracycline derivative, trimethoprim/sulfamethoxazole, or clindamycin, although clindamycin resistance is on the rise.

- Nasal decongestant spray as needed for up to 3 days. Nasal corticosteroid spray may also be added to quicken the resolution of sinusitis.
- Erythromycin or bacitracin ointment q.i.d. for corneal exposure and chemosis if needed.
- If the orbit is tight, an optic neuropathy is present, or the IOP is severely elevated, immediate canthotomy/cantholysis may be needed. See 3.10, TRAUMATIC RETROBULBAR HEMORRHAGE for indications and technique.
- The use of systemic corticosteroids in the management of orbital cellulitis remains controversial. If systemic corticosteroids

are considered, it is probably safest to wait 24 to 48 hours until an adequate intravenous antibiotic load has been given (three to four doses). Studies of pediatric orbital cellulitis with or without abscess found that the concomitant use of systemic corticosteroids with antibiotics shortened the length of intravenous antibiotic therapy and hospital stay.

Follow Up

Re-evaluate at least twice daily in the hospital for the first 48 hours. Severe infections may require multiple daily examinations. Clinical improvement may take 24 to 36 hours.

1. Progress is monitored by:
   - Patient's symptoms.
   - Temperature and white blood cell (WBC) count.
   - Visual acuity and evaluation of optic nerve function.
   - Extraocular motility.
   - Degree of proptosis and any displacement of the globe (significant displacement may indicate an abscess).
   - C-reactive protein (CRP) has been found to be a helpful clinical marker in some studies. One study suggested initiating oral corticosteroids with antibiotic therapy at a threshold CRP of ≤4 mg/dL.

> **NOTE:** If clinical deterioration is noted after an adequate antibiotic load (three to four doses), a CT scan of the orbit and brain with contrast should be repeated to look for abscess formation (see 7.3.2, SUBPERIOSTEAL ABSCESS). If an abscess is found, surgical drainage may be required. Because radiographic findings may lag behind the clinical examination, clinical deterioration may be the only indication for surgical drainage. Other conditions that should be considered when the patient is not improving include cavernous sinus thrombosis, meningitis, resistant organism (HA-MRSA, CA-MRSA), aggressive organism (often from an undiagnosed odontogenic source), or a noninfectious etiology.

2. Evaluate the cornea for signs of exposure.
3. Check IOP.

4. Examine the retina and optic nerve for signs of posterior compression (e.g., chorioretinal folds), inflammation, or exudative retinal detachment.

5. If orbital cellulitis is clearly and consistently improving, then the regimen can be changed to oral antibiotics (depending on the culture and sensitivity results) to complete a 10- to 14-day course. We often use:

- Amoxicillin/clavulanate: 25 to 45 mg/kg/d p.o. in two divided doses for children and a maximum daily dose of 90 mg/kg/d; 875 mg p.o. q12h for adults;

  or

- Cefpodoxime: 10 mg/kg/d p.o. in two divided doses for children and a maximum daily dose of 400 mg; 200 mg p.o. q12h for adults;

  or

- If CA-MRSA is suspected, recommended oral treatment regimens include doxycycline 100 mg p.o. q12h (not in pregnant or nursing women and not in children younger than 8 years), one to two tablets trimethoprim/sulfamethoxazole 160/800 mg p.o. q12h, clindamycin 450 mg p.o. q6h, or linezolid 600 mg p.o. b.i.d. (only with approval from an infectious disease specialist, given current low resistance).

The patient is examined every few days as an outpatient until the condition resolves and instructed to return immediately with worsening signs or symptoms.

NOTE: Medication noncompliance is an extremely common reason for recurrence or failure to improve. The oral antibiotic regimen should be individualized for ease of use and affordability. Effective generic alternatives to brand name antibiotics include doxycycline and trimethoprim/sulfamethoxazole.

References

Yen MT, Yen KG. Effect of corticosteroids in the acute management of pediatric orbital cellulitis with subperiosteal abscess. *Ophthalmic Plast Reconstr Surg.* 2005;21:363-366.

Davies BW, Smith JM, Hink EM, Durairaj VD. C-reactive protein as a marker for initiating steroid treatment in children with orbital cellulitis. *Ophthalmic Plast Reconstr Surg.* 2015;31:364-368.

7.3.2 SUBPERIOSTEAL ABSCESS

Signs and Symptoms

Similar to orbital cellulitis, though may be magnified in scale. Suspect a subperiosteal abscess (SPA) if a patient with orbital cellulitis fails to improve or deteriorates after 48 to 72 hours of intravenous antibiotics.

Differential Diagnosis

- Intraorbital abscess: Rare because the periorbita is an excellent barrier to intraorbital spread. May be seen following penetrating trauma, previous surgery, retained foreign body, extrascleral extension of endophthalmitis, extension of SPA, or from endogenous seeding. Treatment is surgical drainage and intravenous antibiotics. Drainage may be difficult because of several isolated loculations.

- Cavernous sinus thrombosis: Rare in the era of antibiotics. Most commonly seen with zygomycosis (i.e., mucormycosis) (see 10.10, CAVERNOUS SINUS AND ASSOCIATED SYNDROMES [MULTIPLE OCULAR MOTOR NERVE PALSIES]). In bacterial cases, the patient is usually also septic and may be obtunded and hemodynamically unstable. Dental infections have a propensity for aggressive behavior and may spread along the midfacial and skull base venous plexuses into the cavernous sinus. Prognosis is guarded in all cases. Manage with hemodynamic support (possibly in an intensive care unit), broad-spectrum antibiotics, and surgical drainage if an infectious nidus is identified (e.g., paranasal sinuses, tooth abscess, and orbit). Anticoagulation can be considered to limit the propagation of the thrombosis into the central venous sinuses.

Workup

See 7.3.1, ORBITAL CELLULITIS, for workup. In addition:

1. Obtain CT with contrast, which allows for easier identification and extent of an abscess. In cases of suspected cavernous sinus thrombosis, discuss with the radiologist before CT, since special CT techniques and windows may help with diagnosis. MRI may also be indicated in cases of skull base spread of infection.

NOTE: All orbital cellulitis patients who do not improve after 48 to 72 hours of intravenous antibiotic therapy should undergo repeat imaging.

Treatment

1. Microbes involved in SPA formation vary and are to a degree related to the age of the patient. The causative microbes influence response to intravenous antibiotics and the need for surgical drainage. See **Table 7.3.2.1**.

> 📋 **NOTE:** These are guidelines only. All patients with SPA should be followed closely and managed by appropriate subspecialists, often with a combined approach (e.g., otorhinolaryngology). If an optic neuropathy is present or if the abscess is large, emergent drainage of the abscess is required. Adequate drainage may require orbital exploration. In children, a large SPA (>1250 mm^3) with frontal sinus involvement often requires drainage. Simultaneous drainage of both the SPA and the paranasal sinuses appears to decrease the recurrence rate of SPA when compared to SPA drainage alone.

2. Leave an orbital drain in place for 24 to 48 hours to prevent abscess reformation.

3. Intracranial extension necessitates neurosurgical involvement.

4. Expect dramatic and rapid improvement after adequate drainage. Additional imaging, exploration, and drainage may be indicated if improvement does not occur rapidly.

5. Do not reimage immediately unless the patient is deteriorating postoperatively. Imaging usually lags behind clinical response by at least 48 to 72 hours.

TABLE 7.3.2.1 Age and Subperiosteal Abscess

Age (y)	Cultures	Need to Drain
<9	Sterile (58%) or single aerobe	No in 93%
9 to 14	Mixed aerobe and anaerobe	±
>14	Mixed, anaerobes in all	Yes

From Harris GJ. Subperiosteal abscess of the orbit: older children and adults require aggressive treatment. *Ophthal Plast Reconstr Surg.* 2001;17(6):395-397.

REFERENCES

Garcia GH, Harris GJ. Criteria for nonsurgical management of subperiosteal abscess of the orbit: analysis of outcomes 1988-1998. *Ophthalmology.* 2000;107:1454-1458.

Todman MS, Enzer YR. Medical management versus surgical intervention of pediatric orbital cellulitis: The importance of subperiosteal abscess volume as a new criterion. *Ophthalmic Plast Reconstr Surg.* 2011;27:255-259.

Dewan MA, Meyer DR, Wladis EJ. Orbital cellulitis with subperiosteal abscess: demographics and management outcomes. *Ophthalmic Plast Reconstr Surg.* 2011;27:330-332.

7.3.3 ACUTE DACRYOADENITIS: INFECTION/INFLAMMATION OF THE LACRIMAL GLAND

Symptoms

Unilateral pain, redness, and swelling over the outer one-third of the upper eyelid, often with tearing or discharge. Typically occurs in children and young adults.

Signs

(See Figures 7.3.3.1 and 7.3.3.2.)

Critical. Erythema, swelling, and tenderness over the outer one-third of the upper eyelid. May be associated with hyperemia of the palpebral lobe of the lacrimal gland, S-shaped upper eyelid.

Other. Ipsilateral preauricular lymphadenopathy, ipsilateral conjunctival chemosis temporally, fever, and elevated WBC.

Differential Diagnosis

- Hordeolum: Tender eyelid nodule from the blocked gland. See 6.2, CHALAZION/HORDEOLUM.

- Preseptal cellulitis: Erythema and warmth of the eyelids and the surrounding soft tissue. See 6.10, PRESEPTAL CELLULITIS.

- Orbital cellulitis: Proptosis and limitation of ocular motility often accompany eyelid erythema and swelling. See 7.3.1, ORBITAL CELLULITIS.

- IOIS involving the lacrimal gland: May have concomitant proptosis, downward displacement of the globe, or limitation of extraocular

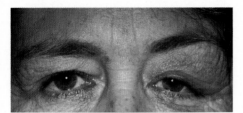

Figure 7.3.3.1 External photograph of dacryoadenitis.

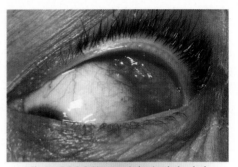

Figure 7.3.3.2 Hyperemic lacrimal gland of dacryoadenitis.

motility. Typically afebrile with a normal WBC. Does not respond to antibiotics but improves dramatically with systemic steroids. See 7.2.2, IDIOPATHIC ORBITAL INFLAMMATORY SYNDROME.

- Leaking dermoid cyst: Dermoid cysts often occur either superolaterally or superomedially. Leakage causes an intense and acute inflammatory reaction.

- Rhabdomyosarcoma: Most common pediatric orbital malignancy. Rapid presentation, but pain and erythema occur in only a minority of cases. See 7.4.1, ORBITAL TUMORS IN CHILDREN.

- Primary malignant lacrimal gland tumor or lacrimal gland metastasis: Commonly produces a displacement of the globe or proptosis. May present with an acute inflammatory clinical picture, but more often presents as a subacute process. Pain is common secondary to perineural spread along sensory nerves. Often palpable, evident on CT scan. See 7.6, LACRIMAL GLAND MASS/CHRONIC DACRYOADENITIS.

- Retained foreign body, with a secondary infectious or inflammatory process. The patient may not remember any history of penetrating trauma.

Etiology

- Inflammatory, noninfectious: By far the most common. A more indolent and painless course is seen in lymphoproliferation, sarcoidosis, IgG4-related disease, etc. More acute and painful presentation in IOIS.

- Bacterial: Rare. Usually due to S. aureus, Neisseria gonorrhoeae, or streptococci.

- Viral: Seen in mumps, infectious mononucleosis, influenza, and varicella zoster. May result in severe dry eye due to lacrimal gland fibrosis. Usually bilateral.

Workup

The following is performed when an acute etiology is suspected. When the disease does not respond to medical therapy or another etiology is being considered, see 7.6, LACRIMAL GLAND MASS/CHRONIC DACRYOADENITIS.

1. History: Acute or chronic? Fever? Discharge? Systemic infection or viral syndrome?

2. Palpate the eyelid and the orbital rim for a mass.

3. Evaluate the resistance of each globe to retropulsion.

4. Check for proptosis by Hertel exophthalmometry.

5. Complete ocular examination, particularly extraocular motility assessment.

6. Obtain smears and bacterial cultures of any discharge.

7. Examine the parotid glands (often enlarged in mumps, sarcoidosis, tuberculosis, lymphoma, and syphilis).

8. Perform a CT scan of the orbit (axial, coronal, and parasagittal views), preferably with contrast (see Figure 7.3.3). CT is preferable to MRI in the assessment of the lacrimal gland because of better detail of the adjacent bony anatomy.

9. If the patient is febrile, a CBC with differential and blood cultures are obtained.

Treatment

If the specific etiology is unclear, it is best to empirically treat the patient with systemic antibiotics (see bacterial etiology below) for 24 hours with careful clinical reassessment. The clinical response to antibiotics can guide further

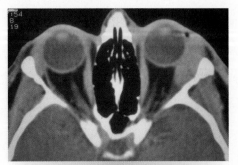

Figure 7.3.3.3 CT of dacryoadenitis.

management and direct one toward a specific etiology.

1. Inflammatory:
   - For treatment, see 7.2.2, IDIOPATHIC ORBITAL INFLAMMATORY SYNDROME. Most often corticosteroid therapy is used. However, preliminary evidence suggests a role for therapeutic debulking and local corticosteroid injection at the time of diagnostic biopsy in improving outcomes and decreasing recurrence.
   - Analgesic as needed.
2. Viral (e.g., mumps and infectious mononucleosis):
   - Cool compresses to the area of swelling and tenderness.
   - Analgesic as needed (e.g., acetaminophen 650 mg p.o. q4h p.r.n.).

NOTE: Aspirin is contraindicated in young children with a viral syndrome because of the risk of Reye's syndrome.

3. Bacterial or infectious (but unidentified) etiology:
   a. If mild to moderate:
      - Amoxicillin/clavulanate: 25 to 45 mg/kg/d p.o. in two divided doses for children, a maximum daily dose of 90 mg/kg/d; 875 mg p.o. q12h for adults; or
      - Cephalexin 25 to 50 mg/kg/d p.o. in two divided doses for children; 500 mg p.o. q6–12h for adults.
   b. If moderate to severe, hospitalize and treat as per 7.3.1, ORBITAL CELLULITIS.

Follow Up

Daily until improvement is confirmed. In patients who fail to respond to antibiotic therapy, judicious use of oral prednisone (see 7.2.2, IDIOPATHIC ORBITAL INFLAMMATORY SYNDROME) is reasonable, as long as close follow up is maintained. Inflammatory dacryoadenitis should respond to oral corticosteroid therapy within 48 hours. Watch for signs of orbital involvement, such as decreased extraocular motility or proptosis, which requires hospital admission for i.v. antibiotic therapy and close monitoring. See 7.6, LACRIMAL GLAND MASS/CHRONIC DACRYOADENITIS.

7.4 Orbital Tumors

7.4.1 ORBITAL TUMORS IN CHILDREN

Signs

Critical. Proptosis or globe displacement.

Other. See the specific etiologies for additional presenting signs. See **Tables 7.4.1.1** and **7.4.1.2** for imaging characteristics.

Differential Diagnosis

- Orbital cellulitis from adjacent ethmoiditis: Most common cause of proptosis in children.

It is of paramount importance to quickly rule out this etiology. See 7.3.1, ORBITAL CELLULITIS.

- Dermoid and epidermoid cysts: Manifest clinically from birth to young adulthood and enlarge slowly. Preseptal dermoid cysts may become symptomatic in childhood and are most commonly found in the temporal upper eyelid or brow, and less often in the medial upper eyelid. The palpable, smooth mass may be mobile or fixed to the periosteum. Posterior dermoids typically become symptomatic in adulthood and may cause proptosis or globe displacement. Dermoid cyst rupture

TABLE 7.4.1.1 Childhood Orbital Lesions

Well circumscribed	Dermoid cyst, rhabdomyosarcoma, optic nerve glioma, plexiform neurofibroma, and hemangioma of infancy
Diffuse and/or infiltrating	Lymphangioma, leukemia, IOIS, hemangioma of infancy, rhabdomyosarcoma, neuroblastoma, teratoma, and Langerhans cell histiocytosis

may mimic orbital cellulitis. The B-scan US, when used, reveals a cystic lesion with good transmission of echoes. Because of the cystic configuration and specific signal properties, CT and MRI are usually diagnostic. See 14.3, MAGNETIC RESONANCE IMAGING.

- Hemangioma of infancy (capillary hemangioma): Seen from birth to 2 years, generally show slow progressive growth over the first 6 to 9 months with slow involution thereafter. May be observed through the eyelid as a bluish mass or be accompanied by a red hemangioma of the skin (strawberry nevus, stork bite), which blanches with pressure **(see Figure 7.4.1.1)**. Proptosis may be exacerbated by crying. It can enlarge over 6 to 12 months, but spontaneously regresses over the following several years. Not to be confused with the unrelated cavernous venous malformation (cavernous hemangioma) of the orbit, typically seen in adults.
- Rhabdomyosarcoma: Average age of presentation is 8 to 10 years, but may occur from infancy to adulthood. May present with explosive proptosis, edema of the eyelids, a palpable eyelid lesion or subconjunctival mass, new-onset ptosis or strabismus, or a history of nosebleeds. Hallmarks are rapid onset and progression. Pain may occur in a minority of cases. Urgent biopsy and referral to a pediatric oncologist is warranted if suspected.
- Metastatic neuroblastoma: Seen during the first few years of life (usually by the age of 5 years). Abrupt presentation with unilateral or bilateral proptosis, eyelid ecchymosis, and globe displacement. The child is usually systemically ill, and 80% to 90% of patients presenting with orbital involvement already

have a known history of neuroblastoma. Note that metastatic neuroblastoma may also present as an isolated Horner syndrome in a child due to metastasis to the lung apex. Prognosis decreases with age.

- Lymphangioma: Usually seen in the first 2 decades of life with a slowly progressive course but may abruptly worsen if the tumor spontaneously bleeds. Proptosis may be intermittent and exacerbated by upper respiratory tract infections. Lymphangioma may present as an atraumatic eyelid ecchymosis. Concomitant conjunctival, eyelid, or oropharyngeal lymphangiomas may be noted (a conjunctival lesion appears as a multicystic mass). MRI is often diagnostic. The B-scan US, when used, often reveals cystic spaces. See **Figure 7.4.1.2**.
- Optic nerve glioma (juvenile pilocytic astrocytoma): Usually first seen at the age of 2 to 6 years and is slowly progressive. The presentation includes painless axial proptosis with decreased visual acuity and a relative afferent pupillary defect. Optic nerve atrophy or swelling may be present. May be associated with neurofibromatosis (types I and II), in which case it may be bilateral. Prognosis decreases with chiasmal or hypothalamic involvement. See 13.13, PHAKOMATOSES.
- Plexiform neurofibroma: Seen in the first decade of life and is pathognomonic for neurofibromatosis type I. Ptosis, eyelid hypertrophy, S-shaped deformity of the upper eyelid, or pulsating proptosis (from the absence of the greater sphenoid wing) may be present. Facial asymmetry and a palpable anterior orbital mass may also be evident. See 13.13, PHAKOMATOSES.
- Leukemia (granulocytic sarcoma): Seen in the first decade of life with rapidly evolving unilateral or bilateral proptosis and, occasionally, swelling of the temporal fossa area due to a mass. Typically, granulocytic sarcoma precedes blood or bone marrow signs of leukemia (usually acute myelogenous leukemia) by several months. Any patient with a biopsy-proven granulocytic sarcoma of the orbit must be closely followed by an oncologist for leukemia development. Acute lymphoblastic leukemia can also produce unilateral or bilateral proptosis.
- Langerhans cell histiocytosis (LCH): May present in the orbit as a rapidly progressive mass with bony erosion on imaging. Three

7

TABLE 7.4.1.2   CT and MRI Characteristics of Pediatric Orbital Lesions

Lesion	CT Characteristics	MRI Features	
		T1 Sequence	**T2 Sequence**
Dermoid or epidermoid cyst	A well-defined lesion that may mold to the bone of the orbital walls. On occasion, bony erosion is noted with the extension of the lesion intracranially or into the temporalis fossa ("dumbbell dermoid").	Hypointense to fat, but usually hyperintense to vitreous. Only capsule enhances with gadolinium. Signal may increase if a large amount of viscous mucus (high protein-to-water ratio) is present within the lesion—an uncommon finding for most orbital masses and helpful in distinguishing this lesion from others.	Iso- or hypointense to fat
Hemangioma of infancy	Irregular, contrast enhancing	Well defined, hypointense to fat, hyperintense to muscle	Hyperintense to fat and muscle
Rhabdomyosarcoma	An irregular, well-defined lesion with possible bone destruction	Isointense to muscle	Hyperintense to muscle
Metastatic neuroblastoma	Poorly defined mass with bony destruction	—	—
Lymphangioma	Nonencapsulated irregular mass, "crabgrass of the orbit"	Cystic, possibly multiloculated, heterogeneous mass. Hypointense to fat, hyperintense to muscle, diffuse enhancement. May show signal of either acute or subacute hemorrhage (hyperintensity on T1).	Markedly hyperintense to fat and muscle
Optic nerve glioma	Fusiform enlargement of the optic nerve	Tubular or fusiform mass, hypointense to gray matter	Homogeneous hyperintensity
Plexiform neurofibroma	Diffuse, irregular soft tissue mass, possible defect in orbital roof	Iso- or slightly hyperintense to muscle	Hyperintense to fat and muscle
Leukemia (granulocytic sarcoma)	Irregular mass with occasional bony erosion	—	—
Langerhans cell histiocytosis	Lytic defect, most commonly in superotemporal orbit or sphenoid wing	Iso-intense to muscle, good enhancement	—

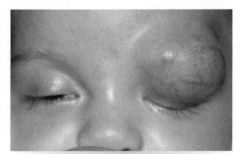

Figure 7.4.1.1 Hemangioma of infancy.

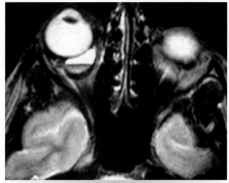

Figure 7.4.1.2 T-2-weighted MRI of orbital lymphangioma with subacute blood cyst.

variants are encountered in the orbit: (1) multifocal, multisystem LCH (Letterer–Siwe disease) occurs in children <2 years old with an aggressive multisystem course and poor prognosis; (2) multifocal unisystem LCH (Hand–Schüller–Christian disease) occurs in children 2 to 10 years of age. The classic triad includes exophthalmos, lytic bone lesions, and diabetes insipidus from pituitary stalk infiltration; (3) unifocal LCH (eosinophilic granuloma) typically causes bony erosion in the superolateral orbit suggestive of malignancy. Occurs in older children and adults. Systemic progression occurs in only a minority of cases.

Workup

1. History: Determine the age of onset and the rate of progression. Does the proptosis vary (e.g., with crying or position)? Nosebleeds? Systemic illness? Fever? Weight loss? Recent URI? Purulent nasal discharge?

2. External examination: Look for an anterior orbital mass, a skin hemangioma, or a temporal fossa lesion. Measure any proptosis (Hertel exophthalmometer) or globe displacement. Refer to a pediatrician for abdominal examination to rule out mass or organomegaly.

3. Complete ocular examination, including visual acuity, pupillary assessment, color vision, IOP, refraction, and optic nerve evaluation. Check the conjunctival cul-de-sacs carefully.

4. Urgent imaging with either CT (axial, coronal, and parasagittal views) or MRI (with gadolinium-DTPA and fat suppression) of brain and orbits to rule out infection or neoplasia.

5. If paranasal sinus opacification is noted in the clinical setting of orbital inflammation, consider immediate systemic antibiotic therapy (see 7.3.1, ORBITAL CELLULITIS).

6. In cases of acute onset and rapid progression with evidence of mass on imaging, an emergency incisional biopsy for frozen and permanent microscopic evaluation is indicated to rule out an aggressive malignancy (e.g., rhabdomyosarcoma).

7. Other tests as determined by the working diagnosis (usually performed in conjunction with a pediatric oncologist):

   • Rhabdomyosarcoma: Physical examination (look especially for enlarged lymph nodes), chest and bone radiographs, bone marrow aspiration, lumbar puncture, and liver function studies.

   • Leukemia: CBC with differential, bone marrow studies, etc.

   • Neuroblastoma: Abdominal imaging (e.g., CT or MRI), urine for vanillylmandelic acid, radioiodinated metaiodobenzylguanidine scintigraphy.

   • LCH: CBC with differential, comprehensive metabolic panel, serum osmolarity, and skeletal survey.

Treatment

1. Dermoid and epidermoid cysts: Complete surgical excision with the capsule intact. If the cyst ruptures, the contents can incite an acute inflammatory response.

2. Hemangioma of infancy: Observe if not causing visual obstruction, astigmatism, and amblyopia. All hemangiomas of infancy will eventually involute. In the presence of visual compromise (e.g., amblyopia and optic neuropathy), several treatment options exist:

a. Systemic ß-blockers: While the exact mechanisms remain unclear, propranolol has become the preferred option in the treatment of refractory and rapidly proliferating infantile hemangiomas. Side effects of propranolol include hypoglycemia, hypotension, and bradycardia. Asthmatics and those with reactive airway disease are at risk for bronchospasm. Therefore, patients should be evaluated by a pediatrician pretreatment and monitored throughout the course of treatment. The initial dose of ß-blocker is typically given in conjunction with cardiopulmonary monitoring. Note that not all lesions respond to this therapy.

b. Oral corticosteroids: Used less frequently since the introduction of ß-blockers. The dose is 2 to 3 mg/kg, tapered over 6 weeks. IOP must be monitored, and patients should be placed on GI prophylaxis.

c. A local corticosteroid injection (e.g., betamethasone 6 mg/mL and triamcinolone 40 mg/mL) is seldom used. Care should be taken to avoid orbital hemorrhage and central retinal artery occlusion during injection. Skin atrophy and depigmentation are other potential complications. Note that periocular injection of triamcinolone is contraindicated by the manufacturer because of the potential risk of embolic infarction. See note in 6.2, CHALAZION/HORDEOLUM.

d. Surgical excision: If the hemangioma is circumscribed and accessible, excision can be performed effectively and is often curative.

e. Interferon therapy: Usually reserved for large or systemic lesions that may be associated with a consumptive coagulopathy or high-output congestive heart failure (Kasabach–Merritt syndrome). There is a risk of spastic diplegia with this therapy. No longer used except in rare cases because of other viable alternatives, including propranolol.

3. Rhabdomyosarcoma: Managed by urgent biopsy and referral to a pediatric oncologist in most cases. Local radiation therapy and systemic chemotherapy are given once the diagnosis is confirmed by biopsy and the patient has been appropriately staged. Significant orbital and ocular complications can occur even with prompt and aggressive management. Overall, the long-term prognosis for orbital rhabdomyosarcoma has greatly improved over the past 50 years due to advances in chemotherapy and radiotherapy, and exenteration is no longer the standard of care. Prognosis depends on the subtype of rhabdomyosarcoma, location of the lesion (orbital lesions have the best prognosis), and stage of the disease. Note that prognosis for orbital lesions decreases with spread to adjacent anatomy (paranasal sinuses or intracranial vault).

4. Lymphangioma: Most are managed by observation. Surgical debulking is performed for a significant cosmetic deformity, ocular dysfunction (e.g., strabismus and amblyopia), or compressive optic neuropathy from acute orbital hemorrhage, but may be difficult because of the infiltrative nature of the tumor. Incidence of hemorrhage into the lesion is increased after surgery. May recur after excision. Aspiration drainage of hemorrhagic cysts ("chocolate cysts") may temporarily improve symptoms. Sclerosing therapy has become the most frequent management option for large, cystic lesions.

5. Optic nerve glioma: Controversial. Observation, surgery, radiation, and/or chemotherapy are used variably on a case-by-case basis.

6. Leukemia: Managed by a pediatric oncologist. Systemic chemotherapy for leukemia. Some physicians administer orbital radiation therapy alone in isolated orbital lesions (chloromas, granulocytic sarcomas) when systemic leukemia cannot be confirmed on bone marrow studies. However, patients need to be monitored closely for eventual systemic involvement.

7. Metastatic neuroblastoma: Managed by a pediatric oncologist in most cases. Local radiation and systemic chemotherapy.

8. Plexiform neurofibroma: Surgical excision is reserved for patients with significant symptoms or disfigurement. The lesions tend to be vascular, infiltrative, and recurrent.

9. LCH: Therapy depends on the extent of the disease. Multisystem involvement requires chemotherapy. With unifocal involvement (eosinophilic granuloma in adults), debulking and curettage are usually curative.

Follow Up

1. Tumors with rapid onset and progression require urgent attention, with appropriate and timely referral to a pediatric oncologist when necessary.
2. Tumors that progress more slowly may be managed less urgently.

7.4.2 ORBITAL TUMORS IN ADULTS

Symptoms

Prominent eye, double vision, and decreased vision, may be asymptomatic.

Signs

Critical. Proptosis, pain, displacement of the globe away from the location of the tumor, orbital mass on palpation, or mass found with neuroimaging. Specific tumors may cause enophthalmos secondary to orbital fibrosis.

Other. A palpable mass, extraocular motility limitation, orbital inflammation, optic disc edema or atrophy, and choroidal folds may be present. See the individual etiologies for more specific findings. See **Tables 7.4.2.1** and **7.4.2.2** for imaging characteristics.

Etiology

- Primarily intraconal/optic nerve:
  1. Cavernous venous malformation (cavernous hemangioma): Most common benign orbital mass in adults. Middle-aged women most commonly affected, with a slow onset of orbital signs. Growth may accelerate during pregnancy **(see Figure 7.4.2.1)**.
  2. Mesenchymal tumors: Orbital lesions with varying degrees of aggressive behavior. The largest group is now labeled solitary fibrous tumor (SFT) and includes fibrous histiocytoma and hemangiopericytoma. These lesions cannot be distinguished clinically or radiographically. May occur at any age. Immunohistochemical staining for STAT6 is usually diagnostic.
  3. Neurilemmoma (schwannoma): Progressive, painless proptosis. Rarely associated with neurofibromatosis type II. Malignant schwannoma has been reported but is rare.

4. Neurofibroma: See 7.4.1, ORBITAL TUMORS IN CHILDREN.
5. Meningioma: Optic nerve sheath meningioma (ONSM) typically occurs in middle-aged women with painless, slowly progressive visual loss, often with mild proptosis. An afferent pupillary defect may be present. Ophthalmoscopy can reveal optic nerve swelling, optic atrophy, or abnormal collateral vessels around the optic nerve head (optociliary shunts).
6. Other optic nerve lesions: Optic nerve glioma, optic nerve sarcoid, malignant optic nerve glioma of adulthood (MOGA). The second most common lesion of the optic nerve (excluding optic neuritis) after ONSM is optic nerve sarcoid, which may be difficult to distinguish from ONSM clinically and radiologically. The ACE level may be normal in cases of isolated optic nerve sarcoid. MOGA is a rapidly progressive optic nerve lesion of the elderly akin to glioblastoma multiforme; it carries a poor prognosis and is often misdiagnosed as a "progressive NAION."
7. Lymphangioma: Usually discovered in childhood. See 7.4.1, ORBITAL TUMORS IN CHILDREN.

- Primarily extraconal:
  1. Mucocele: Often presents with a frontal headache and a history of chronic sinusitis or sinus trauma. Usually located nasally or superonasally, emanating from the frontal and ethmoid sinuses. See **Figure 7.4.2.2**.
  2. Localized neurofibroma: Occurs in young- to middle-aged adults with the slow development of orbital signs. Eyelid infiltration results in an S-shaped upper eyelid. Some have neurofibromatosis type I, but most do not.
  3. SPA or spontaneous hematoma: See 7.3.2, SUBPERIOSTEAL ABSCESS.
  4. Dermoid cyst: See 7.4.1, ORBITAL TUMORS IN CHILDREN.
  5. Others: Tumors of the lacrimal gland (pleomorphic adenoma [well circumscribed], adenoid cystic carcinoma [ACC] [variably circumscribed with adjacent bone destruction]), sphenoid wing meningioma (commonly occurring in middle-aged females and a cause of compressive optic neuropathy), secondary tumors extending from the

TABLE 7.4.2.1 CT and MRI Characteristics of Selected Adult Orbital Lesions

Lesion	CT Characteristics	MRI Features	
		T1 Sequence	**T2 Sequence**
Metastasis	Poorly defined mass conforming to orbital structure; possible bony erosion	Infiltrating mass; hypointense to fat, isointense to muscle; moderate-to-marked enhancement	Hyperintense to fat and muscle
Lymphoid tumors (**Figure 7.6.1C**)	Irregular mass molding to the shape of orbital bones or globe; bone destruction possible in aggressive lesions and HIV	Irregular mass; hypointense to fat, iso- or hyperintense to muscle; moderate-to-marked enhancement	Hyperintense to muscle
Cavernous venous malformation (**Figure 7.4.2.1.**)	Encapsulated mass typically within the muscle cone	Iso- or hyperintense to muscle; delayed, heterogeneous, and diffuse enhancement	Hyperintense to muscle and fat
Optic nerve sheath meningioma	Calcification may be present. Enhancement with contrast.	Three patterns may be seen: fusiform, tubular, and globular; marked enhancement of lesion with gadolinium with sparing of the optic nerve parenchyma.	The typical cuff of CSF around the optic nerve may be effaced by the tumor
Mesenchymal tumors (e.g., SFT)	Well-defined mass anywhere in the orbit	Heterogeneous mass; hypointense to fat, hyper- or isointense to muscle; moderate diffuse or irregular enhancement. May have vascular flow voids.	Variable
Neurilemmoma	Fusiform or ovoid mass often in the superior orbit	Iso- or hyperintense to muscle with variable enhancement	Variable intensity
Neurofibroma	Diffuse, irregular soft tissue mass; a possible defect in orbital roof	Iso- or slightly hyperintense to muscle	Hyperintense to fat and muscle

TABLE 7.4.2.2 CT and MRI Characteristics of Select Adult Extraconal Orbital Lesions

Mucocele (**Figure 7.4.2.2**)	Frontal or ethmoid sinus cyst that extends into orbit	Variable from hypo- to hyperintense, depending on the protein content/viscosity of the lesion	Hyperintense to fat
Localized neurofibroma	Well-defined mass in superior orbit	Well-circumscribed, heterogeneous; iso- or hyperintense to muscle	Hyperintense to fat and muscle

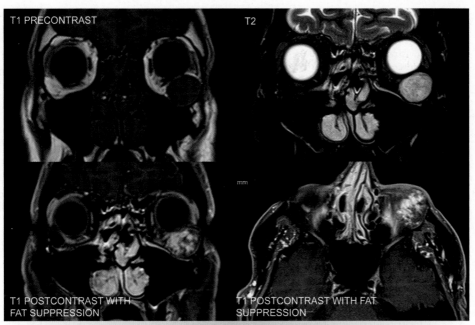

Figure 7.4.2.1 MRI of cavernous venous malformation. Note the heterogeneous contrast enhancement in two lower images.

brain or paranasal sinuses, primary osseous tumors, and vascular lesions (e.g., varix and arteriovenous malformation including CCF).

- Intraconal or extraconal:

  1. Lymphoproliferative disease (lymphoid hyperplasia and lymphoma): More commonly extraconal. About 50% are well circumscribed on imaging, and 50% are

infiltrative. Ocular adnexal lymphoma is typically of the non-Hodgkin B-cell type (NHL), and about 75% to 85% follow an indolent course (extranodal marginal zone lymphoma [EMZL] or mucosa-associated lymphoid tissue lymphoma, grade I or II follicular cell lymphoma, and chronic lymphocytic leukemia [small cell lymphoma]). The remainder are aggressive

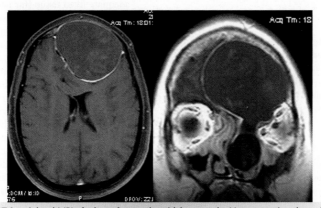

Figure 7.4.2.2 T-1-weighted MRI of a large frontoethmoidal mucocele. Note extension through left orbit and anterior cranial fossa with frontal lobe compression.

lesions (diffuse large B-cell lymphoma and mantle cell lymphoma, among others). May occur at any adult age; orbital NHL is rare in children. Slow onset and progression unless there is an aggressive subtype. Pain may occur in up to 25% of orbital NHL. Typically develops superiorly in the anterior aspect of the orbit, with about 50% occurring in the lacrimal gland. May be accompanied by a subconjunctival salmon-colored lesion. Most orbital NHL (especially if indolent subtype) occurs without evidence of systemic lymphoma (Stage IE). Orbital NHL may be confused with IOIS, especially when it presents more acutely with pain. Note that NHL frequently responds dramatically to systemic corticosteroids, as does IOIS.

2. Metastases: Usually occurs in middle-aged to elderly people with a variable onset of orbital signs. Common primary sources include the breast (most common in women), lung (most common in men), and genitourinary tract (especially prostate). Twenty percent of orbital breast cancer metastases are bilateral and frequently involve extraocular muscles. Enophthalmos (not proptosis) may be seen with scirrhous breast carcinoma. Metastatic prostate adenocarcinoma has a propensity for bone and often involves the zygoma or greater sphenoid wing. Note that uveal metastases are far more common than orbital lesions by a 10 to 1 ratio.

3. Others: Mesenchymal tumors and other malignancies.

Workup

1. History: Determine the age of onset and rate of progression. Headache or chronic sinusitis? History of cancer? Trauma (e.g., mucocele, hematocele, orbital foreign body, or ruptured dermoid)? Classic lymphoma symptoms including fever, night sweats, or unintentional weight loss.

2. Complete ocular examination, particularly visual acuity, pupillary response, ocular motility, dyschromatopsia testing, an estimate of globe displacement and proptosis (Hertel exophthalmometer), IOP, optic nerve evaluation, and automated perimetry of each eye if concerned about an optic neuropathy.

Examine conjunctival surface and cul-de-sacs carefully for salmon patches if lymphoma is suspected.

3. CT (axial, coronal, and parasagittal views) of the orbit and brain or orbital MRI with fat suppression/gadolinium, depending on suspected etiology and age. See 14.2, Computed Tomography and 14.3, MAGNETIC RESONANCE IMAGING.

4. Orbital US with color Doppler imaging as needed to define the vascularity of the lesion. Conventional B-scan has a limited role in the diagnosis of orbital pathology because of the availability and resolution of CT and MRI, but may provide some data on anterior orbital lesions.

5. When a metastasis is suspected and the primary tumor is unknown, the following should be performed:

   • Incisional biopsy to confirm the diagnosis, with estrogen receptor assay if breast adenocarcinoma is suspected.

   • Breast examination and palpation of axillary lymph nodes by the primary physician.

   • Medical workup (e.g., chest imaging, mammogram, prostate examination, PSA testing, and colonoscopy).

   • If the patient has a known history of metastatic cancer and is either a poor surgical candidate or has an orbital lesion that is difficult to access, empiric therapy for the orbital metastasis is a reasonable option.

6. If lymphoproliferative disease (lymphoma or lymphoid hyperplasia) is suspected, a biopsy for definitive diagnosis is indicated. Include adequate fixed tissue (for permanent sectioning and immunohistochemistry) *and fresh tissue (for flow cytometry)*. If lymphoproliferative disease is confirmed, the systemic workup is almost identical for polyclonal (lymphoid hyperplasia) and monoclonal (lymphoma) lesions (e.g., CBC with differential, serum protein electrophoresis, lactate dehydrogenase, and whole-body imaging [CT/MRI or positron emission tomography/CT]). Based on recent data, bone marrow biopsy is indicated in all cases of orbital lymphoma, even indolent subtypes. Close surveillance with serial clinical examination and systemic imaging is indicated over several years in all patients with lymphoproliferative disease, regardless of clonality. A significant percentage of patients

initially diagnosed with orbital lymphoid hyperplasia will eventually develop systemic lymphoma.

Treatment

1. Metastatic disease: Systemic chemotherapy as required for the primary malignancy. Radiation therapy is often used for palliation of the orbital mass; high-dose radiation therapy may result in ocular and optic nerve damage. Hormonal therapy may be indicated in certain cases (e.g., breast and prostate adenocarcinoma).

2. Well-circumscribed lesions: Complete surgical excision is performed when there is compromised visual function, diplopia, rapid growth, or high suspicion of malignancy. Excision for cosmesis can be offered if the patient is willing to accept the surgical risks. An asymptomatic patient can be followed every 6 to 12 months with serial examinations and imaging. Progression of symptoms and rapidly increasing size on serial imaging are indications for exploration and biopsy/excision.

3. Mucocele: Systemic antibiotics (e.g., ampicillin/sulbactam 3 g i.v. q6h) followed by surgical drainage of the mucocele, usually by transnasal endoscopic technique. Orbitotomy for excision is usually unnecessary and contraindicated in most cases as disruption of the mucocele's mucosal lining may lead to recurrent, loculated lesions.

4. Lymphoid tumors: Lymphoid hyperplasia and indolent lymphoma without systemic involvement are treated almost identically. With few exceptions, orbital lymphoproliferations respond dramatically to relatively low doses of radiation (~24 Gy); ocular and optic nerve complications are therefore less common than with other malignancies. Systemic lymphoma or localized aggressive lymphoma are treated with chemotherapy and in many cases with biologics (e.g., rituximab). The vast majority of orbital lymphoma is of B-cell origin and 50% to 60% are EMZL. In older individuals with few symptoms and indolent lesions, more conservative measures may be indicated, including observation alone or brief courses of corticosteroids. To date, there is no clear role for the use of systemic antibiotics in the treatment of orbital lymphoproliferative disease except possibly in certain geographic locations. There is also no clear evidence that orbital EMZL is in any way related to *Helicobacter pylori*-associated gastric EMZL. Remember that the specific subtype of NHL (and therefore level of aggressiveness) and stage of the disease define the ultimate treatment.

5. ONSM: The diagnosis is usually based on slow progression and typical MRI findings. MRI with gadolinium is the preferred imaging modality. CT is occasionally helpful in demonstrating intralesional calcifications. Stereotactic radiation therapy is usually indicated when the tumor is growing and causing significant visual loss. Otherwise, the patient may be followed every 3 to 6 months with serial clinical examinations and imaging studies as needed. Recent studies have shown the significant efficacy of stereotactic radiotherapy in decreasing tumor growth and in visual preservation. Stereotactic radiotherapy is not equivalent to gamma knife therapy ("radiosurgery"). Empiric stereotactic radiotherapy (i.e., without confirmatory biopsy) is a reasonable treatment option, but is reserved for typical cases of ONSM. Atypical or rapidly progressive lesions still require biopsy.

6. Localized neurofibroma: Surgical removal is performed for symptomatic and enlarging tumors. Excision may be difficult and incomplete in infiltrating neurofibromas.

7. Neurilemmoma: Same as for cavernous venous malformation (see above).

8. Mesenchymal tumors (usually SFT): Complete excision when possible. The lesion may be fixed to the surrounding normal anatomy and abut critical structures. In such cases, debulking is reasonable, with long-term follow up and serial imaging to rule out aggressive recurrence or potential malignant transformation. SFT is notoriously difficult to prognosticate. Some lesions will behave in an indolent fashion, while others may present with aggressive recurrence, regional extraorbital extension, or systemic spread.

Follow Up

1. In cases of isolated lesions that can be completely excised (e.g., cavernous venous malformation), routine ophthalmologic follow up is all that is necessary.

2. Other etiologies require long-term follow up at variable intervals.

3. Metastatic disease requires timely workup and management.

REFERENCES

Olsen TG, Heegaard S. Orbital lymphoma. *Surv Ophthalmol.* 2019;64:45-66.

Olsen TG, Holm F, Mikkelsen LH, et al. Orbital lymphoma: an international multicenter retrospective study. *Am J Ophthalmol.* 2019;199:44-57.

Rose GE, Gore SK, Plowman NP. Cranio-orbital resection does not appear to improve survival of patients with lacrimal gland carcinoma. *Ophthalmic Plast Reconstr Surg.* 2019;35:77-84.

NOTE: See 7.6, LACRIMAL GLAND MASS/ CHRONIC DACRYOADENITIS, especially if the mass is in the outer one-third of the upper eyelid, and see 7.4.1, ORBITAL TUMORS IN CHILDREN.

7.5 Traumatic Orbital Disease

ORBITAL BLOWOUT FRACTURE

(See 3.9, ORBITAL BLOWOUT FRACTURE.)

TRAUMATIC RETROBULBAR HEMORRHAGE

(See 3.10, TRAUMATIC RETROBULBAR HEMORRHAGE.)

7.6 Lacrimal Gland Mass/Chronic Dacryoadenitis

Symptoms

Persistent or progressive swelling of the outer one-third of the upper eyelid. Pain or double vision may be present.

Signs

Critical. Chronic eyelid swelling, predominantly in the outer one-third of the upper eyelid, with or without proptosis and displacement of the globe inferiorly and medially. Pain may be present, especially in cases of acute IOIS of the lacrimal gland. Erythema is less common. A dull, aching pain over the forehead or along the temple is an ominous sign, suggestive of malignancy.

Other. A palpable mass may be present in the outer one-third of the upper eyelid. Extraocular motility may be restricted. May have conjunctival injection.

Etiology

• Sarcoidosis: May be bilateral. Typically painless. May have concomitant lung, skin, or renal disease. Lymphadenopathy, parotid gland enlargement, or seventh cranial nerve palsy may be present. Of note, intraocular involvement is uncommon in patients with adnexal sarcoidal inflammation, and vice versa. More common in Americans of African descent, West Africans, and Northern Europeans.

• IOIS: See 7.2.2, IDIOPATHIC ORBITAL INFLAMMATORY SYNDROME. Chronic, painless lacrimal gland enlargement is possible, but atypical for IOIS.

• IgG4-related dacryoadenitis. See NOTE in 7.2.2, IgG4-RELATED ORBITOPATHY.

• Infectious: Enlarged palpebral lobe with surrounding conjunctival injection. Purulent discharge with bacterial dacryoadenitis, which is much less common than noninfectious dacryoadenitis. Bilateral lacrimal gland enlargement may be seen in patients with viral illnesses. CT scan may show fat stranding, abscess.

• Benign mixed tumor (pleomorphic adenoma): Slowly progressive, painless proptosis or inferomedial displacement of the globe in middle-aged adults. Usually involves the orbital lobe of the lacrimal gland. CT may show a well-circumscribed mass with pressure-induced remodeling and enlargement of the lacrimal gland fossa. No true bony erosion occurs **(Figure 7.6.1A).**

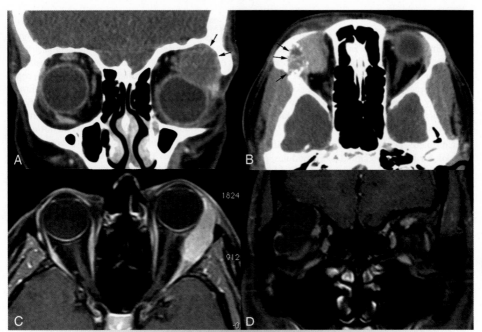

Figure 7.6.1 CT and MRI of lesions involving or near the lacrimal gland. **A:** Pleomorphic adenoma with smooth, pressure induced changes in the lacrimal gland fossa (arrows). **B:** Adenoid cystic carcinoma with bone destruction (arrows) and intralesional calcifications. **C:** Lymphoma involving the lacrimal gland with molding to the globe. **D:** Dermoid cyst arising from the frontoethmoidal suture..

- Lymphoproliferative tumor: Slowly progressive proptosis and globe displacement in an adult. May have a pink "salmon-patch" area of subconjunctival extension. CT usually shows a lacrimal gland lesion that conforms to the native anatomy and is well circumscribed. Indolent forms spare the bone, but bony erosion may be seen in aggressive histopathology (e.g., diffuse large B-cell and mantle cell lymphoma) (**Figure 7.6.1C**).

- ACC: Subacute onset of pain over 1 to 3 months, proptosis, and diplopia, with variable progression. Globe displacement, ptosis, and a motility disturbance are common. This malignant lesion often exhibits perineural invasion, resulting in pain along the temple or forehead and intracranial extension. CT shows an irregular mass, often with bony erosion (**Figure 7.6.1B**).

- Malignant mixed epithelial tumor (pleomorphic adenocarcinoma): Occurs primarily in elderly patients, acutely producing pain and progressing rapidly. May develop primarily or secondarily within a long-standing benign mixed epithelial tumor ("carcinoma

ex pleomorphic adenoma"), or incompletely resected benign mixed tumor. CT findings are similar to those for ACC.

- Lacrimal gland cyst (dacryops): Usually an asymptomatic mass that may fluctuate in size. Typically occurs in a young adult or middle-aged patient.

- Others (may not involve the lacrimal gland, but occur superolaterally in the area of the lacrimal gland and fossa): GPA (formerly Wegener granulomatosis), tuberculosis, leukemia, mumps, mononucleosis, syphilis (exceedingly rare), mucoepidermoid carcinoma, plasmacytoma/multiple myeloma, eosinophilic granuloma, metastasis (especially prostate adenocarcinoma), and dermoid cyst (**Figure 7.6.1D**) (see **Tables 7.4.1.2** and **14.3.2**).

NOTE: Primary, epithelial neoplasms are almost always unilateral; inflammatory disease may be bilateral. Lymphoma is more commonly unilateral, but may be bilateral.

Workup

1. History: Determine the duration of the abnormality and rate of progression. Associated pain, tenderness, or double vision? Weakness, weight loss, fever, or other signs of systemic malignancy? Breathing difficulty, skin rash, or history of uveitis (sarcoidosis)? Any known medical problems? History of lacrimal gland biopsy or surgery?

2. Complete ocular examination: Specifically look for keratic precipitates, iris nodules, posterior synechiae, and old retinal periphlebitis from sarcoidosis. As noted, intraocular sarcoidosis is uncommon in patients with ocular adnexal sarcoidosis, but may occur.

3. Orbital CT (axial, coronal, and parasagittal views). MRI is rarely required unless an intracranial extension is suspected. CT is helpful in defining bony anatomy and abnormality.

4. Consider a chest CT, which may diagnose sarcoidosis, primary malignancy, lymphoproliferative disease, metastatic disease, and, rarely, tuberculosis.

5. Consider CBC with differential, ACE, cANCA, pANCA, SPEP, LDH, IgG4/IgG levels, and purified protein derivative (PPD) or interferon-gamma release assay (IGRA) (e.g., QuantiFERON-TB Gold) if clinical history suggests a specific etiology. In most cases, ACE and LDH suffice.

6. Lacrimal gland biopsy (see Note below) is indicated when a malignant tumor is suspected, or if the diagnosis is uncertain. If possible, avoid treatment with corticosteroids until a biopsy is obtained.

7. Systemic workup by an internist or hematologist/oncologist when lymphoma or other blood dyscrasia is confirmed (e.g., abdominal and head CT scan, PET/CT scan, possible bone marrow biopsy).

NOTE: Do not perform an incisional biopsy on lesions thought to be a benign mixed tumor (pleomorphic adenoma) or dermoid cyst. Incomplete excision of a pleomorphic adenoma may lead to a recurrence with or without malignant transformation. Rupture of a dermoid cyst may lead to a severe inflammatory reaction. These two lesions should be completely excised without violating the capsule or pseudocapsule.

NOTE: If ACC is suspected, some experts recommend avoiding large, debulking biopsies for the preservation of the lacrimal artery. A recent study on the treatment of ACC with an intra-arterial chemotherapeutic protocol concluded that efficacy is compromised if the lacrimal artery is not intact. To avoid iatrogenic injury to the artery, perform an anterior biopsy to confirm the diagnosis of ACC. Other experts do not utilize intraarterial chemotherapy and proceed with complete gross excision of the tumor and obviously involved bone in anticipation of adjunctive radiation therapy.

Treatment

1. Sarcoidosis: Systemic corticosteroids or low-dose antimetabolite therapy. See 12.6, SARCOIDOSIS.

2. IOIS: Systemic corticosteroids. See 7.2.2, IDIOPATHIC ORBITAL INFLAMMATORY SYNDROME.

3. IgG4-related disease: Systemic corticosteroid therapy or low-dose antimetabolite therapy. Biologic therapy may also be used.

4. Benign mixed epithelial tumor (pleomorphic adenoma): Complete surgical removal.

5. Dermoid cyst: Complete surgical removal.

6. Lymphoma confined to the lacrimal gland: Depends on the subtype of lymphoma. Indolent lesions respond well to radiation therapy alone. Aggressive lesions, even when isolated, typically necessitate systemic chemotherapy, including biologic agents (e.g., rituximab). See 7.4.2, ORBITAL TUMORS IN ADULTS.

7. ACC: Consider pretreatment with intra-arterial cisplatinum, followed by wide excision. Orbital exenteration and craniectomy are used less frequently, especially in smaller lesions, since there appears to be no prognostic advantage over more localized excision followed by radiotherapy. Adjunctive radiation is recommended in all patients, possibly with systemic chemotherapy. Proton beam radiotherapy is offered by some centers, but, to date, there is no proven benefit over conventional stereotactic radiotherapy. Regardless of the treatment regimen, the prognosis is guarded and recurrence is the rule. There is no clear evidence

that any specific treatment regimen improves survival. Survival appears to be most dependent on the specific tumor subtype (basaloid or nonbasaloid) and possibly initial tumor size.

8. Malignant mixed epithelial tumor: Similar as for ACC.

9. Lacrimal gland cyst: Excise if symptomatic.

Follow Up

Depends on the specific cause.

7.7 Miscellaneous Orbital Diseases

1. Intracranial disease. Extension of intracranial tumors, usually frontal lobe or sphenoid wing meningiomas, may present with proptosis in addition to cranial neuropathy and decreased vision. Imaging, preferably with MRI, is indicated.

2. Cavernous sinus arteriovenous fistula (AVF) (e.g., carotid–cavernous or dural sinus fistula): AVF is either spontaneous, indirect (usually in older patients, Barrow type B-D) or posttraumatic, direct (in younger patients, Barrow type A). A bruit is sometimes heard by the patient and may be detected if ocular auscultation is performed. Pulsating proptosis, arterialized "corkscrew" conjunctival vessels, increased IOP, retinal venous congestion, and chemosis may be present. May mimic an orbital disease, including TED and IOIS. In the early stages, often misdiagnosed as conjunctivitis, asymmetric glaucoma, etc. CT scan reveals enlarged superior ophthalmic vein(s), sometimes accompanied by enlarged extraocular muscles. An orbital color Doppler US shows reversed, arterialized flow in the superior ophthalmic vein(s). MRA or CTA may reveal AVF but a definitive diagnosis usually requires cerebral arteriography. Evidence of posterior cortical venous outflow on arteriography increases the risk of hemorrhagic stroke. Of note, posterior cortical venous outflow is more common in patients with bilateral orbital signs, but is seen in 10% of patients with unilateral presentation. Also remember that arteriography must be performed on both cerebral hemispheres and include the internal carotid, external carotid, and basilar arteries ("six vessel angio"). The cavernous sinuses are connected by the circular sinus and, on occasion, a carotid–cavernous fistula manifests clinically in the contralateral orbit.

3. Septic cavernous sinus thrombosis: Orbital cellulitis signs, plus dilated and sluggish pupils as well as palsies of the third, fourth, fifth, and/or sixth cranial nerves out of proportion to the degree of orbital edema. Decreasing level of consciousness, nausea, vomiting, and fevers can occur. May be bilateral with rapid progression. See 7.3.1, ORBITAL CELLULITIS.

4. Orbital vasculitis (e.g., GPA and polyarteritis nodosa): Systemic signs and symptoms of vasculitis (especially sinus, renal, pulmonary, and skin disease), fever, markedly increased ESR, and positive cANCA or pANCA. Of note, cANCA may be normal in two-third of patients with the limited sino-orbital variant of GPA.

5. Varix: A large, dilated vein in the orbit that produces proptosis when it fills and dilates (e.g., during a Valsalva maneuver or with the head in a dependent position). When the vein is not engorged, the proptosis disappears. CT demonstrates the dilated vein if an enhanced scan is performed during a Valsalva maneuver. Calcification may be seen in long-standing lesions.

6. Poorly understood processes:
   - Tolosa–Hunt syndrome (THS): NOT equivalent to orbital apical IOIS. Histopathologically, a granulomatous inflammation of the orbital apex and/or carotid siphon within the cavernous sinus. Presents with acute pain, cranial neuropathy, and sometimes proptosis. A diagnosis of exclusion. Difficult to diagnose with CT. MRI shows isolated, ipsilateral enlargement of the cavernous sinus. Usually sensitive to corticosteroid therapy, but pain typically responds much more quickly than external ophthalmoplegia, which may take weeks to resolve. Because confirmatory biopsy is usually not feasible, every patient with presumed THS must be followed long-term, even after rapid response to corticosteroids, to rule out other etiologies. Repeat imaging is usually indicated several months after the initial event to rule out progression. Presumed THS recurs

in about one-third of patients. Remember that other significant pathologies, including sarcoidosis, lymphoma, metastasis, and even aneurysm may show a temporary response to corticosteroids.

- Sclerosing orbital pseudotumor: Likely not a true orbital inflammation or a subtype of IOIS. May be a form of idiopathic multifocal sclerosis. Presents with chronic pain, external ophthalmoplegia, and possibly optic neuropathy. Diagnosis requires biopsy. Histopathology shows wide swaths of monotonous fibrous tissue interspersed with mild inflammation. Treatment is difficult and may necessitate antimetabolite therapy, debulking, and in severe cases, exenteration.

- Orbital amyloid: May be primary (isolated) or secondary to systemic disease. All patients require a systemic workup, including a cardiology consult to rule out cardiomyopathy. Diagnosis is made by judicious orbital biopsy (this lesion is highly vascular and hemostasis is often difficult to obtain). Treatment is highly variable.

Chapter 8

Pediatrics

8.1 Leukocoria

Definition

A white pupillary reflex (see Figure 8.1.1).

Etiology

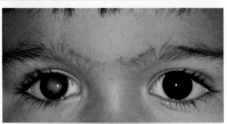

Figure 8.1.1 Leukocoria.

- Retinoblastoma: A malignant tumor of the retina that appears as a white, nodular mass that breaks through the internal limiting membrane into the vitreous (endophytic), as a subretinal mass lesion often underlying a serous retinal detachment (exophytic), or as a diffusely spreading lesion simulating uveitis (diffuse infiltrating). Iris neovascularization is common with large tumors. Aqueous and vitreous seeding may occur. Cataract is uncommon, and the eye is normal in size. May be bilateral, unilateral, or multifocal. Diagnosis is usually made in patients under 5 years of age, with a mean age of 18 months. A family history may be elicited in about 10%.

- Toxocariasis: A nematode infection that may appear as a localized, white, elevated granuloma in the retina or as a diffuse endophthalmitis. Associated with localized inflammation of ocular structures, vitreous traction bands and related macular dragging, traction retinal detachment, and cataract. It is rarely bilateral and is usually diagnosed between 6 months and 10 years of age but may present in adults as well. Paracentesis of the anterior chamber may reveal eosinophils; serum enzyme-linked immunosorbent assay (ELISA) test for Toxocara organisms is positive. The patient may have a history of contact with puppies or of eating dirt. Toxocariasis may also be acquired prenatally and present as a congenital infection.

- Coats disease (see Figure 8.1.2): A retinal vascular abnormality resulting in microaneurysms and macroaneurysms of the retinal vessels, usually in the inferotemporal periphery. Xanthocoria may develop secondary to an exudative, often bullous retinal detachment associated with yellow-colored, lipid-rich subretinal fluid or to extensive, yellow intraretinal and subretinal exudate. Usually develops in boys during the first decade of life; more severe cases occur in early childhood. Coats disease is rarely bilateral. No family history.

- Persistent fetal vasculature (PFV) (previously known as persistent hyperplastic primary vitreous): A developmental ocular abnormality with failure of regression of the fetal hyaloid complex, often with a fibrovascular stalk from the optic nerve to lens and anterior segment. May only present with anterior or posterior findings. It is usually associated with a small eye. Typically there is a membrane behind the lens that places inward traction on elongated ciliary processes. A cataract is noted at birth or early in life. The membrane and lens may rotate anteriorly, shallowing the anterior chamber and resulting in secondary glaucoma. Traction retinal detachment can occur. Usually unilateral. No family history or other risk factors.

- Pediatric cataract: Opacity of the lens present at birth or in first months of life; may be unilateral or bilateral. There may be a family history or an associated systemic disorder. See 8.8, PEDIATRIC CATARACT.

- Retinal astrocytoma: A sessile to slightly elevated, yellow-white retinal mass that may be

183

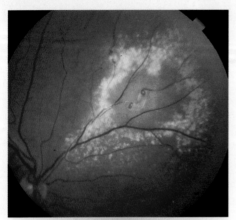

Figure 8.1.2 Coats disease.

calcified and is often associated with tuberous sclerosis complex and rarely neurofibromatosis. May occur on the optic nerve head (giant drusen) in patients with tuberous sclerosis.

- Retinopathy of prematurity (ROP): Predominantly occurs in premature children. Leukocoria is usually the result of a retinal detachment. See 8.2, RETINOPATHY OF PREMATURITY.
- Others: Retinal detachment, retinochoroidal coloboma, familial exudative vitreoretinopathy (FEVR), myelinated nerve fibers, uveitis, toxoplasmosis, trauma, cytomegalovirus retinitis, endophthalmitis, retinal dysplasia, incontinentia pigmenti, Norrie disease, and medulloepithelioma.

Workup

1. History: Age at onset? Family history of one of the conditions mentioned? Prematurity? Contact with puppies or history of eating dirt?
2. Complete ocular examination, including a measurement of corneal diameters (look for a small eye), an examination of the iris (look for neovascularization), and an inspection of the lens (look for a cataract). A dilated fundus examination and an anterior vitreous examination are essential.
3. Any or all of the following may be helpful in diagnosis and planning treatment:
   - B-scan ultrasonography (US), especially if there is no view of the fundus. This can be used to look for calcification within a

suspected tumor, a persistent stalk from the optic disc to the back of the lens, or a retinal detachment.
- Intravenous fluorescein angiogram (useful for evaluation of Coats disease, ROP, retinoblastoma).
- Magnetic resonance imaging (MRI) (or computed tomography [CT]) of the orbit and brain, particularly for bilateral cases of retinoblastoma or those with a family history of retinoblastoma. Also advised in cases of advanced Coats disease. MRI is preferable for retinoblastoma to reduce radiation exposure, given risk of future malignancy.
- Serum ELISA test for Toxocara (positive at 1:8 in the vast majority of infected patients).
- Systemic evaluation by pediatrician, especially if concern for retinal astrocytic hamartoma, retinoblastoma, or cataract secondary to systemic disease.
- Anterior chamber paracentesis and serum ELISA test for evaluation of toxocariasis (serum antibody test positive at 1:8 in the vast majority of patients infected with *Toxocara*). See Appendix 13, ANTERIOR CHAMBER PARACENTESIS.

NOTE: Anterior chamber paracentesis in a patient with a retinoblastoma should be avoided as it could lead to tumor cell dissemination.

4. May need examination under anesthesia (EUA) in young or uncooperative children, particularly when retinoblastoma is being considered as a diagnosis. If there is concern for inherited retinoblastoma, screening examination can be performed in the office within 1 to 2 weeks of birth. See 8.8, PEDIATRIC CATARACT, for a more specific cataract workup.

Treatment

1. Retinoblastoma: Chemoreduction, intra-arterial chemotherapy, intravitreal chemotherapy, cryotherapy, thermotherapy, laser photocoagulation, or plaque radiotherapy. These treatment modalities are typically used in combination. Enucleation is reserved for cases not amenable to the above treatment

options or in advanced unilateral cases. Systemic chemotherapy is used in metastatic disease. External irradiation is rarely used as it is associated with a high incidence of secondary tumors later in life.

2. Toxocariasis:

   • Steroids (topical, periocular, or systemic routes may be used, depending on the severity of the inflammation).

   • Consider vitrectomy when vitreoretinal traction bands form or when the condition does not improve or worsens with medical therapy.

   • Consider laser photocoagulation of the nematode if it is visible.

   • Antihelminth therapy (albendazole) only warranted for systemic disease.

3. Coats disease: Fluorescein angiography–guided laser photocoagulation to leaking vessels and aneurysms and can consider intravitreal anti-VEGF agents in addition to the laser if there is posterior involvement. External drainage

of the subretinal fluid may be beneficial for severe retinal detachment.

4. PFV:

   • Cataract removal and retrolental stalk resection, with posterior vitrectomy depending on extent of posterior involvement.

   • Treat any amblyopia, although visual outcome is often poor secondary to numerous factors such as foveal hypoplasia, anisometropia, optic nerve hypoplasia, and sensory deprivation.

5. Pediatric cataract: See 8.8, PEDIATRIC CATARACT.

6. Retinal astrocytoma: Observation.

7. ROP: See 8.2, RETINOPATHY OF PREMATURITY.

Follow Up

Variable, depending on the diagnosis. If any concern for heritable disorders, consider referral to ophthalmic genetics and screening of family members.

8.2 Retinopathy of Prematurity

Risk Factors

• Prematurity, especially ≤30 weeks of gestation.
• Birth weight ≤1,500 g (3 lb, 5 oz).
• Use of supplemental oxygen, neonatal sepsis, hypoxemia, hypercarbia, failure to thrive, coexisting illness, Caucasian race, and male sex.
• Risk factors mentioned above, when present concurrently, have an additive effect on the risk for development of ROP.

Signs

Critical. Avascular peripheral retina. Demarcation line between vascular and avascular retina.

Other. Extraretinal fibrovascular proliferation, vitreous hemorrhage, retinal detachment, or leukocoria. Commonly bilateral. Association of "plus disease" in more severe cases includes engorgement and tortuosity of the vessels in the posterior pole and/or iris. Poor pupillary dilation despite mydriatic drops. In older children and adults, risk for decreased visual acuity, amblyopia, myopia, strabismus, macular dragging, lattice-like vitreoretinal degeneration, and retinal detachment.

Differential Diagnosis

• FEVR: Can appear similar to ROP, except FEVR is hereditary (although family members may be asymptomatic, and de novo mutations frequently occur) and more often asymmetric; asymptomatic family members often show peripheral retinal vascular abnormalities. There usually is no history of prematurity or oxygen therapy. See 8.3, FAMILIAL EXUDATIVE VITREORETINOPATHY.

• Incontinentia pigmenti: X-linked dominant condition that usually occurs in girls. Often lethal in males. Characterized by skin changes including erythematous maculopapular lesions, vesicles, hypopigmented patches, and alopecia. Associated with eosinophilia. Central nervous system and dental abnormalities also seen.

• See 8.1, LEUKOCORIA, for additional differential diagnoses.

Classification

Location

• **Zone I: Posterior pole:** Twice the disc–fovea distance, centered around the disc (poorest prognosis).

8

> **NOTE:** With the nasal edge of the optic disc at one edge of the field of view with a 28D lens, the limit of zone I is at the temporal field of view.

- **Zone II:** From zone I to the nasal ora serrata; temporally equidistant from the disc.

> **NOTE:** ROP should not be considered zone III until one is sure the nasal side is vascularized to the ora serrata.

- **Zone III:** The remaining temporal periphery.

Extent

- Number of clock hours (30-degree sectors) involved. Of note, the number of clock hours of neovascularization was important in older treatment criteria, but it is not used in the most updated treatment guidelines.

Severity

- **Stage 1:** Flat demarcation line separating the vascular posterior retina from the avascular peripheral retina **(see Figure 8.2.1)**.
- **Stage 2:** Ridged demarcation line.
- **Stage 3:** Ridged demarcation line with fibrovascular proliferation or neovascularization extending from the ridge **(see Figure 8.2.2)**.
- **Stage 4A:** Extrafoveal partial retinal detachment.
- **Stage 4B:** Fovea-involving partial retinal detachment.
- **Stage 5:** Total retinal detachment.

> **NOTE:** Overall stage is determined by the most severe manifestation; however, it is recommended to define each stage and extent.

"Plus" Disease

At least two quadrants of engorged veins and tortuous arteries in the posterior pole; iris vascular engorgement, poor pupil dilatation, and vitreous haze with more advanced plus disease. If plus disease is present, a "+" is placed after the stage (e.g., stage 3+). If vascular dilatation and tortuosity are present but inadequate to diagnose plus

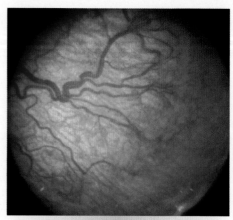

Figure 8.2.1 Retinopathy of prematurity: Stage 1.

disease, it is called "pre-plus" disease and noted after the stage (e.g., stage 3 with pre-plus disease). Rapidly progressing posterior ROP (usually zone I) with extensive plus disease, formerly known as "rush" disease, may progress rapidly to stage 5 ROP without passing through the other stages. This aggressive ROP may also show hemorrhages at the junction between vascular and avascular retina **(see Figure 8.2.3)**.

Type 1 ROP

Defines high-risk eyes that meet the criteria for treatment:

- Zone I, any stage with plus disease.
- Zone I, stage 3 without plus disease.
- Zone II, stage 2 or 3 with plus disease.

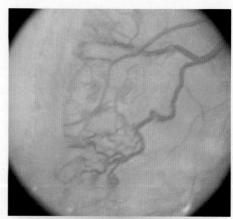

Figure 8.2.2 Retinopathy of prematurity: Stage 3.

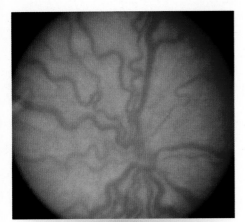

Figure 8.2.3 Retinopathy of prematurity: Plus disease.

Type II ROP

Defines less severely advanced eyes that should be monitored closely for progression to type 1 disease:

- Zone I, stage 1 and 2 without plus disease.
- Zone II, stage 3 without plus disease.

Prethreshold and Threshold Disease

Terminology historically used as part of a classification system based on the CRYO-ROP study. Originally determined treatment criteria, but no longer used as part of standard of care.

Screening Recommendations

- Birth weight ≤1,500 g.
- Gestational age ≤30 weeks.
- Selected infants with birth weight >1,500 g or gestational age ≥31 weeks with unstable clinical course thought to be at high risk.
- Timing of first eye examination is based on postmenstrual (gestational age at birth plus chronologic age) and postnatal (chronologic since birth) age. The first eye examination should start at 31 to 32 weeks postmenstrual age or 4 weeks postnatal age, whichever is later.

NOTE: The American Academy of Pediatrics provides updated guidelines for ROP screening in premature infants. For the latest recommendations, please see their most recent policy statement.

Workup

1. Dilated retinal examination with scleral depression at 31 to 32 weeks after date of mother's last menstrual period or 4 weeks after birth, whichever is later.
2. Can dilate with any two-agent combination from the following: phenylephrine, 1%; tropicamide, 1%; cyclopentolate, 0.2% to 0.5%. A fixed combined drop of phenylephrine 1% and cyclopentolate 0.2% is available. Consider repeating the drops in 30 to 45 minutes if the pupil is not dilated.

Treatment

- Therapeutic goal is ablation of avascular peripheral retina with near-confluent spots. Laser photocoagulation is preferred over cryotherapy. Treatment should be instituted within 48 to 72 hours (see Figure 8.2.4). Use of intravitreal anti-VEGF agents (0.625 mg in 0.025 mL of solution of bevacizumab is the typical dosing) is an emerging treatment modality, especially when photocoagulation is not available or in very posterior zone 1 cases; however, the long-term effects and potential risks of these medications in preterm infants are yet to be determined.
- Type 1 ROP needs treatment.
- Type 2 ROP should be followed closely.
- For acute stages 4 and 5: Surgical repair of retinal detachment by vitrectomy.

Follow Up

- A single ocular examination is sufficient only if it unequivocally shows full retinal vascularization in both eyes.
- One week or less: immature vascularization, zone I, no ROP; immature retina localized to boundary of zones I and II; zone I, stage 1 or 2; zone II, stage 3; or any concern for aggressive posterior ROP.
- One to 2 weeks: immature vascularization localized to posterior zone II; or zone II, stage 2; or zone I, regressing ROP.
- Two weeks: immature vascularization localized to zone II, no ROP; zone II, stage 1; or zone II, regressing ROP.
- Two to 3 weeks: zone III, stage 1 or 2; or zone III, regressing ROP.

1. Children who have had ROP have a higher incidence of myopia, strabismus, amblyopia, macular dragging, cataracts, glaucoma, and

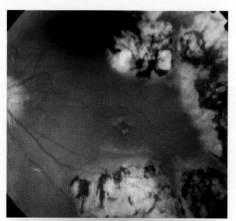

Figure 8.2.4 Retinopathy of prematurity after laser treatment.

retinal detachment. An untreated fully vascularized fundus needs examination at age 6 months to rule out these complications.

NOTE: Because of the possibility of late retinal detachments and other ocular complications, ROP patients should be followed at yearly intervals for life.

2. Acute-phase ROP screening can be discontinued when any of the following signs is present, indicating that the risk of visual loss from ROP is minimal or passed:

- Zone III retinal vascularization attained without previous zone I or II ROP. If there is doubt about the zone or if the postmenstrual age is <35 weeks, confirmatory examinations may be warranted.
- Postmenstrual age of 50 weeks and no ROP disease equivalent to or worse than zone I, any stage or zone II, stage 3.
- Full retinal vascularization in close proximity to the ora serrata (for cases treated with anti-VEGF therapy).
- If treated with anti-VEGF, follow up should be extended due to risk of ROP recurring after 65 to 70 weeks postmenstrual age, if retinal vascularization remains incomplete. Consider prophylactic laser to undeveloped avascular retina if unable to assure follow-up examinations.

8.3   Familial Exudative Vitreoretinopathy

Symptoms

Many are asymptomatic, but patients may report decreased vision depending on the stage.

Signs

(See Figure 8.3.1.)

Critical. Vascular dragging and peripheral retinal nonperfusion, most prominently temporally. Bilateral but often asymmetric. Peripheral retinal vessels have a fimbriated border. Present at birth.

Other. Peripheral neovascularization and/or fibrovascular proliferation at the border of vascular and avascular retina; temporal dragging of macula through contraction of fibrovascular tissue; radial retinal folds; vitreous hemorrhage; tractional, exudative, and/or rhegmatogenous retinal detachment; peripheral intraretinal and subretinal lipid exudation. May present with strabismus or leukocoria in childhood. Cataract,

band keratopathy, neovascular glaucoma, or phthisis possible.

Differential Diagnosis

- ROP: Appears similar to FEVR, but there is lack of family history, and there should be a history of prematurity. See 8.2, RETINOPATHY OF PREMATURITY.
- See 8.1, LEUKOCORIA, for additional diagnoses in the differential including retinoblastoma, Coats disease, PFV, incontinentia pigmenti, Norrie disease, X-linked retinoschisis, and peripheral retinal nonperfusion. Positive family history and bilaterality can help distinguish from others.

Etiology

Due to defects in the Wnt signaling pathway. Often autosomal dominant, but can be autosomal recessive or X-linked. Usually no history of prematurity or oxygen therapy.

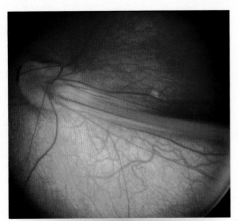

Figure 8.3.1 Familial exudative vitreoretinopathy with a falciform fold.

Workup

1. History: Positive family history? No history of prematurity or oxygen therapy?
2. Complete ocular examination, including dilated retinal examination looking for supernumerary vessels, vascular dragging, macular dragging, neovascularization, and tractional retinal detachment. Fluorescein angiography of both eyes (under general anesthesia if necessary) has become vital for evaluation of diagnosis of anomalous vasculature, retinal nonperfusion, and neovascularization in peripheral retina, which can lead to tractional retinal detachment and result in decreased visual outcomes.
3. All family members suspected of carrying the gene should also have dilated retinal examinations and fluorescein angiography. This may be essential to preventing family members from experiencing permanent vision loss, as this disease is typically asymptomatic.
4. Genetic testing: Commonly affected genes include *FZD4*, *LRP5*, *TSPAN12*, and *NDP*. *LRP5* mutation has been associated with early onset osteoporosis. Many others are included now in genetic panels.

Treatment

Laser of peripheral avascular retina is performed if there is neovascularization and/or exudation. Scleral buckling or vitrectomy can be considered for retinal detachments. Treat amblyopia as needed. Genetic testing and examination of family members recommended.

Follow Up

FEVR is a lifelong disease. All patients should be followed throughout life to monitor for progression.

8.4 Esodeviations

Signs

(See Figure 8.4.1.)

Critical. Either eye is turned inward. The nonfixating eye turns outward to fixate straight ahead when the previously fixating eye is covered during the cover–uncover test. See Appendix 3, COVER/UNCOVER AND ALTERNATE COVER TESTS.

Other. Amblyopia, overaction of the inferior oblique muscles, dissociated vertical deviation, and/or latent nystagmus may be present.

Differential Diagnosis

- Pseudoesotropia: The eyes appear esotropic; however, there is no ocular misalignment detected during cover–uncover testing. Usually, the child has a wide nasal bridge, prominent epicanthal folds, or a small interpupillary distance **(see Figure 8.4.2)**.
- See 8.6, STRABISMUS SYNDROMES.

Types

Comitant Esotropic Deviations

A manifest convergent misalignment of the eyes in which the measured angle of esodeviation is nearly constant in all fields of gaze at distance fixation.

1. Congenital (infantile) esotropia: Manifests by age 6 months. The angle of esodeviation is usually large (>40- to 50-prism diopters) and mostly equal at distance and near fixation. Refractive error is usually normal for age (slightly hyperopic). Amblyopia is uncommon but may be present in those who

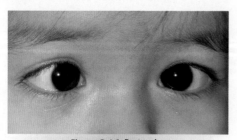

Figure 8.4.1 Esotropia.

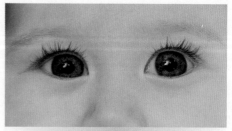

Figure 8.4.2 Pseudoesotropia.

do not cross-fixate. Prohibits development of binocular vision. Family history may be present. Latent nystagmus, inferior oblique overaction, and dissociated vertical deviation may develop as late findings. Congenital esotropia can occur in up to 30% of children with neurologic and developmental disorders (e.g., cerebral palsy, hydrocephalus); however, it is not necessary to perform a neurologic workup in the absence of other findings. Cycloplegic refraction should be considered first, but treatment is often surgical relatively early on in the course of the disease.

2. Acquired nonaccommodative esotropia: Convergent misalignment of the eyes *not* corrected by hyperopic lenses that develops after 6 months of age. Typically starts as intermittent but can become constant over time. Esodeviation is comitant and usually smaller (20 to 35 prism diopters) than that seen in congenital esotropia. Patients may experience diplopia. Usually corrected with strabismus surgery once the angle of the esotropia becomes consistent. In children older than 6 years, this must be assumed to be posterior fossa pathology until proven otherwise and worked up with imaging emergently.

3. Accommodative esotropia: Convergent misalignment of the eyes associated with activation of the accommodative reflex. May present at 6 months to 6 years of age with the average age of onset being 2.5 years. Subtypes of accommodative esotropia:

   • Refractive accommodative esotropia: These children are hyperopic in the range of +3.00 to +10.00 diopters (average, +4.75). The measured angle of esodeviation is usually moderate (20- to 30-prism diopters) and is relatively equal at distance and near fixation. Full hyperopic correction eliminates the esodeviation. The accommodative

convergence–accommodation angle ratio (AC/A) is normal. Amblyopia is common at presentation.

   • Nonrefractive accommodative esotropia (high AC/A ratio): The measured angle of esodeviation is greater at near fixation than at distance fixation. The refractive error may range from normal for age (slight hyperopia) to high hyperopia (may be seen in conjunction with refractive-type accommodative esotropia) or even myopia. Amblyopia is common.

   • Partial or decompensated accommodative esotropia: Refractive and nonrefractive accommodative esotropias that have a reduction in the esodeviation when given full hyperopic correction, but still have a residual esodeviation. When partial, the residual esodeviation is the nonaccommodative component.

4. Sensory-deprivation esotropia: An esodeviation that occurs in a patient with a monocular or binocular condition that prevents good vision.

5. Divergence insufficiency: A convergent ocular misalignment that is greater at distance fixation than at near fixation. This is a diagnosis of exclusion and must be differentiated from divergence paralysis, which, when sudden in onset, can be associated with pontine tumors, neurologic trauma, and elevated intracranial pressure. This can be a benign condition in older patients, requiring only base out prisms in glasses. See 10.8, ISOLATED SIXTH CRANIAL NERVE PALSY.

Incomitant or Noncomitant Esodeviations

The measured angle of esodeviation increases in lateral gaze at distance fixation.

1. Central nervous system pathology causing increased intracranial pressure: Acute and new onset of diplopia secondary to an acquired

sixth cranial nerve palsy, which may be accompanied by nystagmus, headache, or other focal neurologic deficits depending on etiology.

2. Medial rectus restriction (e.g., thyroid disease, medial orbital wall fracture with entrapment).

3. Lateral rectus weakness (e.g., isolated sixth cranial nerve palsy, slipped or detached lateral rectus from trauma or previous surgery).

4. See 8.6, STRABISMUS SYNDROMES and 10.8, ISOLATED SIXTH CRANIAL NERVE PALSY, for additional etiologies.

Other

1. Esophoria: Latent esodeviation controlled by fusion. Eyes are aligned under binocular conditions.

2. Intermittent esotropia: Esodeviation that is intermittently controlled by fusion. Becomes manifest spontaneously, especially with fatigue or illness.

Workup

1. History: Age of onset, frequency of crossing, prior therapy (e.g., glasses, patching).

2. Visual acuity of each eye, with best correction and pinhole. Color vision and stereopsis.

3. Ocular motility examination; observe for restricted movements or oblique overactions.

4. Measure the distance deviation in all fields of gaze and the near deviation in the primary position (straight ahead) using prisms (see Appendix 3, COVER/UNCOVER AND ALTERNATE COVER TESTS). Look specifically for an esotropia increasing in either side gaze.

5. Manifest and cycloplegic refractions especially if <7 years of age.

6. Complete eye examination. Look for any cranial nerve abnormalities and causes of sensory deprivation.

7. If nonaccommodative esotropia, divergence insufficiency or paralysis, muscle paralysis, or incomitant esotropia develops acutely, an MRI brain and orbit is necessary to rule out an intracranial or orbital process, extraocular muscle pathology, bony lesion, etc. MRI should be considered for acute onset comitant esotropia in certain settings.

8. With incomitant esodeviation greater in side gaze, determine whether the lateral rectus function is deficient or the medial rectus is restricted. Forced duction testing (which may require anesthesia for children) may be necessary for that distinction (see Appendix 6, FORCED DUCTION TEST AND ACTIVE FORCE GENERATION TEST). Consider thyroid function tests or a workup for myasthenia gravis. Be sure to look for characteristics of strabismus syndromes (see 8.6, STRABISMUS SYNDROMES).

Treatment

In all cases, correct refractive errors of +2.00 diopters or more. In children, treat any underlying amblyopia (see 8.7, AMBLYOPIA).

1. Congenital esotropia: Almost always requires strabismus surgery. However, prescribe glasses and initiate treatment of any underlying amblyopia prior to surgical intervention as appropriate.

2. Accommodative esotropia: Glasses must be worn full time.

   a. If the patient is <6 years old, correct the hyperopia with the full cycloplegic refraction.

   b. If the patient is >6 years old, attempts should be made to give as close to the full-plus refraction as possible, knowing that some may not tolerate the full prescription. Attempts to push plus lenses during the manifest (noncycloplegic) refraction until distance vision blurs may be tried to give the most plus lenses without blurring distance vision. The goal of refractive correction should be straight alignment without sacrificing visual acuity.

   c. If the patient's eyes are straight at distance with full correction, but still esotropic at near fixation (high AC/A ratio), treatment options include the following:

      • Bifocals (flat-top or executive type) +2.50 or +3.00 diopter add, with top of the bifocal at the lower pupillary border.

      • Echothiophate (phospholine iodide) eyedrops in both eyes nightly.

      • Extraocular muscle surgery targeting the near deviation only may be indicated. This typically requires posterior fixation sutures to the muscle to modify the surgical effect for near only.

      • Wearing full-plus distance glasses only.

 NOTE: There is no universal agreement on the treatment of patients with excess crossing at near only.

3. Nonaccommodative, partially accommodative, or decompensated accommodative esotropia: Muscle surgery is usually performed to correct the nonaccommodative deviation or the significant residual esotropia that remains when glasses are worn.

- Sensory-deprivation esotropia.
- Attempt to identify and correct the cause of poor vision.
- Amblyopia treatment.
- Give the full cycloplegic correction (in fixing eye) if the patient is <6 years of age, otherwise give as much plus as tolerated during manifest refraction.
- Muscle surgery to correct the manifest esotropia.
- All patients with low vision in one eye need to wear protective polycarbonate lens glasses at all times.

Follow Up

At each visit, evaluate for amblyopia and measure the degree of deviation with prisms (with glasses worn).

1. If amblyopia is present, see 8.7, AMBLYOPIA, for management.

2. In the absence of amblyopia, the child is reevaluated in 3 to 6 weeks after a new prescription is given. If no changes are made and the eyes are straight, the patient should be followed up several times a year when young, decreasing to annually when stable.

3. When a residual esotropia is present while the patient wears glasses, an attempt is made to add more plus power to the current prescription. Children <6 years old should receive a new cycloplegic refraction; plus lenses are pushed without cycloplegia in older children. The maximal additional plus lens that does not blur distance vision is prescribed. If the eyes cannot be straightened with more plus power, then a decompensated accommodative esotropia has developed (see above in Section 8.4, Comitant OR Concomitant Esotropic Deviations).

Hyperopia often decreases slowly after age 5 to 7 years of age, and the strength of the glasses may need to be reduced so as not to blur distance vision. If the strength of the glasses must be reduced to improve visual acuity and the esotropia returns, then this is a decompensated accommodative esotropia.

8.5 Exodeviations

Signs

(See Figure 8.5.1.)

Critical. Either eye is constantly or intermittently turned outward. On the cover–uncover test, the uncovered eye moves from the outturned position to the midline to fixate when the previously fixating eye is covered (see Appendix 3, COVER/ UNCOVER AND ALTERNATE COVER TESTS).

Other. Amblyopia, "A" pattern deviation (superior oblique overaction producing an increased deviation in downgaze compared to upgaze), "V" pattern deviation (inferior oblique overaction producing an increased deviation in upgaze compared to downgaze), and dissociated vertical deviations.

Differential Diagnosis

Pseudoexotropia: The patient appears to have an exodeviation, but no movement is noted on cover–uncover testing despite good vision in each eye. A wide interpupillary distance, a naturally large angle k (angle between the pupil center and the visual axis), or temporal dragging of the macula (e.g., from ROP, FEVR, toxocariasis, or other retinal disorders) may be responsible.

Types

1. Exophoria: A latent exodeviation controlled by fusion under conditions of normal binocular vision. Usually asymptomatic, but prolonged strenuous visual activity may cause asthenopia.

   - Intermittent exotropia: A manifest deviation in which one eye demonstrates exodeviation part of the time. The most common type of exodeviation in children. Onset is usually before age 5. Frequency often increases over time. Amblyopia is rare. Usually occurs when the patient is fatigued, sick, or not attentive. Patient often closes one eye or squints in bright sunlight. This

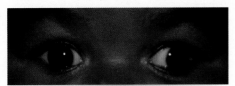

Figure 8.5.1 Exotropia.

is likely due to dissociation and breakdown of their binocular alignment.

A. Clinical evaluation:
- Good control: One eye turns out at only after cover testing and the patient is able to regain fusion quickly without blinking or refixating when the cover is removed.
- Fair control: One eye turns out after cover testing and the patient can only regain fusion with blinking or refixating.
- Poor control: One eye turns out spontaneously and remains manifest for an extended period of time.

B. Good, fair, or poor control can be seen in all four types of intermittent exotropia:
- Basic: Exodeviation is approximately the same with distance and near fixation.
- True divergence excess: Exodeviation that remains greater at distance than near after a period of monocular occlusion.
- Simulated divergence excess: Exodeviation that is initially greater with distance fixation than near that becomes approximately the same after an interval of monocular occlusion.
- Convergence insufficiency: Exodeviation is greater at near than distance. Distinct from isolated convergence insufficiency. See 13.4, CONVERGENCE INSUFFICIENCY.

2. Constant exotropia: Encountered more often in older children. There are three types:
- Congenital exotropia: Also known as infantile exotropia. Presents before age 6 months with a large angle deviation.

Uncommon in otherwise healthy infants and may be associated with a central nervous system or craniofacial disorder.
- Sensory-deprivation exotropia: An eye that does not see well for any reason may turn outward.
- Decompensated intermittent exotropia: A patient with long-standing intermittent exotropia that has decompensated.
- Consecutive exotropia: Follows a diagnosis of esotropia, most commonly after previous surgery for esotropia.

3. Duane syndrome, type 2: Limitation of adduction of one eye, with globe retraction and narrowing of the palpebral fissure on attempted adduction. Rarely bilateral. See 8.6, STRABISMUS SYNDROMES. May present with head turn away from affected eye.

4. Neuromuscular abnormalities:
- Third cranial nerve palsy: See 10.5, ISOLATED THIRD CRANIAL NERVE PALSY.
- Myasthenia gravis: See 10.11, MYASTHENIA GRAVIS.
- Internuclear ophthalmoplegia: See 10.13, INTERNUCLEAR OPHTHALMOPLEGIA.

5. Dissociated horizontal deviation: A change in horizontal ocular alignment caused by a change in the balance of visual input from the two eyes. Not related to accommodation. Seen clinically as a spontaneous unilateral exodeviation or an exodeviation of greater magnitude in one eye during prism and alternate cover testing.

6. Orbital disease (e.g., tumor, idiopathic orbital inflammatory syndrome): Proptosis and restriction of ocular motility are usually evident. See 7.1, ORBITAL DISEASE.

7. Isolated convergence insufficiency: Usually occurs in patients >10 years old. Blurred near vision, asthenopia, or diplopia when reading. An exophoria at near fixation, but straight or small exophoria at distance fixation. Must be differentiated from convergence paralysis. See 13.4, CONVERGENCE INSUFFICIENCY.

8. Convergence paralysis: Similar to convergence insufficiency, but with a relatively acute onset, an exotropia at near, and an inability to overcome base out prism. Often secondary to an intracranial lesion.

8

Workup

1. Evaluate visual acuity of each eye, with correction and pinhole, to evaluate for amblyopia. Color vision and stereopsis.
2. Perform motility examination; observing for restricted eye movements or signs of Duane syndrome.
3. Measure the exodeviation in all cardinal fields of gaze at distance and in primary position (straight ahead) at near, using prisms. See Appendix 3, COVER/UNCOVER AND ALTERNATE COVER TESTS.
4. Perform pupillary, slit lamp, and fundus examinations; check for causes of sensory deprivation (if poor vision).
5. Refraction (cycloplegic or manifest depending on age of the patient).
6. Consider workup for myasthenia gravis when suspected or evidence of fatigability. See 10.11, MYASTHENIA GRAVIS.
7. Consider an MRI of the brain and orbits when neurologic or orbital disease is suspected.

Treatment

In all cases, correct significant refractive errors and treat amblyopia. See 8.7, AMBLYOPIA.

1. Exophoria:
   - No treatment necessary unless it progresses to intermittent exotropia.
2. Intermittent exotropia:
   - Good control: Correct refractive error and treat amblyopia if present. Follow patient closely.
   - Fair control: Correct refractive error and treat amblyopia if present. Nonsurgical treatment may be indicated and include occlusion therapy with alternate daily patching to reduce suppression or additional minus lenses to stimulate accommodative convergence. Muscle surgery may be considered to maintain normal binocular vision.
   - Poor control: Correct refractive error and treat amblyopia if present. Nonsurgical

treatments as described above may be attempted. Muscle surgery is often indicated. Bifixation or peripheral fusion can occasionally be attained.

3. Sensory-deprivation exotropia:
   - Correct the underlying cause, if possible.
   - Treat any amblyopia.
   - Muscle surgery may be performed for manifest exotropia.
   - When one eye has very poor vision, protective glasses (polycarbonate lens glasses) should be worn at all times to protect the good eye.
4. Congenital exotropia:
   - Muscle surgery within a year of onset, as in patients with congenital esotropia.
5. Consecutive exotropia:
   - Additional muscle surgery may be considered.
   - Prism correction in glasses can be used.
   - Over-minus or under-plus correction can stimulate accommodative convergence.
6. Dissociated horizontal deviation:
   - Muscle surgery may be considered.
7. Duane syndrome: See 8.6, STRABISMUS SYNDROMES.
8. Third cranial nerve palsy: See 10.5, ISOLATED THIRD CRANIAL NERVE PALSY.
9. Convergence insufficiency: See 13.4, CONVERGENCE INSUFFICIENCY.
10. Convergence paralysis:
    - Base-in prisms at near to alleviate diplopia.
    - Plus lenses if accommodation is also weakened.

Follow Up

1. If amblyopia is present, see 8.7, AMBLYOPIA.
2. If no amblyopia is present, then reexamine every 3 to 6 months depending on the age of the patient and the control of the deviation. The parents and patient are asked to return sooner if the deviation increases, becomes more frequent, stays out longer, or if the patient begins to close one eye.

8.6 Strabismus Syndromes

Motility disorders that demonstrate typical features of a particular syndrome.

Syndromes

- Duane syndrome: A congenital motility disorder, usually unilateral (85%), characterized by limited abduction, limited adduction, or both. The globe retracts and the eyelid fissure narrows on adduction. In unilateral cases, the strabismus will be incomitant and the patient will often adopt a face turn to allow them to use both eyes together. May be associated with deafness and limb or vertebral abnormalities. Classified into three types:
  - Type 1 (most common): Limited abduction. Primary position frequently esotropia. In unilateral cases, nearly always with face turn toward affected side.
  - Type 2 (least common): Limited adduction. Primary position usually exotropia. In unilateral cases, often with face turn away from affected side.
  - Type 3: Limited abduction and adduction. Esotropia, exotropia, or no primary position deviation. Significant globe retraction.
- Brown syndrome: A motility disorder characterized by limitation of elevation in adduction. Elevation in abduction is normal. Typically, eyes are aligned in primary gaze, although a vertical diplopia with chin-up head position or face turn can be present. Usually congenital, but may be idiopathic or acquired secondary to trauma, surgery, or inflammation in the area of the trochlea. Bilateral in 10% of patients.
- Monocular elevation deficiency (double elevator palsy): Congenital. Unilateral limitation of elevation in all fields of gaze secondary to restriction of the inferior rectus or paresis of the inferior oblique and/or superior rectus. There may be hypotropia of the involved eye that increases in upgaze. Ptosis or pseudoptosis may be present in primary gaze. The patient may assume a chin-up position to maintain fusion if a hypotropia in primary gaze is present.
- Möbius syndrome: Rare congenital condition associated with both sixth and seventh cranial nerve palsies. Esotropia is usually present. Limitation of abduction and/or adduction. A unilateral or bilateral facial nerve palsy is either partial or complete. Other cranial nerve palsies as well as deformities of the limbs, chest, and tongue may occur.
- Congenital fibrosis syndrome: Congenital group of disorders with restriction and fibrous replacement of the extraocular muscles. Usually involves all of the extraocular muscles with total external ophthalmoplegia and ptosis. Most commonly, both eyes are directed downward, so the patient assumes a chin-up position to see. Often autosomal dominant, but other inheritance patterns may be present. Genetic testing is recommended in patients with suspected congenital fibrosis syndrome.

Workup

1. History: Age of onset? History of trauma? Family history? History of other ocular or systemic diseases?
2. Complete ophthalmic examination, including alignment in all fields of gaze. Note head position. Look for retraction of globe and narrowing of interpalpebral fissure in adduction (common in Duane syndrome).
3. Pertinent physical examination, including cranial nerve evaluation.
4. Radiologic studies (e.g., MRI or CT scan) may be indicated for acquired, atypical, or progressive motility disturbances, especially if associated neurologic or developmental abnormalities.
5. Forced duction testing is used to differentiate the two etiologies of monocular elevation deficiency (test will be positive with inferior rectus fibrosis and negative with superior rectus and inferior oblique paresis). Forced ductions can also confirm the diagnosis of Brown syndrome.

Treatment

1. Treatment is usually indicated for a cosmetically significant abnormal head position or if a significant horizontal or vertical deviation exists in primary gaze.
2. Surgery, when indicated, depends on the particular motility disorder, extraocular muscle function, and the degree of abnormal head position.

Follow Up

Follow up depends on the condition or conditions being treated.

8

8.7 Amblyopia

Symptoms

Usually none. Often discovered when decreased vision is detected via visual acuity testing of each eye individually. A history of patching, strabismus, or muscle surgery as a child may be elicited.

> **NOTE:** Amblyopia occasionally occurs bilaterally as a result of bilateral visual deprivation (e.g., congenital cataracts not treated within the earliest months of life).

Signs

Critical. Poorer vision in one eye that is not entirely improved with refraction and not entirely explained by an organic lesion. In anisometropic amblyopia, the involved eye nearly always has a higher refractive error. The decrease in vision develops during the first decade of life. Central vision is primarily affected, while the peripheral visual field usually remains normal.

Other. Individual letters are more easily read than a full line (crowding phenomenon). In reduced illumination, the visual acuity of an amblyopic eye is reduced much less than an organically diseased eye (neutral-density filter effect).

> **NOTE:** Amblyopia, when severe, may cause a trace relative afferent pupillary defect. Care must be taken to be sure that the light is directed along the same axis in each eye, particularly in patients with strabismus. Directing the light off-axis may result in a false-positive result.

Etiology

- Strabismus: Most common form (along with anisometropia). The eyes are misaligned. Vision is worse in the consistently deviating, nonfixating eye. Strabismus can lead to or be the result of amblyopia.
- Anisometropia: Most common form (along with strabismus). A large difference in refractive error (usually ≥1.50 diopters) between the two eyes. Can be seen in cases of eyelid

hemangioma or congenital ptosis inducing astigmatism.
- Media opacity: A unilateral cataract, corneal scar, or PFV may cause a preference for the other eye and thereby cause amblyopia.
- Occlusion: Amblyopia that occurs in the fellow eye as a result of too much patching or excessive use of atropine. Prevented by examining at appropriate intervals (1 week per year of age), patching part-time, or using the full cycloplegic refraction when using atropine.

Workup

1. History: Eye problem in childhood such as misaligned eyes, patching, or muscle surgery?
2. Ocular examination to rule out an organic cause for the reduced vision.
3. Cover–uncover test to evaluate eye alignment. See Appendix 3, COVER/UNCOVER AND ALTERNATE COVER TESTS.
4. Cycloplegic refraction of both eyes.

Treatment

1. Patients younger than 12 years:
   - Appropriate spectacle correction (full cycloplegic refraction or reduce the hyperopia in both eyes symmetrically ≥1.50 diopters). If vision remains reduced after period of refractive adaptation (6 to 12 weeks), begin patching or penalization of fellow eye.
   - Patching: Patch the eye with better corrected vision 2 to 6 hours/day. Follow-up visits should be scheduled for 1 week per year of age (e.g., 3 weeks for a 3-year-old). Adhesive patches placed directly over the eye are most effective. Patches worn over glasses are not ideal due to the risk of children peeking. If a patch causes local irritation, use tincture of benzoin on the skin before applying the patch and use warm water compresses on the patch before removal.
   - Penalization with atropine: Atropine 1% once daily (used with glasses) has been shown to be equally effective as patching in mild-to-moderate amblyopia (20/100 or better). If vision does not improve, the

effect of the atropine can be increased by removing the hyperopic lens from the glasses of the nonamblyopic eye. If the child is experiencing difficulty with school work with the use of atropine, he/she can wear full hyperopic correction with a +2.50 bifocal during school or have the atropine drops instilled on weekends only.

- Optical degradation: Use a high plus lens (e.g., +9.00 diopters or an aphakic contact lens) to blur the image. If the child is highly myopic, the minus lens from the preferred eye may be removed.

2. Continue patching until the vision is equalized or shows no improvement after three compliant cycles of patching. If a recurrence of amblyopia is likely, use part-time patching to maintain improved vision.

3. If occlusion amblyopia (a decrease in vision in the patched eye) develops, patch the opposite eye for a short period (e.g., 1 day per year of age), and repeat the examination.

4. In strabismic amblyopia, delay strabismus surgery until the vision in the two eyes is equal, or maximal vision has been obtained in the amblyopic eye.

5. If treatment of amblyopia fails or the patient presents outside of treatment age range, protective glasses should be worn to prevent accidental injury to the nonamblyopic eye. Any child who does not have vision improved to at least 20/40 needs to wear eye protection during sports (one-eyed athlete rule).

6. Treatment of media opacity: Remove the media opacity and begin patching the nonamblyopic eye.

7. Treatment of anisometropic amblyopia: Give the appropriate spectacle correction at the youngest age possible. If vision remains reduced after period of refractive adaptation (6 to 12 weeks), begin patching or penalization of fellow eye.

Follow Up

Long-term follow up depends on the age of the patient, the amount of prescribed patching, and the severity of the amblyopia.

8.8 Pediatric Cataract

Signs

(See Figure 8.8.1.)

Critical. Opacity of the lens at birth.

Other. A white fundus reflex (leukocoria), absent or asymmetric red pupillary reflex, abnormal eye movements (nystagmus) in one or both eyes, and strabismus. Infants with bilateral cataracts may be noted to be visually inattentive. In patients with a monocular cataract, the involved eye may be smaller. A cataract alone does not cause a relative afferent pupillary defect.

Differential Diagnosis

See 8.1, LEUKOCORIA.

Etiology

- **Idiopathic** (most common)
- **Congenital**
  - Familial: Can be autosomal dominant (most common), autosomal recessive, or rarely part of an X-linked recessive Nance–Horan syndrome. Phenotype varies in terms of cataract morphology and timing of clinical onset.
- Metabolic disease:
  - Galactosemia: Cataract may be the sole manifestation when galactokinase deficiency is responsible. A deficiency of galactose-1-phosphate uridyl transferase may produce mental retardation and symptomatic cirrhosis along with cataracts. The typical oil droplet opacity may or may not be seen. Incidence and onset of cataract may vary according to type of galactosemia (i.e., mutation of uridyl transferase, galactokinase, or epimerase). Cataract may be reversible with appropriate dietary modifications.
- PFV: Usually unilateral, very rarely bilateral. The involved eye is usually slightly smaller than the normal fellow eye. Examination after pupil dilatation may reveal a plaque of fibrovascular tissue behind the lens with elongated ciliary processes extending to it. Progression of the lens opacity often leads to angle-closure glaucoma. If bilateral, 90%

8

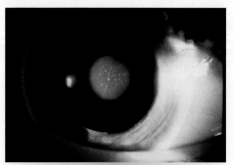

Figure 8.8.1 Pediatric nuclear cataract.

are associated with systemic abnormalities and require further workup.

- Rubella: "Pearly white" nuclear cataract, "salt-and-pepper" chorioretinitis, microphthalmos, corneal clouding, and poorly dilating pupils. Glaucoma may occur with congenital rubella but usually does not occur in the presence of a rubella cataract. Associated hearing defects and heart abnormalities are common.
- Renal syndromes:
  - Lowe syndrome (oculocerebrorenal syndrome): Opaque lens, congenital glaucoma, renal disease, and mental retardation. X-linked recessive. Patients' mothers may have small cataracts.
  - Alport syndrome: Glomerulonephritis, hearing loss, eye abnormalities including cataract, anterior lenticonus, and keratoconus. Most commonly X-linked or autosomal recessive.
  - Others: Intrauterine infection, chromosomal disorders, aniridia, systemic syndromes, metabolic abnormalities, craniofacial syndromes, musculoskeletal disorders, and anterior segment dysgenesis.
- **Acquired:** Trauma, drugs, uveitis, metabolic/endocrine abnormalities, radiation.

Types

1. Zonular (lamellar): Most common type of congenital cataract. White opacities that surround the nucleus with alternating clear and white cortical lamella resembling an onion skin.
2. Polar: Small opacities of the lens capsule and adjacent cortex on the anterior or posterior pole of the lens. Anterior polar cataracts usually are small and tend to grow very little over time. They may be associated with anisometropia and anisometropic amblyopia. Posterior polar cataracts are variable and may grow significantly, causing decreased vision.
3. Nuclear: Opacity within the embryonic/fetal nucleus.
4. Posterior lenticonus: A posterior protrusion, usually opacified, in the posterior capsule.
5. Posterior subcapsular: Opacification of the area immediately anterior to the posterior capsule. Most often acquired due to steroid medications, diabetes, or ionizing radiation.

Workup

1. History: Maternal illness or drug ingestion during pregnancy? Systemic or ocular disease in the infant or child? Radiation exposure or trauma? Family history of congenital cataracts? Steroid use?
2. Visual assessment of each eye individually by using techniques for nonverbal children (Teller cards, following small toys or a light).
3. Ocular examination: Attempt to determine the visual significance of the cataract by evaluating the size and location of the cataract and whether the retina can be seen with a direct ophthalmoscope or retinoscope when looking through an undilated pupil. A blunted retinoscopic reflex suggests the cataract is visually significant. Cataracts ≥3 mm in diameter usually but not always affect vision. Cataracts ≤3 mm may not be inherently visually significant but have been associated with amblyopia secondary to induced anisometropia. Check for signs of associated glaucoma (see 8.11, CONGENITAL/INFANTILE GLAUCOMA) and examine the optic nerve and retina for abnormalities.
4. Cycloplegic refraction.
5. B-scan US may be helpful when the fundus view is obscured. It is essential to rule out posterior PFV in unilateral cataract cases where the fundus is not visible.
6. Ultrasound biomicroscopy can be helpful in cases of anterior segment dysgenesis or PFV.
7. Bilateral cataracts suggest a genetic or metabolic etiology; medical examination by a pediatrician looking for associated abnormalities is recommended.

8. Red blood cell (RBC) galactokinase activity (galactokinase levels) with or without RBC galactose-1-phosphate uridyl transferase activity to rule out galactosemia. The latter test is performed routinely on all infants in the United States as part of the newborn screen.

9. Other tests as suggested by the systemic or ocular examination. The chance that one of these conditions is present in a healthy child is remote.

- Urine: Amino acid quantitation (Alport syndrome), amino acid content (Lowe syndrome).
- Antibody titers for rubella and other suspected intrauterine infections.

Treatment

1. Referral to a pediatrician to treat any underlying disorder.
2. Treat associated ocular diseases.
3. Cataract extraction, usually within days to weeks of discovery to prevent irreversible amblyopia, is performed in the following circumstances:
   - Visual axis is obstructed, and the eye's visual development is at risk.
- Cataract progression threatens the health of the eye (e.g., in PFV).

4. After cataract extraction, treat amblyopia (see 8.7, AMBLYOPIA).

5. A dilating agent (e.g., phenylephrine 2.5% t.i.d. or cyclopentolate 1% b.i.d.) may be used as a temporizing measure, allowing peripheral light rays to pass around the lens opacity and reach the retina. If the cataract is small, and the red reflex is good around the peripheral lens, this may be the only treatment needed.

6. Unilateral cataracts that are not large enough to obscure the visual axis may still result in amblyopia despite not needing cataract extraction. Treat amblyopia as above.

Follow Up

1. Infants and young children who do not undergo surgery are monitored closely for cataract progression and amblyopia.

2. Amblyopia is less likely to develop in older children even if the cataract progresses. Therefore, this age group is followed less frequently.

 NOTE: Children with rubella must be isolated from pregnant women.

8.9 Ophthalmia Neonatorum (Newborn Conjunctivitis)

Signs

Critical. Purulent, mucopurulent, or mucoid discharge from one or both eyes in the first month of life with diffuse conjunctival injection.

Other. Eyelid edema and chemosis.

Differential Diagnosis

- Dacryocystitis: Swelling and erythema just below the inner canthus. See 6.9, DACRYOCYSTITIS/INFLAMMATION OF THE LACRIMAL SAC.
- Nasolacrimal duct obstruction: See 8.10, CONGENITAL NASOLACRIMAL DUCT OBSTRUCTION.
- Congenital glaucoma: See 8.11, CONGENITAL/ INFANTILE GLAUCOMA.

Etiology

- Chemical: Seen within a few hours of instilling a prophylactic agent (e.g., silver nitrate). Lasts no more than 24 to 36 hours. Rarely seen now that erythromycin is used routinely. Gentamicin should be avoided since it may be associated with a toxic reaction.

- *Neisseria gonorrhoeae*: Usually seen within 3 to 4 days after birth. May present with mild conjunctival hyperemia to severe chemosis, copious discharge, rapid corneal ulceration, or corneal perforation. Gram-negative intracellular diplococci seen on Gram stain.

- *Chlamydia trachomatis*: Usually presents within first week or two of birth with mild swelling, hyperemia, tearing, and primarily mucoid discharge. Can progress resulting in increased eyelid swelling and discharge. May form pseudomembranes with bloody discharge. Giemsa stain may show basophilic intracytoplasmic inclusion bodies in conjunctival epithelial cells, polymorphonuclear leukocytes, or lymphocytes. Diagnosis usually made with various molecular tests including immunoassay (e.g., ELISA, enzyme immunoassay, direct antibody tests), polymerase chain reaction (PCR), or DNA hybridization probe.

- Bacteria: Staphylococci (including methicillin-resistant *Staphylococcus aureus*), streptococci, and gram-negative species may be seen on Gram stain.
- Herpes simplex virus: Initially asymptomatic. May present with a cloudy cornea, conjunctival injection, and tearing. Classic herpetic vesicles on the eyelid margins are not always seen. A corneal dendrite which rapidly progresses to a geographic ulcer may occur. Can see multinucleated giant cells on Giemsa stain.

Workup

1. History: Previous or concurrent venereal disease in the mother? Were cervical cultures performed during pregnancy?
2. Ocular examination with use of fluorescein staining to look for corneal involvement.
3. Conjunctival scrapings for two slides: Gram and Giemsa stain.
   - Technique: Irrigate the discharge out of the fornices and place a drop of topical anesthetic (e.g., proparacaine) in the eye. Scrape the palpebral conjunctiva of the lower eyelid with a flame-sterilized spatula (after it cools off) or with a fresh calcium alginate swab (moistened with liquid broth media). Place scrapings on slide (or culture media).
4. Conjunctival cultures with blood and chocolate agars. Chocolate agar should be placed in an atmosphere of 2% to 10% carbon dioxide immediately after being plated. Technique as described above.
5. Scrape the conjunctiva for the chlamydial immunofluorescent antibody test or PCR, if available.
6. Viral culture: Moisten the applicator and roll it along the palpebral conjunctiva. Place the end of the applicator directly into the viral transport medium and mix vigorously to achieve inoculation.

7. Systemic evaluation by primary care provider.

Treatment

Initial therapy is based on the results of the Gram and Giemsa stains if they can be examined immediately. Therapy is then modified according to the culture results and clinical response.

1. No information from stains, no particular organism suspected: Erythromycin ointment q.i.d. plus erythromycin elixir 50 mg/kg/d in four divided doses for 2 to 3 weeks.
2. Suspect chemical (e.g., silver nitrate) toxicity: Discontinue offending agent. No treatment or preservative-free artificial tears q.i.d. Reevaluate in 24 hours.
3. Suspect chlamydial infection: Erythromycin elixir 50 mg/kg/d orally in four divided doses for 14 days, plus erythromycin ointment q.i.d. Alternatively, azithromycin 20 mg/kg orally for 3 days can be used. Topical therapy alone is not effective. If confirmed by culture or immunofluorescent stain, treat the mother and her sexual partners with one of the following:
   - Doxycycline 100 mg p.o. b.i.d. for 7 days (for women who are neither breastfeeding nor pregnant). If breastfeeding or pregnant, one of the following regimens may be used: azithromycin 1 g as a single dose, amoxicillin 500 mg p.o. t.i.d. for 7 days, or erythromycin 250 to 500 mg p.o. q.i.d. for 7 days.

> **NOTE:** Inadequately treated chlamydial conjunctivitis in a neonate can lead to chlamydial otitis or pneumonia.

> **NOTE:** All neonates with chlamydial infection should also be evaluated for *N. gonorrhoeae* infection.

4. Suspect *N. gonorrhoeae*:
   - Saline irrigation of the conjunctiva and fornices until discharge gone.
   - Hospitalize and evaluate for disseminated gonococcal infection with careful physical examination (especially of the joints). Blood and cerebrospinal fluid cultures are obtained if a culture-proven infection is present.

- Ceftriaxone 25 to 50 mg/kg intravenously (i.v.) or intramuscularly (i.m.) (not to exceed 125 mg) as a single dose or cefotaxime 100 mg/kg i.v. or i.m. as a single dose. In penicillin-allergic patients or cephalosporin-allergic patients, an infectious disease consult is recommended. If sensitivities are not initially available, ceftriaxone is the treatment of choice. Systemic antibiotics sufficiently treat gonococcal conjunctivitis, and topical antibiotics are not necessary.
- Topical saline lavage q.i.d. to remove any discharge.
- All neonates with gonorrhea should also be treated for chlamydial infection with erythromycin elixir 50 mg/kg/d in four divided doses for 14 days.

> **NOTE:** If confirmed by culture, the mother and her sexual partners should be treated appropriately for both gonorrhea and chlamydia infections.

5. Gram-positive bacteria with no suspicion of gonorrhea and no corneal involvement: Bacitracin ointment q.i.d. for 2 weeks.
6. Gram-negative bacteria with no suspicion of gonorrhea and no corneal involvement: Gentamicin, tobramycin, or ciprofloxacin ointment q.i.d. for 2 weeks.

7. Bacteria on Gram stain and corneal involvement: Hospitalize, workup, and treat as discussed in 4.11, BACTERIAL KERATITIS.
8. Suspect herpes simplex virus: The neonate (under 1 month of age), regardless of the presenting ocular findings, should be treated with acyclovir intravenously as well as with vidarabine 3% ointment five times per day or ganciclovir 0.15% gel five times per day or trifluridine 1% drops nine times per day. Prompt initiation of intravenous acyclovir may prevent dissemination of the HSV infection and spread to the CNS. Topical therapy is optional when systemic therapy is instituted. In full-term infants, the dosage for acyclovir is 60 mg/kg/d divided into three doses. If infection is limited to the skin, eye, and mouth, it is administered intravenously for 14 days. Treatment duration is extended to 21 days if the disease is disseminated or involves the central nervous system. Consultation with a pediatric infectious disease specialist is recommended. For children with recurrent ocular lesions, oral suppressive therapy with acyclovir (20 mg/kg b.i.d.) may be of benefit.

Follow Up

1. Initially examine daily as an inpatient or outpatient.
2. If the condition worsens (e.g., corneal involvement develops), reculture and hospitalize. Therapy and follow up are tailored according to the clinical response and the culture results.

8.10 Congenital Nasolacrimal Duct Obstruction

Signs

Critical. Wet-looking eye or tears flowing over the eyelid, moist or dried mucopurulent material on the eyelashes (predominantly medially), and reflux of mucoid or mucopurulent material from the punctum when pressure is applied over the lacrimal sac (where the lower eyelid abuts the nose). The eye is otherwise white. Symptoms usually appear in the first 3 months of life.

Other. Erythema of the surrounding skin, redness and swelling of the medial canthus, and increased size of tear meniscus. May become infected and occasionally spread from the nasolacrimal duct, resulting in conjunctivitis (possibly recurrent). Preseptal cellulitis or dacryocystitis may rarely develop.

Differential Diagnosis

- Conjunctivitis: See 5.1, ACUTE CONJUNCTIVITIS.
- Congenital anomalies of the upper lacrimal drainage system: Atresia of the lacrimal puncta or canaliculus.
- Dacryocele: Bluish, cystic, firm mass located just below the medial canthal angle. Caused by both distal and proximal obstruction of the nasolacrimal apparatus. Most often presents within the first week of life.
- Congenital glaucoma: Classic findings are tearing, blepharospasm, corneal clouding, and a large eye (buphthalmos). See 8.11, CONGENITAL/INFANTILE GLAUCOMA.
- Other causes of tearing: Entropion/trichiasis, corneal defects, foreign body under the upper eyelid.

8

Etiology

Usually the result of a congenitally imperforate membrane at the distal end of the nasolacrimal duct over the valve of Hasner.

Workup

1. Exclude other causes of tearing, particularly congenital glaucoma. See 8.11, CONGENITAL/ INFANTILE GLAUCOMA.
2. Palpate over the lacrimal sac; reflux of mucoid or mucopurulent discharge from the punctum confirms the diagnosis. May also use the dye disappearance test. Place fluorescein in both eyes. Check in 10 minutes; fluorescein can be noted in the nose in a normal eye and will remain pooling in the eye with congenital nasolacrimal duct obstruction.

Treatment

1. Digital pressure to lacrimal sac q.i.d. The parent is taught to place his or her index finger over the child's common canaliculus (inner corner of the eye) and apply pressure in an inward and downward fashion.

2. Topical antibiotic (e.g., polymyxin/trimethoprim q.i.d.) as needed to control mucopurulent discharge if present.
3. In the presence of acute dacryocystitis (red, swollen lacrimal sac), a systemic antibiotic is needed. See 6.9, DACRYOCYSTITIS/ INFLAMMATION OF THE LACRIMAL SAC.
4. Most cases open spontaneously with this regimen by 6 months to 1 year of age. Probing should be considered if the nasolacrimal duct obstruction persists beyond a year of age. Probe earlier if recurrent or persistent infections of the lacrimal system develop or at the request of the parents. Most obstructions are corrected after the initial probing, but repeat sessions are sometimes needed. If primary and secondary probings fail, use of balloon dacryoplasty or silicone tubing placement into the nasolacrimal duct (left in place for weeks to months) may be necessary. Consider dacryocystorhinostomy as a last resort.

Follow Up

Routine follow up unless surgery is indicated, sooner if the situation worsens or acute dacryocystitis is present. Monitor for the development of anisometropic amblyopia.

8.11 Congenital/Infantile Glaucoma

Signs

(See Figure 8.11.1.)

Critical. Enlarged globe and corneal diameter (horizontal corneal diameter >12 mm before 1 year of age is suggestive), corneal edema, Haab striae (curvilinear tears in Descemet membrane of the cornea, with scalloped edges with or without associated stromal haze), increased cup/disc ratio, high intraocular pressure (IOP), axial myopia, commonly bilateral (80%). Classic findings are tearing, photophobia, blepharospasm, corneal clouding, and a large eye (buphthalmos).

Other. Corneal stromal scarring or opacification; high iris insertion on gonioscopy; other signs of iris dysgenesis, including heterochromia, may exist.

Differential Diagnosis

• Megalocornea: Bilateral horizontal corneal diameter usually >13 mm, with normal corneal thickness and endothelium, IOP, and cup/disc ratio. Radial iris transillumination defects may be seen. Usually X-linked recessive (boys affected, female carriers may have greater than normal corneal diameters) and may be associated with developmental delay (Neuhauser syndrome, autosomal recessive).
• Trauma from forceps during delivery: May produce tears in the Descemet membrane and localized corneal edema; tears are typically vertical or oblique. Corneal diameter is normal. Usually unilateral and must have history of forceps use to make diagnosis.
• Congenital hereditary endothelial dystrophy: Bilateral full-thickness corneal edema at birth with a normal corneal diameter and axial length. IOP may be falsely elevated by increased corneal thickness and hysteresis but true associated infantile glaucoma has been reported. See 4.25, CORNEAL DYSTROPHIES.

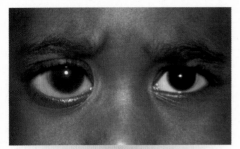

Figure 8.11.1 Buphthalmos of right eye in congenital glaucoma.

- Posterior polymorphous dystrophy: Can present in infancy as bilateral but asymmetric cloudy edematous corneas with characteristic endothelial abnormalities. Normal corneal diameter, axial length, and IOP, but carries lifetime glaucoma risk. Abnormal endothelium may be seen in one parent. See 4.25, CORNEAL DYSTROPHIES.
- Mucopolysaccharidoses and cystinosis: Some inborn errors of metabolism produce cloudy corneas in infancy or early childhood, usually not at birth. The corneal diameter and axial length are normal. IOP is rarely elevated and, if so, usually later in childhood. Always bilateral.
- Nasolacrimal duct obstruction: No photophobia, clear cornea, normal corneal size and axial length, normal IOP. See 8.10, CONGENITAL NASOLACRIMAL DUCT OBSTRUCTION.
- Large eye without other signs of glaucoma can be seen in overgrowth syndromes (e.g., hemihypertrophy) and phakomatoses (e.g., neurofibromatosis, Sturge–Weber) in the absence of glaucoma (although these diagnoses may carry a high risk of glaucoma). May also be autosomal dominant variant without glaucoma.

Etiology

Common

- Primary congenital glaucoma: Not associated with other ocular or systemic disorders. Diagnosed after other causes of glaucoma have been ruled out. Caused by incomplete differentiation of the trabecular meshwork during embryogenesis (e.g., goniodysgenesis).
- Glaucoma following cataract surgery: Most common form of pediatric glaucoma. Typically in older children. All children undergoing cataract surgery are at lifelong risk.

Less Common

- Sturge–Weber syndrome: Usually unilateral (90%); ipsilateral port-wine mark almost always involving eyelid(s), cerebral calcifications/atrophy, and seizures/developmental delay (central nervous system may not be involved at all); not familial. See 13.13, PHAKOMATOSES.

Rare

- Other anterior segment dysgeneses: Axenfeld–Rieger spectrum, Peters anomaly, others. See 8.12, DEVELOPMENTAL ANTERIOR SEGMENT AND LENS ANOMALIES/DYSGENESIS.
- Lowe syndrome (oculocerebrorenal syndrome): Cataract, glaucoma, developmental delay, and renal disease; X-linked recessive.
- Congenital rubella: Glaucoma, cataract, "salt-and-pepper" retinopathy, hearing and cardiac defects (usually peripheral pulmonic stenosis).
- Aniridia: Absence of most of iris, often with only a rudimentary iris stump visible on gonioscopy. Associated with cataracts, glaucoma, macular hypoplasia, and nystagmus. See 8.12, DEVELOPMENTAL ANTERIOR SEGMENT AND LENS ANOMALIES/DYSGENESIS.
- Others: Neurofibromatosis, PFV, Weill–Marchesani syndrome, Rubinstein–Taybi syndrome, covert trauma, steroid-induced infantile glaucoma, complication of ROP, and intraocular tumors.

Workup

1. History: Other systemic abnormalities? Rubella infection during pregnancy? Birth trauma? Family history of congenital glaucoma?
2. Ocular examination, including a visual acuity assessment of each eye separately, measurement of horizontal corneal diameters (measured with calipers or templates), IOP measurement, and a slit lamp or portable slit lamp examination to evaluate for corneal edema and Haab striae. Retinoscopy to estimate refractive error looking for axial myopia. A dilated fundus examination is performed to evaluate the optic disc and retina if able to view through cornea.
3. EUA is performed in cases too difficult to evaluate in the office and in those for

8

whom surgical treatment is considered. Horizontal corneal diameter, IOP measurement, pachymetry, retinoscopy, gonioscopy, and ophthalmoscopy are performed. Axial length is measured with ultrasound (A-scan). At 40 gestational weeks, normal mean axial length is 17 mm. This increases to 20 mm on average by age 1 year. Axial length progression may also be monitored by successive cycloplegic refractions or serial ultrasounds. Disc photos may be taken.

> **NOTE:** IOP may be reduced by general anesthesia, particularly halothane (sevoflurane or desflurane less likely), and over ventilation (low end-tidal CO_2); IOP may be elevated with ketamine hydrochloride, succinylcholine, endotracheal intubation (for 2 to 5 minutes), pressure from the anesthetic mask, speculum use, or inadequate ventilation with elevated end-tidal CO_2.

Treatment

Definitive treatment is surgical, particularly in primary congenital glaucoma. Medical therapy is utilized as a temporizing measure before surgery and to help clear the cornea in preparation for possible goniotomy.

1. Medical:
   • Oral carbonic anhydrase inhibitor (e.g., acetazolamide, 15 to 30 mg/kg/d in three or four divided doses): Most effective.
   • Topical carbonic anhydrase inhibitor (e.g., dorzolamide or brinzolamide b.i.d.): Less effective; better tolerated.
   • Topical beta-blocker (e.g., levobunolol or timolol, 0.25% if <1 year old or 0.5% if older b.i.d.): Important to avoid in asthma patients (betaxolol preferable).
   • Prostaglandin analogs (e.g., latanoprost q.h.s.).

> **NOTE:** Brimonidine is contraindicated in children under the age of 1 year because of the risk of apnea/hypotension/bradycardia/hypothermia from blood–brain permeability. Caution should be used in children under 5 years old or <20 kg or intracranial pathology (such as Sturge–Weber syndrome).

2. Surgical: Nasal goniotomy (incising the trabecular meshwork with a blade or needle under gonioscopic visualization) is the procedure of choice, although some surgeons initially recommend trabeculotomy. Miotics are sometimes used to constrict the pupil before a surgical goniotomy. If the cornea is not clear, trabeculotomy (opening the Schlemm canal from a scleral approach ab externo into the anterior chamber) or endoscopic goniotomy can be performed. If the initial goniotomy is unsuccessful, a temporal goniotomy may be tried. Trabeculectomy or tube shunt may be performed following failed angle incision operations. Cyclodestruction of the ciliary processes through cyclophotocoagulation or cryotherapy may also be an option to decrease aqueous production in certain circumstances.

> **NOTE:** Amblyopia is the most common cause of visual loss in pediatric glaucoma and should be treated appropriately. See 8.7, AMBLYOPIA.

Follow Up

1. Repeated examinations, under anesthesia as needed, to monitor corneal diameter and clarity, IOP, cup/disc ratio, and refraction/axial length.
2. These patients must be followed throughout life to monitor for progression.
3. Other forms of pediatric glaucoma in older children include uveitic glaucoma, traumatic glaucoma, juvenile open-angle glaucoma (autosomal dominant), and others.

8.12 Developmental Anterior Segment and Lens Anomalies/Dysgenesis

Unilateral or bilateral congenital abnormalities of the cornea, iris, anterior chamber angle, and lens.

Specific Entities

- Microcornea: Horizontal corneal diameter small for age. May be isolated or associated with microphthalmia, cataract, or nanophthalmos.

- Posterior embryotoxon: A prominent, anteriorly displaced Schwalbe line. Higher risk for the development of early-onset glaucoma. May be normal or seen in association with Axenfeld–Rieger and Alagille syndromes.

- Axenfeld–Rieger spectrum: Ranges from posterior embryotoxon and iris strands inserting onto Schwalbe line or the cornea to more severe iris malformations including polycoria and corectopia. Glaucoma develops in 50% to 60% of patients. Usually autosomal dominant mutations of PITX2 and FOXC1, although others have been implicated. May be associated with abnormal teeth (e.g., microdontia, conical teeth, hypodontia), skeletal abnormalities, and redundancy of the periumbilical skin. Growth hormone deficiency, cardiac defects, deafness, and mental retardation may be seen **(see Figure 8.12.1)**.

- Peters anomaly: Failure of the lens to form properly from the surface ectoderm and completely detach from surface epithelium during 4 to 7 weeks gestation. Central corneal opacity, usually with iris strands that extend from the collarette to a posterior corneal defect behind the scar. The lens may be clear and normally positioned, cataractous and displaced anteriorly (making the anterior chamber shallow), or adherent to the corneal defect. "Peters plus" syndrome is characterized by an associated skeletal dysplasia with short stature and is more common in bilateral cases. Other malformations may also be seen **(see Figure 8.12.2)**.

- Microspherophakia: The lens is small and spherical in configuration. It can subluxate into the anterior chamber, causing a secondary glaucoma. Can be isolated or seen in association with Weill–Marchesani syndrome **(see Figure 8.12.3)**.

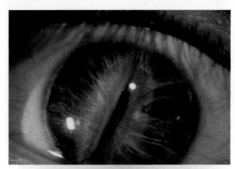

Figure 8.12.1 Axenfeld–Rieger anomaly.

- Anterior and posterior lenticonus: An anterior or posterior ectasia of the lens surface, posterior occurring more commonly than anterior. Often associated with cataract. Unilateral or bilateral. Anterior lenticonus is associated with Alport syndrome. Posterior lenticonus is usually isolated but may be autosomal dominant. It can also be seen with Alport syndrome.

- Ectopia lentis: See 13.10, SUBLUXED OR DISLOCATED CRYSTALLINE LENS.

- Ectopia lentis et pupillae: Lens displacement associated with pupillary displacement in the opposite direction. Usually not associated with glaucoma.

8

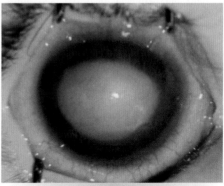

Figure 8.12.2 Peters anomaly.

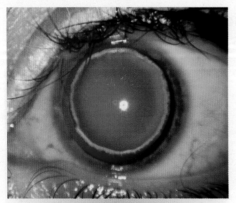

Figure 8.12.3 Microspherophakia.

- Aniridia: Bilateral, near-total absence of the iris. Glaucoma, macular hypoplasia with poor vision, nystagmus, refractive error, and corneal pannus are common. Aniridia is autosomal dominant in two-thirds of patients, a type usually without systemic implications. It occurs sporadically in one-third of cases. May be part of a panocular disorder due to mutations in the master control gene of the eye, PAX6. If PAX6 is deleted as part of a larger chromosomal deletion, it is called WAGR syndrome (Wilms tumor, aniridia, genital abnormalities, retardation). Children with sporadic aniridia have about a 30% chance of Wilms tumor development and require screening, typically with renal ultrasound.
- Sclerocornea: Nonprogressive scleralization of the cornea. Unilateral or bilateral. May be mild and peripheral or severe and diffuse. Associated with severe anterior segment dysgenesis and risk for glaucoma. Often associated with microphthalmia.
- Primary aphakia: Failure of lens development. Usually associated with microphthalmia and severe intraocular dysgenesis including retinal dysplasia and corneal opacity. High risk for glaucoma.

Workup

1. History: Family history of ocular disease? Associated systemic abnormalities?

2. Complete ophthalmic examination, including gonioscopy of the anterior chamber angle and IOP measurement (may require EUA). Fundus photography and A-scan US helpful for serial measurements.
3. Complete physical examination by a primary care physician.
4. In patients with aniridia, obtain chromosomal karyotype with reflex microarray or PAX6 DNA analysis. Until results received, screen with renal ultrasound at diagnosis and no less than every 6 months thereafter until age 7 to 8 years. If deletion involving Wilms tumor gene is found, the frequency of ultrasound should be every 3 months.

Treatment

1. Correct refractive errors and treat amblyopia if present (see 8.7, AMBLYOPIA). Children with unilateral structural abnormalities often have improved visual acuity after amblyopia therapy.
2. Treat glaucoma if present. Beta-blockers, prostaglandin analogs, and carbonic anhydrase inhibitors may be used. Pilocarpine is not effective and is not used in primary therapy (see 9.1, PRIMARY OPEN ANGLE GLAUCOMA). Surgery may be considered initially especially if disease is severe (see 8.11, CONGENITAL/INFANTILE GLAUCOMA).
3. Consider cataract extraction if a significant cataract exists and a corneal transplant if a dense corneal opacity exists.
4. Refer to a specialist for genetic counseling and testing, if desired.
5. Systemic abnormalities (e.g., Wilms tumor) are managed by pediatric specialists.

Follow Up

1. Ophthalmic examination every 6 months throughout life, checking for increased IOP and other signs of glaucoma.
2. If amblyopia exists, follow up may need to be more frequent (see 8.7, AMBLYOPIA).

8.13 Congenital Ptosis

Signs

Critical. Droopy eyelid(s).

Other. Amblyopia, strabismus, astigmatism, and telecanthus. In unilateral ptosis, the involved eye may not open for the first several days of life.

Differential Diagnosis

- Simple congenital ptosis: Either unilateral or bilateral. Present at birth and stable throughout life. May have indistinct or absent upper eyelid crease. The levator muscle is fibrotic resulting in reduced levator function (excursion), less ptosis in downgaze, and often lagophthalmos. May have compensatory brow elevation or chin-up head position. Coexisting motility abnormality if from a third cranial nerve palsy.

- Blepharophimosis syndrome: Blepharophimosis, telecanthus, epicanthal folds, and ptosis. Bilateral and severe. Autosomal dominant with high penetrance **(see Figure 8.13.1)**.

- Marcus Gunn jaw winking: Usually unilateral. Upper eyelid movement with contraction of muscles of mastication, resulting in "winking" while chewing. Upper eyelid crease intact. The ptosis may range from none to severe, but with mastication the levator may lift the eyelid several millimeters above the limbus.

- Acquired ptosis: See 6.1, PTOSIS.

- Horner syndrome: Usually unilateral. Typically 2 to 3 mm of ptosis, associated with anisocoria and lower eyelid reverse ptosis (see 10.2, HORNER SYNDROME). May be congenital (associated with iris heterochromia) or acquired. Acquired forms in children may be related to birth trauma, chest/neck trauma, or metastatic neuroblastoma.

- Pseudoptosis: Dermatochalasis, contralateral proptosis, enophthalmos, hypotropia. See 6.1, PTOSIS.

Etiology

Defective function of either the levator or Müller neuromuscular complexes.

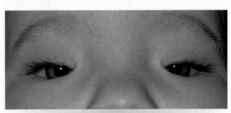

Figure 8.13.1 Blepharophimosis.

Workup

1. History: Age of onset? Duration? Family history? History of trauma or prior surgery? Any crossing of eyes?

2. Visual acuity for each eye separately, with best correction, to evaluate for amblyopia.

3. Refraction checking for anisometropia and astigmatism which is the most common cause for amblyopia with ptosis.

4. Pupillary examination.

5. Ocular motility examination with assessment of head position as well as brow position and action.

6. Measure interpalpebral fissure distance, distance between corneal light reflex and upper eyelid margin, levator function (while manually fixing eyebrow), position and depth of upper eyelid crease. Check for Bell phenomenon and eyelid lag.

7. Slit lamp examination; look for signs of corneal exposure.

8. Dilated fundus examination.

9. If Horner syndrome is suspected, please refer to section 10.2, HORNER SYNDROME and work with a pediatrician for proper systemic evaluation and workup.

Treatment

1. Observation if degree of ptosis is mild, no evidence of amblyopia, and no abnormal head positioning.

2. Simple congenital ptosis: If levator function is poor, consider a frontalis suspension. If levator function is moderate or normal, consider a levator resection.

3. Blepharophimosis syndrome: Ptosis must be repaired by frontalis suspension because of poor levator function. Telecanthus often gets better with time as the head grows and the bridge of the nose grows forward. If the telecanthus is severe, it may be treated with surgery.

4. Marcus Gunn jaw winking: No treatment if mild. Often the jaw winking improves around school age. Any treatment for ptosis with levator resection will increase the excursion during jaw winking.

Follow Up

1. If observing, patients should be reexamined every 3 to 12 months, depending on severity and age, to monitor for occlusion or anisometropic amblyopia.

2. After surgery, patients should be monitored for undercorrection or overcorrection and recurrence. Exposure keratopathy may be a significant problem after ptosis surgery.

8.14 The Bilaterally Blind Infant

Signs

Searching, roving movements of the eyes starting at about 4 to 8 weeks of age. Poor pupillary constriction to light in infants >31 weeks gestation is a key finding. Inability to fix or follow large, bright objects after 4 months of corrected age.

Etiology With an Abnormal Ocular Examination

- Severe ocular disease or malformation.
- ROP. See 8.2, RETINOPATHY OF PREMATURITY.
- Dense bilateral cataracts in children >8 weeks of age. See 8.8, PEDIATRIC CATARACT.
- Aniridia and other severe anterior segment dysgenesis. See 8.12, DEVELOPMENTAL ANTERIOR SEGMENT AND LENS ANOMALIES/ DYSGENESIS.
- Albinism: Iris transillumination defects and foveal hypoplasia. See 13.8, ALBINISM.

> **NOTE:** Ocular abnormalities in patients with albinism and aniridia may be subtle and difficult to assess during an office evaluation.

- Optic nerve hypoplasia: Small optic discs can be difficult to detect when bilateral. When present, a "double-ring" sign (a pigmented ring at the inner and outer edge of a peripapillary scleral ring) is diagnostic. If unilateral, may be seen with strabismus, a relative afferent pupillary defect, and unilateral poor fixation instead of searching nystagmus. Usually idiopathic.

> **NOTE:** Bilateral optic nerve hypoplasia is occasionally associated with septo-optic dysplasia (formerly known as de Morsier syndrome). In contrast, unilateral optic nerve hypoplasia is only rarely associated with this syndrome. Septo-optic dysplasia includes midline abnormalities of the brain as well as growth, thyroid, and other trophic hormone deficiencies. Growth retardation, seizures as a result of hypoglycemia, and diabetes insipidus may develop. If bilateral optic nerve hypoplasia is present, obtain an MRI with attention to the hypothalamic–pituitary area. If unilateral optic nerve hypoplasia is present, imaging studies may be considered as clinically relevant.

- Congenital optic atrophy: Rare. Pale, normal-sized optic disc, often associated with mental retardation or cerebral palsy. Normal electroretinogram (ERG). Autosomal recessive or sporadic.
- Shaken baby syndrome: Multilayered retinal hemorrhages often associated with subdural/ subarachnoid hemorrhage. See 3.21, SHAKEN BABY SYNDROME.
- Extreme refractive error: Diagnosed on cycloplegic refraction.
- Congenital motor nystagmus: Patients with this condition usually have a mild visual deficit (20/60 or better). Binocular conjugate horizontal nystagmus. More than one type of nystagmus may be present, including jerk, pendular, circular, or elliptical. Patients may adopt a face turn to maximize gaze in the direction of the null point. No associated central nervous system abnormalities exist.

Etiologies With a Normal Ocular Examination

- Leber congenital amaurosis: Rod–cone disorder. May have a normal-appearing fundus initially, but by childhood ocular examination reveals narrowing of retinal blood vessels, optic disc pallor, and pigmentary changes. ERG is markedly abnormal or flat which establishes the diagnosis. Autosomal recessive.
- Congenital stationary night blindness: Visual acuity may be close to normal, nystagmus less common, associated with myopia. ERG is abnormal. Autosomal dominant, recessive, and X-linked forms exist. Often have paradoxical pupillary response (pupillary constriction in dim light after exposure to bright light). Retinal pigmentary abnormalities are seen in some types of congenital stationary night blindness.
- Achromatopsia (rod monochromatism): Vision is in the 20/200 range. Marked photophobia. Pupils react normally to light but may have paradoxical pupillary response. Normal fundus, but photopic ERG is markedly attenuated. Absence of response to flicker light stimulus (25 Hz) is diagnostic. Scotopic ERG is normal.
- Cortical visual impairment: One of the most common causes of visual impairment in children from developed countries. Vision is variable. Although the ocular examination is normal, there is an underlying neurologic deficiency causing decreased visual responses.
- Diffuse cerebral dysfunction: Infants do not respond to sound or touch and are neurologically abnormal. Vision may slowly improve with time.
- Delayed maturation of the visual system: Normal response to sound and touch and neurologically normal. The ERG is normal, and vision usually develops between 4 and 12 months of age. More common in patients with some type of albinism (may have nystagmus at presentation).

Workup

1. History: Premature? Normal development and growth? Maternal infection, diabetes, or drug use during pregnancy? Seizures or other neurologic deficits? Family history of eye disease?
2. Evaluate the infant's ability to fixate on an object and follow it.
3. Pupillary examination, noting both equality and briskness.
4. Look carefully for nystagmus (see 10.21, NYSTAGMUS).
5. Examination of the anterior segment; check especially for iris transillumination defects.
6. Dilated retinal and optic nerve evaluation.
7. Cycloplegic refraction.
8. ERG and genetic testing if Leber congenital amaurosis or a retinal dystrophy is suspected.
9. Consider a CT scan or MRI of the brain in cases with other focal neurologic signs, seizures, failure to thrive, developmental delay, optic nerve hypoplasia, or neurologically localizing nystagmus (e.g., seesaw, vertical, gaze paretic, vestibular). If optic atrophy, either unilateral or bilateral, is present, obtain an MRI to evaluate for a glioma of the optic nerve or chiasm and craniopharyngioma.
10. Optical coherence tomography may be helpful to further evaluate optic nerve anomalies.
11. Consider eye movement recordings to evaluate the nystagmus wave form, if available.

Treatment

1. Correct refractive errors and treat known or suspected amblyopia.
2. Parental counseling is necessary in all of these conditions with respect to the infant's visual potential and the likelihood of visual problems in siblings.
3. Referral to educational services for the visually handicapped or blind may be helpful.
4. Provide genetic counseling and testing, if available.
5. If neurologic or endocrine abnormalities are found or suspected, the child should be referred to a pediatrician for appropriate workup and management.

8

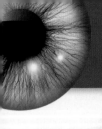
Glaucoma

9.1 Primary Open-Angle Glaucoma

Symptoms

Usually asymptomatic until the later stages. Symptoms may include visual field defects. Usually bilateral, but can present asymmetrically. Severe field damage and loss of central fixation typically do not occur until late in the disease.

Signs

- Intraocular pressure (IOP): Although many patients will have an elevated IOP (normal range of 10 to 21 mm Hg), nearly half have an IOP of 21 mm Hg or lower at any one screening.
- Gonioscopy: Normal-appearing, open anterior chamber angle. No peripheral anterior synechiae (PAS).
- Optic nerve: See **Figure 9.1.1**. Characteristic appearance includes loss of rim tissue (includes notching; increased and/or progressive narrowing most commonly inferiorly followed by superiorly, more rarely nasally or temporally), cupping, nerve fiber layer defect, splinter or nerve fiber layer hemorrhage that crosses the disc margin (Drance hemorrhage), acquired pit, cup/disc (C/D) asymmetry >0.2 in the absence of a cause (e.g., anisometropia, different nerve sizes), bayoneting (sharp angulation of the blood vessels as they exit the nerve), enlarged C/D ratio (>0.6; less specific), progressive enlargement of the cup, and greater disc damage likelihood scale (DDLS) score **(see Figure 9.1.2)**.
- Visual fields: Characteristic visual field loss patterns include nasal step, paracentral scotoma, arcuate scotoma extending from the blind spot nasally (defects usually respect the horizontal midline or are greater in one hemifield than the other), altitudinal defect, or generalized depression **(see Figure 9.1.3)**.

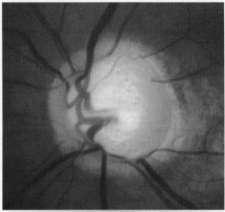

Figure 9.1.1 Primary open-angle glaucoma with advanced optic nerve cupping.

Other. Large fluctuations in IOP, inter-eye IOP asymmetry >5 mm Hg, beta-zone peripapillary atrophy, absence of microcystic corneal edema, and absence of secondary features (e.g., pseudoexfoliation, inflammation).

Differential Diagnosis

If anterior chamber angle open on gonioscopy:

- Ocular hypertension: Normal optic nerve and visual field. See 9.3, OCULAR HYPERTENSION.
- Physiologic optic nerve cupping: Static enlarged C/D ratio without rim notching or visual field loss. Usually normal IOP and large optic nerve (>about 2 mm). Often familial.
- Secondary open-angle glaucoma: Identifiable cause for open-angle glaucoma including inflammatory, exfoliative, pigmentary, steroid-induced, angle recession, traumatic (as a result of direct injury, blood, or debris), and glaucoma related to increased episcleral venous pressure (e.g., Sturge–Weber

	DDLS Stage	Narrowest rim width (rim/disc ratio) [average disc size: 1.50–2.00 mm]	Example
At Risk	1	**0.4** or more	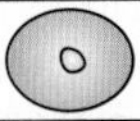
	2	**0.3** to **0.39**	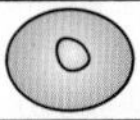
	3	**0.2** to **0.29**	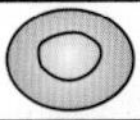
	4	**0.1** to **0.19**	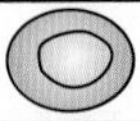
Glaucoma Damage	5	Less than **0.1**	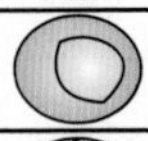
	6	0 (*extension*: less than 45°)	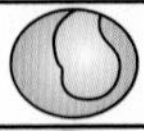
	7	0 (*extension*: 46° to 90°)	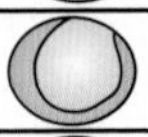
Glaucoma Disability	8	0 (*extension*: 91° to 180°)	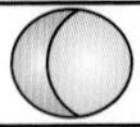
	9	0 (*extension*: 181° to 270°)	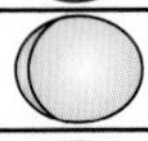
	10	0 (*extension*: more than 270°)	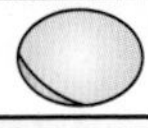

Figure 9.1.2 Disc damage likelihood scale (DDLS).

syndrome, carotid–cavernous fistula), intraocular tumors, degenerated red blood cells (ghost cell glaucoma), lens-induced, degenerated photoreceptor outer segments following chronic rhegmatogenous retinal detachment (Schwartz–Matsuo syndrome), or developmental anterior segment abnormalities.

- Low-tension glaucoma: Same as primary open-angle glaucoma (POAG) except normal IOP. See 9.2, LOW-TENSION PRIMARY OPEN-ANGLE GLAUCOMA (NORMAL PRESSURE GLAUCOMA).
- Previous glaucomatous damage (e.g., from steroids, uveitis, glaucomatocyclitic crisis, trauma) in which the inciting agent has been removed. Nerve appearance now static.
- Optic atrophy: Characterized by disproportionally more optic nerve pallor than cupping. IOP usually normal unless a secondary or unrelated glaucoma is present. Color vision and central vision are often decreased, although not always. Causes include tumors of the optic nerve, chiasm, or tract; syphilis, ischemic optic neuropathy,

drugs, retinal vascular or degenerative disease, and others. Visual field defects that respect the vertical midline are typical of intracranial lesions localized at the chiasm or posterior to it.

- Congenital optic nerve defects (e.g., tilted discs, colobomas, optic nerve pits): Visual field defects may be present but are static.
- Optic nerve drusen: Optic nerves not usually cupped and drusen often visible. Visual field defects may remain stable or progress unrelated to IOP. The most frequent defects include arcuate defects or an enlarged blind spot. Characteristic calcified lesions can be seen on B-scan ultrasonography (US) (as well as on computed tomography [CT]). Autofluorescence can also highlight nerve drusen.

If anterior chamber angle closed or partially closed on gonioscopy:

- Chronic angle closure glaucoma (CACG): Shallow anterior chamber. May present with history of episodic blurred vision or headache. PAS present on gonioscopy. See 9.5, CHRONIC ANGLE CLOSURE GLAUCOMA.

Central 24-2 Threshold test

Fixation monitor: Gaze/Blind spot   Stimulus: III, white   Pupil diameter: 5.1 mm   Date: 03-08-2011
Fixation target: Central   Background: 31.5 ASB   Visual acuity: Time: 12:48 PM
Fixation losses: 2/17   Strategy: SITA-standard   RX: + 1.75 DS   DC X   Age: 70
False POS errors: 5%
False NEG errors: 2%
Test duration: 07:01

Fovea: OFF

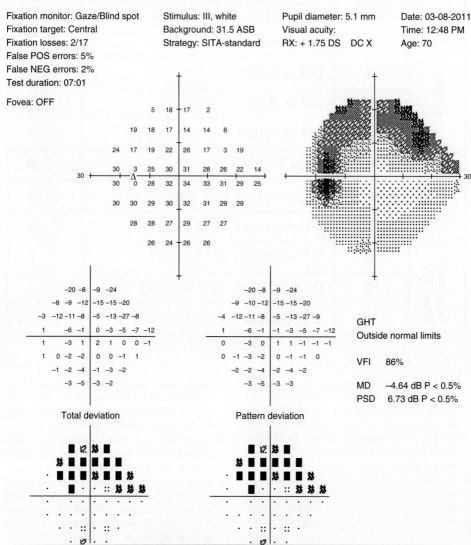

GHT
Outside normal limits

VFI   86%

MD   −4.64 dB P < 0.5%
PSD   6.73 dB P < 0.5%

Total deviation   Pattern deviation

Figure 9.1.3 Humphrey visual field showing a superior arcuate defect or scotoma of the left eye.

Workup

1. History: Presence of risk factors (family history of blindness or visual loss from glaucoma, older age, African descent, diabetes, myopia, hypertension, or hypotension)? Previous history of increased IOP, chronic steroid use, or ocular trauma? Refractive surgery including laser in situ keratomileusis (LASIK) in past (i.e., change in pachymetry)? Review of past medical history to determine appropriate therapy including asthma, chronic obstructive pulmonary disease (COPD), congestive heart failure, heart block or bradyarrhythmia, renal stones, allergies?

2. Baseline glaucoma evaluation: All patients with suspected glaucoma of any type should have the following:

- Complete ocular examination including visual acuity, pupillary assessment for a relative afferent pupillary defect, confrontational visual fields, slit lamp examination, applanation tonometry, gonioscopy, and dilated fundus examination (if the angle is open) with special attention to the optic nerve. Color vision testing is indicated if any suspicion of a neurologic disorder or optic neuropathy.
- Baseline documentation of the optic nerves. May include meticulous drawings, stereoscopic disc photos, red-free photographs, and/or computerized image analysis (e.g., optical coherence tomography [OCT] with analysis of the nerve fiber layer and ganglion cell layer or Heidelberg retina tomography [HRT]) **(see Figure 9.1.4)**. Documentation should include presence or absence of pallor and/or disc hemorrhages.
- Formal visual field testing (e.g., Humphrey or Octopus automated visual field). Goldmann visual field tests may be helpful in patients unable to take the automated tests adequately. Standard visual field testing includes evaluation of peripheral and central field (e.g., Humphrey 24-2 strategy). In cases of paracentral defect or advanced disease, specialized central field testing (e.g., Humphrey 10-2 strategy) is recommended.
- Measure central corneal thickness (CCT). Corneal thickness variations affect apparent IOP as measured with applanation tonometry. Average corneal thickness is 535 to 545 microns. Thinner corneas tend to underestimate IOP, whereas thicker corneas tend to overestimate IOP. Of note, the relationship between corneal thickness and measured IOP is not exactly linear. A thin CCT is an independent risk factor for the development of POAG.
- Evaluation for other causes of optic nerve damage should be considered when any of the following atypical features are present:
  - Optic nerve pallor out of proportion to the degree of cupping.
  - Visual field defects greater than expected based on amount of cupping.
  - Visual field patterns not typical of glaucoma (e.g., defects respecting the vertical midline, hemianopic defects, enlarged blind spot, central scotoma).
  - Unilateral progression despite equal IOP in both eyes.
  - Decreased visual acuity out of proportion to the amount of cupping or field loss.
  - Color vision loss, especially in the red–green axis.

If any of these are present, further evaluation may include:
- History: Acute episodes of eye pain or redness? Steroid use? Acute visual loss? Ocular trauma? Surgery, systemic trauma, heart attack, dialysis, or other event that may lead to hypotension?
- Diurnal IOP curve consisting of multiple IOP checks during the course of the day.
- Consider other laboratory workup for nonglaucomatous optic neuropathy: Heavy metals, vitamin B12/folate, angiotensin-converting enzyme, antinuclear antibody, Lyme antibody, rapid plasma reagin or Venereal Disease Research Laboratory, and fluorescent treponemal antibody absorption or treponemal-specific assay (e.g., MHA-TP). If giant cell arteritis (GCA) is a consideration, check erythrocyte sedimentation rate, C-reactive protein, and platelets (see 10.17, Arteritic Ischemic Optic Neuropathy [Giant Cell Arteritis]).
- In cases where a neurologic disorder is suspected, obtain magnetic resonance imaging (MRI) of the brain and orbits with gadolinium and fat suppression if no contraindications present.
- Check blood pressure, fasting blood sugar, hemoglobin A1c, lipid panel, and CBC (screening for anemia). Refer to an internist for a complete cardiovascular evaluation.

Treatment

General Considerations

1. Who to treat?

   The decision to treat must be individualized. Some general guidelines are suggested.

   Is the glaucomatous process present?

   Glaucomatous damage is likely if any of the following are present: presence of thin or notched optic nerve rim, characteristic

9

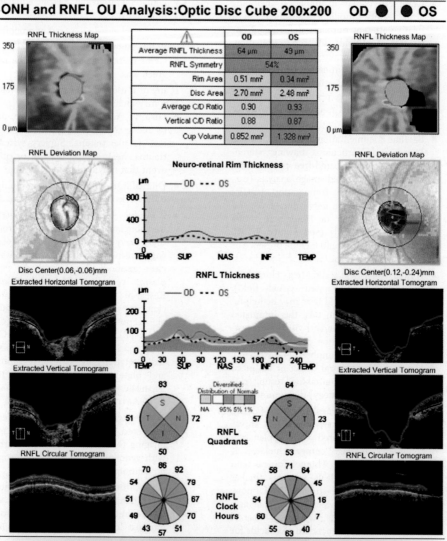

Figure 9.1.4 Optical coherence tomography of the optic nerve head (ONH) and retinal nerve fiber layer (RNFL) thickness.

visual field loss, retinal nerve fiber layer damage, or if DDLS score is >5 (see Figure 9.1.2). Treatment should be considered in the absence of manifest damage if IOP is higher than 30 mm Hg, and/or IOP asymmetry is more than 10 mm Hg.

Is the glaucomatous process active?

Determine the rate of damage progression by careful follow up. Certain causes of optic nerve rim loss may be static (e.g., prior steroid response). Disc hemorrhages suggest active disease.

Is the glaucomatous process likely to cause disability?

Consider the patient's age, overall physical and social health, as well as an estimation of his or her life expectancy.

2. What is the treatment goal?

The goal of treatment is to enhance or maintain the patient's health by halting optic nerve damage while avoiding undue side effects of treatment. The only proven method of stopping or slowing optic nerve damage is reducing IOP. Reduction of IOP by at least 30% appears to have the best chance of preventing further optic nerve damage. An optimal goal may be to reduce the IOP at least 30% below the threshold of progression. If damage is severe, greater reduction in IOP may be necessary.

3. How to treat?

The main treatment options for glaucoma include medications, laser trabeculoplasty (LT) (selective [SLT] more commonly than argon [ALT]), and glaucoma surgery. Medications or LT are appropriate initial therapies. LT may be especially suitable in patients at risk for poor compliance, with medication side effects, and who have significant trabecular meshwork (TM) pigmentation. Surgery may be appropriate initial treatment if damage is advanced in the setting of a rapid rate of progression or difficult follow up. Options include glaucoma filtering surgery (e.g., trabeculectomy, tube shunt), minimally invasive glaucoma surgery (MIGS), laser cyclophotocoagulation of the ciliary body (e.g., with diode laser or endolaser), and cyclocryotherapy. Surgery should always be considered for any patient with advanced/progressive disease or IOP uncontrolled by other methods.

NOTE: MIGS encompasses newer surgical options that offer the advantages of shorter healing times and potentially fewer complications. MIGS is generally considered for patients with mild-to-moderate glaucoma. Some MIGS procedures include trabecular micro-bypass devices, canaloplasty, subconjunctival microstents, deep sclerectomy, endocyclophotocoagulation (ECP), and trabectome trabecular ablation.

Medications

Unless there are extreme circumstances (e.g., IOP >35 mm Hg or impending loss of central fixation), treatment is often started by using one type of drop in one eye (monocular therapeutic trial) with reexamination in 1 to 6 weeks (depending on IOP and individualized risk factors) to check for efficacy.

- Prostaglandin agonists (e.g., latanoprost 0.005% q.h.s., bimatoprost 0.01% or 0.03% q.h.s., travoprost 0.004% q.h.s., tafluprost 0.0015% q.h.s. [preservative free]) are to be used with caution in patients with active uveitis or cystoid macular edema (CME) and are contraindicated in pregnant women or in women wishing to become pregnant. Inform patients of potential pigment changes in iris and periorbital skin, as well as hypertrichosis of eyelashes. Irreversible iris pigment changes rarely occur in blue or dark brown eyes; those at highest risk for iris hyperpigmentation have hazel, gray irides.

- Beta-blockers (e.g., levobunolol or timolol 0.25% to 0.5% daily or b.i.d.) should be avoided in patients with asthma, COPD, heart block, bradyarrhythmia, unstable congestive heart failure, depression, or myasthenia gravis. In addition to bronchospasm and bradycardia, other side effects include hypotension, decreased libido, central nervous system (CNS) depression, and reduced exercise tolerance.

- Selective α2-receptor agonists (brimonidine 0.1%, 0.15%, or 0.2% b.i.d. to t.i.d.) are contraindicated in patients taking monoamine oxidase inhibitors (risk of hypertensive crisis) and relatively contraindicated in children under the age of 5 (risk for cardiorespiratory and CNS depression). See 8.11, CONGENITAL/INFANTILE GLAUCOMA. Apraclonidine 0.5% or 1% is rarely used due to tachyphylaxis and high allergy rate but may be used for short-term therapy (3 months).

- Topical carbonic anhydrase inhibitors (CAIs) (e.g., dorzolamide 2% or brinzolamide 1% b.i.d. to t.i.d.) should be avoided, but are not contraindicated, in patients with sulfa allergy. These medications theoretically could cause the same side effects as systemic CAIs, such as metabolic acidosis, hypokalemia, gastrointestinal symptoms, weight loss, paresthesias, and aplastic anemia. However, systemic symptoms from topical CAIs are extremely rare. There have been no reported cases of aplastic anemia from topical use. Corneal endothelial dysfunction may be exacerbated with topical CAIs; these medications should be used cautiously in patients with Fuchs corneal dystrophy and post keratoplasty.

- Miotics (e.g., pilocarpine q.i.d.) are usually used in low strengths initially (e.g., 1% to 2%) and then built up to higher strengths (e.g.,

9

4%). Commonly not tolerated in patients <40 years because of accommodative spasm. Miotics are usually contraindicated in patients with retinal holes and should be used cautiously in patients at risk for retinal detachment (e.g., high myopes and aphakes).

> **NOTE:** Pilocarpine is not routinely used at Wills Eye due to its adverse side effect profile including associated increased risk for uveitis and retinal detachment, possibility for miosis-induced angle closure, and symptoms such as headache.

- Sympathomimetics (dipivefrin 0.1% b.i.d. or epinephrine 0.5% to 2.0% b.i.d.) rarely reduce IOP to the degree of the other drugs but have few systemic side effects (rarely, cardiac arrhythmias). They often cause red eyes and may cause CME in aphakic patients.

- Systemic CAIs (e.g., methazolamide 25 to 50 mg p.o. b.i.d. to t.i.d., acetazolamide 125 to 250 mg p.o. b.i.d. to q.i.d., or acetazolamide 500 mg sequel p.o. b.i.d.) are relatively contraindicated in patients with renal failure. Potassium levels must be monitored if the patient is taking other diuretic agents or digitalis. Side effects such as fatigue, nausea, confusion, and paresthesias are common. Rare, but severe, hematologic side effects (e.g., aplastic anemia) and Stevens–Johnson syndrome have occurred. Allergy to sulfa drugs is not an absolute contraindication to the use of systemic CAIs, but extra caution should be exercised in monitoring for an allergic reaction. Intravenous forms of systemic CAIs (e.g., acetazolamide 250 to 500 mg i.v.) may be utilized if IOP decrease is urgent or if IOP is refractory to topical therapy. Consider checking baseline creatinine in patients with suspected or confirmed renal disease.

> **NOTE:** Patients should be instructed to press a fingertip into the inner canthus to occlude the punctum for 10 seconds after instilling a drop. Doing so will decrease systemic absorption. If unable to perform punctal occlusion, keeping the eyelids closed without blinking for 1 to 2 minutes after drop administration also reduces systemic absorption.

Argon Laser Trabeculoplasty

In some patients, as previously defined, ALT may be used as first-line therapy. It has an initial success rate of 70% to 80%, dropping to 50% in 2 to 5 years.

Selective Laser Trabeculoplasty

The IOP-lowering effect of SLT is equivalent to ALT. SLT utilizes lower energy and causes less tissue damage, which makes this procedure repeatable.

Guarded Filtration Surgery

Trabeculectomy and tube-shunt surgery may obviate the need for medications. Adjunctive use of antimetabolites (e.g., mitomycin C, 5-fluorouracil) in trabeculectomy surgery may aid in the effectiveness of the surgery but increases the risk of complications (e.g., bleb leaks and hypotony).

Follow Up

1. Patients are reexamined 4 to 6 weeks after starting a new β-blocker or prostaglandin or after ALT/SLT to evaluate efficacy. Topical CAIs, α-agonists, and miotics quickly reach a steady state, and a repeat examination may be performed at any time after 3 days.

2. Closer monitoring (e.g., 1 to 3 days) may be necessary when damage is severe and the IOP is high.

3. Once the IOP has been reduced adequately, patients are reexamined in 3- to 6-months intervals for evaluation of the optic nerve, retinal nerve fiber layer, and IOP.

4. Typically, gonioscopy is performed annually or more often as needed to assess angle anatomy.

5. Formal visual fields and optic nerve imaging (e.g., photographs, OCT, or HRT) are rechecked as needed, often about every 4 to 12 months. If IOP control is not thought to be adequate, visual fields may need to be repeated more often. Once stabilized, formal visual field testing can be repeated annually.

6. Dilated retinal examinations should be performed yearly.

7. If glaucomatous damage progresses, check patient compliance with medications before initiating additional therapy. Consider LT or surgical therapy in setting of progressive damage and poor compliance.

8. Patients must be questioned about side effects associated with their specific agent(s). They often do not associate eye drops with impotence, weight loss, lightheadedness, or other significant systemic symptoms.

REFERENCE

Kass MA, Heuer DK, Higginbotham EJ, et al. The Ocular Hypertension Treatment Study: A randomized trial determines that topical ocular hypotensive medication delays or prevents the onset of primary open angle glaucoma. *Arch Ophthalmol.* 2002;120(6):701-713.

9.2 Low-Tension Primary Open-Angle Glaucoma (Normal Pressure Glaucoma)

Definition

POAG occurring in patients without IOP elevation.

Symptoms

See 9.1, PRIMARY OPEN-ANGLE GLAUCOMA.

Signs

Critical. See Signs in 9.1, PRIMARY OPEN-ANGLE GLAUCOMA, except IOP is consistently below 22 mm Hg. There is a greater likelihood of optic disc hemorrhages. Visual field defects are denser, more localized, and closer to fixation. A dense nasal paracentral defect is typical.

Differential Diagnosis

NOTE: If optic nerve changes and atrophy are unrelated to IOP, it is imperative to investigate potential etiologies of an optic neuropathy other than glaucoma.

- POAG: IOP may be underestimated secondary to large diurnal fluctuations or thin corneas. See 9.1, PRIMARY OPEN-ANGLE GLAUCOMA.
- Shock-related optic neuropathy from previous episode of systemic hypotension (e.g., acute blood loss, myocardial infarction, coronary artery bypass surgery, arrhythmia). Visual field loss should not progress.
- Intermittent IOP elevation (e.g., angle closure glaucoma, glaucomatocyclitic crisis).
- Previous glaucomatous insult with severe IOP elevation that has subsequently resolved. Nonprogressive (e.g., traumatic glaucoma, steroid-induced glaucoma).
- Nonglaucomatous optic neuropathy and others. See DIFFERENTIAL DIAGNOSIS in 9.1, PRIMARY OPEN-ANGLE GLAUCOMA.

Etiology

Controversial. Most investigators believe that IOP plays an important role in low-tension POAG. Other IOP-independent proposed etiologies include vascular dysregulation (e.g., systemic or nocturnal hypotension, vasospasm, or loss of autoregulation), microischemic disease, accelerated apoptosis, and autoimmune disease.

Workup

See Workup in 9.1, PRIMARY OPEN-ANGLE GLAUCOMA. Also consider:

1. History: Evidence of vasospasm (history of migraine or Raynaud phenomenon)? History of hypotensive crisis (recent surgery), anemia, or heart disease? Prior corticosteroid use by any route? Prior ocular trauma or uveitis? Has the vision loss been acute or chronic? GCA symptoms? Additional cardiovascular risk factors such as elevated cholesterol, hypertension, and systemic hypotension (including nocturnal "dippers" in the early morning hours)?
2. Check color plates to rule out optic neuropathy.
3. Check gonioscopy to rule out angle closure, angle recession, or PAS.
4. Consider obtaining a diurnal curve of IOP measurements to help confirm the diagnosis.
5. Consider carotid Dopplers to evaluate ocular blood flow. Check blood pressure (consider 24-hour automated blood pressure home monitor).
6. Consider CT or MRI to rule out compressive lesions of the optic nerve or chiasm especially in cases of decreased visual acuity, color plates, or visual fields suggestive of nonglaucomatous process.

9

Treatment

1. The Collaborative Normal Tension Glaucoma Study (CNTGS) established treatment guidelines for this entity. IOP lowering by at least 30% reduced the 5-year risk of visual field progression from 35% to 12%, thus target IOPs are at least 30% lower than the level at which progressive damage was occurring. Therapies are those for POAG. See 9.1, PRIMARY OPEN-ANGLE GLAUCOMA, for a more in-depth discussion of these therapies. There is evidence that initial therapy with brimonidine 0.2% b.i.d. may be superior to timolol 0.5% b.i.d. in preventing visual field progression in low-tension POAG.

2. Ischemia to the optic nerve head may play a role in the pathogenesis of low-tension POAG. Modification of cardiovascular risk factors is appropriate in managing general health but has not proven beneficial in managing glaucoma. Refer to an internist for control of blood pressure, cholesterol, and optimal management of other comorbid conditions to maximize optic nerve perfusion. If possible, avoid use of antihypertensive drugs at bedtime and use preferentially in the morning.

3. Presence of disc hemorrhages is more common in low-tension glaucoma and is suggestive of progressive disease, warranting more aggressive treatment.

Follow Up

See 9.1, PRIMARY OPEN-ANGLE GLAUCOMA.

REFERENCE

Comparison of glaucomatous progression between untreated patients with normal-tension glaucoma and patients with therapeutically reduced intraocular pressures. Collaborative Normal-Tension Glaucoma Study Group. *Am J Ophthalmol.* 1998;126(4):487-497.

9.3 | Ocular Hypertension

Signs

Critical. Generally defined as IOP >21 on two or more visits. Normal-appearing, open anterior chamber angle with normal anatomy on gonioscopy. Apparently normal optic nerve, retinal nerve fiber layer, and visual field.

Differential Diagnosis

- POAG. See 9.1, Primary Open-Angle Glaucoma.
- Secondary open-angle glaucoma. See 9.1, PRIMARY OPEN-ANGLE GLAUCOMA.
- CACG: PAS are present on gonioscopy with glaucomatous optic nerve and visual field changes. See 9.5, CHRONIC ANGLE CLOSURE GLAUCOMA.

Workup

1. See 9.1, PRIMARY OPEN-ANGLE GLAUCOMA.
2. If any abnormalities are present on formal visual field testing, consider repeat testing in 2 to 4 weeks to exclude the possibility of learning curve artifacts. If the defects are judged to be real, the diagnosis is glaucoma or ocular hypertension along with another pathology accounting for the field loss.

3. OCT and HRT may reveal glaucomatous optic nerve defects. These objective structural tests may show pathology earlier than functional testing (visual fields).

Treatment

1. If there are no suggestive optic nerve or visual field changes and IOP is ≥24 mm Hg, no treatment other than close observation is usually necessary.

2. Patients with an IOP >24 to 30 mm Hg but with normal examinations are candidates for IOP-lowering therapy (threshold varies per glaucoma specialist). A decision to treat a patient should be based on the patient's choice to elect therapy and baseline risk factors such as age, CCT, initial IOP, optic nerve appearance, and family history. The results of the Ocular Hypertension Treatment Study showed that treatment reduced the development of visual field loss from 9.5% to 4.4% at 5 years, with a 20% average reduction of IOP. If treatment is elected, a therapeutic trial in one eye, as described for treatment of POAG, should be used. Some clinicians may elect to monitor these patients with close observation. Risk calculators have been developed to approximate the level of risk

progression to glaucoma if left untreated. These may help guide clinicians and patients as to whether treatment should be initiated. See 9.1, PRIMARY OPEN-ANGLE GLAUCOMA.

Follow Up

Close follow up is required for patients being treated and observed. All patients should initially be followed similarly to POAG; see 9.1, PRIMARY OPEN-ANGLE GLAUCOMA. If there is no progression in the first few years, monitoring frequency can be decreased to every 6 to 12 months. Stopping medication may be considered in patients who have been stable for several years to reassess the need for continued treatment.

REFERENCE

Kass MA, Heuer DK, Higginbotham EJ, et al. The Ocular Hypertension Treatment Study: a randomized trial determines that topical ocular hypotensive medication delays or prevents the onset of POAG. *Arch Ophthalmol.* 2002;120:701-713.

9.4 Acute Angle Closure Glaucoma

Symptoms

Pain, blurred vision, colored halos around lights, frontal headache, nausea, and vomiting.

Signs

(See Figure 9.4.1.)

Critical. Closed angle in the involved eye, acutely increased IOP, and microcystic corneal edema. Narrow or occludable angle in the fellow eye if of primary etiology.

Other. Conjunctival injection; fixed, mid-dilated pupil.

Etiology of Primary Angle Closure

- Pupillary block: Apposition of the lens and the posterior iris at the pupil leads to blockage of aqueous humor flow from the posterior chamber to the anterior chamber. This mechanism leads to increased posterior chamber pressure, forward movement of the peripheral iris, and subsequent obstruction of the TM. Predisposed eyes have a narrow anterior chamber angle recess, anterior insertion of the iris root, or short axial length. Risk factors include increased age, East Asian descent, female sex, hyperopia, and family history. May be precipitated by topical mydriatics or, rarely, miotics; systemic anticholinergics (e.g., antihistamines and antidepressants); accommodation (e.g., reading); or dim illumination. Fellow eye has similar anatomy.
- Angle crowding as a result of an abnormal iris configuration including high peripheral iris roll or plateau iris syndrome angle closure. See 9.13, PLATEAU IRIS.

Etiology of Secondary Angle Closure

- PAS pulling the angle closed: Causes include uveitis, inflammation, and ALT. See 9.5, CHRONIC ANGLE CLOSURE GLAUCOMA.
- Neovascular or fibrovascular membrane pulling the angle closed: See 9.14, NEOVASCULAR GLAUCOMA.
- Membrane obstructing the angle: Causes include endothelial membrane in iridocorneal endothelial syndrome (ICE) and posterior polymorphous corneal dystrophy (PPCD), and epithelial membrane in epithelial downgrowth (may follow penetrating trauma). See 9.15, IRIDOCORNEAL ENDOTHELIAL SYNDROME.
- Lens-induced narrow angles: Iris–TM contact as a result of a large lens (phacomorphic), small lens with anterior prolapse (e.g., microspherophakia), small eye (nanophthalmos), or

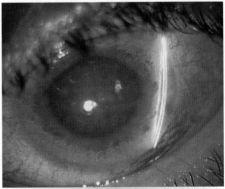

Figure 9.4.1 Acute angle closure glaucoma with mid-dilated pupil, shallow anterior chamber, and corneal edema.

9

zonular loss/weakness (e.g., trauma, advanced pseudoexfoliation, Marfan syndrome).

- Aphakic or pseudophakic pupillary block: Iris bombé configuration secondary to occlusion of the pupil by the anterior vitreous or fibrous adhesions. May also occur with anterior chamber intraocular lenses.

- Topiramate and sulfonamide-induced angle closure: Usually after increase in dose or within first 2 weeks of starting medication. Usually bilateral angle closure due to supraciliary effusion and ciliary body swelling with subsequent anterior rotation of the lens–iris diaphragm. Myopia is induced secondary to anterior displacement of ciliary body and lens along with lenticular swelling.

- Choroidal swelling: Following extensive retinal laser surgery, placement of a tight encircling scleral buckle, retinal vein occlusion, and others.

- Posterior segment tumor: Malignant melanoma, retinoblastoma, ciliary body tumors, and others. See 11.36, CHOROIDAL NEVUS AND MALIGNANT MELANOMA OF THE CHOROID.

- Hemorrhagic choroidal detachment: See 11.27, CHOROIDAL EFFUSION/DETACHMENT.

- Aqueous misdirection syndrome. See 9.17, AQUEOUS MISDIRECTION SYNDROME/ MALIGNANT GLAUCOMA.

- Developmental abnormalities: Axenfeld–Rieger syndrome, Peters anomaly, persistent fetal vasculature, and others. See 8.12, DEVELOPMENTAL ANTERIOR SEGMENT AND LENS ANOMALIES/DYSGENESIS.

Differential Diagnosis of Acute IOP Increase With an Open Angle

- Inflammatory open-angle glaucoma: See 9.7, INFLAMMATORY OPEN-ANGLE GLAUCOMA.

- Traumatic (hemolytic) glaucoma: Red blood cells in the anterior chamber. See 3.6, HYPHEMA AND MICROHYPHEMA.

- Pigmentary glaucoma: Characteristic angle changes (e.g., heavily pigmented TM, Sampaolesi line); vertical pigment deposition on endothelium (Krukenberg spindle); pigment cells floating in the anterior chamber; radial iris transillumination defects (TIDs); pigment line on the posterior lens capsule or anterior hyaloid face. See 9.10, PIGMENT DISPERSION SYNDROME/PIGMENTARY GLAUCOMA.

- Pseudoexfoliation glaucoma: Grayish-white flaky proteinaceous material deposited throughout anterior segment structures and TM (usually irregular pigment most prominent inferiorly). Classically occurs in patients of European descent. Iris TIDs along pupillary margin often present. See 9.11, PSEUDOEXFOLIATION SYNDROME/ EXFOLIATIVE GLAUCOMA.

- Lens-related glaucoma: Leakage of lens material through an intact capsule, usually in the setting of a mature cataract (phacolytic); lens material in the anterior chamber through a violation of the anterior lens capsule after trauma or retained following intraocular surgery (lens particle); or a chronic granulomatous uveitis in response to leaked lens material (phacoantigenic, formerly phacoanaphylaxis). See 9.12, LENS-RELATED GLAUCOMA.

- Glaucomatocyclitic crisis (Posner–Schlossman syndrome): Recurrent IOP spikes in one eye, mild cell, and flare with or without fine keratic precipitates (KP). See 9.8, GLAUCOMATOCYCLITIC CRISIS/POSNER– SCHLOSSMAN SYNDROME.

- Retrobulbar hemorrhage or inflammation. See 3.10, TRAUMATIC RETROBULBAR HEMORRHAGE.

- Carotid–cavernous fistula: See 7.7, MISCELLANEOUS ORBITAL DISEASES.

Workup

1. History: Risk factors including hyperopia or family history? Precipitating events such as being in dim illumination, receiving dilating drops? Retinal problem? Recent laser treatment or surgery? Medications (e.g., topical adrenergics or anticholinergics, oral topiramate, or sulfa medications)?

2. Slit lamp examination: Look for KP, posterior synechiae, iris atrophy or neovascularization (NV), a mid-dilated and sluggish pupil, a swollen lens, anterior chamber cell and flare or iridescent particles, and a shallow anterior chamber. Glaukomflecken (small anterior subcapsular lens opacities) and atrophy of the iris stroma indicate prior attacks. Always carefully examine the other eye and compare.

3. Measure IOP.

4. Gonioscopy of both anterior chamber angles. Corneal edema can be cleared by using

topical hyperosmolar agents (e.g., glycerin). Gonioscopy of the involved eye after IOP reduction is essential in assessment of the persistence and extent of angle closure; also needed to evaluate for the presence of NV.

5. Careful examination of the fundus looking for signs of central retinal vein occlusion, hemorrhage, optic nerve cupping, or spontaneous arterial pulsations which may indicate an exacerbation of IOP elevation. If cupping is pronounced or if there are spontaneous arterial pulsations, treatment is more urgent. Depending on the etiology of angle closure, dilation may be deferred on presentation.

6. When secondary angle closure glaucoma is suspected, B-scan US or US biomicroscopy (UBM) may be helpful.

Treatment

Depends on etiology of angle closure, severity, and duration of attack. Severe, permanent damage may occur within several hours. If visual acuity is hand motion or better, IOP reduction is usually urgent; therapeutic intervention should include all topical glaucoma medications, systemic (preferably intravenous) CAI, and in some cases intravenous osmotic agent (e.g., mannitol) as long as not contraindicated. Paracentesis with a 30-gauge needle on an open tuberculin syringe directed toward the 6 o'clock position will bring down the pressure immediately. See 9.14, NEOVASCULAR GLAUCOMA, 9.16, POSTOPERATIVE GLAUCOMA, and 9.17, AQUEOUS MISDIRECTION SYNDROME/MALIGNANT GLAUCOMA.

1. Compression gonioscopy is essential to determine whether the trabecular blockage is reversible and may break an acute attack.

2. Topical therapy with β-blocker ([e.g., timolol 0.5%] caution with asthma, COPD, and bradycardia), α2 agonist (e.g., brimonidine 0.1%), cholinergic agonist/miotic (pilocarpine 1%), prostaglandin analog (e.g., latanoprost 0.005%), and CAI (e.g., dorzolamide 2%) should be initiated immediately. In urgent cases, three rounds of these medications may be given, with each round being separated by 15 minutes.

3. Topical steroid (e.g., prednisolone acetate 1%) may be useful in reducing corneal edema.

4. Systemic CAI (e.g., acetazolamide 250 to 500 mg i.v. or two 250-mg tablets p.o. in one dose if unable to give i.v.) if reduction in IOP is urgent or if IOP is refractory to topical therapy. Do not use in sulfonamide-induced angle closure or sickle cell disease.

- Recheck the IOP in 1 hour. If IOP reduction is urgent or refractory to therapies listed above, repeat topical medications and give osmotic agent (e.g., mannitol 1 to 2 g/kg i.v. over 45 minutes [note: a 500 mL bag of mannitol 20% contains 100 g of mannitol]). Contraindicated in congestive heart failure, renal disease, and intracranial bleeding.

NOTE: Prior to initiation of systemic CAIs or osmotic agents, consider testing renal function.

5. When acute angle closure glaucoma is the result of:

   a. Phakic pupillary block or angle crowding: Historically, pilocarpine, 1% to 2%, every 15 minutes for two doses was recommended but has fallen out of favor by some physicians due to adverse effects such as headache, accommodative spasm, associated increased risk for uveitis and retinal detachment, and potential for miosis-induced angle closure.

   b. Aphakic or pseudophakic pupillary block or secondary closure of the angle: *Do not use pilocarpine.* Consider a mydriatic and a cycloplegic agent (e.g., cyclopentolate 1% to 2%, and phenylephrine 2.5% every 15 minutes for four doses) when laser or surgery cannot be performed because of corneal edema, inflammation, or both.

   c. Topiramate- or sulfonamide-induced secondary angle closure: Do not use CAIs in sulfonamide-induced angle closure. Immediately discontinue the inciting medication. Consider cycloplegia to induce posterior rotation of the ciliary body (e.g., atropine 1% b.i.d. or t.i.d.). Consider hospitalization and treatment with intravenous hyperosmotic agents and intravenous steroids (e.g., methylprednisolone 250 mg i.v. every 6 hours) for cases of markedly elevated IOP unresponsive to other treatments. Cases involving large ciliochoroidal or choroidal effusions may benefit from intravenous corticosteroids, as inflammation may play a role in their formation. *Peripheral iridotomy (PI) or iridectomy and miotics are not indicated.*

9

6. In phacomorphic glaucoma, the lens should be removed as soon as the eye is quiet and the IOP controlled, if possible. See 9.12.4, PHACOMORPHIC GLAUCOMA.

7. Address systemic problems such as pain and vomiting.

8. For pupillary block (all forms) or primary angle crowding: If the IOP decreases significantly, definitive treatment with yttrium–aluminum–garnet (YAG) laser PI or surgical iridectomy is performed once the cornea is clear and the anterior chamber is quiet, typically 1 to 5 days after attack.

 NOTE: If the affected eye is too inflamed initially for laser PI, perform laser PI of the fellow eye first. An untreated fellow eye has a 40% to 80% chance of acute angle closure in 5 to 10 years. Repeated angle closure attacks with a patent PI may indicate plateau iris syndrome. See 9.13, PLATEAU IRIS.

9. Patients are discharged on a regimen of maintenance dose IOP-lowering drops and oral medications (described above), as well as topical steroids if inflamed. Close monitoring with IOP measurement each day is necessary immediately after an angle closure attack. Once the IOP has been reasonably reduced, follow-up frequency is guided by overall clinical response and stability. On occasion, topical steroids in addition to IOP-lowering medications are necessary for 4 to 7 days to increase the chance of successful iridotomy.

NOTE: If IOP does not decrease after two courses of maximal medical therapy, a laser (YAG) PI should be considered if there is an adequate view of the iris. If IOP still does not decrease after more than one attempt at laser PI, then a laser iridoplasty, surgical PI, or cataract surgery is needed, depending on the etiology. A guarded filtration procedure should also be considered based on the severity of glaucoma and anticipated IOP control after definitive treatment. If IOP remains elevated and the angle remains closed despite a patent iridectomy, surgical treatment of chronic angle closure is indicated.

10. For secondary angle closure: Treat the underlying problem. Consider argon laser gonioplasty to open the angle, particularly in plateau iris syndrome or nanophthalmos. Goniosynechiolysis can be performed for chronic angle closure of <6 months' duration. Systemic steroids may be required to treat serous choroidal detachments secondary to inflammation.

Follow Up

After definitive treatment, patients are reevaluated in weeks to months initially and then less frequently. Visual fields and disc imaging are obtained for baseline purposes.

NOTE

1. Cardiovascular status and electrolyte balance must be considered when contemplating osmotic agents, CAIs, and β-blockers.

2. The corneal appearance may worsen when the IOP decreases.

3. Worsening vision or spontaneous arterial pulsations are signs of increasing urgency for pressure reduction.

4. Since one-third to one-half of first-degree relatives may have occludable angles, patients should be counseled to alert relatives to the importance of screening.

5. Angle closure glaucoma may be seen without an increased IOP. The diagnosis should be suspected in a patient who had episodes of pain and reduced acuity and is noted to have:
   • An edematous, thickened cornea.
   • Normal or markedly asymmetric pressure in both eyes.
   • Shallow anterior chambers in both eyes.
   • Occludable anterior chamber angle in the fellow eye.

9.5 Chronic Angle Closure Glaucoma

Symptoms

Usually asymptomatic, although patients with advanced disease may present with decreased vision or visual field loss. Intermittent eye pain, headaches, and blurry vision may occur.

Signs

(See Figure 9.5.1.)

Critical. Gonioscopy reveals broad bands of PAS in the angle. The PAS block visualization of the underlying angle structures. Glaucomatous optic nerve and visual field defects.

Other. Elevated IOP.

Etiology

Gradual narrowing of the angle with prolonged appositional closure.

Prolonged acute angle closure glaucoma or multiple episodes of subclinical attacks of acute angle closure.

Previous flat anterior chamber from surgery, trauma, or hypotony that resulted in the development of PAS.

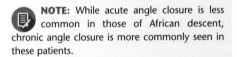 **NOTE:** While acute angle closure is less common in those of African descent, chronic angle closure is more commonly seen in these patients.

Workup

1. History: Presence of symptoms of previous episodes of acute angle closure? History of proliferative diabetic retinopathy, retinal vascular occlusion, or ocular ischemic syndrome? History of prior trauma, hypotony, uveitis, or intraocular surgery?
2. Complete baseline glaucoma evaluation. See 9.1, PRIMARY OPEN-ANGLE GLAUCOMA.

Treatment

See 9.1, PRIMARY OPEN-ANGLE GLAUCOMA.

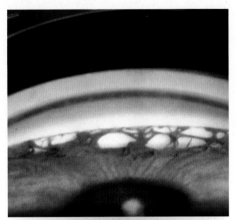

Figure 9.5.1 Chronic angle closure glaucoma with peripheral anterior synechiae.

1. LT contraindicated in CACG and can induce greater scarring of the angle.
2. Laser peripheral iridotomy is indicated to relieve any component of pupillary block and to prevent ongoing development of PAS if closure is not already 360 degrees. Beware of postlaser IOP spikes in these patients whose TM function may be limited.
3. Laser iridoplasty may be performed (and repeated) to decrease the formation of new PAS. This may not be entirely effective and may serve only as a temporizing measure. If iridoplasty fails and other medical therapy has been maximized, the patient may need additional surgery. ECP may be attempted in cases with early glaucoma, but trabeculectomy or tube shunt is usually indicated in more advanced cases. MIGS usually contraindicated due to closed angle.

Follow Up

See 9.1, PRIMARY OPEN-ANGLE GLAUCOMA.

9

9.6 Angle Recession Glaucoma

Symptoms

Usually asymptomatic. Late stages have visual field or acuity loss. History of hyphema or trauma to the glaucomatous eye can often be elicited. Glaucoma due to angle recession (not from the inciting trauma) usually takes many years to develop. Typically unilateral.

Signs

(See Figure 9.6.1.)

Critical. Glaucoma (see 9.1, PRIMARY OPEN-ANGLE GLAUCOMA) in an eye with characteristic gonioscopic findings: an uneven iris insertion, an area of torn or absent iris processes, and a posteriorly recessed iris, revealing a widened ciliary band (may be focal or extend for 360 degrees). Comparison with the contralateral eye can help identify recessed areas.

Other. The scleral spur may appear abnormally white on gonioscopy because of the recessed angle; other signs of previous trauma may be present (e.g., cataract, iris sphincter tears).

Differential Diagnosis

See 9.1, PRIMARY OPEN-ANGLE GLAUCOMA.

Workup

1. History: Trauma? Steroid use? Prior ocular surgery? Family history of glaucoma?
2. Complete baseline glaucoma evaluation. See 9.1, PRIMARY OPEN-ANGLE GLAUCOMA.

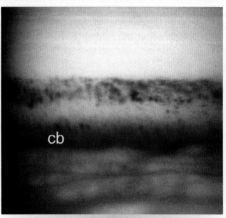

cb

Figure 9.6.1 Angle recession glaucoma with increased width of the ciliary body band.

Treatment

See 9.1, PRIMARY OPEN-ANGLE GLAUCOMA. However, miotics (e.g., pilocarpine) may be ineffective or even cause increased IOP by reduction of uveoscleral outflow. ALT and SLT are rarely effective in this condition. Surgical therapy may be necessary if IOP is uncontrolled with medications.

Follow Up

Both eyes are monitored closely because of high incidence of delayed open-angle glaucoma in the contralateral eye. Patients with angle recession without glaucoma are examined yearly. Those with glaucoma are examined as detailed in 9.1, PRIMARY OPEN-ANGLE GLAUCOMA.

9.7 Inflammatory Open-Angle Glaucoma

Symptoms

Pain, photophobia, and decreased vision; symptoms may be minimal.

Signs

Critical. Elevated IOP with a significant amount of anterior chamber inflammation; open angle on gonioscopy; white blood cells, macrophages, and proteins cause outflow blockage and trabeculitis resulting in elevated IOP. Characteristic glaucomatous optic nerve changes occur late in the disease course.

Other. Miotic pupil, KP, conjunctival injection, ciliary flush, posterior synechiae, and increased TM pigmentation, especially inferiorly. Angle closure glaucoma may occur from progressive PAS formation.

NOTE: Acute IOP increase from any etiology is distinguished from chronic IOP increase by the presence of corneal edema, pain, and visual symptoms.

Differential Diagnosis

- Steroid-response glaucoma: Open angle. Patient on steroid medications (including for uveitis). Can be difficult to differentiate from inflammatory open-angle glaucoma. If significant inflammation is present, pressure elevation should be assumed inflammatory in nature and goal should be to quiet the eye with steroids. See 9.9, STEROID-RESPONSE GLAUCOMA.
- Pigmentary glaucoma: Open angle. Acute increase in IOP, often after exercise or pupillary dilation; pigmented cells in the anterior chamber; 3+ to 4+ trabecular pigmentation; often endopigment in the form of a Krukenberg spindle. Radial iris TIDs are common. See 9.10, PIGMENT DISPERSION SYNDROME/PIGMENTARY GLAUCOMA.
- Neovascular glaucoma. Nonradial, misdirected blood vessels along the pupillary margin, the TM, or both. See 9.14, NEOVASCULAR GLAUCOMA.
- Pseudoexfoliation syndrome: Open angle. Grayish-white flaky material deposited throughout anterior segment structures. Classically in patients of European descent, but not always. Occasionally exfoliative material on cornea can be mistaken for KP. Deposits are more angular, less round than inflammatory KP. See 9.11, PSEUDOEXFOLIATION SYNDROME/EXFOLIATIVE GLAUCOMA.
- Fuchs heterochromic iridocyclitis: Unilateral, more common in middle-aged women. Low-grade inflammation with loss of iris pigmented epithelium causing heterochromia (affected eye typically lighter). Fine bridging vessels in the angle are present and may bleed (Amsler sign). Not neovascular. No PAS. See 12.1, ANTERIOR UVEITIS (IRITIS/IRIDOCYCLITIS).
- Glaucomatocyclitic crisis (Posner–Schlossman syndrome): Open angle and absence of synechiae on gonioscopy. Dramatic IOP elevation with minimal inflammation. Unilateral with recurrent attacks. See 9.8, GLAUCOMATOCYCLITIC CRISIS/POSNER–SCHLOSSMAN SYNDROME.

Etiology

- Uveitis: Anterior, intermediate, posterior, or panuveitis.
- Keratouveitis: Herpetic infections are classically associated with elevated IOP in the setting of early/acute inflammation, whereas other etiologies may cause low IOP from ciliary body shutdown and hyposecretion.
- After trauma or intraocular surgery.

Workup

1. History: Previous attacks? Systemic disease (e.g., juvenile idiopathic arthritis, ankylosing spondylitis, sarcoidosis, acquired immunodeficiency syndrome [AIDS], V1 distribution varicella zoster, toxoplasmosis)? Previous corneal disease, especially herpetic keratitis?
2. Slit lamp examination: Assess the degree of conjunctival injection and aqueous cell and flare. Posterior synechiae present?
3. Complete baseline glaucoma evaluation. See 9.1, PRIMARY OPEN-ANGLE GLAUCOMA.

Treatment

1. Topical steroid (e.g., prednisolone acetate 1%) q1–6h, depending on the severity of the anterior chamber inflammation.

NOTE: Topical steroids are not used, or are used with extreme caution, in patients with an infectious process.

2. Mydriatic/cycloplegic (e.g., cyclopentolate 1% t.i.d.).
3. One or more of the following pressure-reducing agents can be used in addition to the other treatments, depending on the IOP and status of the optic nerve:
   - Topical β-blocker (e.g., timolol 0.5% daily or b.i.d.) if not contraindicated (e.g., asthma, COPD, bradycardia).
   - Topical α2 agonist (e.g., brimonidine 0.1% to 0.2% b.i.d. to t.i.d.).
   - Topical CAI (e.g., dorzolamide 2% t.i.d.) or oral CAI (e.g., methazolamide 25 to 50 mg p.o. b.i.d. to t.i.d. or acetazolamide 500 mg sequel p.o. b.i.d.) if renal function tolerates.
   - Hyperosmotic agent when IOP is acutely increased (e.g., mannitol 20% 1 to 2 g/kg i.v. over 45 minutes) if cardiopulmonary function permits.

9

- Anterior chamber paracentesis if reduction in IOP is urgent or if IOP is refractory to topical therapy (see Appendix 13, ANTERIOR CHAMBER PARACENTESIS).
4. Manage the underlying problem.
5. If IOP remains dangerously elevated despite maximal medical therapy, glaucoma filtering surgery may be indicated. Trabeculectomy surgery has high rates of failure in cases of inflammatory glaucoma. Tube shunt is often the preferred alternative.
6. If HSV suspected, start antiviral coveragse (e.g., acyclovir 400 mg p.o. 5× daily or valacyclovir 500 mg p.o. t.i.d. for 7 to 14 days).

NOTE: Prostaglandin agonists (e.g., latanoprost 0.005%) and miotics (e.g., pilocarpine) should be used with caution in active inflammatory glaucoma, but may be considered once the eye is quiet or if the benefits outweigh the risks.

Follow Up

1. Patients are seen every 1 to 7 days at first. Higher IOP and more advanced glaucomatous cupping warrant more frequent follow up.
2. Antiglaucoma medications are tapered as IOP returns to normal.
3. Steroid-response glaucoma should always be considered if IOP remains high when inflammation has subsided (see 9.9, STEROID-RESPONSE GLAUCOMA). IOP elevation in the presence of significant uveitis suggests the need for more, not less, steroid and additional or alternative pressure lowering therapy.

9.8 Glaucomatocyclitic Crisis/Posner–Schlossman Syndrome

Symptoms

Mild pain, decreased vision, and rainbows around lights. Rare condition. Often a history of previous episodes. Usually unilateral in young to middle-aged patients.

Signs

Critical. Markedly increased IOP (usually 40 to 60 mm Hg), open angle without synechiae on gonioscopy, minimal conjunctival injection (white eye), and very mild anterior chamber reaction (few aqueous cells and little flare).

Other. Corneal epithelial edema, ciliary flush, pupillary constriction, iris hypochromia, few fine KP on the corneal endothelium or TM.

Differential Diagnosis

- Inflammatory open-angle glaucoma: Significant amount of aqueous cells and flare. Synechiae may be present. See 9.7, INFLAMMATORY OPEN-ANGLE GLAUCOMA.
- Pigmentary glaucoma: Acute increase in IOP, often after exercise or pupillary dilation, with pigmented cells in the anterior chamber.

See 9.10, PIGMENT DISPERSION SYNDROME/PIGMENTARY GLAUCOMA.

- Neovascular glaucoma: Abnormal blood vessels along the pupillary margin, the TM, or both. See 9.14, NEOVASCULAR GLAUCOMA.
- Fuchs heterochromic iridocyclitis: Asymmetry of iris color, mild iritis usually present in the eye with the lighter-colored iris. IOP increase is rarely as acute. See 12.1, ANTERIOR UVEITIS (IRITIS/IRIDOCYCLITIS).
- Others: Herpes simplex or varicella zoster keratouveitis, toxoplasmosis, and others.

Etiology

Mechanism unknown, but possible association with a viral etiology (e.g., CMV).

Workup

1. History: Previous attacks? Corneal or systemic disease? Light sensitivity? Pain? Recent exercise?
2. Slit lamp examination: Assess the degree of conjunctival injection and aqueous cell and flare. Careful retinal examination for vasculitis and snowbanking.

3. Gonioscopy: Angle open? Synechiae, neovascular membrane, or KP present?

4. Complete baseline glaucoma evaluation. See 9.1, PRIMARY OPEN-ANGLE GLAUCOMA.

Treatment

Tends to be very responsive to topical steroids and aqueous suppressants.

1. Topical β-blocker (e.g., timolol 0.5% daily or b.i.d.), topical α2 agonist (e.g., brimonidine 0.1% to 0.2% b.i.d. to t.i.d.), and topical CAI (e.g., dorzolamide 2% b.i.d. to t.i.d.).

2. Short course (1-week) of topical steroids (e.g., prednisolone acetate 1% q.i.d.) may decrease inflammation. Longer use may cause an IOP elevation. Oral indomethacin (e.g., 75 to 150 mg p.o. daily) or topical nonsteroidal anti-inflammatory drugs (NSAIDs) (e.g., ketorolac q.i.d.) may also be effective.

3. Consider a systemic CAI (e.g., acetazolamide 500 mg sequel p.o. b.i.d.) if IOP is significantly increased and unresponsive to topical therapy (rare).

4. Hyperosmotic agents (e.g., mannitol 20% 1 to 2 g/kg i.v. over 45 minutes) or anterior

chamber paracentesis can be considered when the IOP is determined to be dangerously high for the involved optic nerve (see Appendix 13, ANTERIOR CHAMBER PARACENTESIS).

5. Consider a cycloplegic agent (e.g., cyclopentolate 1% t.i.d.) if the patient is symptomatic.

Follow Up

1. Patients are seen every few days at first and then weekly until the episode resolves. Attacks usually subside within a few hours to a few weeks.

2. Medical or surgical therapy may be required depending on baseline IOP between attacks.

3. If the IOP decreases to levels not associated with disc damage, no treatment is necessary.

4. Steroids are tapered rapidly if they are used for 1 week or less and slowly if they are used for longer.

5. Both eyes are at risk for the development of chronic open-angle glaucoma. Patients should be followed as if the diagnosis is POAG. See 9.1, PRIMARY OPEN-ANGLE GLAUCOMA.

9

9.9 Steroid-Response Glaucoma

Signs

Critical. Increased IOP with corticosteroid use. Onset typically 2 to 4 weeks after starting ocular (e.g., topical, intravitreal) steroids, though rarely an acute IOP rise can occur within hours in association with systemic use of steroid or adrenocorticotropic hormone.

Other. Signs of POAG may develop. See 9.1, PRIMARY OPEN-ANGLE GLAUCOMA.

> 📝 **NOTE:** Patients with POAG or a predisposition to development of glaucoma (e.g., family history, ocular trauma, diabetes, African descent, high myopia) are more likely to experience a steroid-response and subsequent glaucoma.

Differential Diagnosis

• POAG. See 9.1, PRIMARY OPEN-ANGLE GLAUCOMA.

• Exfoliative glaucoma. See 9.11, PSEUDOEXFOLIATION SYNDROME/EXFOLIATIVE GLAUCOMA.

• Inflammatory open-angle glaucoma: Because steroids are used to treat ocular inflammation, it may be difficult to determine the cause of increased IOP. See 9.7, INFLAMMATORY OPEN-ANGLE GLAUCOMA.

Etiology

Most commonly seen with ophthalmic topical, periocular, or intravitreal steroid therapy. However, elevated IOP can occur with all forms of administration (e.g., oral, intravenous, inhalational, nasal, injected, or dermatologic topical formulations), especially with prolonged use. More potent topical steroids (e.g., dexamethasone, difluprednate) more often cause significant IOP rises compared to those that are less potent (e.g., fluorometholone, loteprednol). IOP typically decreases to pretreatment levels after stopping steroids. The rate of decrease relates to duration of use and severity of the pressure increase. IOP increase is due to reduced outflow facility of the pigmented TM, and when this is severe, the IOP may remain increased for months after steroids are stopped. IOP increase may also be caused by increased inflammation associated with reduction of the steroid medication.

Workup

1. History: Duration of steroid use? Ask about nasal sprays and dermatologic topical medications. Previous intraocular surgery (possible periocular injection)? Previous steroid use or an eye problem from steroid use? Glaucoma or family history of glaucoma? Herpetic keratouveitis? Diabetes? Myopia? Ocular trauma?

2. Complete ocular examination: Look for active or prior inflammation and evaluate the iris and angle (by gonioscopy) to determine the presence NV, pigment suggestive of pigment dispersion syndrome or pseudoexfoliation, blood in Schlemm canal, PAS, etc. Inspect the optic nerve.

3. Complete baseline glaucoma evaluation. See 9.1, PRIMARY OPEN-ANGLE GLAUCOMA.

Treatment

Any or all of the following may be necessary to reduce IOP:

1. Determine if steroid use (in any form) is truly needed. If not needed, stop or taper steroids.

2. Reduce the concentration or dosage of steroid.

3. Change to a steroid with lesser propensity for IOP elevation (e.g., fluorometholone, loteprednol, or rimexolone).

4. Switch to a topical NSAID (e.g., ketorolac 0.4% or 0.5%, diclofenac 0.1%).

5. Start antiglaucoma therapy. See 9.7, INFLAMMATORY OPEN-ANGLE GLAUCOMA, for medical therapy options.

6. Consider anterior chamber paracentesis for rapid control when the IOP is determined to be dangerously high for the involved optic nerve (see Appendix 13, ANTERIOR CHAMBER PARACENTESIS).

7. LT (e.g., SLT) may be effective in treating some patients.

8. For sustained IOP elevation after steroid cessation or in patients at risk of glaucoma progression, treat like POAG, including appropriate surgical options. See 9.1, PRIMARY OPEN-ANGLE GLAUCOMA.

> **NOTE:** For inflammatory glaucoma, if the inflammation is moderate to severe, increase the steroids initially to reduce the inflammation while initiating antiglaucoma therapy.

If a medically uncontrollable dangerously high IOP develops after a depot steroid injection, the steroid may need to be excised. After intravitreal steroid injection, options include glaucoma filtering surgery or a pars plana vitrectomy to remove the steroid.

Steroid-induced glaucoma after LASIK may be difficult to detect using applanation tonometry due to falsely low readings caused by either reduced corneal thickness or interface fluid between the flap and the stromal bed. IOP measurement peripheral to the flap may be more accurate.

Follow Up

Dependent on severity of pressure elevation and glaucomatous damage. Follow patients as if they have POAG. See 9.1, PRIMARY OPEN-ANGLE GLAUCOMA.

9.10 Pigment Dispersion Syndrome/Pigmentary Glaucoma

Definition

Pigment dispersion refers to the release of pigment granules into the anterior chamber. It results from backward bowing of the peripheral iris (reverse pupillary block) with friction between the iris pigment epithelium and the zonular fibers. Pigment is released and may ultimately obstruct the TM, leading to increased IOP and secondary open-angle glaucoma.

Symptoms

Mostly asymptomatic but may have blurred vision, eye pain, and colored halos around lights after exercise or pupillary dilation. More common in young adult, myopic men (age 20 to 45 years). Usually bilateral, but asymmetric. May have lattice degeneration and increased risk of a retinal detachment.

Signs

(See Figures 9.10.1 and 9.10.2.)

Critical. Midperipheral, spoke-like iris TIDs corresponding to iridozonular contact; dense homogeneous pigmentation of the TM for 360 degrees (seen on gonioscopy) in the absence of signs of trauma or inflammation.

Other. A vertical pigment band on the corneal endothelium typically just inferior to the visual axis (Krukenberg spindle); pigment deposition on the posterior equatorial lens surface (Zentmayer line or Scheie line), on the anterior hyaloid face, slightly anterior to Schwalbe line (Sampaolesi line), and sometimes along the iris (which can produce iris heterochromia). Pigment on the posterior lens capsule is nearly pathognomonic. The angle often shows a wide ciliary body band with 3+ to 4+ pigmentation of the posterior TM, homogenous for 360 degrees. Pigmentary glaucoma is characterized by pigment dispersion syndrome plus glaucomatous optic neuropathy. Typically, large fluctuations in IOP can occur, during which pigment cells may be seen floating in the anterior chamber.

Differential Diagnosis

- Exfoliative glaucoma: Iris TIDs may be present, but are near the pupillary margin and are not radial. White, flaky material may be seen on the pupillary border, anterior lens capsule, and corneal endothelium. TM is highly pigmented but in a "splotchy" pattern, often with pigment anterior to Schwalbe line (also seen in PDS). See 9.11, PSEUDOEXFOLIATION SYNDROME/EXFOLIATIVE GLAUCOMA.

- Inflammatory open-angle glaucoma: White blood cells and flare in the anterior chamber; no radial iris TIDs; often PAS on gonioscopy. TM pigment concentrated inferiorly. See 9.7, INFLAMMATORY OPEN-ANGLE GLAUCOMA.

- Iris melanoma: Pigmentation of the angular structures accompanied by either a raised, pigmented lesion on the iris or a diffusely darkened iris. No iris TIDs. See 5.13, MALIGNANT MELANOMA OF THE IRIS.

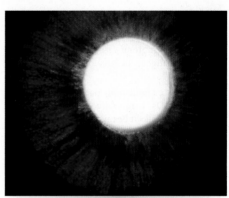

Figure 9.10.1 Pigment dispersion syndrome with spoke-like iris transillumination defects.

- Irradiation: Induces atrophy and depigmentation of the ciliary processes with increased TM pigment deposition.

- Postoperative pigment liberation after posterior chamber intraocular lens implantation.

- Siderosis.

- Iris chafe with sulcus IOL: Iris TIDs outlining the haptics may be seen.

- Bilateral acute depigmentation of the iris: Acute-onset bilateral iris depigmentation, pigment dispersion in the anterior chamber, and heavy pigmentation of the TM. Usually symmetric (versus pigment dispersion syndrome which is typically asymmetric). Alternatively, if accompanied by a mydriatic pupil that is poorly responsive to light with sphincter paralysis, consider bilateral acute iris transillumination.

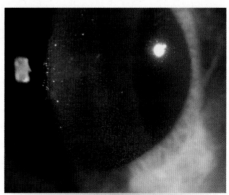

Figure 9.10.2 Pigment dispersion syndrome with a vertical band of endothelial pigment (Krukenberg spindle).

Workup

1. History: Previous episodes of decreased vision or halos? Symptoms associated with exercise? Trauma, surgery, or previous intraocular foreign body?
2. Slit lamp examination, particularly checking for iris TIDs. Large defects may be seen by shining a small slit beam directly into the pupil to obtain a red reflex. Look for Krukenberg spindle on the corneal endothelium. Look for pigment on the posterior lens equator by angling the slit beam nasally and having the patient look temporally (Zentmayer line or Scheie stripe; pathognomonic for pigment dispersion). Examine the angle looking for dense, evenly dispersed TM pigmentation. Careful retinal examination because of increased incidence of lattice degeneration and retinal detachment.
3. Perform baseline glaucoma evaluation. See 9.1, PRIMARY OPEN-ANGLE GLAUCOMA.

Treatment

Similar to POAG. Depends on IOP, optic nerve damage, and symptom extent. Usually patients with pigment dispersion without ocular hypertension, glaucoma, or symptoms are observed carefully. A stepwise approach to control IOP is usually taken when mild-to-moderate glaucomatous changes are present. When advanced glaucoma is discovered on initial examination, maximal medical therapy may be instituted initially. See 9.1, PRIMARY OPEN-ANGLE GLAUCOMA.

1. Decrease mechanical iridozonular contact. Two methods have been proposed:
   - Miotic agents: A theoretical first-line therapy because they minimize iridozonular contact. However, because most patients are young and myopic, the resulting fluctuation in myopia may not be tolerated. In addition, approximately 14% of patients have lattice retinal degeneration and are thus predisposed to retinal detachment from the use of miotics. In some cases, pilocarpine 4% gel q.h.s. may be tolerated.
   - Peripheral laser iridotomy: Laser PI has been recommended to reduce pigment dispersion by decreasing iridozonular contact, but remains controversial. It may be best suited in early-stage disease and ill-advised in more advanced stages.
2. Other antiglaucoma medications. See 9.1, PRIMARY OPEN-ANGLE GLAUCOMA.
3. SLT or ALT. Due to greater risk of postlaser IOP spikes, lower energy should be used, and only 180 degrees of treatment is advised initially. Careful postlaser monitoring is needed to detect early IOP rise.
4. Consider MIGS surgery, guarded filtration procedure, or tube shunt when medical and laser therapies fail. These young myopic patients are at greater risk for hypotony maculopathy and surgical technique should aim to avoid early overfiltration.

Follow Up

Same as POAG. See 9.1, PRIMARY OPEN-ANGLE GLAUCOMA.

9.11 Pseudoexfoliation Syndrome/Exfoliative Glaucoma

Definition

A systemic disorder in which grayish-white exfoliation material, along with pigment released from the iris sphincter region, block the TM and raise the IOP. Diagnosis confers a 25% risk of glaucoma, which can be poorly responsive to therapy. Pseudoexfoliation is the most common secondary glaucoma in those of European descent, but can be seen in nearly all ethnic groups.

Symptoms

Usually asymptomatic in its early stages. Unlike POAG, more often asymmetric/unilateral at presentation.

Signs

(See Figures 9.11.1 and 9.11.2.)

Critical. White, flaky material on the pupillary margin; anterior lens capsular changes (central zone of exfoliation material, often with rolled-up edges, middle clear zone, and a peripheral cloudy zone); peripupillary iris TIDs; and glaucomatous optic neuropathy. Bilateral, but often asymmetric.

Other. Irregular black pigment deposition on the TM more marked inferiorly than superiorly; black scalloped deposition of pigment anterior to Schwalbe line (Sampaolesi line) seen on gonioscopy, especially inferiorly. White, flaky material may be seen on the corneal endothelium,

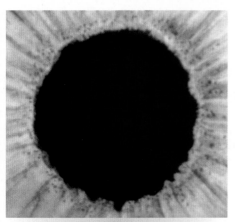

Figure 9.11.1 Pseudoexfoliation syndrome with white material on pupillary margin.

which often has a lower than normal endothelial cell density; can look like angular, irregular KP. Iris atrophy. Poor pupillary response to dilation (with more advanced cases, believed to be secondary to iris dilator muscle atrophy). Incidence increases with age. Zonular laxity can lead to anterior lens dislocation, angle narrowing, and secondary angle closure.

Differential Diagnosis

- Inflammatory glaucoma: Corneal endothelial deposits can be present in both exfoliative and uveitic glaucoma. Typically, IOP is highly volatile in both. The ragged volcano-like PAS of some inflammatory glaucomas are not seen in the exfoliation syndrome, but angle

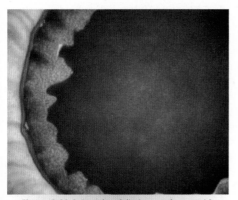

Figure 9.11.2 Pseudoexfoliation syndrome with white material on anterior lens capsule.

closure due to zonular instability can occur. Photophobia is common with uveitis. See 9.7, INFLAMMATORY OPEN-ANGLE GLAUCOMA.

- Pigmentary glaucoma: Midperipheral iris TIDs. Pigment on corneal endothelium and posterior equatorial lens surface. Deep anterior chamber angle. Myopia. See 9.10, PIGMENT DISPERSION SYNDROME/PIGMENTARY GLAUCOMA.

- Capsular delamination (true exfoliation): Trauma, exposure to intense heat (e.g., glass blower), or severe uveitis can cause a thin membrane to peel off the anterior lens capsule. Glaucoma uncommon.

- Primary amyloidosis: Amyloid material can deposit along the pupillary margin or anterior lens capsule. Glaucoma can occur.

- Uveitis/glaucoma/hyphema (UGH) syndrome: Prior surgery. See 9.16.3, UVEITIS, GLAUCOMA, HYPHEMA SYNDROME.

Workup

1. History: Family history.
2. Slit lamp examination. Look for white, flaky material along the pupillary margin, peripapillary TIDs; often need to dilate the pupil to see anterior lens capsular changes.
3. Perform baseline glaucoma evaluation. See 9.1, PRIMARY OPEN-ANGLE GLAUCOMA.

Treatment

1. For medical and surgical therapy, see 9.1, PRIMARY OPEN-ANGLE GLAUCOMA. LT can be particularly effective, possibly related to higher laser uptake due to pigmentation.
2. The course of exfoliative glaucoma is nonlinear. Early, the condition may be benign. However, pseudoexfoliation is associated with highly volatile IOP. Once IOP becomes difficult to control, the glaucoma may progress rapidly (e.g., within months).

NOTE: Cataract extraction does not eradicate the glaucoma. Cataract extraction may be complicated by weakened zonular fibers and synechiae between the iris and peripheral anterior lens capsule with increased risk of intraoperative vitreous loss and zonular dehiscence. Postoperative intraocular lens dislocation may occur with time.

Follow Up

Every 1 to 3 months as with POAG, but with the awareness that damage can progress very rapidly.

> **NOTE:** Many patients have pseudoexfoliation syndrome without glaucoma. These patients are reexamined every 6 to 12 months because of glaucoma risk; treatment is initiated with evidence of IOP elevation and glaucomatous damage.

9.12 Lens-Related Glaucoma

9.12.1 PHACOLYTIC GLAUCOMA

Definition

Leakage of lens material through an intact lens capsule leads to outflow obstruction (typically in presence of a hypermature cataract).

Symptoms

Unilateral pain, decreased vision (despite poor vision from cataract, increased blurring may be noticeable), tearing, injection, and photophobia.

Signs

Critical. Markedly increased IOP, accompanied by iridescent particles and white material in the anterior chamber or on anterior surface of lens capsule. A hypermature (liquefied, Morgagnian) or mature cataract is typical. May occur less commonly in presence of an immature cataract with liquefaction of the posterior cortex. Pain is usually severe.

Other. Microcystic corneal edema, anterior chamber cell and flare (cells may be larger than typical uveitic white blood cells), pseudohypopyon, and severe conjunctival injection. Gonioscopy reveals an open anterior chamber angle. Clumps of macrophages may be seen in the inferior angle.

Differential Diagnosis

All of the following can produce an acute increase in IOP to high levels, but none display iridescent particles in the anterior chamber:

- Inflammatory glaucoma. See 9.7, INFLAMMATORY OPEN-ANGLE GLAUCOMA.
- Glaucomatocyclitic crisis. See 9.8, GLAUCOMATOCYCLITIC CRISIS/POSNER–SCHLOSSMAN SYNDROME.
- Acute angle closure glaucoma. See 9.4, ACUTE ANGLE CLOSURE GLAUCOMA.
- Lens particle glaucoma. See 9.12.2, LENS PARTICLE GLAUCOMA.
- Endophthalmitis. See 12.13, POSTOPERATIVE ENDOPHTHALMITIS.
- Glaucoma secondary to intraocular tumor: May have unilateral cataract.
- Others: Traumatic glaucoma, ghost cell glaucoma, phacomorphic glaucoma, phacoantigenic (formerly phacoanaphylaxis) glaucoma, neovascular glaucoma, and others.

Workup

1. History: Longstanding poor vision (chronic/mature cataract)? Recent trauma or ocular surgery? Recurrent episodes? Prior uveitis?
2. Slit lamp examination: Look for iridescent or white particles as well as cell and flare in the anterior chamber. Check IOP. Evaluate for cataract and corneal edema. Look for signs of trauma. Note, the lens capsule is intact in this diagnosis.
3. Gonioscopy of the anterior chamber angles of both eyes: Topical glycerin may be placed on the cornea, after topical anesthesia, to temporarily clear any edema.
4. Retinal and optic disc examination if possible. Otherwise, B-scan US before cataract extraction to rule out intraocular tumor or retinal detachment.
5. If the diagnosis is in doubt, an anterior chamber paracentesis can be performed to detect macrophages bloated with lens material on microscopic examination (see Appendix 13, ANTERIOR CHAMBER PARACENTESIS).

Treatment

The immediate goal of therapy is to reduce the IOP and inflammation. The cataract should be removed promptly (within several days).

- Medical therapy options include:
  - Topical β-blocker (e.g., timolol 0.5% daily or b.i.d.), α2 agonist (e.g., brimonidine 0.1% to 0.2% b.i.d. to t.i.d.), and/or topical CAI (e.g., dorzolamide 2% t.i.d.).
  - Systemic CAI (e.g., acetazolamide 500 mg sequel p.o. b.i.d.). Benefit of maintaining topical CAI in addition to a systemic agent is controversial.
  - Topical cycloplegic (e.g., cyclopentolate 1% t.i.d.).
  - Topical steroid (e.g., prednisolone acetate 1% every 15 minutes for four doses then q1h).
  - Hyperosmotic agent if necessary and no contraindications are present (e.g., mannitol, 1 to 2 g/kg i.v. over 45 minutes).
- The IOP usually does not respond adequately to medical therapy. In cases where IOP cannot be managed medically, cataract removal is usually performed within 24 to 48 hours. In patients who have noticed a sudden decrease in vision, the urgency of cataract surgery is increased, especially in those whose vision has progressed to NLP over a few hours. In such cases, lowering the IOP immediately with an anterior chamber paracentesis is necessary prior to cataract extraction (see Appendix 13, ANTERIOR CHAMBER PARACENTESIS). Glaucoma surgery is usually not necessary at the same time as cataract surgery.

Follow Up

1. If patients are not hospitalized, they should be reexamined the day after surgery. Patients may be hospitalized for 24 hours after cataract surgery for IOP monitoring.
2. If the IOP returns to normal, the patient should be rechecked within 1 week.

9.12.2 LENS PARTICLE GLAUCOMA

Definition

Lens material liberated by trauma or surgery obstructs aqueous outflow channels.

Symptoms

Pain, blurred vision, red eye, tearing, and photophobia. History of recent ocular trauma or intraocular surgery.

Signs

Critical. White, fluffy pieces of lens cortical material in the anterior chamber, combined with increased IOP.

Other. Anterior chamber cell and flare, conjunctival injection, or corneal edema. The anterior chamber angle is open on gonioscopy.

Differential Diagnosis

- See 9.12.1, PHACOLYTIC GLAUCOMA. In phacolytic glaucoma, the lens capsule is intact.
- Infectious endophthalmitis: Usually a normal or low IOP. Unless lens cortical material can be unequivocally identified in the anterior chamber, and there is nothing atypical about the presentation, endophthalmitis must be excluded. See 12.13, POSTOPERATIVE ENDOPHTHALMITIS and 12.15, TRAUMATIC ENDOPHTHALMITIS.
- Phacoantigenic (formerly phacoanaphylaxis): Requires prior sensitization to lens material. Follows trauma or intraocular surgery, producing anterior chamber inflammation and sometimes a high IOP. The inflammation is often granulomatous, and fluffy lens material is not present in the anterior chamber. See 9.12.3, PHACOANTIGENIC (FORMERLY PHACOANAPHYLAXIS).

Workup

1. History: Recent trauma or intraocular surgery?
2. Slit lamp examination: Search the anterior chamber for lens cortical material and measure the IOP.
3. Gonioscopy of the anterior chamber angle.
4. Optic nerve evaluation: Degree of optic nerve cupping helps determine how long the increased IOP can be tolerated.

Treatment

See 9.12.1, PHACOLYTIC GLAUCOMA, for medical treatment. If medical therapy fails to control the IOP, the residual lens material must be removed surgically.

Follow Up

Depending on the IOP and health of the optic nerve, patients are reexamined in 1 to 7 days.

9.12.3 PHACOANTIGENIC GLAUCOMA (FORMERLY PHACOANAPHYLAXIS)

Formerly known as "phacoanaphylaxis," this rare condition presents with chronic granulomatous uveitis in response to prior sensitization of lens material liberated by trauma or intraocular surgery. It may have associated glaucomatous optic neuropathy, although this is rare at presentation. After lens material is liberated, there is a latent period where an immune sensitivity develops. Inflammatory cells surround lens material, and glaucoma may result from blockage of the TM by these cells and lens particles. Other forms of uveitis should be considered, including sympathetic ophthalmia. Other forms of lens-induced glaucoma must be considered including lens particle and phacolytic glaucoma. Treatment is with topical steroids and antiglaucoma medications. The lens should be removed surgically, particularly if IOP or inflammation cannot be adequately controlled with medications.

9.12.4 PHACOMORPHIC GLAUCOMA

Phacomorphic glaucoma is caused by closure of the anterior chamber angle by a large intumescent cataract. A pupillary block mechanism may play a role. The initial treatment includes topical antiglaucoma medication(s), although a systemic CAI and hyperosmotic agent may be necessary as well (see 9.4, ACUTE ANGLE CLOSURE GLAUCOMA). Can be mistaken for pupillary ACG; however, the anterior chamber may be more uniformly shallow than in a purely pupillary block mechanism where iris bombé is prominent. A laser iridectomy may be effective in relieving any part of pupillary block, although this may only be a temporizing measure. Cataract extraction is the definitive treatment.

9.12.5 GLAUCOMA CAUSED BY LENS DISLOCATION OR SUBLUXATION

Lens dislocation/subluxation may be caused by trauma, pseudoexfoliation syndrome, or congenital zonular dysgenesis (e.g., Marfan syndrome, spherophakia). Mechanisms for glaucoma in dislocated/subluxed lenses include an inflammatory reaction caused by the lens material itself, pupillary block, or damage to the anterior chamber angle sustained during trauma. A dislocated lens may become hypermature and cause a phacolytic glaucoma (see 9.12.1, PHACOLYTIC GLAUCOMA). In addition, a dislocated or subluxed lens can lead to sensitization of lens proteins if associated with capsule violation (see 9.12.3, PHACOANTIGENIC GLAUCOMA [FORMERLY PHACOANAPHYLAXIS]). Pupillary block is the most common mechanism and can occur secondary to anterior displacement of the lens or vitreous plugging the pupil. Treatment is aimed at relieving the pupillary block. Iridectomy is usually indicated and necessary to prevent future attacks. Cycloplegics are helpful along with face up/supine head positioning to allow lens to fall back. IOP-lowering medications are employed. Avoid miotics. Surgical lens removal often needed, occasionally through a pars plana approach. See 13.10, SUBLUXED OR DISLOCATED CRYSTALLINE LENS, for a more in-depth discussion.

9.13 Plateau Iris

Symptoms

Usually asymptomatic, unless acute angle closure glaucoma develops. See 9.4, ACUTE ANGLE CLOSURE GLAUCOMA.

Signs

Critical. Persistent appositional angle after laser iridotomy (see 9.4, ACUTE ANGLE CLOSURE GLAUCOMA).

Differential Diagnosis

• Acute angle closure glaucoma associated with pupillary block: The central anterior chamber depth is decreased, but more pronounced peripheral shallowing with iris bombé, giving the iris a convex appearance. See 9.4, ACUTE ANGLE CLOSURE GLAUCOMA.

• Aqueous misdirection syndrome: Marked diffuse shallowing of the anterior chamber both centrally and peripherally, often after cataract extraction or glaucoma surgery. See 9.17, AQUEOUS MISDIRECTION SYNDROME/ MALIGNANT GLAUCOMA.

- For other disorders, see 9.4, ACUTE ANGLE CLOSURE GLAUCOMA.

Types

1. Plateau iris configuration: Because of the anatomic configuration of the angle, acute angle closure glaucoma develops from only a mild degree of pupillary block. These angle closure attacks may be treated with a laser PI to break any component of pupillary block but this is not curative.

2. Plateau iris syndrome: The peripheral iris can bunch up in the anterior chamber angle and obstruct aqueous outflow without any element of pupillary block. The plateau iris syndrome is present when the angle closes and the IOP rises after dilation, despite a patent PI, and in the absence of phacomorphic glaucoma. UBM findings are characterized by an anteriorly rotated ciliary body. See **Figure 9.13.1**.

Workup

1. Slit lamp examination: Specifically check for the presence of a patent PI and the critical signs listed previously.

2. Measure IOP.

3. Gonioscopy of both anterior chamber angles. "Double hump sign" on indentation gonioscopy is critical where the iris drapes over the lens and is anterior near the pupil and then falls back over the zonular area and is again forward and appositional in the angle.

4. Undilated optic nerve evaluation.

5. Can be assessed by UBM.

> **NOTE:** If dilation must be performed in a patient suspected of having a plateau iris, warn the patient that this may provoke an acute angle closure attack. The preferred agent is 0.5% tropicamide. Recheck the IOP every few hours until the pupil returns to normal size. Have the patient notify you immediately if symptoms of acute angle closure develop.

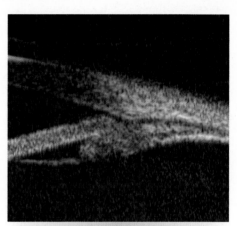

Figure 9.13.1 Ultrasonography biomicroscopy of a plateau iris.

Treatment

If acute angle closure is present:

1. Treat medically. See 9.4, ACUTE ANGLE CLOSURE GLAUCOMA.

2. A laser PI is performed within 1 to 3 days if the angle closure attack can be broken medically. If the attack cannot be controlled, a laser or surgical PI may need to be done as an emergency procedure. Consider a laser iridoplasty to break an acute attack not responsive to medical treatment and PI.

3. One week after the laser PI, gonioscopy should be repeated prior to dilating the eye with a weak mydriatic (e.g., tropicamide 0.5%). If the IOP increases or a spontaneous angle closure episode occurs, plateau iris syndrome is diagnosed and should be treated with an iridoplasty. Second-line therapy includes chronic instillation of a weak miotic agent (e.g., pilocarpine 0.5% to 1% t.i.d. to q.i.d.).

4. If the patient's IOP does respond to a laser PI (e.g., plateau iris configuration), then a prophylactic laser PI may be indicated in the contralateral eye within 1 to 2 weeks.

If acute angle closure is not present:

1. Laser PI to relieve any pupillary block component; also done to prove pupillary block is not the primary mechanism.

2. Check gonioscopy every 4 to 6 months to evaluate the angle.

- Most do well with close observation alone. Perform iridoplasty if new PAS or further narrowing of the angle develops.
- If the angle continues to develop new PAS or becomes narrower despite iridoplasty, then consider lens extraction. Can consider ECP at the time of phacoemulsification to shrink ciliary processes. If uncontrolled IOP, treat as CACG (see 9.5, CHRONIC ANGLE CLOSURE GLAUCOMA).

Follow Up

1. Similar to performing a PI in acute angle closure. Reevaluate in 1 week, 1 month, and 3 months, and then yearly if no problems have developed.

2. Patients with a plateau iris configuration without previous acute angle closure are examined every 6 months.

3. Every examination should include IOP measurement and gonioscopy looking for PAS formation, narrowing angle recess, or increasing angle closure. The PI should be examined for patency. Dilation should cautiously be performed periodically (approximately every 2 years) to ensure that the PI remains adequate to prevent angle closure. If the patient needs more frequent dilation due to retinal pathology, consider cataract surgery to help open the angle.

4. Ophthalmoscopic disc evaluation is essential.

5. Recommend examination of immediate family members.

9.14 Neovascular Glaucoma

Definition

Glaucoma caused by a fibrovascular membrane overgrowing the anterior chamber angle structures. Initially, despite an open appearance on gonioscopy, the angle may be blocked by the membrane. The fibrovascular membrane eventually contracts, causing PAS formation and secondary angle closure glaucoma. Rarely, it may have NV of the angle without NV of the iris (NVI) at the pupillary margin. Ischemia-driven vascular endothelial growth factor (VEGF) release from a variety of causes results in the formation of the fibrovascular membrane.

Symptoms

May be asymptomatic or include pain, redness, photophobia, and decreased vision.

Signs

(See Figures 9.14.1 and 9.14.2.)

Critical
- Stage 1: Nonradial, misdirected blood vessels along the pupillary margin, the TM, or both. No signs of glaucoma. Normal iris blood vessels run radially and are typically symmetric.
- Stage 2: Stage 1 plus increased IOP (open-angle neovascular glaucoma).
- Stage 3: Partial or complete angle closure glaucoma caused by a fibrovascular membrane pulling the iris well anterior to the TM

(usually at the level of Schwalbe line). NVI is common.

Other. Mild anterior chamber cell and flare, conjunctival injection, corneal edema with acute IOP increase, hyphema, eversion of pupillary margin allowing visualization of iris pigment epithelium (ectropion uveae), optic nerve cupping, and visual field loss.

Differential Diagnosis

- Inflammatory glaucoma: Anterior chamber cell and flare, dilated normal iris blood vessels

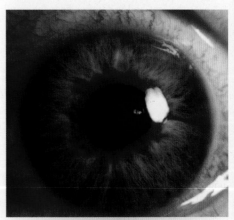

Figure 9.14.1 Iris neovascularization.

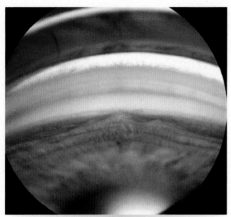

Figure 9.14.2 Neovascularization of the angle.

may be seen. Open angle with no NV. See 9.7, INFLAMMATORY OPEN-ANGLE GLAUCOMA.

- Primary acute angle closure glaucoma. See 9.4, ACUTE ANGLE CLOSURE GLAUCOMA.

Etiology

- Diabetic retinopathy with retinal ischemia. See 11.12, DIABETIC RETINOPATHY.
- Central retinal vein occlusion, particularly the ischemic type. See 11.8, CENTRAL RETINAL VEIN OCCLUSION.
- Central retinal artery occlusion. See 11.6, CENTRAL RETINAL ARTERY OCCLUSION.
- Ocular ischemic syndrome (carotid occlusive disease). See 11.11, OCULAR ISCHEMIC SYNDROME/CAROTID OCCLUSIVE DISEASE.
- Others: Branch retinal vein occlusion, branch retinal artery occlusion, chronic uveitis, chronic retinal detachment, intraocular tumors, trauma, other ocular vascular disorders, radiation therapy, and chronic long-standing increased IOP (e.g., neglected angle closure glaucoma). See specific sections.

Workup

1. History: Determine underlying etiology.
2. Complete ocular examination, including IOP measurement and gonioscopy to evaluate degree of angle closure, if any. A dilated retinal examination is essential in determining the etiology and for disc evaluation.

3. Fluorescein angiography as needed to identify an underlying retinal abnormality or in preparation for panretinal photocoagulation (PRP).
4. Carotid Doppler studies to rule out stenosis when no retinal etiology is identified.
5. B-scan US is indicated when the retina cannot be visualized to rule out an intraocular tumor or retinal detachment.

Treatment

1. Reduce inflammation and pain: Topical steroid (e.g., prednisolone acetate 1% q1–6h) and a cycloplegic (e.g., atropine 1% t.i.d.).
2. Reduce the IOP if it is increased (markedly high IOP is not uncommon). Where visual potential is good and cupping advanced, a lower target IOP may be appropriate. Any or all of the following medications are used:
   - Topical β-blocker (e.g., timolol 0.5% daily or b.i.d.).
   - Topical α2 agonists (e.g., brimonidine 0.1% to 0.2% b.i.d. to t.i.d.).
   - Topical and/or systemic CAI (e.g., dorzolamide 2% b.i.d. to t.i.d. and/or acetazolamide 500 mg sequel p.o. b.i.d.).
   - Prostaglandins may help lower IOP, but may increase inflammation and are usually avoided in the acute phase.
   - If need for IOP reduction is urgent or refractory to therapies listed above, consider an osmotic agent (e.g., mannitol 1 to 2 g/kg i.v. over 45 minutes).

> **NOTE:** Miotics (e.g., pilocarpine) are contraindicated because of their effects on the blood–aqueous barrier. Epinephrine compounds (e.g., dipivefrin) are usually ineffective.

3. In the acute stages, after a rapid rise in IOP, an anterior chamber paracentesis may be helpful. Caution should be exercised as this may also result in a hyphema. See Appendix 13, ANTERIOR CHAMBER PARACENTESIS.
4. If retinal ischemia is thought to be responsible for the NV, then treat with PRP and/or anti-VEGF intravitreal injections. If the retina cannot be visualized, lower the IOP and treat the retina once the cornea clears. These procedures are used if the angle is open as it may be

possible to reverse the angle NV and restore normal aqueous outflow.

5. Glaucoma filtration surgery may be performed when the NV is inactive and the IOP cannot be controlled with medical therapy. Tube-shunt procedures may be helpful to control IOP in some patients with active NV, but may be complicated by postoperative bleeding. They should not be performed unless there is useful vision to preserve. Transscleral cyclophotocoagulation is an option but is more often reserved for cases with poor visual potential.

6. Intravitreal anti-VEGF agents (e.g., ranibizumab, bevacizumab, or aflibercept) may be used to promote regression of iris NV prior to, or in conjunction with, filtering surgery or PRP. Their effect is temporary, and their use for treatment of NV is currently off-label. They are particularly useful in stage 1 and 2 neovascular glaucoma, where the angle is still open, to prevent angle closure during the interval required for PRP to take effect. Caution should be used when no view of

the retina is possible. (See 11.12, DIABETIC RETINOPATHY and 11.17, NEOVASCULAR OR EXUDATIVE (WET) AGE-RELATED MACULAR DEGENERATION, for a discussion on anti-VEGF agents.)

7. In eyes without useful vision, topical steroids and cycloplegics may be adequate therapy for pain control. The pain in chronic neovascular glaucoma is not primarily a function of the IOP itself; thus, reducing IOP may not be necessary if the goal is pain control and comfort measures only. See 13.12, BLIND, PAINFUL EYE.

Follow Up

The presence of NVI, especially with high IOP, requires urgent therapeutic intervention, usually within 1 to 2 days. Angle closure can proceed rapidly (days to weeks).

 NOTE: NVI without glaucoma is managed similarly, but there is no need for pressure-reducing agents unless IOP increases.

9.15 Iridocorneal Endothelial Syndrome

Definition

Three overlapping syndromes—essential iris atrophy, Chandler, and iris nevus (Cogan–Reese)—that share an abnormal corneal endothelial cell layer, which can grow across the anterior chamber angle. Secondary angle closure can result from contraction of this membrane.

Symptoms

Asymptomatic early. Later, the patient may note an irregular pupil or iris appearance, blurred vision, monocular diplopia, or pain if IOP increases or corneal edema develops. Usually unilateral and most common in patients 20 to 50 years of age. More common in women. Sporadic in presentation.

Signs

(See Figure 9.15.1.)

Critical. Corneal endothelial changes (fine, beaten-bronze appearance); microcystic corneal edema; localized, irregular, high PAS that often

extend anterior to Schwalbe line; deep central anterior chamber; iris alterations as follows:

• Essential iris atrophy: Marked iris thinning leading to iris holes with displacement and distortion of the pupil (corectopia). Usually good prognosis.

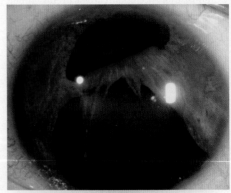

Figure 9.15.1 Essential iris atrophy.

- Chandler syndrome: Mild iris thinning and corectopia. The corneal and angle changes are most marked in this variant. Degree of findings is highly variable. Patients often have corneal edema even at normal IOP. Accounts for about 50% of ICE syndrome cases. Variable prognosis.

- Iris nevus/Cogan–Reese syndrome: Pigmented nodules (not true nevi) on the iris surface, variable iris atrophy. Similar changes may be seen in Chandler syndrome and essential iris atrophy, resulting from contraction of the membrane over the iris, constricting around small islands of iris tissue. Usually poor prognosis.

Other. Corneal edema, elevated IOP, optic nerve cupping, or visual field loss. Glaucoma is nearly always unilateral; occasional mild corneal changes may be seen in the fellow eye.

Differential Diagnosis

- Axenfeld–Rieger spectrum: Bilateral. Prominent, anteriorly displaced Schwalbe line (posterior embryotoxon); peripheral iris strands extending to (but not anterior to) Schwalbe line; iris thinning with atrophic holes. See 8.12, DEVELOPMENTAL ANTERIOR SEGMENT AND LENS ANOMALIES/ DYSGENESIS.
- PPCD: Bilateral. Endothelial vesicles or band-like lesions, occasionally associated with iridocorneal adhesions, corneal edema, and glaucoma. No PAS. Autosomal dominant. See 4.25, CORNEAL DYSTROPHIES.
- Fuchs endothelial dystrophy: Bilateral corneal edema and endothelial guttae. Normal iris and angle. See 4.26, FUCHS ENDOTHELIAL DYSTROPHY.
- Prior uveitis with pigmented KP and posterior synechiae.
- Iridoschisis: Usually bilateral separation of iris into an anterior and posterior layer.

Workup

1. Family history: ICE syndrome is not inherited, Axenfeld–Rieger spectrum and PPCD are usually autosomal dominant.

2. Perform baseline glaucoma evaluation. See 9.1, PRIMARY OPEN-ANGLE GLAUCOMA. Careful attention should be given to cornea and iris evaluation.

3. Consider slit lamp photos and corneal endothelial specular microscopy.

Treatment

No treatment is needed unless glaucoma or corneal edema is present, at which point one or more of the following treatments may be used:

1. IOP-reducing medications. See 9.1, PRIMARY OPEN-ANGLE GLAUCOMA. The IOP may need to be reduced dramatically to eliminate corneal edema. This critical level may become lower as the patient ages.

2. Hypertonic saline solutions (e.g., sodium chloride 5% drops q.i.d. and ointment q.h.s.) may reduce corneal edema.

3. LT and laser PI are ineffective. Newer glaucoma surgical techniques and devices such as iStent are not indicated due to angle disorder. May consider filtering procedure (trabeculectomy) when medical therapy fails; however, there is higher rate of failure for glaucoma filtering surgery. Tube-shunt surgery preferred. If tube-shunt procedure is performed, place tube far into the anterior chamber to lessen the likelihood of occlusion with the endothelial membrane.

4. Consider an endothelial transplant or full-thickness corneal transplant in cases of advanced chronic corneal edema in the presence of good IOP control.

Follow Up

Varies according to the IOP and optic nerve damage. If asymptomatic with healthy optic nerve, may see every 6 to 12 months. If glaucoma is present, then every 1 to 4 months, depending on the severity.

9

9.16 Postoperative Glaucoma

9.16.1 EARLY POSTOPERATIVE GLAUCOMA

IOP tends to increase approximately 1 hour after cataract extraction and usually returns to normal within 1 week. Etiologies include retained viscoelastic material or lens particle(s), pupillary block, hyphema, pigment dispersion, and generalized inflammation. Patients at greatest risk include those with ocular hypertension, glaucoma, preoperative IOP >22 mm Hg, and intraoperative complications. Most healthy eyes can tolerate an IOP up to 30 mm Hg for many months. However, eyes with preexisting optic nerve damage require IOP-lowering medications for any significant pressure increase. Prostaglandin analogs are generally avoided postoperatively because of their proinflammatory characteristics and delayed onset of action. Most eyes with an IOP >30 mm Hg should be treated. If inflammation is excessive, increase the topical steroid dose to every 2 hours while awake and consider a topical NSAID (e.g., ketorolac, flurbiprofen or diclofenac q.i.d., bromfenac b.i.d., or nepafenac daily). See 9.7, INFLAMMATORY OPEN-ANGLE GLAUCOMA.

9.16.2 POSTOPERATIVE PUPILLARY BLOCK

Differential Diagnosis

Early Postoperative Period (Within 2 Weeks)

- Aqueous misdirection syndrome (malignant glaucoma). See 9.17, AQUEOUS MISDIRECTION SYNDROME/MALIGNANT GLAUCOMA.
- Suprachoroidal hemorrhage.
- Anterior chamber lens with vitreous loss: Vitreous plugs the pupil if iridectomy is not performed. Can also occur if patient is aphakic.
- Silicone oil or expansile intraocular gas (e.g., sulfur hexafluoride [SF6] and perfluoropropane [C3F8]) after retinal detachment repair. Can occur via open angle or closed angle mechanisms.

- After endothelial keratoplasty, air or gas can migrate behind iris and cause pupillary block.
- Angle closure after scleral buckling procedure.

Late Postoperative Period (After 2 Weeks)

- Pupillary block glaucoma. See 9.4, ACUTE ANGLE CLOSURE GLAUCOMA.
- Suprachoroidal hemorrhage.
- UGH syndrome. See 9.16.3, UVEITIS, GLAUCOMA, HYPHEMA SYNDROME.
- Aqueous misdirection syndrome (malignant glaucoma): When cycloplegics are stopped. See 9.17, AQUEOUS MISDIRECTION SYNDROME/MALIGNANT GLAUCOMA.
- Steroid-induced glaucoma. See 9.9, STEROID-RESPONSE GLAUCOMA.

Signs

Increased IOP, shallow or partially flat anterior chamber with anterior iris bowing (iris bombé), absence of a patent PI. Posterior iris adhesions to lens, anterior capsule, or intraocular lens usually present.

Treatment

1. If the cornea is clear and the eye is not significantly inflamed, a PI is performed, usually by YAG laser. Because the PI tends to close, it is often necessary to perform two or more iridotomies. See Appendix 15, YAG LASER PERIPHERAL IRIDOTOMY.

2. If the cornea is hazy, the eye is inflamed, or a PI cannot be performed immediately, then:
   - Mydriatic agent (e.g., cyclopentolate 2% and phenylephrine 2.5%, every 15 minutes for four doses).
   - Topical therapy with β-blocker (e.g., timolol 0.5%), α2 agonist (e.g., brimonidine 0.1% to 0.2%), and CAI (dorzolamide 2%) should be initiated immediately if no contraindication. In urgent cases, three rounds of these medications may be given, with each round being separated by 15 minutes.
   - Systemic CAI (e.g., acetazolamide 250 to 500 mg i.v. or two 250-mg tablets p.o.

in one dose if unable to give i.v.) if IOP decrease is urgent or if IOP is refractory to topical therapy.

- Topical steroid (e.g., prednisolone acetate 1%) every 15 to 30 minutes for four doses.
- PI, preferably YAG laser, when the eye is less inflamed. If the cornea is not clear, topical glycerin may help clear it temporarily.
- A surgical PI may be needed.
- A guarded filtration procedure or tube shunt may be needed if the angle has become closed.

9.16.3 UVEITIS, GLAUCOMA, HYPHEMA SYNDROME

Signs

Anterior chamber cell and flare, increased IOP, hyphema, and possible iris TIDs. Usually secondary to irritation from a malpositioned anterior or posterior chamber intraocular lens with adjacent iris and ciliary body chafe. UBM may help to confirm diagnosis by demonstrating IOL haptic contact to ciliary body in the sulcus.

Treatment

1. Atropine 1% b.i.d.
2. Topical steroid (e.g., prednisolone acetate 1% four to eight times per day or difluprednate 0.05% four to six times per day) and consider topical NSAID (e.g., ketorolac q.i.d., bromfenac b.i.d., or nepafenac daily).
3. Systemic CAI (e.g., acetazolamide 500 mg sequel p.o. b.i.d.) or may consider topical CAI (e.g., dorzolamide 2% t.i.d.).
4. Topical β-blocker (e.g., timolol 0.5% daily or b.i.d.) and α2 agonist (e.g., brimonidine 0.1% to 0.2% b.i.d. to t.i.d.).
5. Consider laser ablation if bleeding site can be identified.
6. Consider surgical repositioning, replacement, or removal of the intraocular lens, especially if patient experiences recurrent episodes, formation of PAS, or persistent CME.
7. Consider YAG vitreolysis if vitreous strands can be seen.

9

9.17 Aqueous Misdirection Syndrome/Malignant Glaucoma

Symptoms

May be very mild early in course. Moderate pain, red eye, and photophobia may develop. Classically follows incisional (e.g., cataract, glaucoma, retinal) or laser surgery in eyes with small anterior segments (e.g., hyperopia, nanophthalmos) or with primary angle closure glaucoma. May occur spontaneously or be induced by miotics.

Signs

Critical. Diffusely shallow or flat anterior chamber and increased IOP in the presence of a patent PI and in the absence of both a choroidal detachment and iris bombé. IOP may not be significantly elevated, especially early in the presentation.

Differential Diagnosis

- Pupillary block glaucoma: Iris bombé, adhesions of iris to other anterior chamber structures. See 9.16.2, POSTOPERATIVE PUPILLARY BLOCK.
- Acute angle closure glaucoma: See 9.4, ACUTE ANGLE CLOSURE GLAUCOMA.

- Overfiltration after surgery:
  - Choroidal detachment: Shallow or flat anterior chamber, but the IOP is typically low. See 11.27, CHOROIDAL EFFUSION/ DETACHMENT.
  - Postoperative wound leak: Shallow or flat anterior chamber often with positive Seidel test. IOP is typically low. See 13.11, HYPOTONY SYNDROME. See Appendix 5, SEIDEL TEST TO DETECT A WOUND LEAK.
- Suprachoroidal hemorrhage: Shallow or flat anterior chamber. IOP typically high. See 11.27, CHOROIDAL EFFUSION/DETACHMENT.

Etiology

Believed to result from anterior rotation of the ciliary body with posterior misdirection of the aqueous; aqueous then accumulates in the vitreous resulting in forward displacement of the ciliary processes, crystalline lens, intraocular implant, or the anterior vitreous face, causing secondary angle closure. Newer theories point toward choroidal expansion, reduced conductivity of fluid through vitreous, and reduced trans-scleral fluid movement as factors in development.

Workup

1. History: Previous eye surgery?
2. Slit lamp examination: Determine if a patent PI or iris bombé is present. Pupillary block is unlikely in the presence of a patent PI unless it is plugged, bound down, or plateau iris syndrome is present.
3. Gonioscopy and IOP measurement.
4. Dilated retinal examination unless phakic angle closure is likely.
5. Perform B-scan US to rule out choroidal detachment and suprachoroidal hemorrhage.
6. Seidel test to detect postoperative wound leak if clinically indicated.

Treatment

1. If an iridectomy is not present or an existing PI is not clearly patent, pupillary block cannot be ruled out, and a PI should be performed. See 9.4, ACUTE ANGLE CLOSURE GLAUCOMA. If signs of aqueous misdirection are still present with a patent PI, attempt medical therapy to control IOP and return aqueous flow to the normal pathway.
2. Atropine 1% and phenylephrine 2.5% q.i.d. topically. Miotics can worsen condition and are contraindicated.
3. Systemic CAI (e.g., acetazolamide 500 mg i.v. or two 250-mg tablets p.o.).
4. Topical β-blocker (e.g., timolol 0.5% daily or b.i.d.).
5. Topical α2 agonist (e.g., apraclonidine 1.0% or brimonidine 0.1% to 0.2% b.i.d.).

6. If needed, hyperosmotic agent (e.g., mannitol 20% 1 to 2 g/kg i.v. over 45 minutes).

If the attack is broken (anterior chamber deepens and IOP normalizes), continue atropine 1% daily, indefinitely. At a later date, perform PI in the contralateral eye if the angle is occludable.

If steps 1 through 6 are unsuccessful, consider one or more of the following surgical interventions to disrupt the anterior hyaloid face in an attempt to restore the normal anatomic flow of aqueous. Ultimately, the goal is to create a unicameral eye:

- YAG laser disruption of the anterior hyaloid face and posterior capsule if aphakic or pseudophakic. If phakic, may attempt through a preexisting large PI.

NOTE: An undetected anterior choroidal detachment may be present. Therefore, a sclerotomy to drain a choroidal detachment may be considered before vitrectomy.

- Pars plana vitrectomy combined with iridozonulo-hyaloidectomy: Performing vitrectomy with localized excision of iris, lens capsule, zonules, and anterior hyaloid face plus reformation of the anterior chamber has been shown to be helpful.
- Lensectomy with disruption of the anterior hyaloid or vitrectomy.
- Argon laser of the ciliary processes.

Follow Up

Variable, depending on the therapeutic modality used. PI is usually performed in an occludable contralateral eye within a week after treatment of the involved eye.

9.18 Postoperative Complications of Glaucoma Surgery

BLEB INFECTION (BLEBITIS)

See 9.19, BLEBITIS.

INCREASED POSTOPERATIVE IOP AFTER FILTERING PROCEDURE

Grade of Shallowing of Anterior Chamber

I. Peripheral iris–cornea contact.

II. Entire iris in contact with cornea.

III. Lens (or lens implant or vitreous face)–corneal contact.

NOTE: Please be sure to differentiate anterior chamber shallowing grading from both the Shaffer grading classification of angle depth and the Van Herick method for angle chamber estimation, all of which use numerical systems for grading. See Appendix 14, ANGLE CLASSIFICATION.

Differential Diagnosis

(See **Table 9.18.1**.)

If the anterior chamber is flat or shallow and IOP is increased, consider the following:

- Suprachoroidal hemorrhage: Sudden onset of excruciating pain (commonly 1 to 5 days after surgery), variable IOP (typically high), hazy cornea, and shallow chamber. See 11.27, CHOROIDAL EFFUSION/DETACHMENT.
- Aqueous misdirection/malignant glaucoma: See 9.17, AQUEOUS MISDIRECTION SYNDROME/MALIGNANT GLAUCOMA.
- Postoperative pupillary block: See 9.16.2, POSTOPERATIVE PUPILLARY BLOCK.

If the anterior chamber is deep, consider the following:

- Internal filtration occlusion by an iris plug, hemorrhage, fibrin, and vitreous or viscoelastic material.
- External filtration occlusion by a tight trabeculectomy flap (sutured tightly or scarred).

- Occluded tube shunt or increased IOP prior to tube ligature release.
- Obstruction of Schlemm canal and collector channels by blood after goniotomy procedure or MIGS implant.

Treatment

Initial gonioscopy to assist in diagnosis is essential before starting any treatment.

1. If the bleb is not formed and the anterior chamber is deep, light ocular pressure should be applied to determine if the sclerostomy will drain (Carlo Traverso Maneuver). In fornix-based procedures, take great care to not disrupt the limbal wound.

NOTE: If the sclerostomy is blocked with iris, any pressure on the globe is contraindicated due to potential for further iris incarceration.

TABLE 9.18.1   Postoperative Complications of Glaucoma Surgery

Diagnosis	Intraocular Pressure	Anterior Chamber	Iris Bombé	Pain	Bleb
Inflammation	Variable; may be low	Deep	No	Possible	Varies
Hyphema	Mild to moderately elevated	Varies	Not early	Possible	Varies
Failure to filter	Moderately elevated	Deep	No	Possible	Flat
Aqueous misdirection/ malignant glaucoma	Early: moderately elevated Late: moderately to markedly elevated	Diffusely shallow, Grade 2 or 3	No	Moderate	Flat
Suprachoroidal hemorrhage	Early: markedly elevated Late: mild to moderately elevated	Grade 1 and 2	No	Excruciating	Flat
Pupillary block	Early: moderately elevated, may become markedly elevated	Grade 1 to 3	Yes	Possible if markedly elevated pressure	None
Serous choroidal detachment	Low	Grade 1 to 3	No	Ache frequently present	Usually elevated; may flatten with time

2. Laser suture lysis or removal of releasable sutures may be indicated to increase filtration around the scleral flap.

3. Topical pilocarpine or slow intracameral injection of acetylcholine can pull the iris out of the sclerostomy if iris incarceration developed within the past 2 to 3 days. If this fails, and the sclerostomy is completely blocked by iris, transcorneal mechanical retraction of the iris may work. In rare cases, argon laser iridoplasty may be useful to pull the iris enough to restore filtration. If the sclerostomy is blocked with vitreous, photodisruption of the sclerostomy with a YAG laser may be attempted. Blood or fibrin at the sclerostomy may clear with time or tissue plasminogen activator (10 μg) injected intracamerally may reestablish aqueous flow through the sclerostomy.

4. Iris-tube obstruction may be treated in a similar fashion as above. A stent suture may be removed or ligature suture may be lysed to open a valveless tube, but care must be taken as the IOP may drop dramatically if the tube is opened prior to postoperative month one.

5. Additional medical therapy may be necessary if these measures are not successful. See 9.1, PRIMARY OPEN-ANGLE GLAUCOMA.

6. For suprachoroidal effusion or hemorrhage, if the IOP is mildly increased and the chamber is formed, observation with medical management is indicated. Surgical drainage is indicated for persistent chamber flattening or IOP elevation, corneal–lenticular touch, chronic retinal fold apposition, and/or intolerable pain. If possible, delay drainage for at least 10 days in cases of suprachoroidal hemorrhage.

7. If the above measures fail, reoperation may be necessary.

LOW POSTOPERATIVE IOP AFTER FILTERING PROCEDURE

Low pressures (<7 to 8 mm Hg) can be associated with complications such as flat anterior chamber, choroidal detachment, and suprachoroidal hemorrhage. An IOP <4 mm Hg is more likely associated with complications including macular hypotony and corneal edema.

Differential Diagnosis and Treatment

1. Large bleb with a deep chamber (overfiltration): It is often beneficial to have a large bleb in the first few weeks after trabeculectomy. However, treatment is appropriate if it is still present 6 to 8 weeks after surgery, the patient is symptomatic, IOP is decreasing, or the anterior chamber is shallowing. Treatment includes topical atropine 1% b.i.d., intracameral viscoelastic, and possibly autologous blood injection into the bleb. Observation is recommended if the IOP is low but stable, the vision is stable, and the anterior chamber is deep.

2. Large bleb with a flat chamber (Grade I or II): Treatment includes cycloplegics (atropine 1% t.i.d.) and careful observation. If the anterior chamber becomes more shallow (e.g., Grade I becoming Grade II), the IOP decreases as the bleb flattens, or choroidal detachment develops, the anterior chamber may be reformed with a viscoelastic material.

3. No bleb with flat chamber: Check carefully for a wound leak by Seidel testing (see Appendix 5, SEIDEL TEST TO DETECT A WOUND LEAK). If positive, aqueous suppressants, antibiotic ointment, bandage contact lens, patching, or surgical closure may be necessary. If negative, look for a cyclodialysis cleft (by gonioscopy and UBM) or serous choroidal detachments. Cyclodialysis clefts are managed by cycloplegics, laser or cryotherapy (to close the cleft), or surgical closure. Serous choroidal detachments are often observed, since in most cases they resolve when the IOP normalizes. See 11.27, CHOROIDAL EFFUSION/DETACHMENT.

4. Grade III flat chamber: This is a surgical emergency and demands prompt correction. Office-based reformation with viscoelastic is appropriate. Surgical treatments include drainage of a choroidal detachment and reformation of the anterior chamber with or without revision of the scleral flap or tube, reformation of the anterior chamber with viscoelastic, and cataract extraction with or without other procedures.

COMPLICATIONS OF ANTIMETABOLITES (5-FLUOROURACIL, MITOMYCIN C)

Corneal epithelial defects, corneal edema, conjunctival wound leaks, bleb overfiltration, bleb rupture, scleral thinning and perforation, and increased risk of blebitis.

COMPLICATIONS OF CYCLODESTRUCTIVE PROCEDURES

Pain, uveitis, decreased vision, cataract, hypotony, scleral thinning, choroidal effusion, suprachoroidal hemorrhage, sympathetic ophthalmia, and phthisis.

MISCELLANEOUS COMPLICATIONS OF FILTERING PROCEDURES

Cataracts, corneal edema, corneal delle, endophthalmitis, uveitis, hyphema, and bleb dysesthesia (discomfort).

MISCELLANEOUS COMPLICATIONS OF TUBE-SHUNT PROCEDURES

Cataracts, corneal edema, endophthalmitis, hyphema, scleral perforation, diplopia, and tube/implant erosion.

9.19 Blebitis

Definition

Infection of a filtering bleb. May occur any time after glaucoma filtering procedures (days to years). Greater incidence with use of antimetabolites during initial surgery, multiple surgeries, and postoperative complications including flat anterior chamber and wound leak.

- Grade 1 (mild): Bleb infection, hyperemia or purulence, but no anterior chamber or vitreous involvement.
- Grade 2 (moderate): Bleb infection with anterior chamber inflammation but no vitreous involvement.
- Grade 3 (severe): Bleb infection with anterior chamber and vitreous involvement. See 12.13, POSTOPERATIVE ENDOPHTHALMITIS.

Symptoms

Red eye and discharge early. Later, aching pain, photophobia, decreased vision, and mucous discharge.

Signs

(See Figure 9.19.1.)

- Grade 1: Bleb appears milky with loss of translucency, microhypopyon in loculations of the bleb, may have frank purulent material in or leaking from the bleb, intense conjunctival injection. IOP is usually unaffected.
- Grade 2: Grade 1 plus anterior chamber cell and flare, possibly an anterior chamber hypopyon, with no vitreous inflammation.

- Grade 3: Grade 2 plus vitreous involvement. Same appearance as endophthalmitis except with bleb involvement.

Differential Diagnosis

- Episcleritis: Sectoral inflammation, rarely superior. No bleb involvement. Minimal/mild pain. See 5.6, EPISCLERITIS.
- Conjunctivitis: Minimal decrease in vision, no pain or photophobia. Bacterial conjunctivitis can progress to blebitis if not promptly treated. See 5.1, ACUTE CONJUNCTIVITIS.
- Anterior uveitis: Anterior chamber inflammation without bleb involvement. Photophobia. See 12.1, ANTERIOR UVEITIS (IRITIS/IRIDOCYCLITIS).

9

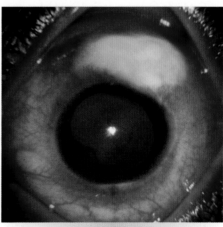

Figure 9.19.1 Blebitis.

- Endophthalmitis: Similar findings as severe blebitis without bleb involvement. May have more intense pain, eyelid edema, chemosis, greater decrease in vision, and hypopyon. See 12.13, POSTOPERATIVE ENDOPHTHALMITIS.
- Ischemic bleb: Seen after the use of antimetabolites in immediate postoperative period. Conjunctiva is opaque with sectoral conjunctival injection.

Workup

1. Slit lamp examination with careful evaluation of the bleb, anterior chamber, and vitreous. Search for bleb leak by performing a Seidel test (see Appendix 5, SEIDEL TEST TO DETECT A WOUND LEAK). Look for microhypopyon with gonioscopy.
2. Culture bleb or perform anterior chamber tap for moderate blebitis. If severe, see 12.13, POSTOPERATIVE ENDOPHTHALMITIS.

NOTE: The most frequent organisms in the early postoperative period include *Staphylococcus epidermidis, Staphylococcus aureus,* and other Gram-positive organisms. If blebitis occurs months to years later, *Streptococcus, Haemophilus influenzae, S. aureus, Moraxella, Pseudomonas,* and *Serratia* are more common.

3. B-scan US will help identify vitritis if visualization is difficult.

Treatment

1. Grade 1: Intensive topical antibiotics with either of the two regimens:

- Fortified cefazolin or vancomycin *and* fortified tobramycin or gentamicin alternating every half-hour for the first 24 hours. May begin with a loading dose of one drop of each every 5 minutes and then repeated four times.

or

- Fluoroquinolones q1h around the clock after a loading dose.
- Reevaluate in 6 to 12 hours and again at 12 to 24 hours. Must not be getting worse.
- May treat bleb leak with aqueous suppressants and cycloplegia.

2. Grade 2: Same approach as mild blebitis, plus cycloplegics, and more careful monitoring. May consider use of oral fluoroquinolones as well (e.g., ciprofloxacin 500 mg p.o. b.i.d. or moxifloxacin 400 mg daily).

3. Grade 3: Treat as endophthalmitis with some preference for early pars plana vitrectomy, as bleb-associated endophthalmitis appears to be more fulminant than infection following cataract surgery. See 12.13, POSTOPERATIVE ENDOPHTHALMITIS.

Follow Up

Daily until infection is resolving. Hospital admission may be indicated.

REFERENCE

Razeghinejad MR, Havens S, Katz LJ. Trabeculectomy bleb-associated infection. *Surv Ophthalmol.* 2017;62(5):591-610.

Chapter 10

Neuro-ophthalmology

10.1 | Anisocoria

Eyelid position, globe position (e.g., to rule out proptosis), and extraocular motility MUST be evaluated when anisocoria is present **(see Figure 10.1.1)**.

Classification

1. The abnormal pupil is constricted.
   - Unilateral exposure to a miotic agent (e.g., pilocarpine).
   - Iritis: Eye pain, redness, and anterior chamber cell and flare.

> **NOTE:** In cases of inflammation resulting in posterior synechiae formation, the abnormal pupil may appear irregular, nonreactive, and/or larger.

   - Horner syndrome: Mild ptosis on the side of the small pupil. See 10.2, HORNER SYNDROME.
   - Argyll Robertson (i.e., syphilitic) pupil: Always bilateral, irregularly round miotic pupils, but a mild degree of anisocoria is often present. See 10.3, ARGYLL ROBERTSON PUPILS.
   - Long-standing Adie pupil: The pupil is initially dilated, but over time may constrict. Hypersensitive to pilocarpine 0.125%. See 10.4, ADIE (TONIC) PUPIL.
2. The abnormal pupil is dilated.
   - Iris sphincter muscle damage from trauma or surgery: Torn pupillary margin or iris transillumination defects seen on slit lamp examination.
   - Adie (tonic) pupil: The pupil may be irregular, reacts minimally to light, and slowly and tonically to accommodation. Hypersensitive to pilocarpine 0.125%. See 10.4, ADIE (TONIC) PUPIL.

   - Third cranial nerve palsy: Always has associated ptosis and/or extraocular muscle palsies. See 10.5, ISOLATED THIRD CRANIAL NERVE PALSY.
   - Unilateral exposure to a mydriatic agent: Cycloplegic drops (e.g., atropine), scopolamine patch for motion sickness, ill-fitting mask in patients on nebulizers (using ipratropium bromide), and possible use of sympathetic medications (e.g., pseudoephedrine). If the mydriatic exposure is recent, pupil will not react to pilocarpine 1%.
3. Physiologic anisocoria: Pupil size disparity is the same in light as in dark, and the pupils react normally to light. The size difference is usually, but not always, <2 mm in diameter.

Workup

1. History: When was the anisocoria first noted? Associated symptoms or signs? Ocular trauma? Eye drops or ointments? Syphilis history (or risk factors)? Old photographs?
2. Ocular examination: Try to determine which pupil is abnormal by comparing pupil sizes in light and in dark. Anisocoria greater in light suggests the larger pupil is abnormal; anisocoria greater in dark suggests the smaller pupil is abnormal. Test the pupillary reaction to both light and near. Evaluate for the presence of an afferent pupillary defect. Look for ptosis, evaluate ocular motility, and examine the pupillary margin with a slit lamp.
   - If the abnormal pupil is small, a diagnosis of Horner syndrome may be confirmed by a cocaine or apraclonidine test (see 10.2, HORNER SYNDROME).
   - If the abnormal pupil is large and there is no sphincter muscle damage or signs

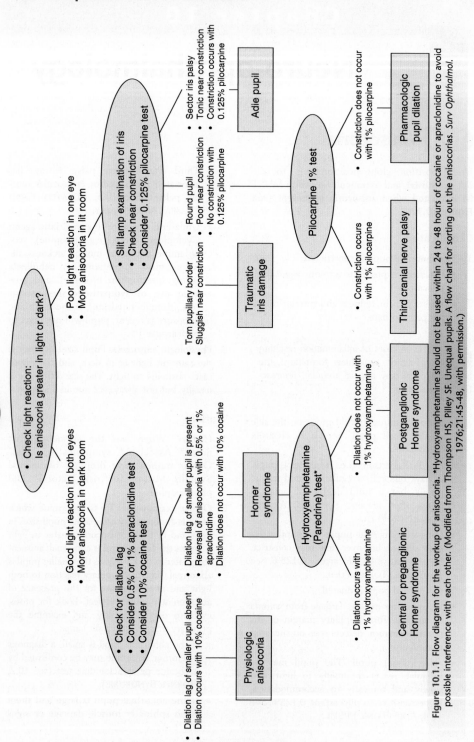

Figure 10.1.1 Flow diagram for the workup of anisocoria. *Hydroxyamphetamine should not be used within 24 to 48 hours of cocaine or apraclonidine to avoid possible interference with each other. (Modified from Thompson HS, Pilley SF. Unequal pupils. A flow chart for sorting out the anisocorias. *Surv Ophthalmol.* 1976;21:45-48, with permission.)

of third cranial nerve palsy (e.g., extra-ocular motility deficit, ptosis), the pupils are tested with one drop of pilocarpine 0.125%. Within 10 to 15 minutes, an Adie pupil will constrict significantly more than the fellow pupil (see 10.4, ADIE [TONIC] PUPIL).

 NOTE: For an acute Adie pupil, the pupil may not react to a weak cholinergic agent.

- If the pupil does not constrict with pilo-carpine 0.125%, or pharmacologic dilation is suspected, pilocarpine 1% is instilled in both eyes. A normal pupil constricts sooner and to a greater extent than the pharmaco-logically dilated pupil. An eye that recently received a strong mydriatic agent such as atropine usually will not constrict at all.

See 10.2, HORNER SYNDROME, 10.3, ARGYLL ROBERTSON PUPILS, 10.4, ADIE (TONIC) PUPIL, and 10.5, ISOLATED THIRD CRANIAL NERVE PALSY.

10.2 Horner Syndrome

Symptoms

Ptosis and anisocoria. May have anhydrosis. Often asymptomatic.

Signs

(See Figure 10.2.1.)

Critical. Anisocoria that is greater in dim illumination (especially during the first few seconds after the room light is dimmed). The abnormal small pupil dilates less than the normal, larger pupil. Mild ptosis (2 mm) and lower eyelid elevation ("reverse ptosis") occur on the side of the small pupil.

Other. Lower intraocular pressure, lighter iris color in congenital cases (iris heterochromia), loss of sweating (anhydrosis, distribution depends on the site of lesion), and transient increase in accommodation (older patients hold their reading card closer in the Horner eye). Involved eye may have conjunctival hyperemia due to decreased episcleral vascular tone. Light and near reactions are intact.

Differential Diagnosis

See 10.1, ANISOCORIA.

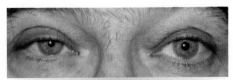

Figure 10.2.1 Right Horner syndrome with ptosis and miosis.

Etiology

- First-order neuron disorder: Stroke (e.g., ver-tebrobasilar artery insufficiency or infarct), tumor, multiple sclerosis (MS). Rarely, severe osteoarthritis of the neck with bony spurs.
- Second-order neuron disorder: Tumor (e.g., lung carcinoma, metastasis, thyroid adenoma, neurofibroma), aortic aneurysm (e.g., tertiary syphilis). Patients with pain in the arm or scapular region should be suspected of having a Pancoast tumor. In children, consider neuro-blastoma, lymphoma, or metastasis.
- Third-order neuron disorder: Headache syn-drome (e.g., cluster, migraine, Raeder paratri-geminal syndrome), internal carotid dissection, varicella zoster virus, otitis media, Tolosa–Hunt syndrome, neck trauma/tumor/inflam-mation, cavernous sinus pathology.
- Congenital Horner syndrome: May also be caused by birth trauma.
- Other rare causes: Cervical paraganglioma, ectopic cervical thymus.

Workup

1. Diagnosis confirmed by a relative reversal in anisocoria with apraclonidine (0.5% or 1%). The miotic pupil with Horner syndrome will appear larger than the normal pupil after apraclonidine instillation. Alternatively, 10% cocaine may be used. Place one drop of either medication in both eyes. Check in 15 minutes. If no change in pupillary size is noted, repeat drops and recheck the pupils in 15 minutes (repeat until normal pupil dilates). A Horner pupil dilates less than the normal pupil.

10

> **NOTE:** There may be a high false-negative rate to pharmacologic testing in an acute Horner syndrome.

2. A third-order neuron disorder may be distinguished from a first-order and second-order neuron disorder with hydroxyamphetamine. Place one drop of 1% hydroxyamphetamine in both eyes. Check in 15 minutes and repeat if no change in pupillary size is noted. Failure of the Horner pupil to dilate to an equivalent degree as the fellow eye indicates a third-order neuron lesion, which may help guide the workup. However, most experts feel the entire sympathetic pathway should be imaged in Horner syndrome regardless of the results of pharmacologic testing. Additionally, hydroxyamphetamine is often unavailable even from compounding pharmacies.

> **NOTE:** The hydroxyamphetamine test has a sensitivity of up to 93% and a specificity of 83% for identifying a third-order neuron lesion. Hydroxyamphetamine should not be used within 24 to 48 hours of cocaine or apraclonidine to avoid possible interference with each other. Both drops require an intact corneal epithelium and preferably no prior eye drops (including anesthetic drops) for accurate results.

3. Determine the duration of the Horner syndrome from the patient's history and an examination of old photographs. New-onset Horner syndrome requires a more urgent diagnostic workup to exclude life-threatening etiologies (e.g., internal carotid artery dissection, which can present with transient visual loss, head/neck/face pain, pulsatile tinnitus, or dysgeusia [foul taste in the mouth]). An old Horner syndrome is more likely to be benign.

4. History: Headaches? Arm pain? Previous stroke? Previous surgery that may have damaged the sympathetic chain, including cardiac, thoracic, thyroid, or neck surgery? History of head or neck trauma? Ipsilateral neck pain?

5. Physical examination (especially check for supraclavicular nodes, thyroid enlargement, or a neck mass).

6. Complete blood count (CBC) with differential.

7. Computed tomography (CT) or magnetic resonance imaging (MRI) of the chest to evaluate lung apex for possible mass (e.g., Pancoast tumor).

8. MRI of the brain and neck.

9. Magnetic resonance angiography (MRA) or CT angiography (CTA) of the head/neck to evaluate for carotid artery dissection (especially with neck pain). Obtain carotid angiogram if MRA or CTA yield equivocal results.

10. Lymph node biopsy when lymphadenopathy is present.

Treatment

1. Treat the underlying disorder if possible.

> **NOTE:** Carotid dissection usually requires antiplatelet therapy to prevent carotid occlusion and hemispheric stroke in consultation with neurology and neurosurgery. Anticoagulation is occasionally used. Rarely, ischemic symptoms in the distribution of the dissection persist despite antiplatelet therapy. In these cases, surgical intervention may be considered.

2. Ptosis surgery may be performed electively.

Follow Up

1. Workup acute Horner syndromes as soon as possible to rule out life-threatening causes. Neuroimaging (as above) should be performed immediately for dissection. Remaining workup may be performed within 1 to 2 days.

2. Chronic Horner syndrome can be evaluated with less urgency. There are no ocular complications that necessitate close follow up.

10.3 Argyll Robertson Pupils

Symptoms

Usually asymptomatic.

Signs

Critical. Small, irregular pupils that exhibit "light-near" dissociation (react poorly or not at all to light but constrict normally during accommodation/convergence). By definition, vision must be intact.

Other. The pupils dilate poorly in darkness. Always bilateral, although may be asymmetric.

Differential Diagnosis of "Light-Near" Dissociation

- Bilateral optic neuropathy or severe retinopathy: Reduced visual acuity with normal pupil size.
- Adie (tonic) pupil: Unilateral or bilateral irregularly dilated pupil that constricts slowly and unevenly to light. Normal vision. See 10.4, ADIE (TONIC) PUPIL.
- Dorsal midbrain (Parinaud) syndrome: Associated with eyelid retraction (Collier sign), supranuclear upgaze palsy, and convergence retraction nystagmus. See 10.4, ADIE (TONIC) PUPIL AND "CONVERGENCE-RETRACTION" in 10.21, NYSTAGMUS.
- Rarely caused by third cranial nerve palsy with aberrant regeneration. See 10.6, ABERRANT REGENERATION OF THE THIRD CRANIAL NERVE.
- Others: Diabetes, alcoholism, etc.

Etiology

- Tertiary syphilis.

Workup

1. Test the pupillary reaction to light and convergence: To test the reaction to convergence, patients are asked to look first at a distant target and then at their own finger, which the examiner holds in front of them and slowly brings in toward their face.
2. Slit lamp examination: Look for interstitial keratitis (see 4.17, INTERSTITIAL KERATITIS).
3. Dilated fundus examination: Search for chorioretinitis, papillitis, and uveitis.
4. Fluorescent treponemal antibody absorption (FTA-ABS) or treponemal-specific assay (e.g., microhemagglutination assay–*Treponema pallidum* [MHA-TP]) and rapid plasma reagin (RPR) or Venereal Disease Research Laboratory (VDRL) test.
5. If the diagnosis of syphilis is established, lumbar puncture (LP) may be indicated. See 12.12, SYPHILIS, for specific indications.

Treatment

1. Treatment is based on the presence of active disease and previous appropriate treatment.
2. See 12.12, SYPHILIS, for treatment indications and specific antibiotic therapy.

Follow Up

Pupillary findings alone are not an emergency. Diagnostic workup and determination of syphilitic activity should be undertaken within a few days.

10

10.4 Adie (Tonic) Pupil

Symptoms

Difference in size of pupils, blurred near vision, and photophobia. May be asymptomatic.

Signs

Critical. An irregularly dilated pupil that has minimal or no reactivity to light. Slow, tonic constriction with convergence, and slow redilation. May have vermiform iris movement and/or sectoral iris sphincter paresis.

 NOTE: Typically presents unilaterally and more commonly in young women.

Other. May have an acute onset and become bilateral. The involved pupil may become smaller than the normal pupil over time.

Differential Diagnosis

See 10.1, ANISOCORIA.

• Parinaud syndrome/dorsal midbrain lesion: Bilateral mid-dilated pupils that react poorly to light but constrict normally with convergence (not tonic). Associated with eyelid retraction (Collier sign), supranuclear upgaze paralysis, and convergence retraction nystagmus. An MRI should be performed to rule out pinealoma and other midbrain pathology.

• Holmes–Adie syndrome: Tonic pupil and tendon areflexia. May be associated with autonomic and peripheral neuropathy.

• Argyll Robertson pupils: See 10.3, ARGYLL ROBERTSON PUPILS.

Etiology

Idiopathic most commonly. Orbital trauma, surgery, and varicella zoster virus infection are seen frequently. Early syphilis, parvovirus B19, herpes simplex virus, botulism, paraneoplastic syndrome, giant cell arteritis (GCA), panretinal photocoagulation, and neurologic Lyme disease less commonly. Rare associations reported with endometriosis, seminomas, and Sjögren syndrome.

Workup

See 10.1, ANISOCORIA, for a general workup when the diagnosis is uncertain.

1. Evaluate pupils and iris at slit lamp or with a muscle light for irregular slow constriction or abnormal movement.
2. Test for cholinergic hypersensitivity. Instill 0.125% pilocarpine in both eyes and recheck pupils in 10 to 15 minutes. An Adie pupil constricts while the normal pupil does not.
3. If bilateral simultaneous Adie pupils, consider further laboratory investigations including testing for the aforementioned etiologies. For unilateral involvement, no further laboratory investigations are necessary.

NOTE: The dilute pilocarpine test may occasionally be positive in familial dysautonomia. Hypersensitivity may not be present with an acute Adie pupil and may need to be retested a few weeks later.

4. If Adie pupil is present in a patient younger than 1 year, consult a pediatric neurologist to rule out familial dysautonomia (Riley–Day syndrome).

Treatment

Pilocarpine 0.125% b.i.d. to q.i.d. may be considered for cosmesis and to aid in accommodation.

Follow Up

If the diagnosis is certain, follow up is routine.

10.5 Isolated Third Cranial Nerve Palsy

Symptoms

Binocular diplopia and ptosis; with or without pain.

NOTE: Pain does not distinguish between microvascular infarction and compression.

Signs

(See Figures 10.5.1 to 10.5.4.)

Critical

1. External ophthalmoplegia.
   • Complete palsy: Limitation of ocular movement in all fields of gaze except abduction.

• Incomplete palsy: Partial limitation of ocular movement.
• Superior division palsy: Ptosis and poor eye elevation.

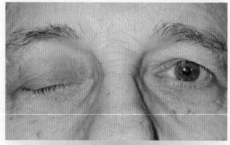

Figure 10.5.1 Isolated right third cranial nerve palsy with complete ptosis.

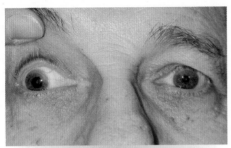

Figure 10.5.2 Isolated right third cranial nerve palsy: Primary gaze showing right exotropia and dilated pupil.

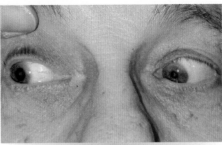

Figure 10.5.4 Isolated right third cranial nerve palsy: Right gaze showing normal abduction of right eye.

- Inferior division palsy: Inability to adduct or depress the eye.
2. Internal ophthalmoplegia.
   - Pupil-involving: A fixed, dilated, poorly reactive pupil.
   - Pupil-sparing: Pupil not dilated and normally reactive to light.
   - Relative pupil-sparing: Pupil partially dilated and sluggishly reactive to light.

Other. An exotropia or hypotropia. Aberrant regeneration. See 10.6, ABERRANT REGENERATION OF THE THIRD CRANIAL NERVE.

Differential Diagnosis

- Myasthenia gravis: Diurnal variation of symptoms and signs, pupil never involved, increased eyelid droop after sustained upgaze.
- Thyroid eye disease: Eyelid lag, eyelid retraction, injection over the rectus muscles, proptosis, positive forced duction testing. See 7.2.1, THYROID EYE DISEASE.

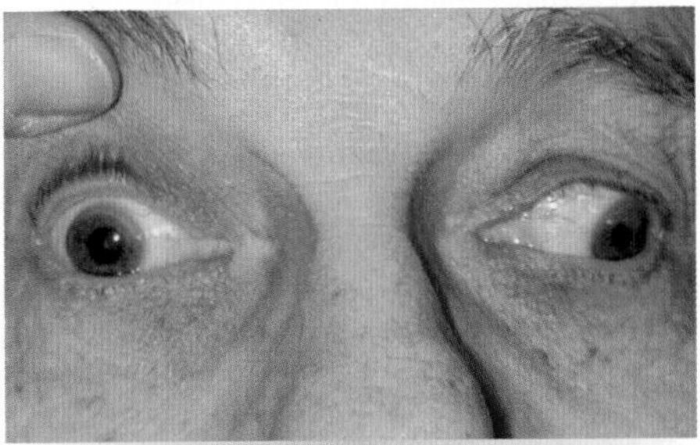

Figure 10.5.3 Isolated right third cranial nerve palsy: Left gaze showing inability to adduct right eye.

- Chronic progressive external ophthalmoplegia (CPEO): Bilateral, slowly progressive ptosis and motility limitation. Pupil spared, often no diplopia. See 10.12, CHRONIC PROGRESSIVE EXTERNAL OPHTHALMOPLEGIA.
- Idiopathic orbital inflammatory syndrome: Pain and proptosis common. See 7.2.2, IDIOPATHIC ORBITAL INFLAMMATORY SYNDROME.
- Internuclear ophthalmoplegia (INO): Unilateral or bilateral adduction deficit with horizontal nystagmus of opposite abducting eye. No ptosis. See 10.13, INTERNUCLEAR OPHTHALMOPLEGIA.
- Skew deviation: Supranuclear brainstem lesion producing asymmetric, mainly vertical ocular deviation not consistent with single cranial nerve defect. See DIFFERENTIAL DIAGNOSIS in 10.7, ISOLATED FOURTH CRANIAL NERVE PALSY.
- Parinaud syndrome/dorsal midbrain lesion: Bilateral mid-dilated pupils that react poorly to light but constrict normally with convergence (not tonic). Associated with eyelid retraction (Collier sign), supranuclear upgaze paralysis, and convergence retraction nystagmus. No ptosis.
- GCA: Extraocular muscle ischemia due to involvement of the long posterior ciliary arteries. Any extraocular muscle may be affected, resulting in potentially complex horizontal and vertical motility deficits. Pupil typically not involved. Age ≥55 years. See 10.17, ARTERITIC ISCHEMIC OPTIC NEUROPATHY (GIANT CELL ARTERITIS).

Etiology

- Pupil-involving:
  - More common: Aneurysm, particularly posterior communicating artery aneurysm.

• Less common: Tumor, trauma, congenital, uncal herniation, cavernous sinus mass lesion, pituitary apoplexy, orbital disease, varicella zoster virus, ischemia (e.g., diabetic), GCA, and leukemia. In children, ophthalmoplegic migraine.

• Pupil-sparing: Ischemic microvascular disease; rarely cavernous sinus syndrome or GCA.

• Relative pupil-sparing: Ischemic microvascular disease; less likely compressive.

• Aberrant regeneration present: Trauma, aneurysm, tumor, congenital. Not microvascular. See 10.6, ABERRANT REGENERATION OF THE THIRD CRANIAL NERVE.

Workup

1. History: Onset and duration of diplopia? Recent trauma? Pertinent medical history (e.g., diabetes, hypertension, known cancer or central nervous system [CNS] mass, recent infections). If ≥55 years old, ask specifically about GCA symptoms.

2. Complete ocular examination: Check for pupillary involvement, the directions of motility restriction (in both eyes), ptosis, a visual field defect (visual fields by confrontation), proptosis, resistance to retropulsion, orbicularis muscle weakness, and eyelid fatigue with sustained upgaze. Look carefully for signs of aberrant regeneration. See 10.6, ABERRANT REGENERATION OF THE THIRD CRANIAL NERVE.

3. Neurologic examination: Carefully assess the other cranial nerves on both sides.

NOTE: The ipsilateral fourth cranial nerve can be assessed by focusing on a superior conjunctival blood vessel and asking the patient to look down. The eye should intort, and the blood vessel should turn down and toward the nose even if the eye cannot be adducted.

4. Immediate CNS imaging to rule out mass/aneurysm is indicated for all third cranial nerve palsies whether pupil-involving or pupil-sparing. One possible exception is a patient with *complete* sparing of the pupil and *complete* involvement of the other muscles (i.e., complete ptosis and complete paresis of extraocular muscles innervated by cranial nerve three).

NOTE: Most sensitive modality to identify aneurysm is contrast-enhanced CTA, though MRA is also very sensitive and can be done if CTA is contraindicated or unavailable. Gadolinium-enhanced MRI is most sensitive for identifying mass lesions and inflammatory etiologies. Choice of imaging should be made in conjunction with neuroradiology. If initial imaging studies are negative but clinical suspicion remains high, catheter angiography may be indicated.

5. Cerebral angiography is indicated for all patients >10 years of age with pupil-involving third cranial nerve palsies and whose imaging study is not definitively negative or shows a mass consistent with an aneurysm.

6. CBC with differential in children.

7. Ice test, rest test, or edrophonium chloride test when myasthenia gravis is suspected.

8. For suspected ischemic disease: Check blood pressure, fasting blood sugar, and hemoglobin A1c.

9. Immediate erythrocyte sedimentation rate (ESR), C-reactive protein (CRP), and platelet count if GCA is suspected. See 10.17, ARTERITIC ISCHEMIC OPTIC NEUROPATHY (GIANT CELL ARTERITIS).

Treatment

1. Treat the underlying abnormality.

2. If the third cranial nerve palsy is causing symptomatic diplopia, an occlusion patch or prism may be placed over the involved eye. Patching is usually not performed in children <11 years of age because of the risk of amblyopia. Children should be monitored closely for the development of amblyopia in the deviated eye.

3. Strabismus surgery may be considered for persistent significant misalignment.

Follow Up

1. Follow-up intervals vary depending on underlying disorder and stability of examination findings. Comanagement with medicine, neurosurgery, and/or neurology may be necessary.

2. If secondary to ischemia, function should return within 3 months. Refer to internist for management of vasculopathic disease risk factors.

3. If pupil-involving and imaging/angiography are negative, an LP should be considered.

10.6 Aberrant Regeneration of the Third Cranial Nerve

Symptoms

See 10.5, ISOLATED THIRD CRANIAL NERVE PALSY.

Signs

(See Figures 10.6.1 and 10.6.2.)

The most common signs of aberrant third cranial nerve regeneration include the following:

- Eyelid-gaze dyskinesis: Elevation of involved eyelid on downgaze (Pseudo-von Graefe sign) or adduction.
- Pupil-gaze dyskinesis: Pupil constricts on downgaze or adduction.
- Other signs may include limitation of elevation and depression of eye, adduction of involved eye on attempted elevation or depression, absent optokinetic response, or pupillary light-near dissociation.

Etiology

Thought to result from misdirection of the third cranial nerve fibers from their original destination to alternate third cranial nerve controlled muscles (e.g., inferior rectus to the pupil).

- Aberrancy from congenital third cranial nerve palsies: Can be seen in up to two-thirds of these patients.
- Aberrancy from prior acquired third cranial nerve palsies: Seen most often in patients recovering from third cranial nerve damage by trauma or compression by a posterior communicating artery aneurysm.

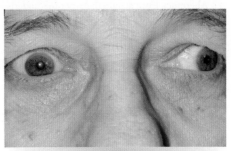

Figure 10.6.2 Aberrant regeneration of right third cranial nerve showing right upper eyelid retraction on attempted left gaze.

- Primary aberrant regeneration: A term used to describe the presence of aberrant regeneration in a patient who has no history of a third cranial nerve palsy. Usually indicates the presence of a progressively enlarging parasellar lesion such as a carotid aneurysm or meningioma within the cavernous sinus.

Workup

1. Aberrancy from congenital: None. Document workup of prior congenital third cranial nerve palsy.
2. Aberrancy from acquired: See 10.5, ISOLATED THIRD CRANIAL NERVE PALSY. Document workup of prior acquired third cranial nerve palsy if previously obtained.
3. Primary aberrancy: All patients must undergo neuroimaging to rule out slowly compressive lesion or aneurysm.

NOTE: Ischemic third cranial nerve palsies DO NOT produce aberrancy. If aberrant regeneration develops in a presumed ischemic palsy, neuroimaging should be performed.

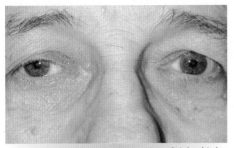

Figure 10.6.1 Aberrant regeneration of right third cranial nerve showing right-sided ptosis in primary gaze.

Treatment

1. Treat the underlying disorder.
2. Consider strabismus surgery if significant symptoms are present.

Follow Up

1. Aberrancy from congenital: Routine.
2. Aberrancy from acquired: As per the underlying disorder identified in the workup.

3. Primary aberrancy: As per neuroimaging and clinical examination findings. Patients are instructed to return immediately for any changes (e.g., ptosis, diplopia, sensory abnormality).

10.7 Isolated Fourth Cranial Nerve Palsy

Symptoms

Binocular vertical (or oblique) diplopia, difficulty reading, sensation that objects appear tilted; may be asymptomatic.

Signs

(See Figures 10.7.1 and 10.7.2.)

Critical. Deficient inferior movement of an eye when attempting to look down and in. The three-step test isolates a palsy of the superior oblique muscle (see #3 under Workup, Perform the three-step test).

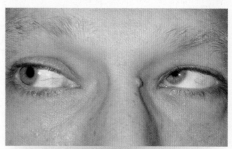

Figure 10.7.2 Isolated left fourth cranial nerve palsy: Right gaze with left inferior oblique overaction.

Other. The involved eye is higher (hypertropic) in primary gaze. The hypertropia increases when looking in the direction of the uninvolved eye or tilting the head toward the ipsilateral shoulder. The patient often maintains a head tilt toward the contralateral shoulder to eliminate diplopia.

Differential Diagnosis

All of the following may produce binocular vertical diplopia, hypertropia, or both:

- Myasthenia gravis: Variable symptoms with fatigability. Ptosis common. Orbicularis oculi weakness often present.
- Thyroid eye disease: May have proptosis, eyelid lag, eyelid retraction, or injection over

the involved rectus muscles. Positive forced duction test. See 7.2.1, THYROID EYE DISEASE and Appendix 6, FORCED DUCTION TEST AND ACTIVE FORCE GENERATION TEST.

- Idiopathic orbital inflammatory syndrome: Pain and proptosis are common. See 7.2.2, IDIOPATHIC ORBITAL INFLAMMATORY SYNDROME.
- Orbital fracture: History of trauma. Positive forced duction test. See 3.9, ORBITAL BLOWOUT FRACTURE.
- Skew deviation: The three-step test does not isolate a particular muscle. Rule out a posterior fossa or brainstem lesion with neuroimaging. See 10.13, INTERNUCLEAR OPHTHALMOPLEGIA.
- Incomplete third cranial nerve palsy: Inability to look down and in, usually with adduction weakness. Intorsion on attempted downgaze. Three-step test does not isolate the superior oblique. See 10.5, ISOLATED THIRD CRANIAL NERVE PALSY.
- Brown syndrome: Limitation of elevation in adduction due to restriction of superior oblique tendon. May be congenital or acquired (e.g., trauma, inflammation). Positive forced duction test. See 8.6, STRABISMUS SYNDROMES.
- GCA: Extraocular muscle ischemia causing nonspecific motility deficits or neural

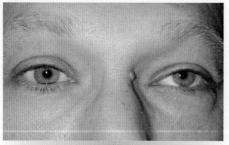

Figure 10.7.1 Isolated left fourth cranial nerve palsy: Primary gaze showing left hypertropia.

ischemia mimicking a cranial nerve palsy. Age ≥55 years, usually associated with systemic symptoms. See 10.17, ARTERITIC ISCHEMIC OPTIC NEUROPATHY (GIANT CELL ARTERITIS).

Etiology

More Common. Trauma, vascular infarct (often the result of underlying diabetes or hypertension), congenital, or demyelinating disease.

Rare. Tumor, hydrocephalus, aneurysm, GCA.

Workup

1. History: Onset and duration of the diplopia? Misaligned eyes or head tilt since early childhood? Trauma? Stroke?
2. Examine old photographs to determine whether the head tilt is long-standing, indicating a chronic or congenital fourth cranial nerve palsy.
3. Perform the three-step test:

   Step 1: Determine which eye is deviated upward in primary gaze. This is best seen with the cover–uncover test (see Appendix 3, COVER/UNCOVER AND ALTERNATE COVER TESTS). The higher eye comes down after being uncovered.

   Step 2: Determine whether the upward deviation is greater when the patient looks to the left or to the right.

   Step 3: Determine whether the upward deviation is greater when tilting the head to the left shoulder or right shoulder.

   - Patients with a superior oblique muscle paresis have a hyperdeviation that is worse on contralateral gaze and when tilting the head toward the shoulder ipsilateral to the affected eye.
   - In addition to the findings on the three-step test, the hypertropia should be greater in downgaze than in upgaze.
   - Patients with bilateral fourth cranial nerve palsies demonstrate hypertropia of the right eye when looking left, hypertropia of the left eye when looking right, and a "V"-pattern esotropia (the eyes cross more when looking down due to a decrease of the abducting effect of the superior oblique muscles in depression as well as overaction of the inferior oblique muscles).

4. Perform the double Maddox rod test if bilateral fourth cranial nerve palsies are suspected to measure total excyclotorsion.

   - A white Maddox rod is placed before one eye and a red Maddox rod is placed before the other eye in a trial frame or phoropter, aligning the axes of each rod along the 90 degrees vertical mark. While looking at a white light in the distance, the patient is asked if both the white and red lines seen through the Maddox rods are horizontal and parallel to each other. If not, the patient is asked to rotate the Maddox rod(s) until they are parallel. If he or she rotates the top of this vertical axis outward (away from the nose) for more than 10 degrees total for the two eyes, then a bilateral superior oblique muscle paresis is likely present.

NOTE: The double Maddox rod test (or variations thereof) can be used to evaluate any suspected underlying strabismus and can help the practitioner measure ocular misalignment and subtle deviations.

5. Measure vertical fusional amplitudes with a vertical prism bar to distinguish a congenital from an acquired palsy.

   - A patient with an acquired fourth cranial nerve palsy has a normal vertical fusional amplitude of 6 prism diopters or less. A patient with a congenital fourth cranial nerve palsy has greater than 6 prism diopters of fusional amplitude.

6. Ice test, rest test, or less commonly edrophonium chloride test if myasthenia gravis is suspected.
7. CT scan of head and orbits (axial, coronal, and parasagittal views) for suspected orbital disease.
8. Blood pressure measurement, fasting blood sugar, and hemoglobin A1c. Immediate ESR, CRP, and platelets if GCA is suspected.
9. MRI of the brain for:

   - A fourth cranial nerve palsy accompanied by other cranial nerve or neurologic abnormalities.
   - All patients <45 years of age with no history of significant head trauma, and patients aged 45 to 55 years with no vasculopathic risk factors or trauma.

10

Treatment

1. Treat the underlying disorder.
2. An occlusion patch may be placed over one eye or fogging plastic tape can be applied to one lens of patient's spectacles to relieve symptomatic double vision. Patching is usually not performed in children <11 years of age because of the risk of amblyopia.
3. Prisms in spectacles may be prescribed for small, stable hyperdeviations.
4. Strabismus surgery may be indicated for bothersome double vision in primary or reading position or for a cosmetically significant head tilt. Defer surgery for at least 6 months after onset of the palsy to allow for deviation stabilization or possible spontaneous resolution.

Follow Up

1. Congenital fourth cranial nerve palsy: Routine.
2. Acquired fourth cranial nerve palsy: As per the underlying disorder. If the workup is negative, the lesion is presumed vascular or idiopathic and the patient is reexamined in 1 to 3 months. If the palsy does not resolve in 3 months or if an additional neurologic abnormality develops, appropriate imaging studies of the brain are indicated. Patients are instructed to return immediately for any changes (e.g., ptosis, worsening diplopia, sensory abnormality, pupil abnormality).

10.8 Isolated Sixth Cranial Nerve Palsy

Symptoms

Binocular horizontal diplopia, worse for distance than near, most pronounced in the direction of the paretic lateral rectus muscle.

Signs

(See Figures 10.8.1 and 10.8.2..)

Critical. Deficient lateral movement of an eye with negative forced duction testing (see Appendix 6, FORCED DUCTION TEST AND ACTIVE FORCE GENERATION TEST).

Other. No proptosis.

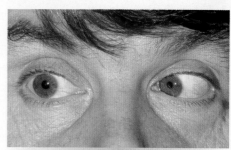

Figure 10.8.2 Isolated right sixth cranial nerve palsy: Right gaze showing limited abduction.

Differential Diagnosis of Limited Abduction

- Thyroid eye disease: May have proptosis, eyelid lag, eyelid retraction, injection over the involved rectus muscles, and positive forced duction testing. See 7.2.1, THYROID EYE DISEASE.
- Myasthenia gravis: Variable symptoms with fatigability. Ptosis common. Positive ice test, rest test, or less commonly edrophonium chloride test.
- Idiopathic orbital inflammatory syndrome: Pain and proptosis are common. See 7.2.2, IDIOPATHIC ORBITAL INFLAMMATORY SYNDROME.

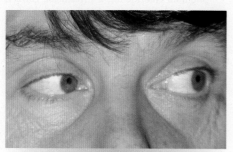

Figure 10.8.1 Isolated right sixth cranial nerve palsy: Left gaze showing full adduction.

- Orbital trauma: Fracture causing medial rectus entrapment, positive forced duction testing. See 3.9, ORBITAL BLOWOUT FRACTURE.
- Duane syndrome, type 1: Congenital; narrowing of the palpebral fissure and retraction of the globe on adduction (usually no diplopia). See 8.6, STRABISMUS SYNDROMES.
- Möbius syndrome: Congenital; bilateral facial paralysis present. See 8.6, STRABISMUS SYNDROMES.
- Convergence spasm: Intermittent, variable episodes of convergence and miosis. May appear to have abduction deficit when assessing versions; however, ductions are full. Miotic pupils help to differentiate since pupils are not affected in an isolated sixth cranial nerve palsy.
- Primary divergence insufficiency: Usually acquired and benign; esotropia and diplopia only at distance and single binocular vision at near. Symptoms may improve spontaneously without treatment or may be corrected with base-out prisms or surgery. If the history reveals sudden onset, trauma, infection (e.g., meningitis, encephalitis), MS, or malignancy, divergence paralysis should be considered and a neurologic workup with MRI of the brain and brainstem obtained. MRI rarely reveals pathology in true divergence-insufficiency.
- GCA: Less common; however, may occur with extraocular muscle ischemia in patients age ≥55 years. May be associated with systemic symptoms. See 10.17, ARTERITIC ISCHEMIC OPTIC NEUROPATHY (GIANT CELL ARTERITIS).

Etiology

Adults

More Common. Vasculopathic (e.g., diabetes, hypertension, other atherosclerotic risk factors), trauma, idiopathic.

Less Common. Increased intracranial pressure, cavernous sinus mass (e.g., meningioma, aneurysm, metastasis), MS, sarcoidosis, vasculitis, after myelography or LP, stroke (usually with other neurologic deficits), meningeal inflammation/infection (e.g., Lyme disease, neurosyphilis), and GCA.

Children

Benign and usually self-limited after viral infection or vaccination, trauma, increased intracranial pressure (e.g., obstructive hydrocephalus),

pontine glioma, and Gradenigo syndrome (petrositis causing sixth and often seventh cranial nerve involvement, with or without eighth and fifth cranial nerve involvement on the same side; associated with complicated otitis media).

Workup

Adults

1. History: Do the symptoms fluctuate during the day? Cancer, diabetes, or thyroid disease? Symptoms of GCA (in the appropriate age group)?
2. Complete neurologic and ophthalmic examinations; pay careful attention to the function of the other cranial nerves and the appearance of the optic disc. Because of the risk of corneal damage, it is especially important to evaluate the fifth cranial nerve. Corneal sensation (supplied by the first division) can be tested by touching a wisp of cotton or a tissue to the corneas before applying topical anesthetic. Ophthalmoscopy looking for papilledema is required because increased intracranial pressure from any cause can result in unilateral or bilateral sixth cranial nerve palsies.
3. Check blood pressure, fasting blood sugar, and hemoglobin A1c.
4. MRI of the brain is indicated for the following patients:
   - Younger than 45 years of age (if MRI is negative, consider LP).
   - Patients aged 45 to 55 years with no vasculopathic risk factors.
   - Sixth cranial nerve palsy accompanied by severe pain or any other neurologic or neuro-ophthalmic signs.
   - Any history of cancer.
   - Bilateral sixth cranial nerve palsies.
   - Papilledema is present.
5. Immediate ESR, CRP, and platelet count if GCA is suspected. See 10.17, ARTERITIC ISCHEMIC OPTIC NEUROPATHY (GIANT CELL ARTERITIS).
6. Consider Lyme antibody.

Children

1. History: Recent illness or trauma? Neurologic symptoms, lethargy, or behavioral changes? Chronic ear infections?
2. Complete neurologic and ophthalmic examinations as described for adults.

10

3. Otoscopic examination to rule out complicated otitis media.
4. MRI of the brain in all children.

Treatment

1. Treat any underlying problem revealed by the workup.
2. An occlusion patch may be placed over one eye or fogging plastic tape applied to one spectacle lens to relieve symptomatic diplopia. In patients <11 years, patching is avoided, and these patients are monitored closely for the development of amblyopia. See 8.7, AMBLYOPIA.

3. Prisms in glasses may be fit acutely for temporary relief or for chronic stable deviations (e.g., after stroke). Consider strabismus surgery for a stable deviation that persists >6 months.

Follow Up

Reexamine every 6 weeks after the onset of the palsy until it resolves. MRI of the head is indicated if any new neurologic signs or symptoms develop, the abduction deficit increases, or the isolated sixth cranial nerve palsy does not resolve in 3 to 6 months.

10.9 Isolated Seventh Cranial Nerve Palsy

Symptoms

Weakness or paralysis of one side of the face, inability to close one eye, excessive drooling.

Signs

(See Figures 10.9.1 and 10.9.2.)

Critical. Unilateral weakness or paralysis of the facial musculature.

- Central lesion: Weakness or paralysis of lower facial musculature only. Upper eyelid closure and forehead wrinkling intact.
- Peripheral lesion: Weakness or paralysis of upper and lower facial musculature.

Other. Flattened nasolabial fold, droop of corner of the mouth, ectropion, and lagophthalmos. May have ipsilateral decreased taste on anterior two-thirds of tongue, decreased basic tear production, or hyperacusis. May have an injected

eye with a corneal epithelial defect. Synkinesis, a simultaneous movement of muscles supplied by different branches of the facial nerve or simultaneous stimulation of visceral efferent fibers of facial nerve (e.g., corner of mouth contracts when eye closes, excessive lacrimation when eating ["crocodile" tears]), secondary to aberrant regeneration implying chronicity.

Etiology

Central Lesions

- Cortical: Lesion of contralateral motor cortex or internal capsule (e.g., stroke, tumor). Loss of voluntary facial movement; emotional facial movement sometimes intact. May also have ipsilateral hemiparesis.
- Extrapyramidal: Lesion of basal ganglia (e.g., parkinsonism, tumor, vascular lesion of basal ganglia). Loss of emotional facial movement;

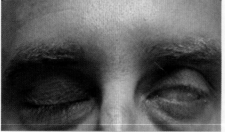

Figure 10.9.1 Isolated peripheral left seventh cranial nerve palsy demonstrating lagophthalmos.

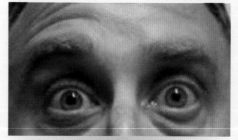

Figure 10.9.2 Isolated peripheral left seventh cranial nerve palsy demonstrating paralysis of upper facial muscles.

volitional facial movement intact. Not a true facial paralysis.

- Brainstem: Lesion of ipsilateral pons (e.g., MS, stroke, tumor). Often with ipsilateral sixth cranial nerve palsy, contralateral hemiparesis. Occasionally with cerebellar signs.

Peripheral Lesions

- Cerebellopontine angle (CPA) masses (e.g., acoustic neuroma, facial neuroma, meningioma, cholesteatoma, metastasis): Gradual progressive onset, although sometimes acute. May have facial pain, twitching, or a characteristic nystagmus. This is small-amplitude rapid jerk nystagmus in which the fast phase is directed away from the side of the lesion (peripheral vestibular) in conjunction with a slow, gaze-evoked nystagmus directed toward the side of the lesion (from brainstem compression). May have eighth cranial nerve dysfunction, including hearing loss, tinnitus, vertigo, or dysequilibrium.
- Temporal bone fracture: History of head trauma. May have Battle sign (ecchymoses over mastoid region), cerebrospinal fluid otorrhea, hearing loss, vertigo, or vestibular nystagmus.
- Other trauma: Accidental or iatrogenic (e.g., facial laceration, local anesthetic block, parotid or mastoid surgery).
- Acute or chronic suppurative otitis media.
- Malignant otitis externa: *Pseudomonas* infection in diabetic or elderly patients. Begins in external auditory canal but may progress to osteomyelitis, meningitis, or abscess.
- Ramsay–Hunt syndrome (varicella zoster virus oticus): Viral prodrome followed by ear pain; vesicles on pinna, external auditory canal, tongue, face, or neck. Progresses over 10 days. May have sensorineural hearing loss, tinnitus, or vertigo.
- Guillain–Barré syndrome: Viral syndrome followed by progressive motor weakness or paralysis or cranial nerve palsies or both. Loss of deep tendon reflexes. May have bilateral facial palsies.
- Lyme disease: May have rash, fever, fatigue, arthralgias, myalgias, or nausea. There may or may not be a history of tick bite. See 13.3, LYME DISEASE.
- Sarcoidosis: May have uveitis, parotitis, skin lesions, or lymphadenopathy. May have bilateral facial palsies. See 12.6, SARCOIDOSIS.

- Parotid neoplasm: Slowly progressive paralysis of all or portion of facial musculature. Parotid mass with facial pain.
- Metastasis: History of primary tumor (e.g., breast, lung, prostate). Multiple cranial nerve palsies in rapid succession may be seen. Can be the result of basilar skull metastasis or carcinomatous meningitis.
- Bell palsy: Idiopathic seventh cranial nerve palsy. Most common, but other etiologies must be ruled out. May have viral prodrome followed by ear pain, facial numbness, decreased tearing or taste. Facial palsy may be complete or incomplete and progress over 10 days. May be recurrent, rarely bilateral. Possible familial predisposition.
- Others: Diabetes mellitus, botulism, human immunodeficiency virus, syphilis, Epstein–Barr virus, acute porphyrias, nasopharyngeal carcinoma, collagen–vascular disease, and others.

Workup

1. History: Onset and duration of facial weakness? First episode or recurrence? Facial or ear pain? Trauma? Stroke? Recent infection? Hearing loss, tinnitus, dizziness, or vertigo? History of sarcoidosis or cancer?
2. Examine old photographs to determine chronicity of facial droop.
3. Complete neurologic examination: Determine if facial palsy is central or peripheral, complete or incomplete. Look for motor weakness and cerebellar signs. Carefully assess other cranial nerves, especially the fifth, sixth, and seventh. Consider assessing taste on anterior two-thirds of the tongue on affected side.
4. Complete ocular examination: Check ocular motility and look for nystagmus. Assess orbicularis strength bilaterally, degree of ectropion, and Bell phenomenon. Examine cornea carefully for signs of exposure (superficial punctate keratopathy, epithelial defect, or ulcer). Perform Schirmer test (see 4.3, DRY EYE SYNDROME) to assess basic tear production. Check for signs of uveitis.
5. Otolaryngologic examination: Examine ear and oropharynx for vesicles, masses, or other lesions. Palpate parotid for mass or lymphadenopathy. Check hearing.

10

6. CT scan if history of trauma to rule out basilar skull fracture: Axial, coronal, and parasagittal cuts with attention to temporal bone.

7. MRI or CT scan of the brain if any other associated neurologic signs, history of cancer, or duration >3 months. Sixth cranial nerve involvement warrants attention to the brainstem. Eighth cranial nerve involvement warrants attention to the CPA. Multiple cranial nerve involvement warrants attention to the skull base and cavernous sinus.

8. CT chest or chest radiograph and angiotensin-converting enzyme (ACE) level if sarcoidosis suspected.

9. Consider CBC with differential, Lyme antibody, FTA-ABS or treponemal-specific assay, and RPR or VDRL tests depending on suspected etiology.

10. Consider rheumatoid factor, ESR, antinuclear antibody, and antineutrophil cytoplasmic antibody if collagen–vascular disease suspected.

11. Echocardiogram, Holter monitor, and carotid noninvasive studies in patients with a history of stroke.

12. LP in patients with history of primary neoplasm to rule out carcinomatous meningitis (may repeat if negative to increase sensitivity).

Treatment

1. Treat the underlying disease as follows:
   - Stroke: Refer to neurologist.
   - CPA masses, temporal bone fracture, nerve laceration: Refer to neurosurgeon.
   - Otitis: Refer to otolaryngologist.
   - Ramsay–Hunt syndrome: If seen within 72 hours of onset, start acyclovir 800 mg five times per day for 7 to 10 days (contraindicated in pregnancy and renal failure). Refer to otolaryngologist.
   - Guillain–Barré syndrome: Refer to neurologist. May require urgent hospitalization for rapidly progressive motor weakness or respiratory distress.
   - Lyme disease: Refer to infectious disease specialist. May need LP. Treat with oral doxycycline, penicillin, or intravenous (i.v.) ceftriaxone. See 13.3, LYME DISEASE.

- Sarcoidosis: Treat uveitis if present. Consider brain MRI, LP, or both to rule out CNS involvement; if present, refer to neurologist. Refer to internist for systemic evaluation. May require systemic prednisone for extraocular or CNS disease. See 12.6, SARCOIDOSIS.

- Metastatic disease: Refer to oncologist. Systemic chemotherapy, radiation, or both may be required.

2. Bell palsy: 86% of patients recover completely with observation alone within 2 months. Options for treatment include the following:
   - Physical therapy with facial massage and/or electrical stimulation of facial musculature.
   - For new-onset Bell palsy, steroids (e.g., prednisone 60 mg p.o. daily for 7 days, followed by a taper of 5 to 10 mg per day) have been shown to increase the likelihood of facial nerve recovery. Antiviral agents, in combination with prednisone, may be offered to patients although the benefit has not been well established.

3. The primary ocular complication of facial palsy is corneal exposure, which is managed as follows (also see 4.5, EXPOSURE KERATOPATHY):
   - Mild exposure keratitis: Artificial tears q.i.d. with lubricating ointment q.h.s.
   - Moderate exposure keratitis: Preservative-free artificial tears, gel or ointment q1–2h or moisture chamber with lubricating ointment during the day; moisture chamber with lubricating ointment or tape tarsorrhaphy q.h.s. Consider a temporary tarsorrhaphy.
   - Severe exposure keratitis: Temporary or permanent tarsorrhaphy. For expected chronic facial palsy, consider eyelid gold weight to facilitate eyelid closure.

Follow Up

1. Recheck all patients at 1 and 3 months and more frequently if corneal complications arise.

2. If not resolved after 3 months, order MRI of the brain to rule out mass lesion.

In nonresolving facial palsy with repeatedly negative workup, consider referral to neurosurgeon or plastic surgeon for facial nerve graft, cranial nerve reanastomosis, or temporalis muscle transposition for patients who desire improved facial motor function.

10.10 Cavernous Sinus and Associated Syndromes (Multiple Ocular Motor Nerve Palsies)

Symptoms

Double vision, eyelid droop, pain in the distribution of the V-1 and V-2 branches of the ipsilateral trigeminal nerve, or numbness.

Signs

Critical

Limitation of eye movement corresponding to any combination of a third, fourth, or sixth cranial nerve palsy on one side; facial pain or numbness or both corresponding to first or second branches of the fifth cranial nerve; ptosis and a small pupil (Horner syndrome); the pupil also may be dilated if the third cranial nerve is involved. Any combination of the above may be present simultaneously because of the anatomy of the cavernous sinus. All signs involve the same side of the face when one cavernous sinus/superior orbital fissure is involved. The circular sinus connects the cavernous sinuses, and its involvement can cause contralateral signs. Consider orbital apex syndrome when proptosis and optic neuropathy are present.

Other

Proptosis may be present when the superior orbital fissure is involved.

Differential Diagnosis

- Myasthenia gravis: Fatigable ptosis, orbicularis weakness, and limited motility. Pupils never involved and never any sensory symptoms. No proptosis. See 10.11, MYASTHENIA GRAVIS.
- CPEO: Progressive, painless, bilateral motility limitation with ptosis. Normal pupils. Orbicularis always weak. See 10.12, CHRONIC PROGRESSIVE EXTERNAL OPHTHALMOPLEGIA.
- Orbital lesions (e.g., tumor, thyroid disease, inflammation). Proptosis and increased resistance to retropulsion are usually present, in addition to motility restriction. Results of forced duction tests are abnormal (see Appendix 6, FORCED DUCTION TEST AND ACTIVE FORCE GENERATION TEST). May have an afferent pupillary defect if the optic nerve is involved.

NOTE: Orbital apex syndrome combines the superior orbital fissure syndrome with optic nerve dysfunction, and most commonly results from an orbital lesion.

- Brainstem disease: Tumors and vascular lesions of the brainstem produce ocular motor nerve palsies, particularly the sixth cranial nerve. MRI of the posterior fossa and brainstem is best for making this diagnosis.
- Carcinomatous meningitis: Diffuse seeding and infiltration of the leptomeninges by metastatic tumor cells can produce a rapidly sequential bilateral cranial nerve disorder. Workup includes neuroimaging and LP.
- Skull base tumors, especially nasopharyngeal carcinoma or clivus lesions: Most commonly affects the sixth cranial nerve, but the second, third, fourth, and fifth cranial nerves may be involved as well. Typically, one cranial nerve after another is affected by invasion of the skull base. The patient may have cervical lymphadenopathy, nasal obstruction, ear pain, or popping caused by serous otitis media or blockage of the Eustachian tube, weight loss, or proptosis.

  Clivus tumors may produce fluctuating symptoms of double vision with an incomitant esotropia and only very mildly limited abduction deficits. These tumors also may produce relatively comitant esotropias due to involvement of both sixth cranial nerves as they ascend the clivus.

- Progressive supranuclear palsy (PSP): Vertical limitation of eye movements, typically beginning with downward gaze. Postural instability, dementia, and rigidity of the neck and trunk may be present. All eye movements are eventually lost. Significant cognitive impairment is often present and can progress rapidly. See 10.12, CHRONIC PROGRESSIVE EXTERNAL OPHTHALMOPLEGIA.

- Rare: Myotonic dystrophy, bulbar variant of the Guillain–Barré syndrome (Miller–Fisher variant), intracranial sarcoidosis, others.

Etiology

- Arteriovenous fistula (AVF) (carotid–cavernous ["high-flow"] or dural–cavernous ["low-flow"]): Proptosis, chemosis, increased IOP, and dilated

10

and tortuous ("corkscrew") episcleral and conjunctival blood vessels are usually present (see Figure 10.10.1). Enhanced ocular pulsation ("pulsatile proptosis") may occur, usually discernible on slit lamp examination during applanation. A bruit may be heard in high flow fistulas by the physician, and sometimes by the patient, with auscultation around the globe or temple. Reversed, arterialized flow in the superior ophthalmic vein is detectable with orbital color Doppler US. Orbital CT or MRI may show an enlarged superior ophthalmic vein. MRA or CTA may occasionally reveal the fistula, but definitive diagnosis usually requires arteriography. High-flow fistulas have an abrupt onset, often following trauma or rupture of an intracavernous aneurysm. Low-flow fistulas have a more insidious presentation, most commonly in hypertensive women >50 years of age, and are due to dural arteriovenous malformations. The Barrow classification is used for preoperative planning and subdivides carotid–cavernous fistulas as follows:

A. Direct fistula.

B. Indirect with branches solely from internal carotid artery (rare).

C. Indirect with branches solely from external carotid artery.

D. Indirect with branches from both internal and external carotid arteries (most common).

- Tumors within the cavernous sinus: May be primary intracranial neoplasms with local invasion of the cavernous sinus (e.g., meningioma, pituitary adenoma, craniopharyngioma); or metastatic tumors to the cavernous sinus, either local (e.g., nasopharyngeal carcinoma, perineural spread of a periocular squamous cell carcinoma) or distant metastasis (e.g., breast, lung, lymphoma).

NOTE: Previously resected tumors may invade the cavernous sinus years after resection.

- Intracavernous aneurysm: Usually not ruptured. If aneurysm does rupture, the signs of a carotid–cavernous fistula develop.

- Zygomycosis (such as mucormycosis): Must be suspected in all diabetic patients, particularly those in ketoacidosis or recent poor sugar control and any debilitated or immunocompromised individual, especially patients on chemotherapy for cancer, with multiple cranial nerve palsies, with or without proptosis. Onset is typically acute. Bloody nasal discharge may be present, and nasal examination may reveal black, crusty material. This condition may produce massive hemispheric strokes and is always life threatening.

- Pituitary apoplexy: Acute onset of the critical signs listed previously; often bilateral with severe headache, decreased vision, and possibly bitemporal hemianopsia or blindness. A pre-existing pituitary adenoma may enlarge during pregnancy and predispose to apoplexy. Peripartum hemorrhage/shock can cause an infarction of the pituitary gland, leading to apoplexy of a nontumorous pituitary gland (Sheehan syndrome). An enlarged sella turcica or an intrasellar mass, usually with acute hemorrhage, is seen on CT scan or MRI of the brain. Note that this may be clinically and radiographically indistinguishable from lymphocytic hypophysitis.

- Varicella zoster virus: Patients with the typical zoster rash may develop ocular motor nerve palsies as well as a mid-dilated pupil that reacts better to convergence than to light.

- Cavernous sinus thrombosis: Proptosis, chemosis, and eyelid edema. Usually bilateral. Fever, nausea, vomiting, and an altered level of consciousness often develop. May result from spread of infection from the face, mouth, throat, sinus, or orbit. Less commonly noninfectious, resulting from trauma or surgery. These patients are deathly ill.

- Tolosa–Hunt syndrome: Acute idiopathic inflammation of the superior orbital fissure or anterior cavernous sinus. Orbital pain often precedes restriction of eye movements. Recurrent episodes are common. This is a diagnosis of exclusion after high resolution MRI and CT scans with and without contrast of the cavernous sinus area. Lymphomas often are mis-diagnosed as Tolosa-Hunt syndrome.

- Others: Sarcoidosis, granulomatosis with polyangiitis (formerly Wegener granulomatosis), mucocele, tuberculosis, and other infectious and inflammatory conditions.

Work-Up

1. History: Diabetes? Hypertension? Recent significant head trauma? Prior cancer (including skin cancer)? Weight loss? Ocular bruit? Recent infection? Severe headache? Diurnal variation of symptoms?

2. Ophthalmic examination: Careful attention to pupils, extraocular motility, Hertel exophthalmometry, and resistance to retropulsion.

3. Examine the periocular skin for malignant or locally invasive lesions.

4. CT scan (axial, coronal, and parasagittal views) or MRI of the sinuses, orbit, and brain.

5. Orbital color doppler imaging is a dynamic evaluation, distinct from the static images of CT, MRI, and MRA. It is quick, painless, non-invasive and may be diagnostic when the other imaging studies are unrevealing. For some ateriovenous malformations (AVMs) and CCFs, cerebral angiography is required for diagnosis, and often for treatment.

6. LP to rule out carcinomatous meningitis in patients with a history of primary carcinoma. More than one LP might be required in some cases.

7. Nasopharyngeal examination with or without a biopsy to rule out nasopharyngeal carcinoma or infectious process.

8. Lymph node biopsy when lymphadenopathy is present.

9. CBC with differential, ESR, ANA, rheumatoid factor to rule out infection, malignancy, and systemic vasculitis. Antineutrophilic cytoplasmic antibody if granulomatosis with polyangiitis is suspected.

10. Cerebral arteriography is rarely required to rule out an aneurysm or AVM because most of these are seen by noninvasive imaging studies.

NOTE: Patients suspected of having dural arteriovenous fistulas are recommended to undergo arteriography to look for cortical venous drainage. If present, this puts the patient at greater risk for intracranial hemorrhage. These AVMs may present with a variable double vision syndrome involving partial paresis of the third, fourth and sixth cranial nerves. These lesions do not produce proptosis or any of the other external signs of cavernous sinus vascular lesions. The eyes are white and quiet. These lesions are especially difficult to diagnose and can produce large stroke syndromes.

11. If cavernous sinus thrombosis is being considered, obtain two to three sets of peripheral blood cultures and also culture the presumed primary source of the infection. Lemierre's syndrome refers to an infectious thrombophlebitis of the internal jugular vein that is a result of spread from an oropharyngeal infection. This rare and potentially fatal entity may present in young, otherwise healthy individuals with neck pain, signs of sepsis, proptosis, and extraocular motility deficits.

Treatment and Follow-Up

Arteriovenous Fistula

1. Many dural fistulas close spontaneously or after arteriography. Others may require treatment via interventional neuroradiologic techniques.

2. Resolution of the fistula usually results in normalization of the intraocular pressure. However, medical treatment with aqueous suppressants for secondary glaucoma may be necessary. Drugs that increase outflow facility (e.g., latanoprost and pilocarpine) are usually not as effective because the intraocular pressure is increased as a result of increased episcleral venous pressure. See 9.1, PRIMARY OPEN ANGLE GLAUCOMA.

Metastatic Disease to the Cavernous Sinus

Often requires systemic chemotherapy (if a primary is found) with or without radiation therapy to the metastasis. Refer to an oncologist.

Intracavernous Aneurysm

Refer to a neurosurgeon for work-up and possible treatment.

Zygomycosis (Mucormycosis)

1. Immediate hospitalization because this is a rapidly progressive, life-threatening disease.

2. Emergent CT scan of the sinuses, orbit, and brain.

3. Consult infectious disease, neurosurgery, otolaryngology, and endocrinology as indicated.

4. Begin amphotericin B 0.25 to 0.30 mg/kg i.v. in D5W slowly over 3 to 6 hours on the first day, 0.5 mg/kg i.v. on the second day, and then up to 0.8 to 1.0 mg/kg i.v. daily. The duration of treatment is determined by the clinical condition.

10

NOTE: Renal status and electrolytes must be checked before initiating therapy with amphotericin B and then monitored closely during treatment. Liposomal amphotericin has significantly less renal toxicity.

5. A biopsy should be obtained from any necrotic tissue (e.g., nasopharynx, paranasal sinuses) if zygomycosis/mucormycosis is suspected.

6. Early surgical debridement of all necrotic tissue (possibly including orbital exenteration), plus irrigation of the involved areas with amphotericin B, is often necessary to eradicate the infection.

7. Treat the underlying medical condition (e.g., diabetic ketoacidosis), with appropriate consultation as required.

Pituitary Apoplexy

These patients may be quite ill and require immediate systemic steroid therapy. Refer emergently to neurosurgery for surgical consideration.

Varicella Zoster Virus

See 4.16, HERPES ZOSTER OPHTHALMICUS/ VARICELLA ZOSTER VIRUS.

Cavernous Sinus Thrombosis

1. For possible infectious cases (usually caused by *Staphylococcus aureus*), hospitalize the patient for treatment with intravenous antibiotics for several weeks. Consult infectious disease for antibiotic management.

2. Intravenous fluid replacement is usually required.

3. For aseptic cavernous sinus thrombosis, consider systemic anticoagulation (heparin followed by warfarin) or aspirin 325 mg p.o. daily in collaboration with a medical internist.

4. Exposure keratopathy is treated with preservative-free lubricating ointment or drops (see 4.5, EXPOSURE KERATOPATHY).

5. Treat secondary glaucoma. See 9.1, PRIMARY OPEN ANGLE GLAUCOMA.

Tolosa–Hunt Syndrome

Prednisone 80 to 100 mg p.o. daily for 1 week, and then decrease dose by 10 mg per week until discontinued. If pain persists after 72 hours, stop steroids and initiate reinvestigation to rule out other disorders. This condition requires a very gradual steroid taper.

NOTE: Other infectious or inflammatory disorders may also respond to steroids initially, so these patients need to be monitored closely.

10.11 Myasthenia Gravis ▶

Symptoms

Painless, droopy eyelid or double vision that is variable throughout the day or worse when the individual is fatigued; may have weakness of facial muscles, proximal limb muscles, and difficulty swallowing or breathing.

Signs

Critical

Worsening of ptosis with sustained upgaze or diplopia with continued eye movements, weakness of the orbicularis muscle (cannot close the eyelids forcefully to resist examiner's opening them). No pupillary abnormalities or pain.

Other

Upward twitch of ptotic eyelid when shifting gaze from inferior to primary position (Cogan eyelid twitch). Can have complete limitation of all ocular movements.

Differential Diagnosis

• Eaton–Lambert syndrome: A myasthenia-like paraneoplastic condition associated with carcinoma, especially lung cancer. Isolated eye signs do not occur, although eye signs may accompany systemic signs of weakness. Unlike myasthenia, muscle strength increases after exercise. Electromyography (EMG) distinguishes between the two conditions.

- Myasthenia-like syndrome due to medication (e.g., penicillamine, aminoglycosides).
- CPEO: No diurnal variation of symptoms or relation to fatigue; usually a negative intravenous edrophonium chloride test. Typically no diplopia. See 10.12, CHRONIC PROGRESSIVE EXTERNAL OPHTHALMOPLEGIA.
- Kearns–Sayre syndrome: CPEO and retinal pigmentary degeneration in a young person; heart block develops. See 10.12, CHRONIC PROGRESSIVE EXTERNAL OPHTHALMOPLEGIA.
- Third cranial nerve palsy: Pupil may be involved, no orbicularis weakness, no fatigability, no diurnal variation. See 10.5, ISOLATED THIRD CRANIAL NERVE PALSY.

> **NOTE:** Myasthenia may mimic cranial nerve palsies, but the pupil is never involved.

- Horner syndrome: Miosis accompanies the ptosis. Pupil does not dilate well in darkness. See 10.2, HORNER SYNDROME.
- Levator muscle dehiscence or disinsertion: High eyelid crease on the side of the droopy eyelid, no variability of eyelid droop, no orbicularis weakness.
- Thyroid eye disease: No ptosis. May have eyelid retraction or eyelid lag, may or may not have exophthalmos, no diurnal variation of diplopia. Graves disease occurs in 5% of patients with myasthenia gravis. See 7.2.1, THYROID EYE DISEASE.
- Idiopathic orbital inflammatory syndrome: Proptosis, pain, ocular injection. See 7.2.2, IDIOPATHIC ORBITAL INFLAMMATORY SYNDROME.
- Myotonic dystrophy: May have ptosis and rarely, gaze restriction. After a handshake, these patients are often unable to release their grip (myotonia). Polychromatic lenticular deposits ("Christmas tree" cataract) and pigmentary retinopathy present.

Etiology

Autoimmune antibody-mediated disease; sometimes associated with underlying thyroid dysfunction. May be associated with thymic enlargement, representing either a benign thymoma or rarely a malignant thymoma. Increased incidence of other autoimmune disease (e.g., systemic lupus erythematosus, MS, rheumatoid arthritis). All age groups may be affected.

Work-Up

1. History: Do the signs fluctuate throughout the day and worsen with fatigue? Any systemic weakness? Difficulty swallowing, chewing, or breathing? Medications (worsened by beta-blockers, macrolides)?
2. Assess for presence of fatigability: Measure the degree of ptosis in primary gaze. Have the patient focus on your finger in upgaze for 1 minute. Observe whether the ptosis worsens.
3. Assess orbicularis strength by asking the patient to squeeze the eyelids shut while you attempt to force them open.
4. Test pupillary function. This will always be normal in myasthenia gravis.
5. Blood test for acetylcholine receptor antibodies (binding, blocking, and modulating). An elevated antibody titer establishes the diagnosis of myasthenia. However, values may be positive in only 60% to 88% of patients with myasthenia and are less likely to be positive in purely ocular myasthenia gravis. Anti muscle–specific kinase (MUSK) antibodies are found in some patients who are negative for acetylcholine receptor antibodies, but those patients usually have systemic findings and have signs/symptoms that are not isolated to extraocular muscle function.
6. In adults, ice test (see later), rest test (see later), or, if cardiac monitoring present, edrophonium chloride or neostigmine test may confirm the diagnosis.

> **NOTE:** Cholinergic crisis, syncopal episode, and respiratory arrest, although rare, may be precipitated by the edrophonium chloride test. Treatment includes atropine 0.4 mg i.v., while monitoring vital signs. Consider pretreating with atropine to prevent problems.

> **NOTE:** Intramuscular neostigmine may be used instead of edrophonium chloride in children or in patients where injecting intravenous medication is problematic. The effect has a longer onset and lasts for approximately 2 to 4 hours.

10

7. For the ice test, an ice pack is placed over closed ptotic eye(s) for 2 minutes. Improvement of ptosis by at least 2 mm is a positive test for myasthenia gravis (see Figures 10.11.1 and 10.11.2).

8. In children, observation for improvement immediately after a 1- to 2-hour nap (sleep test) is a safe alternative. A similar rest test (keeping eyes closed) for 30 minutes in adults may be similarly diagnostic.

9. Check swallowing and breathing function as well as proximal limb muscle strength to rule out systemic involvement.

10. Thyroid function tests (including thyroid-stimulating hormone [TSH]).

11. CT scan of the chest to rule out thymoma.

12. Consider ANA, rheumatoid factor, and other tests to rule out other autoimmune disease.

13. A single-fiber EMG including the orbicularis muscle may be performed if other testing is negative and the diagnosis is still suspected. May be the most sensitive test for involvement of the ocular muscles.

Treatment

Refer to a neurologist familiar with this disease.

1. If the patient is having difficulty swallowing or breathing, urgent hospitalization for plasmapheresis, intravenous immunoglobulin (IVIG), neuromuscular disease specialist consult, and respiratory support may be indicated.

2. If the condition is mild, purely ocular, and is not disturbing to the patient, therapy need not be instituted (the patient may patch one eye as needed).

3. If the condition is disturbing or more severe, an oral anticholinesterase agent such as pyridostigmine should be given (often starting with 30 mg p.o. t.i.d. gradually increasing to an approximate dose of 60 mg p.o. q.i.d. for an adult). The dosage must be adjusted according to the response. Patients rarely benefit from >120 mg p.o. q3h of pyridostigmine. Overdosage may produce cholinergic crisis.

4. If symptoms persist, consider systemic steroids. There is no uniform agreement concerning the dosage. One option is to start with prednisone 20 mg p.o. daily, increasing the dose slowly until the patient is receiving 100 mg/d. These patients may require hospitalization for several days when a high-dose regimen of steroids is employed.

NOTE: Steroid use in myasthenia may precipitate respiratory crisis in the first 2 weeks of treatment. Therefore, in patients with systemic symptoms, hospitalization to begin steroids is required.

5. Azathioprine (2-3 mg/kg/d) may be helpful in older patients. Other medications to consider include mycophenolate mofetil and cyclosporine. Some patients with systemic myasthenia are treated with regularly scheduled IVIG or plasmapheresis.

6. Treat any underlying thyroid disease or infection.

7. Surgical removal of the thymus can be performed. This is indicated for anyone with thymoma. It may also improve symptoms in patients with generalized myasthenia without thymoma.

Follow-Up

1. If systemic muscular weakness is present, patients need to be monitored every 1 to 4 days by an appropriate medical specialist until improvement is demonstrated.

2. Patients who have had their isolated ocular abnormality for an extended time (e.g., months) should be seen every 4 to 6 months and if proven to be stable, every 6 to 12 months.

3. Patients should always be warned to return immediately if swallowing or breathing difficulties arise. After isolated ocular myasthenia has been present for 2 to 3 years, progression to systemic involvement is unlikely.

NOTE: Newborn infants of myasthenic mothers should be observed carefully for signs of myasthenia because acetylcholine receptor antibodies may cross the placenta. Poor sucking reflex, ptosis or decreased muscle tone may be seen.

10.12 Chronic Progressive External Ophthalmoplegia

Symptoms

Slowly progressive, symmetric ophthalmoplegia and droopy eyelids. Almost never have diplopia. Usually bilateral; there is no diurnal variation; there may be a family history.

Signs

Critical. Ptosis, limitation of ocular motility (sometimes complete limitation), normal pupils, and orthophoric.

Other. Weak orbicularis oculi muscles, weakness of limb and facial muscles, and exposure keratopathy.

Differential Diagnosis

The following syndromes must be ruled out when CPEO is diagnosed:

- Kearns–Sayre syndrome: Onset of CPEO before age 20 years associated with retinal pigmentary degeneration (classically exhibiting a salt-and-pepper appearance) and heart block that usually occurs years after the ocular signs and may cause sudden death. Other signs may include hearing loss, mental retardation, cerebellar signs, short stature, delayed puberty, nephropathy, vestibular abnormalities, increased cerebrospinal fluid protein, and characteristic "ragged red fiber" findings on muscle biopsy. Although some are inherited maternally, the vast majority are due to spontaneous mitochondrial deletions.

- Progressive supranuclear palsy (Steele–Richardson–Olszewski syndrome): Rare progressive neurodegenerative disorder affecting the brainstem that causes early gait instability and ophthalmoplegia. Often downgaze affected first followed by other gaze limitations; vertical more than horizontal. Other eye movement problems include abnormalities in the saccadic and pursuit subsystems of horizontal gaze. Often the eyelids are held wide open resulting in a "staring" type of facial expression. Neck and axial rigidity is an important sign.

- Abetalipoproteinemia (Bassen–Kornzweig syndrome): Retinal pigmentary degeneration similar to retinitis pigmentosa, diarrhea, ataxia, and other neurologic signs. Acanthocytosis of red blood cells is seen on peripheral blood smear and LP demonstrates increased cerebrospinal fluid protein. See 11.28, RETINITIS PIGMENTOSA AND INHERITED CHORIORETINAL DYSTROPHIES.

- Refsum disease: Retinitis pigmentosa and increased blood phytanic acid level. May have polyneuropathy, ataxia, hearing loss, anosmia, and others. See 11.28, RETINITIS PIGMENTOSA AND INHERITED CHORIORETINAL DYSTROPHIES.

- Oculopharyngeal dystrophy: Difficulty swallowing, sometimes leading to aspiration of food; may have autosomal dominant inheritance.

- Mitochondrial myopathy and encephalopathy, lactic acidosis, and stroke-like episodes: Occurs in children and young adults. May have headache, transient hemianopsia, hemiparesis, nausea, and vomiting. Elevated serum and cerebrospinal fluid lactate levels and may have abnormalities on MRI.

Workup

1. Careful history: Determine the rate of onset (gradual versus sudden, as in cranial nerve disease).
2. Family history.
3. Carefully examine the pupils and ocular motility.
4. Test orbicularis oculi strength.
5. Fundus examination: Look for diffuse pigmentary changes.
6. Check swallowing function.
7. Ice test, rest test, or edrophonium chloride test to check for myasthenia gravis.

> **NOTE:** Some patients with CPEO are supersensitive to edrophonium chloride which may precipitate heart block and arrhythmias.

8. Prompt referral to a cardiologist for full cardiac workup (including yearly electrocardiograms) if Kearns–Sayre syndrome is suspected.
9. If neurologic signs and symptoms develop, consult a neurologist for workup (including possible LP).

10

10. Lipoprotein electrophoresis and peripheral blood smear if abetalipoproteinemia suspected.

11. Serum phytanic acid level if Refsum disease suspected.

12. Consider genetic testing.

Treatment

There is no cure for CPEO, but associated abnormalities are managed as follows:

1. Treat exposure keratopathy with lubricants at night and artificial tears during the day. See 4.5, EXPOSURE KERATOPATHY.

2. Single vision reading glasses or base-down prisms within reading glasses may help reading when downward gaze is restricted.

3. In Kearns–Sayre syndrome, a pacemaker may be required.

4. In oculopharyngeal dystrophy, dysphagia and aspirations may require cricopharyngeal surgery.

5. In severe ptosis, consider ptosis crutches or surgical repair, but watch for worsening exposure keratopathy.

6. Genetic counseling as needed.

Follow Up

Depends on ocular and systemic findings.

10.13 Internuclear Ophthalmoplegia

Definition

Ophthalmoplegia secondary to lesion in the medial longitudinal fasciculus (MLF).

Symptoms

Double vision, blurry vision, or vague visual complaints.

Signs

(See Figures 10.13.1 and 10.13.2.).

Critical. Weakness or paralysis of adduction, with horizontal jerk nystagmus of the abducting eye.

 NOTE: INO is localized to the side with the weak adduction.

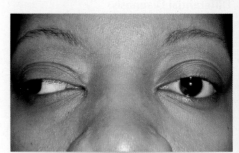

Figure 10.13.2 Left internuclear ophthalmoplegia: Right gaze with severe adduction deficit.

Other. May be unilateral or bilateral (WEBINO: "wall-eyed," bilateral INO). Upbeat nystagmus on upgaze may occur when INO is unilateral or bilateral. The involved eye can sometimes turn in when attempting to read (intact convergence). A skew deviation (relatively comitant vertical deviation not caused by neuromuscular junction disease or intraorbital pathology) may be present; brainstem and posterior fossa pathology should be ruled out. With skew deviation, the three-step test cannot isolate a specific muscle. See 10.7, ISOLATED FOURTH CRANIAL NERVE PALSY. In addition, presence of other neurologic signs, including gaze-evoked nystagmus, gaze palsy, dysarthria, ataxia, and hemiplegia, favors skew deviation rather than fourth cranial nerve palsy.

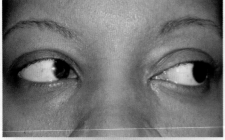

Figure 10.13.1 Left internuclear ophthalmoplegia: Left gaze showing full abduction.

Differential Diagnosis of Attenuated Adduction

- Myasthenia gravis: May closely mimic INO; however, ptosis and orbicularis oculi weakness are common. Nystagmus of INO is faster; myasthenia gravis is more gaze paretic. Symptoms vary throughout the day.
- Orbital disease (e.g., tumor, thyroid disease, idiopathic orbital inflammatory syndrome): Proptosis, globe displacement, or pain may be present. Nystagmus is usually not present. See 7.1, ORBITAL DISEASE.
- One-and-a-half syndrome: Pontine lesion that includes the ipsilateral MLF and horizontal gaze center (sixth cranial nerve nucleus). The only preserved horizontal movement is abduction of the eye contralateral to the lesion. This is because of an ipsilateral adduction deficit (from the MLF lesion) and a horizontal gaze paresis in the direction of the lesion (from the horizontal gaze center lesion). Causes include stroke and pontine neoplasia.

Etiology

- MS: More common in young patients, usually bilateral.
- Brainstem stroke: More common in elderly patients, usually unilateral.
- Brainstem mass lesion.
- Rare causes: CNS cryptococcosis, tuberculosis granuloma, pyoderma gangrenosum (all shown to cause WEBINO).

Workup

1. History: Age? Are symptoms constant or only toward the end of the day with fatigue? Prior optic neuritis, urinary incontinence, numbness or paralysis of an extremity, or another unexplained neurologic event (concerning for MS)?
2. Complete evaluation of eye movement to rule out other eye movement disorders (e.g., sixth cranial nerve palsy, skew deviation).

NOTE: Ocular motility can appear to be full, but a muscular weakness can be detected by observing slower saccadic eye movement in the involved eye compared with the contralateral eye. The adducting saccade is assessed by having the patient fix on the examiner's finger held laterally and then asking the patient to make a rapid eye movement from lateral to primary gaze. If an INO is present, the involved eye will show a slower adducting saccade than the uninvolved eye. The contralateral eye may be tested in a similar fashion.

3. Ice test, rest test, or edrophonium chloride test when the diagnosis of myasthenia gravis cannot be ruled out.
4. MRI of the brainstem and midbrain.

Treatment/Follow Up

1. If an acute stroke is diagnosed, admit to the hospital for neurologic evaluation and observation.
2. If concern for demyelinating disease, consider treatment recommendations described in 10.14, OPTIC NEURITIS.
3. Patients are managed by physicians familiar with the underlying disease.

10.14 | Optic Neuritis

Symptoms

Typical optic neuritis associated with MS causes vision loss over hours to days, with the nadir approximately 1 week after onset. Visual loss may be subtle or profound. Usually unilateral, rarely bilateral. Age typically 18 to 45 years. Retroorbital pain, especially with eye movement. Acquired loss of color vision. Reduced perception of light intensity. May have other focal neurologic symptoms (e.g., weakness, numbness, tingling in extremities). May have antecedent flulike viral syndrome. Occasionally altered perception of moving objects (Pulfrich phenomenon) or a worsening of symptoms with exercise or increase in body temperature (Uhthoff sign).

More recently, immune-mediated disorders of the CNS, such as neuromyelitis optica spectrum disorder (NMOSD), have been described as causes of atypical optic neuritis. Atypical features include advanced patient age, severe vision loss with poor recovery, and simultaneous or rapidly sequential bilateral optic neuritis.

Signs

Critical. Relative afferent pupillary defect in unilateral or asymmetric cases; decreased color vision; central, cecocentral, or arcuate visual field defects.

Other. Swollen disc (in one-third of patients) usually without peripapillary hemorrhages (papillitis most commonly seen in children and young adults) or a normal disc (in two-thirds of patients; retrobulbar optic neuritis more common in adults). Posterior vitreous cells possible.

Differential Diagnosis

- Ischemic optic neuropathy: Visual loss is sudden but in up to 35% of patients may progress over 4 weeks. Typically, no pain with ocular motility, though pain may be present in 10% of cases (compared to 92% of patients with optic neuritis). Optic nerve swelling due to nonarteritic ischemic optic neuropathy (NAION) is initially hyperemic and then becomes pale. Optic nerve swelling in GCA is diffuse and chalk white. Patients tend to be older (40 to 60 for NAION and ≥55 in arteritic ischemic optic neuropathy). See 10.17, ARTERITIC ISCHEMIC OPTIC NEUROPATHY (GIANT CELL ARTERITIS) and 10.18, NONARTERITIC ISCHEMIC OPTIC NEUROPATHY.
- Acute papilledema: Bilateral disc edema, usually no decreased color vision, minimal to no decreased visual acuity, no pain with ocular motility, and no vitreous cells. See 10.15, PAPILLEDEMA.
- Severe systemic hypertension: Bilateral disc edema, increased blood pressure, flame-shaped retinal hemorrhages, and cotton–wool spots. See 11.10, HYPERTENSIVE RETINOPATHY.
- Orbital tumor compressing the optic nerve: Unilateral and usually associated with proptosis, resistance to retropulsion, and/or restriction of extraocular motility. See 7.4, ORBITAL TUMORS.
- Intracranial mass compressing the afferent visual pathway: Normal or pale disc, afferent pupillary defect, decreased color vision, and mass evident on CT scan or MRI of the brain.
- Leber hereditary optic neuropathy: Usually occurs in males in the second or third decade of life. Patients may have a family history and present with rapid visual loss of one and then the other eye within days to months. Early examination of the disc may reveal peripapillary telangiectasias followed by optic atrophy.
- Toxic or metabolic optic neuropathy: Progressive painless bilateral visual loss that may be secondary to alcohol, malnutrition, various toxins (e.g., ethambutol, chloroquine, isoniazid, chlorpropamide, heavy metals), anemia, and others.

Etiology

- MS: Frequently optic neuritis is the initial manifestation of MS.
- NMOSD should be considered in all first-time optic neuritis patients.
- Childhood infections or vaccinations: Measles, mumps, chickenpox, and others.
- Other viral infections: Mononucleosis, varicella zoster, encephalitis, and others.
- Contiguous inflammation of the meninges, orbit, or sinuses.
- Granulomatous inflammations/infections: Tuberculosis, syphilis, sarcoidosis, cryptococcus, and others.
- Idiopathic.

Workup

1. History: Determine the patient's age and rapidity of onset of the visual loss. Previous episode? Pain with eye movement? Intractable hiccups, nausea/vomiting, and severe itching are features strongly suggestive of NMOSD.
2. Complete ophthalmic and neurologic examinations, including pupillary and color vision assessment, evaluation for vitreous cells, and dilated retinal examination with attention to the optic nerve.
3. For all cases, MRI of the brain and orbits with gadolinium and fat suppression should be obtained **(see Figure 10.14.1)**. While a short segment of optic nerve is involved in typical optic neuritis, lesions in NMOSD may be longitudinally extensive. In addition, patients with NMOSD should have MRI of the spine to look for signs of transverse myelitis. Antibodies for anti-aquaporin 4 (anti-AQP4) and anti-myelin oligodendrocyte glycoprotein (anti-MOG) should be drawn.

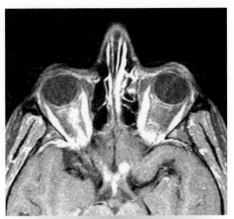

Figure 10.14.1 MRI of optic neuritis showing enhancement of the right optic nerve.

4. Check blood pressure.

5. Visual field test, preferably automated (e.g., Humphrey).

6. Consider the following: CBC, ESR, anti-AQP4 and anti-MOG antibodies for NMOSD, ACE level, Lyme antibody, FTA-ABS or treponemal-specific assay and RPR or VDRL tests, and chest x-ray or CT.

Treatment

Typical Optic Neuritis

If patient seen acutely with no prior history of MS or optic neuritis:

1. Offer pulsed i.v. steroid in the following regimen within 14 days of decreased vision:

   - Methylprednisolone 1 g/day i.v. for 3 days, then
   - Prednisone 1 mg/kg/d p.o. for 11 days, then
   - Taper prednisone over 4 days (20 mg on day 1, 10 mg on days 2 through 4).
   - Antiulcer medication (e.g., omeprazole 20 mg p.o. daily or ranitidine 150 mg p.o. b.i.d.) for gastric prophylaxis.

> **NOTE:** The Optic Neuritis Treatment Trial (ONTT) found steroid treatment reduced initial progression to clinically definite multiple sclerosis (CDMS) for 2 years. Steroid therapy only increases the rapidity of visual return but does not improve final visual outcome.

2. If MRI shows two or more characteristic demyelinating lesions, treat with the aforementioned steroid regimen and refer to neurologist or neuro-ophthalmologist for further management. Currently, there are fourteen drugs that have been FDA approved for treatment of MS. These include agents that are given orally, by injection, or by infusion. The most commonly used medications include interferon-beta, glatiramer acetate, fingolimod, dimethyl fumarate, teriflunomide, alemtuzumab, natalizumab, ocrelizumab, and dalfampridine.

3. Patients with one or more typical signal changes on MRI have a 72% chance of developing CDMS over 15 years.

> **NOTE:** NEVER use oral prednisone as a primary treatment because of increased risk of recurrence found in ONTT. Disease-modifying drugs as listed above have been shown to reduce probability of progression to CDMS in high-risk patients.

4. With a negative MRI, the risk of MS is low, 25% at 15 years. Thus, observation was an acceptable option in the past. However, in the current era of NMOSD, negative MRI should arouse suspicion for this condition. Pulsed i.v. steroid should be administered in all patients, and additional serological studies for antibodies should be obtained.

In a patient with a diagnosis of prior MS or typical optic neuritis:

1. Observation or pulsed i.v. steroids, as above. We usually treat with i.v. pulsed steroids.

Atypical Optic Neuritis

NMOSD (anti-AQP4 positive, anti-MOG positive, or seronegative disease):

1. For acute optic neuritis, high-dose i.v. steroids are used first.

2. Plasmapheresis should be performed if response to steroids is poor.

3. Referral to a neurologist/neuroimmunologist for long-term immunosuppression with agents such as rituximab, azathioprine, or mycophenolate. Eculizumab was recently approved by the FDA for anti-AQP4 positive NMOSD.

10

Follow Up

Diagnosis of Prior MS or Typical Optic Neuritis

1. Reexamine the patient approximately 4 to 6 weeks after presentation and then every 3 to 6 months.
2. Clinically isolated syndromes without features of MS need repeat MRI brain every 6 months initially and then annually to monitor for development of MS lesions.
3. Patients at high risk for MS, including patients with CNS demyelination on MRI or a positive neurologic examination, should be referred to a neurologist or neuro-ophthalmologist for evaluation and management of possible MS.

Atypical Optic Neuritis

NMOSD: Even closer follow up initially may be necessary due to frequency of relapses and severity of vision loss. Follow up within 2 weeks of initial treatment with rapid referral to neurologist experienced in treating NMOSD.

REFERENCES

Beck RW, Cleary PA, Anderson MM Jr, et al. A randomized, controlled trial of corticosteroids in the treatment of acute optic neuritis. The Optic Neuritis Study Group. *N Engl J Med*. 1992;326:581-588.

Beck RW, Cleary PA, Trobe JD, et al. The effect of corticosteroids for acute optic neuritis on the subsequent development of multiple sclerosis. The Optic Neuritis Study Group. *N Engl J Med*. 1993;329:1764-1769.

Chen J, Pittock S, Flanagan E, et al. Optic neuritis in the era of biomarkers. *Surv Ophthalmol*. 2020;65(1): 12-17.

Jacobs LD, Beck RW, Simon JH, et al. Intramuscular interferon beta-1a therapy initiated during a first demyelinating event in multiple sclerosis. CHAMPS Study Group. *N Engl J Med*. 2000;343:898-904.

Optic Neuritis Study Group. Multiple sclerosis risk after optic neuritis: final follow-up from the Optic Neuritis Treatment Trial. *Arch Neurol*. 2008;65:727-732.

10.15 Papilledema

Definition

Optic disc swelling produced by increased intracranial pressure.

Symptoms

Episodes of transient, usually bilateral visual loss (lasting seconds), often precipitated after rising from a lying or sitting position (altering intracranial pressure); headache; double vision; nausea; vomiting; and, rarely, a decrease in visual acuity (a mild decrease in visual acuity can occur in the acute setting if associated with a macular disturbance). Visual field defects and severe loss of central visual acuity occur more often with chronic papilledema.

Signs

(See Figure 10.15.1.)

Critical. Bilaterally swollen, hyperemic discs (in early papilledema, disc swelling may be asymmetric) with nerve fiber layer edema causing blurring of the disc margin, often obscuring the blood vessels.

Other. Papillary or peripapillary retinal hemorrhages (often flame shaped); loss of venous pulsations (20% of the normal population do not have venous pulsations); dilated, tortuous retinal veins; normal pupillary response and color vision; an enlarged physiologic blind spot or other visual field defects by formal visual field testing.

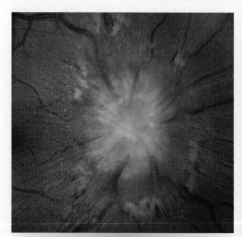

Figure 10.15.1 Swollen optic disc with obscured blood vessels and blurring of the disc margin. Flame-shaped hemorrhages may occur.

In chronic papilledema, the hemorrhages and cotton–wool spots resolve, disc hyperemia disappears, and the disc becomes gray in color. Peripapillary gliosis and narrowing of the peripapillary retinal vessels occur, and optociliary shunt vessels may develop on the disc. Loss of color vision, loss of central visual acuity, and visual field defects (especially inferonasally) may be observed.

> **NOTE:** Unilateral or bilateral sixth cranial nerve palsy may result from increased intracranial pressure.

Differential Diagnosis of Disc Edema or Elevation

- Pseudopapilledema (e.g., optic disc drusen or congenitally anomalous disc): Not true disc swelling. Vessels overlying the disc are not obscured, the disc is not hyperemic, and the surrounding nerve fiber layer is normal. Spontaneous venous pulsations (SVPs) are often present. Buried drusen may be present and can be identified with B-scan ultrasonography or autofluorescence; will also be visible on CT imaging.
- Papillitis: An afferent pupillary defect and decreased color vision are present; decreased visual acuity occurs in most cases, usually unilateral. See 10.14, OPTIC NEURITIS.
- Hypertensive optic neuropathy: Extremely high blood pressure, narrowed arterioles, arteriovenous crossing changes, hemorrhages with or without cotton–wool spots extending into the peripheral retina. See 11.10, HYPERTENSIVE RETINOPATHY.
- Central retinal vein occlusion: Hemorrhages extend far beyond the peripapillary area; dilated and tortuous veins, generally unilateral; acute loss of vision in most cases. See 11.8, CENTRAL RETINAL VEIN OCCLUSION.
- Ischemic optic neuropathy: Disc swelling is pale but may be hyperemic; initially unilateral unless due to GCA, with sudden visual loss. See 10.17, ARTERITIC ISCHEMIC OPTIC NEUROPATHY (GIANT CELL ARTERITIS) and 10.18, NONARTERITIC ISCHEMIC OPTIC NEUROPATHY.
- Infiltration of the optic disc (e.g., sarcoid or tuberculous granuloma, leukemia, metastasis,

other inflammatory disease or tumor): Other ocular or systemic abnormalities may be present. Usually unilateral.
- Leber hereditary optic neuropathy: Usually occurs in males in the second or third decade of life. Patients may have a family history and present with rapid visual loss of one and then the other eye within days to months. Early examination of the disc may reveal peripapillary telangiectasias followed by optic atrophy.
- Orbital optic nerve tumors: Unilateral disc swelling, may have proptosis.
- Diabetic papillopathy: Benign disc edema in one or both eyes of a diabetic patient, most commonly with mild visual loss. No correlation with diabetic retinopathy. In addition to disc edema, disc hyperemia due to telangiectasias of the disc vessels may occur, simulating neovascularization. More common in patients with juvenile-onset diabetes. No treatment is indicated. Spontaneous resolution usually occurs after 3 to 4 months but may take even longer.
- Thyroid-related optic neuropathy: May have eyelid lag or retraction, ocular misalignment, resistance to retropulsion. See 7.2.1, THYROID EYE DISEASE.
- Uveitis (e.g., syphilis or sarcoidosis): Pain or photophobia, anterior chamber/vitreous cells. See 12.3, POSTERIOR UVEITIS.
- Amiodarone toxicity: May present with subacute visual loss and disc edema.

> **NOTE:** Optic disc swelling in a patient with leukemia is often a sign of leukemic optic nerve infiltration. Urgent initiation of therapy including corticosteroids and chemotherapy/radiation is required to achieve best visual outcomes.

Etiology

- Primary and metastatic intracranial tumors.
- Hydrocephalus.
- Idiopathic intracranial hypertension: Often occurs in young, overweight females. See 10.16, IDIOPATHIC INTRACRANIAL HYPERTENSION/ PSEUDOTUMOR CEREBRI.
- Subdural and epidural hematomas.
- Subarachnoid hemorrhage: Severe headache, may have preretinal hemorrhages (Terson syndrome).

- Arteriovenous malformation.
- Brain abscess: Often produces high fever and mental status changes.
- Meningitis: Fever, stiff neck, headache (e.g., syphilis, tuberculosis, Lyme disease, bacterial, inflammatory, neoplastic).
- Encephalitis: Often produces mental status abnormalities.
- Cerebral venous sinus thrombosis.

Workup

1. History and physical examination, including blood pressure measurement.
2. Ocular examination, including a pupillary examination and assessment for dyschromatopsia, posterior vitreous evaluation for white

blood cells, and a dilated fundus examination. The optic disc is best examined with a slit lamp and a 60-diopter (or equivalent), Hruby, or fundus contact lens.

3. Emergency MRI with gadolinium and magnetic resonance venography (MRV) of the head are preferred. CT scan (axial, coronal, and parasagittal views) may be done if MRI not available emergently.
4. If MRI/MRV or CT is unrevealing, perform LP with CSF analysis and opening pressure measurement if no contraindication.

Treatment

Treatment should be directed at the underlying cause of the increased intracranial pressure.

10.16 Idiopathic Intracranial Hypertension/ Pseudotumor Cerebri

Definition

A syndrome in which patients present with symptoms and signs of elevated intracranial pressure, the nature of which may be either idiopathic or due to various causative factors.

Symptoms

Headache, transient episodes of visual loss (typically lasting seconds) often precipitated by changes in posture, double vision, pulsatile tinnitus, nausea, or vomiting accompanying the headache. Occurs predominantly in obese women.

Signs

Critical. By definition, the following findings are present:

- Papilledema due to increased intracranial pressure.
- Negative MRI/MRV of the brain.
- Increased opening pressure on LP with normal CSF composition.

Other. See 10.15, PAPILLEDEMA. Unilateral or bilateral sixth cranial nerve palsy may be present. There are no other neurologic signs on examination aside from possible sixth cranial nerve palsy.

Differential Diagnosis

See 10.15, PAPILLEDEMA.

Associated Factors

Obesity, significant weight gain, and pregnancy are often associated with the idiopathic form. Possible causative factors include various medications such as oral contraceptives, tetracyclines (including semisynthetic derivatives, e.g., doxycycline), cyclosporine, vitamin A (>100,000 U/d), amiodarone, sulfa antibiotics, lithium, and historically nalidixic acid (now rarely used). Systemic steroid intake and withdrawal may also be causative.

Workup

1. History: Inquire specifically about medications.
2. Ocular examination, including pupillary examination, ocular motility, assessment for dyschromatopsia (e.g., color plates), and optic nerve evaluation.
3. Systemic examination, including blood pressure and temperature.
4. MRI/MRV of the orbit and brain. Any patient with papilledema needs to be imaged immediately. If normal, the patient should have an LP, to rule out other causes of optic nerve

edema and to determine the opening pressure (see 10.15, PAPILLEDEMA).

5. Visual field test is the most important method for following these patients (e.g., Humphrey).

Treatment

Idiopathic intracranial hypertension may be a self-limited process. Treatment is indicated in the following situations:

- Severe, intractable headache.
- Evidence of progressive decrease in visual acuity or visual field loss.
- Some ophthalmologists suggest treating all patients with papilledema.

Methods of treatment include the following:

1. Weight loss if overweight.
2. Acetazolamide 250 mg p.o. q.i.d. initially, building up to 500 to 1000 mg q.i.d. if tolerated. Use with caution in sulfa-allergic patients.
3. Discontinuation of any causative medication.
4. Consider short course of systemic steroids, especially if any plans for surgical intervention.

If treatment by these methods is unsuccessful, consider a surgical intervention:

1. A neurosurgical shunt (ventriculoperitoneal or lumboperitoneal) or venous sinus stenting procedure should be considered if intractable headache is a prominent symptom.

2. Optic nerve sheath decompression surgery or neurosurgical shunt (ventriculoperitoneal or lumboperitoneal) is often effective if vision is threatened.

Special Circumstances

1. Pregnancy: Incidence of idiopathic intracranial hypertension does not increase during pregnancy beyond what would be expected from the weight gain. No increased risk of fetal loss. Acetazolamide may be used after 20 weeks of gestation (in consultation with OB/GYN). Intense weight loss is contraindicated during pregnancy. Without visual compromise, close observation with serial visual fields is recommended. With visual compromise, consider steroids, optic nerve sheath decompression, shunting, or repeat LPs.

2. Children/adolescents: A secondary cause is identifiable in 50% patients.

Follow Up

1. If acute, patients can be monitored every 3 months in the absence of visual field loss. If chronic, initially follow patient every 3 to 4 weeks to monitor visual acuity and visual fields and then every 3 months depending on the response to treatment.

2. In general, the frequency of follow up depends on the severity of visual loss. The more severe, the more frequent the follow up.

10

10.17 Arteritic Ischemic Optic Neuropathy (Giant Cell Arteritis)

Symptoms

Sudden, painless visual loss. Initially unilateral, but may rapidly become bilateral. Occurs in patients ≥55 years of age. Antecedent or simultaneous headache, jaw claudication (pain with chewing), scalp tenderness especially over the superficial temporal arteries (e.g., tenderness with hair combing), proximal muscle and joint aches (polymyalgia rheumatica), anorexia, weight loss, or fever may occur.

Signs

(See Figure 10.17.1.)

Critical. Afferent pupillary defect; visual loss (often counting fingers or worse); pale, swollen disc, at times with flame-shaped hemorrhages.

Later, optic atrophy and cupping occur as the edema resolves. The ESR, CRP, and platelet count may be markedly increased.

Other. Visual field defect (commonly altitudinal or involving the central field); a palpable, tender, and often nonpulsatile temporal artery; and a central retinal artery occlusion or a cranial nerve palsy (especially a sixth cranial nerve palsy) may occur.

Differential Diagnosis

- NAION: Patients may be younger. Visual loss often less severe, do not have the accompanying symptoms of GCA listed previously, and usually have a normal ESR and CRP. See 10.18, NONARTERITIC ISCHEMIC OPTIC NEUROPATHY.

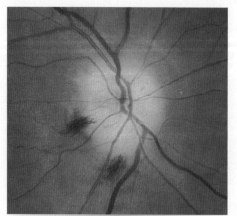

Figure 10.17.1 Chalky, pale, swollen optic disc with flame-shaped hemorrhages in giant cell arteritis.

- Inflammatory optic neuritis: Younger age group. Pain with eye movements. Optic disc swelling, if present, is more hyperemic. See 10.14, OPTIC NEURITIS.
- Compressive optic nerve tumor: Optic nerve pallor or atrophy may be seen; disc heme unlikely. Slowly progressive visual loss. Few to no symptoms common with GCA.
- Central retinal vein occlusion: Severe visual loss may be accompanied by an afferent pupillary defect and disc swelling, but the retina shows diffuse retinal hemorrhages extending out to the periphery. See 11.8, CENTRAL RETINAL VEIN OCCLUSION.
- Central retinal artery occlusion: Sudden, painless, severe visual loss with an afferent pupillary defect. No disc swelling. Retinal edema with a cherry-red spot frequently observed. See 11.6, CENTRAL RETINAL ARTERY OCCLUSION.

Workup

1. History: GCA symptoms present? Age is critical.
2. Complete ocular examination, particularly pupillary assessment, dyschromatopsia evaluation (e.g., color plates), dilated retinal examination to rule out retinal causes of severe visual loss, and optic nerve evaluation.
3. Immediate ESR (Westergren is the most reliable method), CRP (does not rise with age), and platelet count (may have thrombocytosis). A guideline for top-normal ESR calculation: men, age/2; women, (age + 10)/2. ESR

may not be increased. CRP and platelet upper limit values are based on laboratory-specific standards.

4. Perform a temporal artery biopsy if GCA is suspected.

NOTE: The biopsy should be performed within 1 week after starting systemic steroids, but a positive result may be seen up to 1 month later. Biopsy is especially important in patients in whom steroids are relatively contraindicated (e.g., diabetics).

Treatment

1. Systemic steroids should be given immediately once GCA is suspected. Methylprednisolone 250 mg i.v., q6h for 12 doses, and then switch to prednisone 80 to 100 mg p.o. daily. A temporal artery biopsy specimen should be obtained within 1 week of systemic steroid initiation.
2. If the temporal artery biopsy is positive for GCA (or clinical presentation/therapeutic response warrants continued therapy), the patient must be maintained on prednisone, about 1 mg/kg initially. Oral steroids are tapered on an individual basis with the goal of using the lowest required dose necessary for disease suppression (see below).
3. If the biopsy is negative on an adequate (2 to 3 cm) section, the likelihood of GCA is small. However, in highly suggestive cases, biopsy of the contralateral artery is performed.
4. Steroids are usually discontinued if the disease is not found in adequate biopsy specimens, *unless the clinical presentation is classic and a response to treatment has occurred.*

NOTE

1. Without steroids (and occasionally on adequate steroids), the contralateral eye can become involved within 1 to 7 days.
2. Concurrent antiulcer (e.g., proton-pump inhibitor [e.g., omeprazole 20 mg p.o. daily] or histamine type 2 receptor blocker [e.g., ranitidine 150 mg p.o. b.i.d.]) should be used for gastrointestinal prophylaxis while on steroids.
3. A medication to help prevent osteoporosis should be used as directed by an internist, particularly given the long-term need for steroids.

Follow Up

1. Patients suspected of having GCA must be evaluated and treated immediately.

2. After the diagnosis is confirmed by biopsy, the initial oral steroid dosage is maintained until the symptoms resolve and lab values normalize. The dosage is then tapered slowly, repeating bloodwork with each dosage change and/or monthly (whichever appropriate based on disease stability) to ensure that the new steroid dosage is enough to suppress the disease.

3. If the ESR or CRP increase or symptoms return, the dosage must be increased.

4. Treatment should last at least 6 to 12 months. The smallest steroid dose that suppresses disease is used.

Tocilizumab, a novel humanized IL-6 receptor antagonist, has been recently approved by the FDA for long-term management of GCA. Addition of subcutaneous tocilizumab to standardized steroid regimens helps achieve remission faster and significantly reduces the dose and toxicity of corticosteroids.

10.18 Nonarteritic Ischemic Optic Neuropathy

Symptoms

Sudden, painless visual loss of moderate degree, initially unilateral, but may become bilateral. Typically occurs in patients 40 to 60 years of age, but well-documented cases have been reported in patients in their teenage years. In younger patients, NAION should be suspected when painless visual loss develops with a contralateral "disc at risk" (i.e., crowded disc with small or absent optic cup [cup:disc ratio less than 0.3]) and normal MRI scan. The visual deficit may improve. Hyperlipidemia, labile hypertension, and sleep apnea are the common risk factors for younger patients.

Signs

(See Figure 10.18.1.)

Critical. Afferent pupillary defect, pale disc swelling (often segmental), flame-shaped hemorrhages, normal ESR and CRP.

- Nonprogressive NAION: Sudden initial decrease in visual acuity and visual field, which stabilizes.

- Progressive NAION: Sudden initial decrease in visual acuity and visual field followed by worsening in visual acuity or visual field days to weeks later. As many as 35% of NAION cases may be progressive.

Other. Reduced color vision, altitudinal or central visual field defect, optic atrophy without cupping (segmental or diffuse) after the edema resolves. Crowded or congenitally anomalous disc with small or absent cup in fellow eye.

Differential Diagnosis

See 10.17, ARTERITIC ISCHEMIC OPTIC NEUROPATHY (GIANT CELL ARTERITIS).

Etiology

Idiopathic: Arteriosclerosis, diabetes, hypertension, hyperlipidemia, hyperhomocysteinemia, anemia, and sleep apnea are associated risk factors, but causation has never been proven. Relative nocturnal hypotension may play a role, especially in patients taking antihypertensive medication. Nocturnal hypotension may be related to sleep apnea.

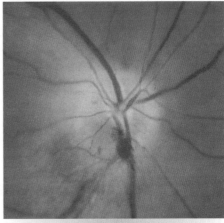

Figure 10.18.1 Nonarteritic ischemic optic neuropathy with segmental disc edema and hemorrhage.

NOTE: Currently, phosphodiesterase-5 inhibitors (e.g., sildenafil, vardenafil, and tadalafil) often used for erectile dysfunction have not been proven to cause NAION. However, the FDA has issued a warning regarding a possible association with these medications and NAION. It is recommended that patients with risk factors for NAION (listed previously) be counseled against the use of these medications.

Workup

1. Same as 10.17, ARTERITIC ISCHEMIC OPTIC NEUROPATHY (GIANT CELL ARTERITIS).
2. Consult internist to rule out cardiovascular disease, diabetes, hypertension, and sleep apnea.

Treatment

1. Observation.
2. Cardiovascular risk factor modification.
3. Consider avoiding blood pressure medication at bedtime to help avoid nocturnal hypotension.

Follow Up

1. One month.
2. Up to 40% of patients show mild improvement in vision over 3 to 6 months in some studies. Optic nerve edema resolves within 8 weeks.
3. Patients should be counseled of risk to the contralateral eye (variable).

10.19 Posterior Ischemic Optic Neuropathy

Symptoms

Painless visual loss. Most commonly occurs in the postoperative setting at any time from upon awakening from anesthesia to 4 to 7 days thereafter. May be unilateral or bilateral, with a partial or complete deficit.

Signs

See 10.18, NONARTERITIC ISCHEMIC OPTIC NEUROPATHY. Optic discs may appear normal initially in acute posterior ischemic optic neuropathy, but eventually pale disc edema, followed by pallor, develops.

Etiology

• Postoperative: May occur after head and neck surgery, spinal surgery, gastrointestinal surgery, open heart surgery, or any procedure associated with hypotension, anemia, increased surgical time, large amounts of blood loss, increased central venous pressure, or positioning of head in a dependent, down-tilt position.

History of peripheral vascular disease, diabetes, and anemia may increase risk.

NOTE: Operative planning in high-risk patients should include attention to head positioning and length of surgical time, balance of risk and benefits of hypotensive anesthesia, aggressive replacement of blood loss, monitoring vision early in the postoperative period, and prompt ophthalmic consultation if patient describes visual disturbances.

• Inflammatory/infectious: GCA, varicella zoster virus, systemic lupus erythematosus, and others.

Treatment

1. Although no controlled studies exist for postoperative posterior ischemic optic neuropathy, it has been suggested that prompt blood transfusion with correction of hypotension and anemia may be beneficial and should be considered.
2. Treat any inflammatory or infectious etiology as appropriate.

10.20 Miscellaneous Optic Neuropathies

TOXIC/METABOLIC OPTIC NEUROPATHY

Symptoms

Painless, progressive, bilateral loss of vision.

Signs

Critical. Bilateral cecocentral or central visual field defects, signs of alcoholism, tobacco/substance use, certain medication use, heavy metal exposure, or poor nutrition.

Other. Visual acuity of 20/50 to 20/200, reduced color vision, temporal disc pallor, optic atrophy, or normal-appearing disc initially.

Etiology

- Tobacco/alcohol or other substance abuse.
- Severe malnutrition with thiamine (vitamin B1) deficiency.
- Pernicious anemia: Usually due to vitamin B12 malabsorption.
- Toxic: Exposure to medications such as chloramphenicol, ethambutol, linezolid, isoniazid, digitalis, streptomycin, chlorpropamide, ethchlorvynol, disulfiram, amiodarone, and lead. Methanol can cause an acute optic neuropathy.

Workup

- History: Drug or substance abuse? Medications? Diet?
- Complete ocular examination, including pupillary assessment, dyschromatopsia evaluation, and optic nerve examination.
- Formal visual field test.
- CBC with differential and peripheral smear.
- Serum vitamin B1, B12, and folate levels.
- Consider a heavy metal (e.g., lead, thallium) screen.
- If disc is swollen, consider blood test for Leber hereditary optic neuropathy.

Treatment

- Thiamine 100 mg p.o. b.i.d.
- Folate 1.0 mg p.o. daily.
- Multivitamin tablet daily.
- Eliminate any causative agent (e.g., alcohol, medication).
- Coordinated care with an internist, including vitamin B12 1,000 mg intramuscularly every month for pernicious anemia.

Follow Up

Every month at first and then every 6 to 12 months.

COMPRESSIVE OPTIC NEUROPATHY

Symptoms

Slowly progressive visual loss, although occasionally acute or noticed acutely.

Signs

Critical. Central visual field defect, relative afferent pupillary defect.

Other. The optic nerve can be normal, pale, or, occasionally, swollen; proptosis; optociliary (collateral) shunt vessels. Collateral vessels occur only with intrinsic lesions of the nerve (never with extrinsic lesions).

Etiology

- Optic nerve glioma: Age usually <20 years, often associated with neurofibromatosis.
- Optic nerve meningioma: Usually adult women. Orbital imaging may show an optic nerve mass, diffuse optic nerve thickening, or a railroad-track sign (increased contrast of the periphery of the nerve).
- Any intraorbital or intracranial mass (e.g., hemangioma, schwannoma).

Workup

All patients with progressive visual loss and optic nerve dysfunction should have an MRI of the orbit and brain.

Treatment

1. Depends on the etiology.
2. Treatment for optic nerve glioma is controversial. These lesions are often monitored unless there is evidence of intracranial involvement, at which point surgical excision may be indicated. Most of these patients are young children, who are very susceptible to cognitive complications of radiotherapy. Chemotherapy may be considered if there is progressive visual loss.
3. For optic nerve sheath meningiomas, fractionated stereotactic radiotherapy treatment should be considered. Serial MRIs may be used to monitor tumor control.

LEBER HEREDITARY OPTIC NEUROPATHY

Symptoms

Painless progressive visual loss in one and then the other eye within days to months of each other. Visual loss is bilateral at onset in approximately 25% of cases.

Signs

Critical. Mild swelling of optic disc progressing over weeks to optic atrophy; small, telangiectatic blood vessels near the disc that do not leak on i.v. fluorescein angiography often present acutely; usually occurs in young men aged 15 to 30 years, and less commonly in women who are often older.

Other. Visual acuity 20/200 to counting fingers, cecocentral visual field defect.

Transmission

By mitochondrial DNA (transmitted by mothers to all offspring). However, 50% to 70% of sons and 10% to 15% of daughters manifest the disease. All daughters are carriers, and none of the sons can transmit the disease.

Workup

Genetic testing is available for the most frequent base-pair nucleotide substitutions at positions 11778, 3460, and 14484 in the mitochondrial gene for the NADH dehydrogenase protein.

Treatment

1. Idebenone is used in Canada and the United Kingdom but is not available in the United States. Studies thus far have shown variable results regarding its effectiveness. Phase 3 clinical trials of gene replacement are ongoing.
2. Tobacco (or exposure to smoke) and alcohol avoidance are recommended.

3. Genetic counseling should be offered.
4. Consider cardiology consult because of increased incidence of cardiac conduction defects.

DOMINANT OPTIC ATROPHY

Mild-to-moderate bilateral visual loss (20/40 to 20/200) usually presenting at approximately age 4 years old. Slow progression, temporal disc pallor, cecocentral visual field defect, tritanopic (blue-yellow) color defect on Farnsworth–Munsell 100-hue test, strong family history, and no nystagmus. OPA1 and other mutations are responsible.

COMPLICATED HEREDITARY OPTIC ATROPHY

Bilateral optic atrophy with spinocerebellar degenerations (e.g., Friedreich, Marie, Behr), polyneuropathy (e.g., Charcot–Marie–Tooth), or inborn errors of metabolism.

RADIATION OPTIC NEUROPATHY

Delayed effect (usually 1 to 5 years) after radiation therapy to the eye, orbit, sinus, nasopharynx, and brain with acute or gradual stepwise visual loss that is commonly severe. Disc swelling, radiation retinopathy, or both may be present. Enhancement of optic nerve or chiasm on MRI.

10.21 Nystagmus

Nystagmus is divided into congenital and acquired forms.

Symptoms

Congenital and acquired nystagmus may be symptomatic with decreased visual acuity. The environment may be noted to oscillate horizontally, vertically, or torsionally in cases of acquired nystagmus, but only occasionally in congenital cases.

Signs

Critical. Repetitive, rhythmic oscillations of the eye horizontally, vertically, or torsionally.

• Jerk nystagmus: The eye repetitively slowly drifts in one direction (slow phase) and then rapidly returns to its original position (fast phase).

• Pendular nystagmus: Drift occurs in two phases of equal speed, giving a smooth back-and-forth slow movement of the eye.

CONGENITAL FORMS OF NYSTAGMUS

INFANTILE NYSTAGMUS

Onset by age 2 to 3 months with wide, swinging eye movements. At age 4 to 6 months, small pendular eye movements are added. At age 6 to 12 months, jerk nystagmus and a null point (a position of gaze where the nystagmus is minimized) develop. Compensatory head positioning may develop at any point up to 20 years of age. Infantile nystagmus is usually horizontal and uniplanar (same direction in all gazes) and typically dampens with convergence. May have a latent component (worsens when one eye is occluded).

Differential Diagnosis

- Opsoclonus/saccadomania: Repetitive, conjugate, multidirectional rapid saccadic eye movements associated with cerebellar or brainstem disease, postviral encephalitis, visceral carcinoma, or neuroblastoma.
- Spasmus nutans: Head nodding and head turn with vertical, horizontal, or torsional nystagmus appearing between 6 months and 3 years of age and resolving between 2 and 8 years of age. Unilateral or bilateral (but asymmetric) rapid "shimmering nystagmus." Spasmus nutans is a benign condition; however, gliomas of the anterior visual pathway may produce an identical clinical picture and need to be ruled out with MRI.
- Latent nystagmus (see below).
- Nystagmus blockage syndrome (see below).

Etiology

- Idiopathic.
- Albinism: Iris transillumination defects and foveal hypoplasia. See 13.8, ALBINISM.
- Aniridia: Bilateral, near-total congenital iris absence. See 8.12, DEVELOPMENTAL ANTERIOR SEGMENT AND LENS ANOMALIES/DYSGENESIS.
- Leber congenital amaurosis: Markedly abnormal or flat electroretinogram (ERG).
- Others: Bilateral optic nerve hypoplasia, bilateral congenital cataracts, rod monochromatism, or optic nerve or macular disease.

Workup

1. History: Age of onset? Head nodding or head positioning? Known ocular or systemic abnormalities? Medications? Family history?
2. Complete ocular examination: Observe the head position and eye movements, perform iris transillumination, and carefully inspect the optic disc and macula.
3. Consider obtaining an eye movement recording if the diagnosis is uncertain.

4. If opsoclonus is present, obtain abdominal and chest imaging (e.g., ultrasound, CT, MRI) to rule out neuroblastoma and visceral carcinoma. Refer to primary medical doctor or pediatrician for additional workup (e.g., urinary vanillylmandelic acid) as appropriate.
5. In selected cases and in all cases of suspected spasmus nutans, obtain an MRI of the brain (axial, coronal, and parasagittal views) to rule out an anterior optic pathway lesion.

Treatment

1. Maximize vision by refraction.
2. Treat amblyopia if indicated.
3. If small face turn: Prescribe prism in glasses with base toward direction of face turn.
4. If large face turn: Consider muscle surgery.

LATENT NYSTAGMUS

Occurs when only one eye is viewing. Conjugate horizontal nystagmus with fast phase beating toward viewing eye.

Manifest latent nystagmus occurs in children with strabismus or decreased vision in one eye, in whom the nonfixating or poorly seeing eye behaves as an occluded eye.

NOTE: When testing visual acuity in one eye, fog (e.g., add plus lenses in front of) rather than occlude the opposite eye to minimize induction of latent nystagmus.

Treatment

1. Maximize vision by refraction.
2. Treat amblyopia if indicated.
3. Consider muscle surgery if symptomatic strabismus or cosmetically significant head turn exists.

NYSTAGMUS BLOCKAGE SYNDROME

Any nystagmus that decreases when the fixating eye is in adduction and demonstrates an esotropia to dampen the nystagmus.

Treatment

For large face turn, consider muscle surgery.

ACQUIRED FORMS OF NYSTAGMUS

Etiology

- Visual loss (e.g., dense cataract, trauma, cone dystrophy): Usually monocular and vertical nystagmus (Heimann–Bielschowsky phenomenon).
- Toxic/metabolic: Alcohol intoxication, lithium, barbiturates, phenytoin, salicylates, benzodiazepines, phencyclidine, other anticonvulsants or sedatives, Wernicke encephalopathy, and thiamine deficiency.
- CNS disorders in brainstem or cerebellum: Hemorrhage, tumor, stroke, trauma, MS, and others.
- Peripheral vestibular disease: Typically worsened by head movements and positional, often accompanied by tinnitus, hearing loss. Fast phase is contralateral to pathology.
- Nonphysiologic: Voluntary, rapid, horizontal, small oscillatory movements of the eyes that usually cannot be sustained >30 seconds without fatigue.

Nystagmus With Localizing Neuroanatomic Significance

- Seesaw: One eye rises and intorts while the other descends and extorts. Lesion typically involves the parasellar region and chiasm. Typically pendular when chiasmal region involved and jerk if involving the midbrain. One proposal suggests a unilateral lesion of the interstitial nucleus of Cajal or its connections are responsible for this nystagmus subtype. May have a bitemporal hemianopsia resulting from chiasmal compression. May be congenital or associated with septo-optic dysplasia.
- Convergence retraction: Not a true nystagmus, but convergence movements accompanied by globe retraction when the patient attempts an upward saccade. May be associated with limitation of upward gaze, eyelid retraction, and bilateral mid-dilated pupils that react poorly to light but constrict better with convergence. Usually, a pineal region tumor or other dorsal midbrain abnormality is responsible. See 10.4, ADIE (TONIC) PUPIL.
- Downbeat: The fast phase of nystagmus is down and most prominent looking down and to the right and left. Most commonly, either a manifestation of cerebellar degeneration or associated with a lesion at the cervicomedullary junction (e.g., Arnold–Chiari malformation).
- Periodic alternating: In primary position, fast eye movements are in one direction for 60 to 90 seconds and then reverse direction for 60 to 90 seconds. The cycle repeats continuously. Patients may attempt to minimize nystagmus with periodic head turning. May be congenital. Acquired forms are most commonly the result of lesions of the cervicomedullary junction and posterior fossa. Other causes include MS, medication side effects, and rarely blindness.
- Gaze evoked: Absent in primary gaze, but appears as the eyes look to the side. Nystagmus increases when looking in the direction of fast phase. Slow frequency. Most commonly the result of alcohol intoxication, sedatives, and cerebellar or brainstem disease.
- Peripheral vestibular: Horizontal or horizontal-rotary nystagmus. May be accompanied by vertigo, tinnitus, or deafness. May be due to dysfunction of vestibular end organ (inner ear disease), eighth cranial nerve, or eighth cranial nerve nucleus in brainstem. Destructive lesions produce fast phases opposite to lesion. Irritative lesions (e.g., Meniere disease) produce fast phase in the same direction as the lesion. Vestibular nystagmus associated with interstitial keratitis is called Cogan syndrome.
- Spasmus nutans: See above.
- Others: Rebound nystagmus (cerebellar lesions), Bruns nystagmus (CPA), oculomasticatory myorhythmia (Whipple disease), oculopalatal myoclonus (prior brainstem stroke).

Differential Diagnosis

- Superior oblique myokymia: Small, unilateral, vertical, and torsional movements of one eye can be seen with a slit lamp or ophthalmoscope. Patients complain of unilateral oscillopsia. Symptoms and signs are more pronounced when the involved eye looks inferonasally. Usually benign, resolving spontaneously, but rarely due to a mass lesion so requires neuroimaging. Consider treating with carbamazepine.
- Opsoclonus/saccadomania: Rapid, chaotic conjugate saccades in multiple directions. Etiology in children is a paraneoplastic effect of neuroblastoma or encephalitis. In adults, in addition to paraneoplastic or infectious, it can be seen with drug intoxication or following infarction.

Workup

1. History: Nystagmus, strabismus, or amblyopia in infancy? Oscillopsia? Drug or alcohol use? Vertigo? Episodes of weakness, numbness, or decreased vision in the past? MS?
2. Family history: Nystagmus? Albinism? Eye disorder?
3. Complete ocular examination: Careful motility examination. Slit lamp or optic disc observation may be helpful in subtle cases. Iris transillumination should be performed to rule out albinism.
4. Consider an eye movement recording if diagnosis unclear.
5. Visual field examination, particularly with seesaw nystagmus.
6. Consider a drug/toxin/nutritional screen of the urine, serum, or both.
7. CT scan or MRI as needed with careful attention to appropriate area of interest.

NOTE: The cervicomedullary junction and cerebellum are best evaluated with sagittal MRI.

Treatment

1. The underlying etiology must be treated.
2. The nystagmus of periodic alternating nystagmus may respond to baclofen. Baclofen is not recommended for pediatric use. Other medications may be tried empirically for other nystagmus types.
3. Severe and disabling nystagmus can rarely be treated with retrobulbar injections of botulinum toxin.

Follow Up

Appropriate follow-up time is dictated by the condition responsible for the nystagmus.

10.22 Transient Visual Loss/Amaurosis Fugax

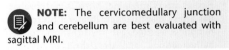

Symptoms

Monocular visual loss that usually lasts seconds to minutes, but may last up to 1 to 2 hours. Vision returns to normal.

Signs

Critical. May see an embolus within an arteriole or the ocular examination may be normal.

Other. Signs of ocular ischemic syndrome (see 11.11, OCULAR ISCHEMIC SYNDROME/CAROTID OCCLUSIVE DISEASE), an old branch retinal artery occlusion (sheathed arteriole), or neurologic signs and symptoms caused by cerebral ischemia (e.g., transient ischemic attacks [TIAs] with contralateral arm or leg weakness).

Differential Diagnosis of Transient Visual Loss

- Papilledema: Optic disc swelling is evident. Visual loss lasts seconds, is usually bilateral, and is often associated with postural change or Valsalva maneuver. See 10.15, PAPILLEDEMA.

- GCA: ESR, CRP, and platelet count typically elevated. GCA symptoms often present. Transient visual loss may precede an ischemic optic neuropathy or central retinal artery occlusion. See 10.17, ARTERITIC ISCHEMIC OPTIC NEUROPATHY (GIANT CELL ARTERITIS).

- Impending central retinal vein occlusion: Dilated, tortuous retinal veins are observed, though the fundus may be normal. See 11.8, CENTRAL RETINAL VEIN OCCLUSION.

- Migraine with aura: Visual loss/disturbance from 10 to 50 minutes, often with history of carsickness or migraine headache (personal or family). Vision loss is associated with "positive phenomena (e.g., scintillating scotoma)." See 10.27, MIGRAINE.

- Acephalgic migraine: Visual aura without migraine headache. Usually a diagnosis of exclusion. Often have recurrent episodes. See 10.27, MIGRAINE.

- Vertebrobasilar artery insufficiency: Transient, bilateral blurred vision. Associated with vertigo, dysarthria or dysphasia, perioral numbness, and hemiparesis or hemisensory loss. History of drop attacks. See 10.23, VERTEBROBASILAR ARTERY INSUFFICIENCY.

10

- Basilar artery migraine: Mimics vertebrobasilar artery insufficiency. Bilateral blurring or blindness, vertigo, gait disturbances, formed hallucinations, and dysarthria or dysphasia in a patient with migraine. See 10.23, VERTEBROBASILAR ARTERY INSUFFICIENCY and 10.27, MIGRAINE.
- Vertebral artery dissection: After trauma or resulting from atherosclerotic disease.
- Intermittent intraocular hemorrhage (e.g., vitreous hemorrhage, uveitis-glaucoma-hyphema [UGH] syndrome).
- Others: Optic nerve head drusen, intermittent angle closure, intermittent pigment dispersion.

Etiology

1. Embolus from the carotid artery (most common), heart, or aorta.
2. Vascular insufficiency as a result of arteriosclerotic disease of vessels anywhere along the path from the aorta to the globe causing hypoperfusion often precipitated by a postural change or cardiac arrhythmia.
3. Hypercoagulable/hyperviscosity state.
4. Rarely, an intraorbital mass may compress the optic nerve or a nourishing vessel in certain gaze positions, causing gaze-evoked transient visual loss.
5. Vasospasm.

Workup

1. Amaurosis fugax is considered by the American Heart Association to be a form of TIA. Current guidelines recommend MRI with diffusion weighted imaging, urgent carotid and cardiac studies, and neurology consultation. If patient is seen within days of the event, emergent referral to a stroke center or emergency room is required.
2. Immediate ESR, CRP, and platelet count when GCA is suspected.
3. History: Monocular visual loss or homonymous hemianopsia (verified by covering each eye)? Duration of visual loss? Previous episodes of transient visual loss or TIA? Cardiovascular disease risk factors? Oral contraceptive use? Smoker? Vascular surgeries?

4. Ocular examination, including a confrontation visual field examination and a dilated retinal evaluation. Look for an embolus or signs of other aforementioned disorders.
5. Medical examination: Cardiac and carotid auscultation.
6. Noninvasive carotid artery evaluation (e.g., duplex Doppler US). Consider orbital color Doppler US, if available, which may reveal a retrolaminar central retinal artery stenosis or embolus proximal to the lamina cribrosa. MRA or CTA may also be considered, but cannot evaluate flow like a duplex Doppler US.
7. CBC with differential, fasting blood sugar, hemoglobin A1c, and lipid profile (to rule out polycythemia, thrombocytosis, diabetes, and hyperlipidemia).
8. Cardiac evaluation including an echocardiogram.

Treatment

1. Carotid disease.
   - Consider aspirin 81 mg or 325 mg p.o. daily.
   - Consult vascular surgery in select patients if a surgically accessible, high-grade carotid stenosis is present for consideration of carotid endarterectomy or endovascular stent.
   - Control hypertension, diabetes, and dyslipidemia (follow up with a medical internist).
   - Lifestyle modification (e.g., smoking cessation).
2. Cardiac disease.
   - Consider aspirin 325 mg p.o. daily.
   - In presence of a thrombus, coordinate care with internal medicine and/or cardiology with likely hospitalization and anticoagulation (e.g., heparin therapy).
   - Consider referral to cardiac surgery as needed.
   - Control arteriosclerotic risk factors (follow up with medical internist).
3. If carotid and cardiac diseases are ruled out, a vasospastic etiology can be considered (extremely rare). Treatment with a calcium channel blocker may be beneficial.

10.23 Vertebrobasilar Artery Insufficiency

Symptoms

Transient, bilateral blurred vision, sometimes accompanied by flashing lights. Ataxia, vertigo, dysarthria or dysphagia, perioral numbness, and hemiparesis or hemisensory loss may accompany the visual symptoms. History of drop attacks (the patient suddenly falls to the ground without warning or loss of consciousness). Recurrent attacks are common.

Signs

May have a hemianopsia, ocular motility deficits, or nystagmus, but often presents with a normal ocular examination.

Differential Diagnosis of Transient Visual Loss

See DIFFERENTIAL DIAGNOSIS in 10.22, TRANSIENT VISUAL LOSS/AMAUROSIS FUGAX.

Workup

1. History: Associated symptoms of vertebrobasilar insufficiency? History of carsickness or migraine? Symptoms of GCA? Smoker?
2. Dilated fundus examination to rule out retinal emboli or papilledema.
3. Blood pressure in each arm to rule out subclavian steal syndrome.
4. Cardiac auscultation to rule out arrhythmia.
5. CBC to rule out anemia and polycythemia, with immediate ESR, CRP, and platelet count if GCA is considered.
6. Electrocardiography, echocardiography, and cardiac monitoring to rule out dysrhythmia.
7. Consider noninvasive carotid flow studies.
8. MRA, CTA, or transcranial/vertebral artery Doppler US to evaluate posterior cerebral blood flow.

Treatment

1. Coordinated care with internal medicine or neurology with initiation of antiplatelet and/or anticoagulation therapy.
2. Consult internist for hypertension, diabetes, and dyslipidemia control if present.
3. Lifestyle modification (e.g., smoking cessation).
4. Correct any underlying problem revealed by the workup.

Follow Up

If outpatient, 1 week to check test results. Thereafter follow-up time is dictated by identified underlying causative condition(s).

10

10.24 Cortical Blindness

Symptoms

Bilateral complete or severe loss of vision. Patients may deny they are blind (Anton syndrome) or may perceive moving targets but not stationary ones (Riddoch phenomenon).

Signs

Critical. Markedly decreased vision and visual field in both eyes (sometimes no light perception) with normal pupillary responses.

Etiology

- Most common: Bilateral occipital lobe infarctions.
- Other: Toxic, postpartum (amniotic embolus), posterior reversible encephalopathy syndromes.
- Rare: Neoplasm (e.g., metastasis, meningioma), incontinentia pigmenti.

Workup

1. Test vision at distance (patients with bilateral occipital lobe infarcts may appear completely blind, but actually have a very small residual visual field). Patients will do much worse with near-card testing than distance if only a small island remains.
2. Complete ocular and neurologic examinations.
3. MRI of the brain.
4. Rule out nonphysiologic visual loss by appropriate testing (see 10.25, NONPHYSIOLOGIC VISUAL LOSS).
5. Cardiac auscultation and electrocardiography to rule out arrhythmia.
6. Check blood pressure.
7. Consult neurologist or internist for evaluation of stroke risk factors.

Treatment

1. Patients diagnosed with a stroke within 72 hours of symptom onset are admitted to the hospital for neurologic evaluation and observation.
2. If possible, treat the underlying condition.

3. Arrange for services to help the patient optimize function at home and their surrounding environment.

Follow Up

As per the internist or neurologist.

10.25 Nonphysiologic Visual Loss

Symptoms

Loss of vision. Malingerers frequently are involved with an insurance claim or are looking for other forms of financial gain. Those with psychogenic visual loss truly believe they have lost vision.

Signs

Critical. No ocular or neuro-ophthalmic findings that would account for the decreased vision. Normal pupillary light reaction.

Differential Diagnosis

- Amblyopia: Poor vision in one eye since childhood, rarely both eyes. Patient often has strabismus or anisometropia. Vision is no worse than counting fingers, especially in the temporal periphery of an amblyopic eye. See 8.7, AMBLYOPIA.
- Cortical blindness: Bilateral complete or severe visual loss with normal pupils. See 10.24, CORTICAL BLINDNESS.
- Retrobulbar optic neuritis: Afferent pupillary defect is present. See 10.14, OPTIC NEURITIS.
- Cone–rod or cone dystrophy: Positive family history, decreased color vision, abnormal results on dark adaptation studies and multifocal ERG. See 11.29, CONE DYSTROPHIES.
- Chiasmal tumor: Visual loss may precede optic atrophy. Pupils usually react sluggishly to light, and an afferent pupillary defect is often present. Visual fields are abnormal.
- Cancer-associated retinopathy or melanoma-associated retinopathy: Immune-mediated attack of photoreceptors. Fundus often appears normal. Abnormal macular ocular coherence tomography (OCT) and ERG.

Workup

The following tests may be used to diagnose a patient with nonphysiologic visual loss (to prove the malingerer or hysteric can see better than he or she admits).

Two codes are used in the list below:

U: This test may be used in patients feigning unilateral decreased vision.

B: This test may be used in patients feigning bilateral vision loss.

Patients Claiming No Light Perception

Determine whether each pupil reacts to light (U or B): The presence of a normal pupillary reaction suggests that anterior visual pathways are intact but do *not* prove nonorganic visual loss (pupillary response is maintained in cortical blindness). When only one eye has no light perception, its pupil will not react to light. The pupil should not appear dilated unless the patient has bilateral lack of light perception or third cranial nerve involvement. If a patient responds aversely to light stimulus, one can establish some level of afferent input.

Patients Claiming Counting Fingers to No Light Perception

1. Test for an afferent pupillary defect (U): A defect should be present in unilateral or asymmetric visual loss to this degree. If not, the likelihood of nonphysiologic visual loss substantially increases.
2. Mirror test (U or B): If the patient claims unilateral visual loss, cover the better-seeing eye; with bilateral complaints leave both eyes uncovered. Ask the patient to hold eyes still and slowly tilt a large mirror from side to side in front of the eyes, holding it beyond the patient's range of hand motion vision. If the eyes move, the patient can see better than hand motion.
3. Optokinetic test (U or B): Patch the uninvolved eye when unilateral visual loss is claimed. Ask the patient to look straight ahead

and slowly move an optokinetic tape in front of the eyes (or rotate an optokinetic drum). If nystagmus can be elicited, vision is better than counting fingers. Note: Some patients can purposely minimize or suppress an ocular response by diverting focus past the drum.

4. Base-out prism test (U): Place a 4 to 6 diopter prism base-out in front of the supposedly poorly seeing eye. If there is an inward shift of the eye (or a convergent movement of the opposite eye), this indicates vision better than what the patient claims.

5. Vertical prism dissociation test (U): Hold a 4 diopter prism base-down or base-up in front of the supposedly good-seeing eye. If the patient sees two separate images (one above another), this suggests nearly symmetric vision in both eyes.

6. Worth four-dot test (U): Place red-green glasses on patient and quickly turn on four-dot pattern and ask the patient how many dots are seen. If the patient closes one eye (cheating), try reversing the glasses and repeating test. If all four dots are seen, vision is better than hand motion.

Patients Claiming 20/40 to 20/400 Vision

1. Visual acuity testing (U or B): Start with the 20/10 line and ask the patient to read it. When the patient claims inability to read it, look amazed and then offer reassurance. Inform the patient you will go to a larger line and show the 20/15 line. Again, force the patient to work to see this line. Slowly proceed up the chart, asking the patient to read each line as you pass it (including the three or four 20/20 lines). It may help to express disbelief that the patient cannot read such large letters. By the time the 20/30 or 20/40 lines are reached, the patient may in fact read one or two letters correctly. The visual acuity can then be recorded.

2. Fog test (U): Dial the patient's refractive correction into the phoropter. Add +4.00 to the normally seeing eye. Put the patient in the phoropter with both eyes open. Tell the patient to use both eyes to read each line, starting at the 20/15 line and working up the chart slowly, as described previously. Record visual acuity with both eyes open (this should be visual acuity of supposedly poorly seeing eye) and document the vision of the "good

eye" through the +4.00 lens to prove the vision obtained was from the "bad eye."

3. Retest visual acuity in the supposedly poorly seeing eye at 10 feet from the chart (U or B): Vision should be twice as good (e.g., a patient with 20/100 vision at 20 feet should read 20/50 at 10 feet). If it is better than expected, record the better vision. If the vision is worse, this suggests nonphysiologic visual loss.

4. Test near vision (U or B): If normal near vision can be documented, nonphysiologic visual loss or myopia has been documented.

5. Visual field testing (U or B): Goldmann visual field tests often reveal inconsistent responses and nonphysiologic field losses.

Children

1. Tell the child that there is an eye abnormality, but the strong drops about to be administered will cure it. Dilate the child's eyes (e.g., tropicamide 1%) and retest the visual acuity after approximately 30 minutes. Children, as well as adults, sometimes need a "way out." Provide a reward (bribe them).

2. Test as described previously.

Treatment

1. Patients are usually told that no ocular abnormality can be found that accounts for their decreased vision. In general, they should not be told that they are faking the visual loss.

2. Hysterical patients often benefit from being told that their vision can be expected to return to normal by their next visit. Psychiatric referral is sometimes indicated.

Follow Up

1. If nonphysiologic visual loss is highly suspected but cannot be proven, reexamine in 1 to 2 weeks.

2. Consider obtaining an ERG, visual-evoked response, macular OCT, or an MRI of the brain.

3. If functional visual loss can be documented, have the patient return as needed.

 NOTE: Always try to determine the patient's actual visual acuity if possible and carefully document your findings.

10.26 Headache

Most headaches are not dangerous or ominous; however, they can be symptoms of a life-threatening or vision-threatening problem. Accompanying signs and symptoms that may indicate a life-threatening or vision-threatening headache and some of the specific signs and symptoms of various headaches are listed below.

Warning Symptoms and Signs of a Serious Disorder

- Scalp tenderness, weight loss, pain with chewing, muscle pains, or malaise in patients at least 55 years of age (GCA).
- Optic nerve swelling.
- Fever.
- Altered mentation or behavior.
- Stiff neck.
- Decreased vision.
- Neurologic signs.
- Subhyaloid (preretinal) hemorrhages on fundus examination.

Suggestive Symptoms and Signs

- Onset in a previously headache-free individual.
- A different, more severe headache than the usual headache.
- A headache that is always in the same location.
- A headache that awakens the person from sleep.
- A headache that does not respond to pain medications that previously relieved it.
- Nausea and vomiting, particularly projectile vomiting.
- A headache followed by migraine-like visual symptoms (abnormal time course of events).

Etiology

Life or Vision Threatening

- GCA: Age ≥55 years. May have high ESR, CRP, and platelet count. See 10.17, ARTERITIC ISCHEMIC OPTIC NEUROPATHY (GIANT CELL ARTERITIS).
- Acute angle closure glaucoma: Decreased vision, painful eye, fixed mid-dilated pupil, and high intraocular pressure. See 9.4, ACUTE ANGLE CLOSURE GLAUCOMA.
- Ocular ischemic syndrome: Periorbital eye pain. See 11.11, OCULAR ISCHEMIC SYNDROME/CAROTID OCCLUSIVE DISEASE.
- Malignant hypertension: Marked increase of blood pressure, often accompanied by retinal cotton–wool spots, hemorrhages, and, when severe, optic nerve swelling. See 11.10, HYPERTENSIVE RETINOPATHY.
- Increased intracranial pressure: May have papilledema and/or a sixth cranial nerve palsy. Headaches usually worse in the morning and with Valsalva. See 10.15, PAPILLEDEMA.
- Infectious CNS disorder (meningitis or brain abscess): Fever, stiff neck, mental status changes, photophobia, and neurologic signs.
- Structural abnormality of the brain (e.g., tumor, aneurysm, arteriovenous malformation): Mental status change, signs of increased intracranial pressure, or neurologic signs during, and often after, the headache episode.
- Subarachnoid hemorrhage: Extremely severe headache, stiff neck, mental status change; rarely, subhyaloid hemorrhages seen on fundus examination, usually from a ruptured aneurysm.
- Epidural or subdural hematoma: Follows head trauma; altered level of consciousness; may produce anisocoria or cranial neuropathy.

Others

- Migraine (see 10.27, MIGRAINE).
- Cluster headache (see 10.28, CLUSTER HEADACHE).
- Tension headache.
- Varicella zoster virus: Headache or pain may precede the herpetic vesicles (see 4.16, HERPES ZOSTER OPHTHALMICUS/VARICELLA ZOSTER VIRUS).
- Sinus disease.

NOTE: A "sinus" headache may be a serious headache in diabetic patients and immunocompromised hosts given the possibility of zygomycosis infection (e.g., mucormycosis).

- Tolosa–Hunt syndrome.
- Cervical spine disease.
- Temporomandibular joint syndrome.
- Dental disease.
- Trigeminal neuralgia (tic douloureux).
- Anterior uveitis: See 12.1, ANTERIOR UVEITIS (IRITIS/IRIDOCYCLITIS).
- Status post LP.
- Paget disease.
- Depression/psychogenic.
- Convergence insufficiency: See 13.4, CONVERGENCE INSUFFICIENCY.
- Accommodative spasm: See 13.5, ACCOMMODATIVE SPASM.

Workup

1. History: Location, intensity, frequency, possible precipitating factors, and timing? Determine age of onset, exacerbating/relieving factors, and whether there are any associated signs or symptoms. Specifically ask about concerning symptoms and signs listed above. Also ask about trauma, medications including birth-control pills, personal or family history of migraine, and motion sickness or cyclic vomiting as a child?

2. Complete ocular examination, including pupillary, motility, and visual field evaluation; intraocular pressure measurement, optic disc and venous pulsation assessment, and a dilated retinal examination. Manifest and cycloplegic refractions may be helpful.

NOTE: The presence of SVPs classically indicates a normal intracranial pressure. However, about 20% of normal individuals do not have SVPs and thus their absence has little significance.

3. Neurologic examination (check neck flexibility and other meningeal signs).
4. Palpate the temporal arteries for tenderness, swelling, and hardness. Ask specifically about fever, jaw claudication, scalp tenderness, temporal headaches, and unexpected weight loss. Immediate ESR, CRP, and platelet count when GCA is suspected (see 10.17, ARTERITIC ISCHEMIC OPTIC NEUROPATHY [GIANT CELL ARTERITIS]).
5. Temperature and blood pressure.
6. Refer the patient to a neurologist, neurosurgeon, otolaryngologist, or internist, as indicated.

Treatment/Follow Up

See individual sections.

10.27 | Migraine

Symptoms

Typically unilateral (although it may occur behind both eyes or across the entire front of the head), throbbing or boring head pain accompanied at times by nausea, vomiting, mood changes, fatigue, photophobia, or phonophobia. An aura with visual disturbances, including flashing (zig-zagging or kaleidoscopic) lights, blurred vision, or a visual field defect lasting 15 to 50 minutes, may precede the migraine. May experience temporary or rarely permanent neurologic deficits, such as paralysis, numbness, tingling, or others. A family history is common. Motion sickness or cyclic vomiting as a child is also common. Migraine in children may be seen as recurrent abdominal pain and malaise. Of these patients, 60% to 70% are girls.

Migraine prevalence is highest between ages 30 and 39 years and progressively declines after age 40. Migraine attacks may be shorter and less typical with advancing age. New-onset migraines are uncommon after the age of 50, and these patients should be worked up for secondary causes such as vascular lesions, intracranial hemorrhages, infarcts, masses, or GCA.

NOTE: Most unilateral migraine headaches at some point change sides of the head. Headaches always on the same side of the head may have another cause of headache (e.g., intracranial structural lesions).

Determine if headache precedes visual symptoms, which is more common with arteriovenous malformations, mass lesions with cerebral edema, or seizure foci.

10

Signs

Usually none. Complicated migraines may have a permanent neurologic or ocular deficit (see the following discussion).

Differential Diagnosis

See 10.26, HEADACHE.

International Classification

Consult International Classification of Headache Disorders, 3rd edition, for further information.

- Migraine without aura (common migraine; 80%): Lasts 4 to 72 hours. Unilateral location, pulsating quality, moderate-to-severe pain, and/or aggravation by physical activity. Nausea, vomiting, photophobia, and/or phonophobia are the characteristics.
- Migraine with typical aura (classic migraine; 10%): Fully reversible binocular visual symptoms that may be perceived as monocular (e.g., flickering lights, spots, lines, loss of vision) or fully reversible unilateral sensory symptoms (e.g., numbness, "pins and needles"). Symptoms gradually develop over 5 minutes and last between 5 and 60 minutes. No motor symptoms are present.
- Typical aura without headache (acephalgic migraine): Visual or sensory symptoms as above without accompanying or subsequent headache.
- Familial hemiplegic and sporadic hemiplegic migraine: Migraine with aura as above with accompanying motor weakness with (familial) or without (sporadic) history in a first-degree or second-degree relative. Sporadic cases always require neuroimaging.
- Retinal migraine: Fully reversible monocular visual phenomenon (e.g., scintillations, scotoma, blindness) accompanied by headache fulfilling migraine definition. Appropriate investigations to exclude other causes of transient monocular blindness should be completed. Existence of retinal migraine is controversial.
- Basilar-type migraine: Aura symptoms mimic vertebrobasilar artery insufficiency in a patient with migraine. See 10.23, VERTEBROBASILAR ARTERY INSUFFICIENCY.
- Ophthalmoplegic migraine: Onset in childhood. Headache with third cranial nerve palsy.

Likely an inflammation, rather than migraine, as MRI shows enhancement of CNIII.

Associations or Precipitating Factors

Birth control or other hormonal pills, puberty, pregnancy, menopause, foods containing tyramine or phenylalanine (e.g., aged cheeses, wines, chocolate, cashew nuts), nitrates or nitrites, monosodium glutamate, alcohol, aspartame, caffeine withdrawal, weather changes, fatigue, emotional stress, or bright lights.

Workup

See 10.26, HEADACHE, for a general headache workup.

1. History: May establish the diagnosis.
2. Ocular and neurologic examinations, including refraction.
3. CT scan or MRI of the head is indicated for:
   - Atypical migraines: New onset migraines in patients over 50 years old. Migraines that are always on the same side of the head or those with an unusual sequence such as visual disturbances persisting into or occurring after the headache phase.
   - Complicated migraines.
4. Consider checking for uncontrolled blood pressure or low blood sugar (hypoglycemic headaches are almost always precipitated by stress or fatigue).

Treatment

1. Avoid agents that precipitate the headaches (e.g., stop using birth control pills; avoid alcohol and any foods that may precipitate attacks; reduce stress).
2. Referral to neurologist or internist for pharmacologic management.
   a. Abortive therapy: Medications used at onset of the headache. Best for infrequent headaches.
      i. Initial therapy: Aspirin or nonsteroidal anti-inflammatory agents.
      ii. More potent therapy (when initial therapy fails): Ergotamines or selective serotonin receptor agonists (triptans). More recently FDA-approved medications include rimegepant and ubrogepant (calcitonin gene–related peptide

[CGRP] antagonists) and lasmiditan (selective serotonin agonist without vasoconstrictor activity). Check contraindications for specific agents.

 NOTE: Opioid drugs should be avoided.

b. Prophylactic therapy: Used in patients with frequent or severe headache attacks (e.g., two or more headaches per month)

or those with neurologic changes. Includes beta-blockers, calcium channel blockers, antidepressants, anti-CGRP monoclonal antibodies, and others.

c. Antinausea medication as needed during an acute episode.

Follow Up

Reevaluate in 4 to 6 weeks to assess the efficacy of the therapy.

10.28 Cluster Headache

Symptoms

Typically unilateral, very painful (stabbing), periorbital, frontal, or temporal headache associated with ipsilateral tearing, rhinorrhea, sweating, nasal stuffiness, and/or a droopy eyelid. Usually lasts for minutes to hours. Typically recurs once or twice daily for several weeks, followed by a headache-free interval of months to years. The cycle may repeat. Predominantly affects men. Headache awakens patients, whereas migraine does not.

Signs

Ipsilateral conjunctival injection, facial flush, or Horner syndrome (third-order neuron etiology) may be present. Ptosis may become permanent.

Precipitating Factors

Alcohol, nitroglycerin.

Differential Diagnosis

- Migraine headache: Typically unilateral headache possibly associated with visual and neurologic symptoms. See 10.27, MIGRAINE.
- Chronic paroxysmal hemicrania: Several attacks of pain and cranial autonomic features (e.g., tearing, ocular injection, rhinorrhea) occurring throughout the day and typically lasting no more than 30 minutes. Patients have dramatic improvement with indomethacin.
- Idiopathic stabbing "ice pick" headache: Episodic, momentary sharp pain, or stabbing sensations lasting less than a second that may occur in patients with preexisting migraine or cluster headache history. Lack the classic autonomic features of cluster headaches.

- Short-lasting unilateral neuralgiform headache attacks with conjunctival injection and tearing: A trigeminal autonomic cephalgia that presents with burning or stabbing pain felt unilaterally, primarily around the eye. Pain lasts for seconds to minutes and may occur >100 times per day. May have tearing, ptosis, eyelid edema, and conjunctival injection. Episodes last days to months and often recur. Distinguish from cluster headaches due to shorter duration, increased frequency, and more prominent autonomic findings.
- Others: See 10.26, HEADACHE.

Workup

1. History and complete ocular examination.
2. Neurologic examination, particularly a cranial nerve evaluation.
3. If Horner syndrome present, consider imaging studies to eliminate other causes. See 10.2, HORNER SYNDROME.
4. Obtain an MRI of the brain when the history is atypical or a neurologic abnormality is present.

Treatment

1. Avoid alcoholic beverages or cigarette smoking during a cluster cycle.
2. Refer patient to neurologist to help coordinate pharmacologic therapy.
3. Abortive therapy for acute attack:
   - Oxygen, 5 to 8 L/min by face mask for 10 minutes at onset of attack. Relieves pain in 70% of adults.

10

- Sumatriptan used subcutaneously (6 mg) or intranasally (20 mg) is often effective in relieving pain.
- Zolmitriptan 5 or 10 mg intranasally also appears to be effective.
- Less frequent medications used include ergotamine inhalation, dihydroergotamine, or corticosteroids.

4. When headaches are moderate to severe and are unrelieved by nonprescription medication, one of the following drugs may be an effective prophylactic agent during cluster periods:

- Calcium channel blockers (e.g., verapamil 360 to 480 mg/day p.o. in divided doses).
- Lithium 600 to 900 mg p.o. daily is administered in conjunction with the patient's medical doctor. Baseline renal (blood urea nitrogen, creatinine, urine electrolytes) and thyroid function tests (triiodothyronine, thyroxine, TSH) are obtained. Lithium intoxication may occur in patients using indomethacin, tetracycline, or methyldopa.
- Ergotamine 1 to 2 mg p.o. daily.
- Methysergide 2 mg p.o. b.i.d. with meals. Do not use for longer than 3 to 4 months because of the significant risk of retroperitoneal fibrosis. Methysergide is not recommended in patients with coronary artery or peripheral vascular disease, thrombophlebitis, hypertension, pregnancy, or hepatic or renal disease.
- Oral steroids (e.g., prednisone 40 to 80 mg p.o. for 1 week, tapering rapidly over an additional week if possible) and an antiulcer agent (e.g., omeprazole 20 mg p.o. daily or ranitidine 150 mg p.o. b.i.d.).
- Galcanezumab is a monoclonal antibody to CGRP, which received FDA approval for prevention of cluster headaches and migraines.

5. If necessary, an acute, severe attack can be treated with i.v. diazepam.

Follow Up

1. Patients started on systemic steroids are seen within a few days and then every several weeks to evaluate the effects of treatment and monitor intraocular pressure.

2. Patients taking methysergide or lithium are reevaluated in 7 to 10 days. Plasma lithium levels are monitored in patients taking this agent.

10

Chapter 11

Retina

11.1 | Posterior Vitreous Detachment

Symptoms

Floaters, blurred vision, and/or flashes of light which are more common in dim illumination or with eye movement. Symptoms usually present acutely and progress over hours to days.

Signs

Critical. One or more discrete near-translucent or light gray vitreous opacities, one often in the shape of a ring ("Weiss ring") or broken ring, suspended over the optic disc (see Figure 11.1.1).

Other. Retinal break/tear (RT), retinal detachment (RD), or vitreous hemorrhage (VH) may occur with or without a posterior vitreous detachment (PVD), with similar symptoms. Peripheral retinal and disc margin hemorrhages, released retinal pigment epithelial cells in the anterior vitreous ("tobacco dust" or Shafer sign).

> **NOTE:** Approximately 8% to 26% of all patients with acute symptomatic PVD have a retinal break. The presence of pigmented cells in the anterior vitreous or VH in association with an acute PVD indicates a high probability (>70%) of a coexisting retinal break. See 11.2, RETINAL BREAK.

Differential Diagnosis

- Uveitis: In vitritis, vitreous cells may be found in both the posterior and anterior vitreous, the condition may be bilateral, and the cells are not typically pigmented. Many uveitides, particularly white dot syndromes, will also present with floaters and photopsias. See 12.3, POSTERIOR UVEITIS.
- Migraine: Multicolored photopsias in a zig-zag pattern that obstructs vision lasts approximately 20 minutes. A headache may or may not follow, and symptoms may be bilateral. Normal fundus examination. See 10.27, MIGRAINE.

Workup

1. History: Duration of symptoms? Distinguish retinal photopsias from the visual distortion of migraine, which may be accompanied by new floaters. Location of photopsias does not correlate with location of retinal break(s), if present. Risk factors for retinal break (trauma, previous intraocular surgery, yttrium aluminum garnet [YAG] laser capsulotomy, high myopia, personal or family history of RT/RD)?

2. Complete ocular examination, including evaluation of the anterior vitreous for pigmented cells and a dilated fundus examination with indirect ophthalmoscopy and scleral depression to rule out a retinal break and detachment. Optical coherence tomography (OCT) can be helpful in confirming the presence or absence of a PVD. Hyperreflective dots in the vitreous ("falling ash sign"), when present,

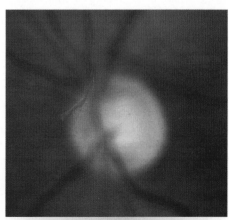

Figure 11.1.1 Posterior vitreous detachment.

have a high correlation with peripheral retinal breaks. Pseudophakic patients may have smaller anterior breaks compared to phakic patients. Examine the fellow eye to assess for presence of PVD and peripheral retinal pathology.

3. Visualize the PVD at the slit lamp with a 60- or 90-diopter lens by identifying a gray-to-black strand suspended in the vitreous. If not visible, have the patient make rapid saccades and then look straight to float the PVD into view.

4. If VH obscures visualization of the retina, ultrasonography (US) is indicated to identify the PVD and rule out a retinal break, RD, or other causes of vitreous hemorrhage. Inferior layering vitreous hemorrhage may mimic a retinal break on US. See 11.13, VITREOUS HEMORRHAGE.

Treatment

No treatment is indicated for PVD unless an acute retinal break or dense vitreous hemorrhage is found; see 11.2, RETINAL BREAK.

> **NOTE:** In the setting of acute PVD symptoms, chronic retinal breaks (pigmented) or lattice degeneration usually warrant treatment.

Follow Up

- The patient should be given a list of RD symptoms (a significant increase in floaters or flashing lights, worsening vision, or the appearance of a persistent curtain or shadow anywhere in the field of vision) and told to return immediately if these symptoms develop. The timing of symptoms could be anywhere from days to years later.

- Patients should be informed that they will also likely develop a PVD in their fellow eye, if not already present.

- If no retinal break or hemorrhage is found, the patient should be scheduled for repeat examination with scleral depression in 4 to 6 weeks. There is a 2% to 5% risk of developing new retinal breaks in patients with PVD and no retinal break at presentation.

- If no retinal break is found, but mild VH or peripheral punctate retinal hemorrhages are present (indicating increased vitreous traction), repeat examinations are performed in 2 weeks.

- If no retinal break is found but significant VH or anterior pigmented vitreous cells are present, repeat examination should be performed within 24 hours by a retina specialist because of the high likelihood of a retinal break.

11.2 Retinal Break (Tear)

Symptoms

Acute retinal break: Flashes of light, floaters ("cobwebs," "hair," or "film" that changes position with eye movement) with or without visual acuity changes. Can be identical to PVD symptoms, though may be more profound.

Chronic retinal breaks or atrophic retinal holes: Usually asymptomatic.

Signs

(See Figure 11.2.1.)

Critical. A full-thickness retinal defect, usually seen in the periphery.

Other. Acute retinal break: Pigmented cells in the anterior vitreous, VH, PVD, retinal flap, subretinal fluid (SRF), or an operculum (a free-floating piece of retina suspended above a RT).

Chronic retinal break: Surrounding pigmentation ring or demarcation line between attached and detached retina and signs (but not necessarily symptoms) of an acute retinal break.

Predisposing Conditions

Lattice degeneration, high myopia, aphakia, pseudophakia, age-related retinoschisis, vitreoretinal tufts, meridional folds, history of previous retinal break or detachment in the fellow eye, family history of retinal break or detachment, collagen vascular disorders, and trauma.

Differential Diagnosis

- Lattice degeneration.
- White without pressure: Abrupt changes in retinal pigmentation that may mimic a break or subretinal fluid. Benign findings, etiology unclear.

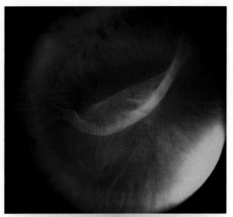

Figure 11.2.1 Giant retinal tear.

- Choroidal rupture or retinal hemorrhage (all layers): May occur without retinal break or obscure retinal break.
- Meridional fold: Small radial fold of retina perpendicular to the ora serrata and overlying an oral tooth; may have small retinal hole at the base.
- Vitreoretinal tuft: Focal area of vitreous traction causing elevation of the retina.

Workup

Complete ocular examination with a slit lamp and indirect ophthalmoscopy of both eyes with scleral depression. After trauma, scleral depression may be gently performed once open globe injury has been ruled out. B-scan US may be helpful when the retina is not visible (e.g., vitreous hemorrhage, dense cataract, etc.)

Treatment

In general, laser therapy or cryotherapy is required within 24 hours for acute retinal breaks. Treatment may be less urgent for chronic breaks. However, each case must be individualized based on patient risk factors. We follow these general guidelines:

1. Treatment recommended:
   - Acute symptomatic break (e.g., a horseshoe or operculated tear).
   - Acute traumatic break (including a dialysis).
   - Acute symptoms and presence of lattice degeneration.
2. Treatment to be considered:
   - Asymptomatic retinal break that is large (e.g., ≥1.5 mm), above the horizontal meridian, or both, particularly in the absence of PVD.
   - Asymptomatic retinal break in an aphakic or pseudophakic eye, a highly myopic eye, or an eye in which the involved or contralateral eye has had an RD.

Follow Up

1. Patients with predisposing conditions or retinal breaks that do not require treatment are followed at 3 months and then every 6 to 12 months if stable.
2. Patients treated for a retinal break are reexamined in 2 weeks, 6 weeks, 3 months, and then every 6 to 12 months.
3. RD symptoms (a dramatic increase in floaters or flashing lights, worsening visual acuity, or the appearance of a curtain, shadow, or bubble anywhere in the field of vision) are explained and patients are told to return immediately if these symptoms develop.

11

11.3 Retinal Detachment

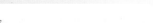

There are three distinct types of RD.

RHEGMATOGENOUS RETINAL DETACHMENT

Symptoms

Flashes of light, floaters, a curtain or shadow moving over the field of vision, peripheral or central visual loss, or both.

Signs

(See Figures 11.3.1 to 11.3.3.)

Critical. Elevation of the retina from the retinal pigment epithelium (RPE) by fluid in the subretinal space due to an accompanying full-thickness retinal break or breaks. See 11.2, RETINAL BREAK.

Other. Anterior vitreous pigmented cells; VH; PVD; may have low (due to increased fluid

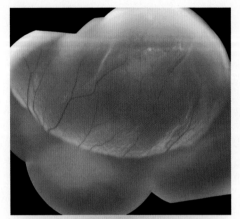

Figure 11.3.1 Rhegmatogenous retinal detachment.

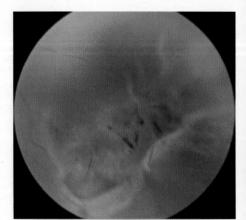

Figure 11.3.2 Retinal detachment with retinal break in lattice degeneration.

pumping through the RPE), high (Schwartz–Matsuo syndrome, released photoreceptors clogging trabecular meshwork), or normal intraocular pressure (IOP) in the affected eye. SRF is clear and does not shift with gravity. The detached retina is often corrugated and partially opaque in appearance. A mild relative afferent pupillary defect (RAPD) may be present in large RDs.

NOTE: A chronic rhegmatogenous retinal detachment (RRD) often shows a pigmented demarcation line at the posterior extent of the RD, intraretinal cysts, fixed folds, and/or subretinal precipitates or a combination of these with a relative visual field defect. It should be differentiated from retinoschisis, which is typically smooth and dome-shaped, translucent, and produces an absolute visual field defect. Underlying choroidal vasculature appears normal (unlike RRD, where it is obscured).

Etiology

A retinal break allows fluid to move through the hole and separate the overlying retina from the RPE.

Workup

1. Slit lamp examination to assess for signs of uveitis, lens status, presence of vitreous pigment/hemorrhage, and PVD.
2. Indirect ophthalmoscopy with scleral depression of both eyes. Slit lamp examination of the periphery with a 90-diopter or widefield lens may help in finding small breaks.
3. B-scan US may be helpful if media opacities are present.

EXUDATIVE/SEROUS RETINAL DETACHMENT

Symptoms

Visual field defect with varying degrees of vision loss; visual changes may vary with changes in head position.

Signs

(See Figure 11.3.4.)

Critical. Serous elevation of the retina with shifting SRF with patient positioning. While sitting, the SRF accumulates inferiorly, detaching the inferior retina; while in the supine position, the fluid accumulates in the posterior pole, detaching the macula. There is no retinal break; fluid accumulation is due to breakdown of the normal blood–retinal barrier. The detachment typically does not extend to the ora serrata.

Other. The detached retina is smooth and may become quite bullous. A mild RAPD may be present in large RDs.

Etiology

- Neoplastic: Choroidal malignant melanoma, metastasis, choroidal hemangioma, multiple myeloma, retinal capillary hemangioblastoma, etc.

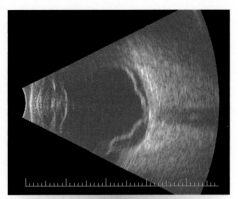

Figure 11.3.3 B-scan ultrasonography of retinal detachment.

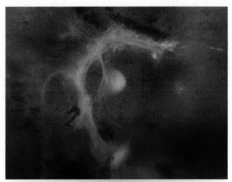

Figure 11.3.5 Tractional retinal detachment.

in patients with high hyperopia, particularly nanophthalmic eyes.

Workup

1. Intravenous fluorescein angiography (IVFA) may demonstrate leakage or pooling and identify the SRF source.
2. OCT may help identify the source of SRF (e.g., CNV).
3. B-scan US may help delineate the underlying cause.
4. Systemic workup to rule out the above causes.

TRACTIONAL RETINAL DETACHMENT

Symptoms

Visual loss or visual field defect; may be asymptomatic.

Signs

(See Figure 11.3.5.)

Critical. A traction retinal detachment (TRD) appears concave with a smooth surface; cellular and vitreous membranes exerting traction on the retina are present; retinal striae extending from these areas may also be seen. Detachment may become a convex RRD if a tractional RT develops (combined RRD/TRD).

Other. The retina is immobile, and the detachment rarely extends to the ora serrata. A mild RAPD may be present in large RDs.

Etiology

Fibrocellular bands in the vitreous (e.g., resulting from proliferative diabetic retinopathy [PDR],

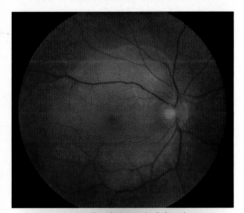

Figure 11.3.4 Exudative retinal detachment.

- Inflammatory disease: Vogt–Koyanagi–Harada syndrome, posterior scleritis, sympathetic ophthalmia, other chronic inflammatory processes.
- Congenital abnormalities: Optic pit, morning glory syndrome, and choroidal coloboma (although these may have an associated retinal break).
- Vascular: Choroidal neovascularization (CNV), Coats disease, malignant hypertension (HTN), preeclampsia, and familial exudative vitreoretinopathy (FEVR). See specific sections.
- Idiopathic central serous chorioretinopathy (CSCR): May rarely present with bullous RD. See 11.15, CENTRAL SEROUS CHORIORETINOPATHY.
- Uveal effusion syndrome: Bilateral detachments of the peripheral choroid, ciliary body, and retina; leopard-spot RPE changes; vitreous cells; dilated episcleral vessels. More common

11

sickle cell retinopathy, retinopathy of prematurity, FEVR, toxocariasis, trauma, proliferative vitreoretinopathy) contract and detach the retina.

Workup

1. Slit lamp examination to assess lens status, sequelae of retinal vascular disease (e.g., neovascularization of the iris), and PVD.
2. Indirect ophthalmoscopy with scleral depression of both eyes. Slit lamp examination of the periphery with a 90-diopter or widefield lens may help in finding small breaks.
3. B-scan US may be helpful if media opacities are present.
4. OCT is useful in identifying tractional membranes and can be useful in differentiating tractional membranes from detached retina.

Differential Diagnosis for All Three Types of Retinal Detachment

- Acquired/age-related degenerative retinoschisis: Commonly bilateral, smooth, bullous, usually inferotemporal. No pigmented cells or hemorrhage are present in the vitreous. Inner or outer retinal holes may be present. See 11.4, RETINOSCHISIS.
- X-linked retinoschisis: Petaloid foveal changes are present over 90% of the time. Dehiscence occurs in the nerve fiber layer (NFL) 50% of the time. See 11.4, RETINOSCHISIS.
- Choroidal detachment: Serous choroidal detachment: Orange-brown, more solid in appearance than an RD, often extends 360 degrees. Often secondary to hypotony

or inflammation. See 11.27, CHOROIDAL EFFUSION/DETACHMENT.

Treatment

1. Patients with an acute RRD that threatens the macula should have surgical repair performed urgently. The visual prognosis is significantly worse in detachments that progress to involve the macula. Surgical options include laser photocoagulation, cryotherapy, pneumatic retinopexy, vitrectomy, and/or scleral buckle.
2. RRDs that are macula-off should be repaired, but are not necessarily urgent. Multiple studies suggest that visual outcomes for macula-off detachments do not change if surgery is performed within 7 to 10 days of the onset.
3. Chronic macula-off RDs are treated within 1 week if possible.
4. TRDs may or may not require intervention depending on etiology, status of the fellow eye, and the extent/location of retinal traction.
5. For exudative RDs, successful treatment of the underlying condition often leads to resolution of the detachment.

Follow Up

All patients with RRD require urgent follow up with a retina specialist. After surgery, these patients are typically followed at 1 day, 1 week, 1 month, 2 to 3 months, and then every 6 to 12 months. Follow up for serous RD and TRD depends on underlying etiology and individual patient factors.

11.4 Retinoschisis

Retinoschisis, a splitting of the retina, occurs in X-linked (juvenile) and age-related (degenerative) forms.

X-LINKED (JUVENILE) RETINOSCHISIS

Symptoms

Decreased vision due to macular involvement. Sometimes VH. Can be asymptomatic. The condition is congenital but may not be detected at birth if an examination is not performed. A family history may or may not be elicited (X-linked recessive).

Signs

Critical. Foveal schisis seen as stellate maculopathy: Cystoid foveal changes with retinal folds that radiate from the center of the fovea (petaloid pattern). Unlike the cysts of cystoid macular edema (CME), they do not stain or leak on IVFA, but can be seen with indocyanine green angiography (ICGA) and on OCT. The macular appearance changes in adulthood and the petaloid pattern may disappear.

Other. Classically taught as separation of the NFL from the outer retinal layers in the retinal periphery (bilaterally in the inferotemporal quadrant, most commonly) with the development of NFL breaks; this peripheral retinoschisis occurs in 50% of patients. However, schisis may occur between any two retinal layers, and recent evidence suggests that the outer plexiform layer is frequently separated in X-linked forms. RD, VH, and pigmentary changes may also occur. Pigmented demarcation lines may be seen (indicating previous RD) even in the absence of active detachment, unlike acquired age-related degenerative retinoschisis.

Differential Diagnosis

- Age-related (degenerative) retinoschisis. See Age-Related (Degenerative) Retinoschisis.
- RRD: Usually unilateral, acquired, and associated with a RT. Pigment in the anterior vitreous is seen. See 11.3, RETINAL DETACHMENT.

Workup

1. Family history.
2. Dilated retinal examination with scleral depression to rule out retinal break or detachment.
3. OCT can help determine the layer of schisis and help to differentiate schisis from an RD.
4. IVFA will show no leakage.
5. Fundus autofluorescence (FAF) may help delineate areas of schisis.
6. Electroretinography (ERG) is not necessary for diagnosis but can show a reduced b-wave with a preserved a-wave.

Treatment

1. No definitive treatment for stellate maculopathy. Topical carbonic anhydrase inhibitors have been shown to decrease foveal thickness and improve visual acuity in some patients.
2. For nonclearing VH, consider vitrectomy.
3. Surgical repair of an RD should be performed.
4. Superimposed amblyopia may be present in children younger than 11 years of age when one eye is more severely affected, and a trial of patching should be considered. See 8.7, AMBLYOPIA.

Follow Up

Every 6 months; more frequently if treating amblyopia.

AGE-RELATED (DEGENERATIVE) RETINOSCHISIS

Symptoms

Usually asymptomatic; may have decreased vision.

Signs

(See Figure 11.4.1.)

Critical. The schisis cavity is dome-shaped with a smooth surface and is usually located temporally, typically inferotemporally. The findings are usually bilateral and may show sheathing of retinal vessels and "snowflakes" or "frosting" (persistent Mueller fibers) on the elevated inner wall of the schisis cavity. Splitting usually occurs at the level of the outer plexiform layer. The area of schisis is not mobile and there is no associated RPE pigmentation in contrast to an RD, which may have corrugations and a pigmented demarcation line.

Other. Prominent cystoid degeneration near the ora serrata, an absolute scotoma corresponding to the area of schisis, hyperopia is common, no pigment cells or hemorrhage in the vitreous, and absence of a demarcation line. An RRD may occasionally develop.

Differential Diagnosis

- RRD: Surface is corrugated in appearance and moves more with eye movements. A long-standing RD may resemble retinoschisis, but intraretinal cysts, demarcation lines between attached and detached retina, and

11

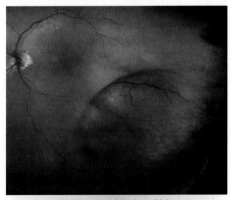

Figure 11.4.1 Retinoschisis.

white subretinal dots may be seen. Only a relative scotoma is present. See 11.3, RETINAL DETACHMENT.

- X-linked juvenile retinoschisis (see above).

Workup

1. Slit lamp evaluation for anterior chamber inflammation and pigmented anterior vitreous cells; neither should be present in isolated retinoschisis.
2. Dilated retinal examination with scleral depression to rule out a concomitant RD or an outer layer retinal hole, which may lead to an RD.
3. A slit lamp examination using a 90-diopter lens or fundus contact lens as needed to aid in recognizing outer layer retinal breaks.
4. OCT can help determine which layer of the retina is split.

5. Visual field testing will reveal an absolute scotoma in the area of schisis.

Treatment

1. Surgery is indicated when a clinically significant RD develops.
2. A small RD walled off by a demarcation line is usually not treated. This may take the form of pigmentation at the posterior border of outer layer breaks.

Follow Up

Every 6 months. RD symptoms (an increase in floaters or flashing lights, blurry vision, or the appearance of a curtain or shadow anywhere in the field of vision) are explained to all patients, and patients are told to return immediately if these symptoms develop.

11.5 Cotton–Wool Spot

Symptoms

Visual acuity usually normal. Often asymptomatic.

Signs

(See Figure 11.5.1.)

Critical. Localized whitening in the superficial retinal NFL with fluffy appearance to margins

NOTE: The presence of even a single cotton–wool spot (CWS) is not normal. In a patient without diabetes mellitus, acute changes in blood pressure (most commonly hypertension), or a retinal vein occlusion, a workup for an underlying systemic condition should be performed.

Differential Diagnosis

- Retinal whitening secondary to infectious retinitis, such as that seen in toxoplasmosis, herpes simplex virus, varicella zoster virus, and cytomegalovirus. These entities typically have vitritis and retinal hemorrhages associated with them. See 12.5, TOXOPLASMOSIS and 12.8, ACUTE RETINAL NECROSIS (ARN).
- Myelinated NFL: Develops postnatally. Usually peripapillary but may be in retinal areas remote from the disc **(see Figure 11.5.2)**.

Etiology

Thought to be an acute obstruction of a precapillary retinal arteriole causing blockage of axoplasmic flow and subsequent buildup of axoplasmic debris in the NFL.

- Diabetes mellitus: Most common cause. Often associated with microaneurysms, dot-blot hemorrhages, and hard exudates. See 11.12, DIABETIC RETINOPATHY.
- Chronic or acute HTN: May see retinal arteriolar narrowing and flame hemorrhages in

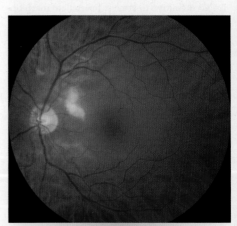

Figure 11.5.1 Cotton–wool spot.

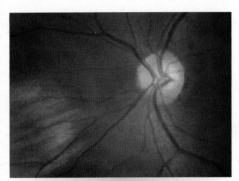

Figure 11.5.2 Myelinated nerve fiber layer.

chronic HTN. Acute HTN may have hard exudates, optic nerve swelling, exudative RD. See 11.10, HYPERTENSIVE RETINOPATHY.

• Retinal vein occlusion: Unilateral, multiple hemorrhages, venous dilation, and tortuosity. Multiple CWSs, usually ≥6, seen in ischemic varieties. See 11.8, CENTRAL RETINAL VEIN OCCLUSION and 11.9, BRANCH RETINAL VEIN OCCLUSION.

• Retinal emboli: Often from carotid arteries or heart with resulting ischemia and subsequent CWS distal to arterial occlusion. Patients require carotid Doppler examination and echocardiography. See 10.22, TRANSIENT VISUAL LOSS/AMAUROSIS FUGAX.

• Collagen vascular disease: Systemic lupus erythematosus (most common), granulomatosis with polyangiitis (formerly Wegener granulomatosis), polyarteritis nodosa, scleroderma, etc.

• Giant cell arteritis (GCA): Age ≥55 years. Symptoms include vision loss, scalp tenderness, jaw claudication, proximal muscle aches, etc. See 10.17, ARTERITIC ISCHEMIC OPTIC NEUROPATHY (GIANT CELL ARTERITIS).

• HIV retinopathy: Single or multiple CWSs in the posterior pole. See 12.10, NONINFECTIOUS RETINAL MICROVASCULOPATHY/HIV RETINOPATHY.

• Other infections: Toxoplasmosis, orbital zygomycosis, Lyme disease, leptospirosis, Rocky Mountain spotted fever, onchocerciasis, subacute bacterial endocarditis, others.

• Hypercoagulable state: Polycythemia, multiple myeloma, cryoglobulinemia, Waldenström macroglobulinemia, antiphospholipid syndrome, factor V Leiden, activated protein C resistance, hyperhomocysteinemia, protein C

and S deficiency, antithrombin III mutation, prothrombin mutation, etc.

• Radiation retinopathy: Follows radiation therapy to the eye or periocular structures when the eye is irradiated inadvertently. May occur any time after radiation, but occurs most commonly within a few years. Maintain a high suspicion even in patients in whom the eye was reportedly shielded. Usually, 3,000 cGy is necessary, but it has been noted to occur with 1,500 cGy. Resembles diabetic retinopathy.

• Interferon therapy.

• Purtscher and pseudo-Purtscher retinopathy: Multiple CWSs and/or superficial hemorrhages in a peripapillary configuration. Typically bilateral but can be unilateral and asymmetric. See 3.20, PURTSCHER RETINOPATHY.

• Cancer: Metastatic carcinoma, leukemia, lymphoma, others.

• Others: Migraine, hypotension, intravenous drug use, papilledema, papillitis, severe anemia, sickle cell, acute blood loss, etc.

Workup

1. History: Diabetes or HTN? Prior ocular or periocular radiation? GCA symptoms in appropriate age group? Symptoms of collagen vascular disease including joint pain, rashes, etc.? HIV risk factors? Hematologic abnormalities?

2. Complete ocular examination, including dilated retinal examination with a slit lamp and a 60- or 90-diopter lens and indirect ophthalmoscopy. Look for concurrent hemorrhages, vascular occlusion, vasculitis, hard exudates.

3. Check blood pressure.

4. Check fasting blood sugar and hemoglobin A1c.

5. Consider erythrocyte sedimentation rate (ESR), C-reactive protein (CRP), and platelets if GCA suspected.

6. Consider blood and urine cultures, chest x-ray, carotid and orbital Doppler examination, chest computed tomography (CT), and echocardiography if emboli are suspected.

7. Consider HIV testing.

8. Fluorescein angiography is generally not helpful for an isolated CWS without concomitant pathology. IVFA reveals areas of capillary nonperfusion adjacent to CWS location.

11

Treatment

Identify and treat underlying etiology.

Follow Up

Depends on underlying etiology. If concern for infectious process, serial dilated examinations are recommended. CWSs typically fade in 5 to 7 weeks but can remain longer if associated with diabetic retinopathy.

11.6 Central Retinal Artery Occlusion

Symptoms

Unilateral, painless, acute vision loss (counting fingers to light perception in 94% of eyes) occurring over seconds; may have a history of transient visual loss (amaurosis fugax).

Signs

(See Figure 11.6.1.)

Critical. Superficial opacification or whitening of the retina in the posterior pole and a cherry-red spot in the center of the macula (may be subtle).

Other. Marked RAPD. Narrowed retinal arterioles; boxcarring or segmentation of the blood column in the arterioles. Occasionally, retinal arteriolar emboli or cilioretinal artery sparing of the foveola is evident. If visual acuity is light perception or worse, strongly suspect ophthalmic artery occlusion.

Differential Diagnosis

- Acute ophthalmic artery occlusion: Usually no cherry-red spot; the entire retina appears whitened. Increased concern for GCA.

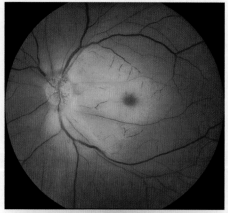

Figure 11.6.1 Central retinal artery occlusion.

- Commotio retinae: Retinal whitening from intracellular edema and fragmentation of the photoreceptor outer segments and RPE. Follows blunt trauma, resolves spontaneously. May result in permanent retinal damage. May mimic a cherry-red spot when the posterior pole is involved (Berlin edema). See 3.17, COMMOTIO RETINAE.

- Other causes of a cherry-red spot: Tay–Sachs, Niemann–Pick disease type A, others. These conditions present early in life with other, often severe, systemic manifestations. Ophthalmic findings are usually bilateral.

Etiology

- Embolus: Three main types include cholesterol, calcium, and platelet-fibrin emboli. All are seen within a vessel. Cholesterol emboli (Hollenhorst plaque) are typically refractile, yellow, and seen at retinal vessel bifurcations. They arise from ulcerated atheromas, usually from the carotid arteries. Calcium emboli are white and frequently cause distal retinal infarction. They typically arise from cardiac valves. Platelet-fibrin emboli are a dull white and typically arise from atheromas in the carotid arteries.

- Thrombosis.

- GCA: May produce central retinal artery occlusion (CRAO), branch retinal artery occlusion (BRAO), ophthalmic artery occlusion, or an ischemic optic neuropathy. See 10.17, ARTERITIC ISCHEMIC OPTIC NEUROPATHY (GIANT CELL ARTERITIS).

- Other collagen vascular disease: Systemic lupus erythematosus, polyarteritis nodosa, others.

- Hypercoagulable state: Polycythemia, multiple myeloma, cryoglobulinemia, Waldenström macroglobulinemia, antiphospholipid syndrome, factor V Leiden, activated protein C resistance, hyperhomocysteinemia, protein C

and S deficiency, antithrombin III mutation, prothrombin mutation, etc.
- Rare causes: Migraine, Behçet disease, syphilis, sickle cell disease.
- Trauma.

Workup

1. Should be treated as an acute stroke. The American Academy of Ophthalmology (AAO) 2018 guidelines suggest that all these patients should be sent immediately to an emergency department, preferably affiliated with a stroke center, for evaluation and workup.
2. Immediate ESR, CRP, and platelets to rule out GCA if the patient is 55 years of age or older and no embolus seen on examination. Query GCA review of systems. If the patient's history, laboratories, or both are consistent with GCA, start high-dose systemic steroids. See 10.17, ARTERITIC ISCHEMIC OPTIC NEUROPATHY (GIANT CELL ARTERITIS).
3. Check the blood pressure.
4. Other blood tests: Fasting blood sugar and hemoglobin A1c, complete blood count (CBC) with differential, prothrombin time/activated partial thromboplastin time (PT/PTT). In patients younger than 50 years or with appropriate risk factors or positive review of systems, consider lipid profile, antinuclear antibody (ANA), rheumatoid factor, syphilis testing (RPR or VDRL and FTA-ABS or treponemal-specific assay), serum protein electrophoresis, hemoglobin electrophoresis, and further evaluation for hypercoagulable state (see above).
5. Carotid artery evaluation by duplex Doppler US.
6. Cardiac evaluation with electrocardiography (ECG), echocardiography, and possibly Holter monitoring or bubble study.
7. OCT can be very helpful in making the diagnosis. Can also consider IVFA. Less commonly ERG is used.

Treatment

CRAO is treated as an acute stroke and immediate referral to an emergency department with an affiliated stroke center is warranted. If GCA suspected, see 10.17, ARTERITIC ISCHEMIC OPTIC NEUROPATHY (GIANT CELL ARTERITIS) for treatment recommendations.

For specific management of ocular signs and symptoms, there are anecdotal reports of improvement after the following treatments, if instituted within 90 to 120 minutes of the occlusive event. None of these treatments have been proven effective in randomized, controlled clinical trials and should not be considered standard of care.

1. Immediate ocular massage with fundus contact lens or digital massage.
2. Anterior chamber paracentesis: See Appendix 13, ANTERIOR CHAMBER PARACENTESIS.
3. IOP reduction with acetazolamide, 500 mg i.v. or two 250-mg tablets p.o. or a topical beta-blocker (e.g., timolol or levobunolol, 0.5% daily or b.i.d.).

Follow Up

1. Follow as directed by managing internist and/or neurologist.
2. Repeat eye examination in 1 to 4 weeks, checking for neovascularization of the iris/disc/angle/retina (NVI/NVD/NVA/NVE), which develops in up to 20% of patients at a mean of 4 weeks after onset. If neovascularization develops, perform panretinal photocoagulation (PRP) and/or administer an anti-vascular endothelial growth factor (anti-VEGF) agent.

11

11.7 Branch Retinal Artery Occlusion

Symptoms

Unilateral, painless, abrupt change in vision, usually partial visual field loss; may have a history of transient visual loss (amaurosis fugax).

Signs

(See Figure 11.7.1.)

Critical. Superficial opacification or whitening along the distribution of a branch retinal artery. The affected retina becomes edematous.

Other. Narrowed branch retinal artery; boxcarring, segmentation of the blood column, or emboli are sometimes seen in the affected branch retinal artery. Cholesterol emboli appear as bright,

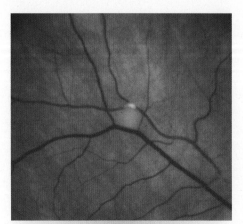

Figure 11.7.1 Branch retinal artery occlusion with Hollenhorst plaque.

reflective crystals, usually at a vessel bifurcation. CWSs may appear in the involved area.

Etiology

See 11.6, CENTRAL RETINAL ARTERY OCCLUSION.

Workup

See 11.6, CENTRAL RETINAL ARTERY OCCLUSION. Unlike in CRAO, an ERG is not helpful.

> **NOTE:** When a BRAO is accompanied by optic nerve edema or retinitis, obtain appropriate serologic testing to rule out cat-scratch disease (*Bartonella [Rochalimaea] hense-lae*), syphilis, Lyme disease, and toxoplasmosis.

Treatment

1. The AAO 2018 guidelines suggest that all these patients should be sent immediately to an emergency department, preferably affili-ated with a stroke center, for evaluation and workup. See treatment in 11.6, CENTRAL RETINAL ARTERY OCCLUSION.
2. No ocular therapy of proven value is available.
3. Treat any underlying medical problem.

Follow Up

1. Patients need immediate evaluation to treat any underlying disorders (especially GCA).
2. Reevaluate every 3 to 6 months initially to monitor progression. Ocular neovasculariza-tion after BRAO is rare.

11.8 Central Retinal Vein Occlusion

Symptoms

Painless loss of vision, usually unilateral.

Signs

(See Figure 11.8.1.)

Critical. Diffuse retinal hemorrhages in all four quadrants of the retina; dilated, tortuous retinal veins.

Other. CWSs; disc edema and hemorrhages; macular edema (ME); optociliary collateral vessels on the disc (later finding); NVD, NVI, NVA, and NVE.

Differential Diagnosis

- Ocular ischemic syndrome (OIS) or carotid occlusive disease: Dilated and irregular veins without tortuosity. Midperipheral retinal

hemorrhages are typically present, but disc edema and disc hemorrhages are not charac-teristic. NVD is present in one-third of cases. Patients may have a history of transient visual loss (amaurosis fugax), transient ischemic attacks, or orbital pain. IOP may be decreased. May have pain or intraocular inflammation. Can have abnormal ophthalmodynamometry. See 11.11, OCULAR ISCHEMIC SYNDROME/CAROTID OCCLUSIVE DISEASE.

- Diabetic retinopathy: Hemorrhages and microaneurysms concentrated in the pos-terior pole. Typically bilateral. IVFA differ-entiates this condition from central retinal vein occlusion (CRVO). See 11.12, DIABETIC RETINOPATHY.

- Papilledema: Bilateral disc swelling with flame-shaped hemorrhages surrounding the disc. Would not expect as extensive and diffuse

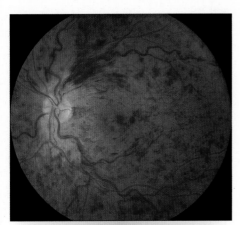

Figure 11.8.1 Central retinal vein occlusion with dilated, tortuous vasculature, diffuse retinal hemorrhages in all four quadrants, and macular edema.

retinal hemorrhage and vascular tortuosity. See 10.15, PAPILLEDEMA.

- Radiation retinopathy: History of irradiation. Disc swelling with radiation papillopathy and retinal neovascularization may be present. Generally, CWSs are a more prominent feature than hemorrhages.

Etiology

- Atherosclerosis of the adjacent central retinal artery: The artery compresses the central retinal vein in the region of the lamina cribrosa, secondarily inducing thrombosis in the vein lumen.
- HTN: Most common systemic disease associated with CRVO.
- Optic disc edema.
- Glaucoma: Most common ocular disease associated with CRVO.
- Optic disc drusen.
- Hypercoagulable state: Polycythemia, multiple myeloma, cryoglobulinemia, Waldenström macroglobulinemia, antiphospholipid syndrome, factor V Leiden, activated protein C resistance, hyperhomocysteinemia, protein C and S deficiency, antithrombin III mutation, prothrombin mutation, and others.
- Vasculitis: Sarcoidosis, syphilis, systemic lupus erythematosus, and others.
- Drugs: Oral contraceptives, diuretics, and others.

- Abnormal platelet function.
- Orbital disease: Thyroid eye disease, orbital tumors, arteriovenous fistula, and others.
- Migraine: Rare.

Types

- Ischemic CRVO: Vision typically worse (<20/200) with RAPD and visual field defects. Extensive retinal hemorrhage, CWSs, venous tortuosity, and widespread capillary nonperfusion on IVFA (often >10 disc diameters). ERG shows decreased b-wave amplitude. Higher risk of neovascularization.
- Nonischemic CRVO: Vision often better than 20/200, mild or no RAPD, mild fundus changes. Lower risk of neovascularization.

Workup

Ocular

1. Complete ocular examination, including IOP measurement, careful slit lamp examination and gonioscopy to rule out NVI and NVA (both of which are best observed before dilation), and dilated fundus examination.
2. IVFA: Risk of neovascularization proportional to degree of capillary nonperfusion.
3. OCT: Used to help detect presence and extent of ME as well as to monitor response to therapy.
4. If the diagnosis is uncertain, oculopneumoplethysmography or ophthalmodynamometry may help to distinguish CRVO from carotid disease (but are infrequently performed). Ophthalmic artery pressure is low in carotid disease but is normal to increased in CRVO.

Systemic

1. History: Medical problems, medications (especially antihypertensive medications, oral contraceptives, diuretics), eye diseases?
2. Check blood pressure.
3. Blood tests: Fasting blood sugar and hemoglobin A1c, CBC with differential, platelets, PT/PTT, lipid profile.
4. If clinically indicated, particularly in younger patients, consider hemoglobin electrophoresis, RPR or VDRL, FTA-ABS or treponemal-specific assay, ANA, cryoglobulins, antiphospholipid antibodies, factor V Leiden mutation, protein C and S levels, antithrombin III

11

mutation, prothrombin mutation, homocysteine levels, serum protein electrophoresis, and chest radiograph.

5. Complete medical evaluation, with careful attention to cardiovascular disease or hypercoagulability.

Treatment

1. Discontinue oral contraceptives; change diuretics to other antihypertensive medications if possible.

2. Reduce IOP if increased in either eye. See 9.1, PRIMARY OPEN-ANGLE GLAUCOMA.

3. Treat underlying medical disorders.

4. If NVI or NVA is present, perform PRP promptly. Consider PRP if NVD or retinal neovascularization is present. Prophylactic PRP for nonperfusion is usually not recommended unless follow up is in doubt. Intravitreal VEGF inhibitors are very effective in temporarily halting or reversing anterior and posterior segment neovascularization. They may be a useful adjunct to PRP, particularly when rapid reversal of neovascularization is needed.

5. Aspirin 81 to 325 mg p.o. daily is often recommended, but no clinical trials have demonstrated efficacy to date, and it may increase the risk of hemorrhage.

CRVO-Related Macular Edema

1. Intravitreal ranibizumab 0.5 mg and aflibercept 2 mg are US Food and Drug Administration (FDA)–approved for treating RVO-related ME. Intravitreal bevacizumab has been used off-label in a similar fashion. Risks of intravitreal injections are low but include VH and endophthalmitis, among others.

2. Dexamethasone intravitreal implant, a biodegradable 0.7 mg implant, is FDA-approved for the treatment of ME associated with retinal vein occlusion. Off-label intravitreal steroid (e.g., triamcinolone 40 mg/mL, injecting 1 to 4 mg) can also be considered and has been effective in both improving vision and reducing vision loss in patients with ME secondary to CRVO. Complications include cataract formation and elevated IOP.

NOTE: In a large, prospective, randomized trial (SCORE-CRVO), a 1 mg dose of intravitreal triamcinolone was found to be equally as effective as a 4 mg dose, but with fewer side effects (elevated IOP and cataract formation).

Follow Up

1. Every month initially, with gradual interval taper based on vision, presence of ME, and response to treatment.

2. At each follow-up visit, evaluate anterior segment for NVI and assess presence/absence of NVA with undilated gonioscopy, followed by careful dilated fundus examination looking for NVD or other retinal neovascularization. Evidence of early NVI or NVA should prompt immediate PRP and/or anti-VEGF therapy and monthly follow up until stabilized or regressed.

3. Patients should be informed that there is an 8% to 10% risk for the development of a branch retinal vein occlusion (BRVO) or CRVO in the fellow eye.

REFERENCES

Brown DM, Campochiaro PA, Singh RP, et al. Ranibizumab for macular edema following central retinal vein occlusion: six-month primary end point results of a phase III study. *Ophthalmology.* 2010;117(6):1124-1133.

Haller JA, Bandello F, Belfort R Jr, et al. Randomized sham-controlled trial of dexamethasone intravitreal implant in patients with macular edema due to retinal vein occlusion. *Ophthalmology.* 2010;117(6):1134-1146.

Ip MS, Scott IU, VanVeldhuisen PC, et al. A randomized trial comparing the efficacy and safety of intravitreal triamcinolone with observation to treat vision loss associated with macular edema secondary to central retinal vein occlusion: the Standard Care vs Corticosteroid for Retinal Vein Occlusion (SCORE) study report 5. *Arch Ophthalmol.* 2009;127(9):1101-1114.

Boyer D, Heier J, Brown DM, et al. Vascular endothelial growth factor Trap-Eye for macular edema secondary to central retinal vein occlusion: six-month results of the Phase III COPERNICUS Study. *Ophthalmology.* 2012;119:1024-1032.

11.9 Branch Retinal Vein Occlusion

Symptoms

Blind spot in the visual field or loss of vision, usually unilateral.

Signs

(See Figure 11.9.1.)

Critical. Superficial hemorrhages in a sector of the retina along a retinal vein. The hemorrhages usually do not cross the horizontal raphe (midline).

Other. CWSs, retinal edema, a dilated and tortuous retinal vein, narrowing and sheathing of the adjacent artery, retinal neovascularization, VH.

Differential Diagnosis

- Diabetic retinopathy: Dot-blot hemorrhages and microaneurysms extend across the horizontal raphe. Nearly always bilateral. See 11.12, DIABETIC RETINOPATHY.
- Hypertensive retinopathy: Narrowed retinal arterioles. Hemorrhages are not confined to a sector of the retina and usually cross the horizontal raphe. Bilateral in most. See 11.10, HYPERTENSIVE RETINOPATHY.

Etiology

Disease of the adjacent arterial wall (usually secondary to HTN, arteriosclerosis, or diabetes) compresses the venous wall at a crossing point.

Workup

1. History: Systemic disease, particularly HTN or diabetes?
2. Complete ocular examination, including dilated retinal examination with indirect ophthalmoscopy to look for retinal neovascularization and ME.
3. OCT: Used to help detect presence and extent of ME as well as monitor response to therapy.
4. Check blood pressure.
5. Blood tests: Fasting blood sugar and hemoglobin A1c, lipid profile, CBC with differential and platelets, PT/PTT. If clinically indicated, consider a more comprehensive workup. See 11.8, CENTRAL RETINAL VEIN OCCLUSION.
6. Medical examination: Performed by an internist to check for cardiovascular disease.
7. An IVFA is obtained after the hemorrhages clear or sooner if neovascularization is suspected.

Treatment

1. Retinal neovascularization: Sector PRP to the ischemic area, which corresponds to area of capillary nonperfusion on IVFA.
2. Prompt and appropriate treatment of underlying medical conditions (e.g., HTN).

BRVO-Related Macular Edema

1. Anti-VEGF treatment is now the gold standard. Intravitreal ranibizumab 0.5 mg and aflibercept 2 mg are FDA-approved for treating RVO-associated ME. Intravitreal bevacizumab has also been used off-label. Risks of intravitreal injection are low but include VH and endophthalmitis.
2. Focal retinal laser photocoagulation has historically been the gold-standard treatment if edema is present for 3 to 6 months duration, and visual acuity is below 20/40 with macular capillary perfusion. However, anti-VEGF treatment is now largely favored. Limitations of focal laser include length of time before effect (often several months) and the need to wait until retinal hemorrhages clear.

11

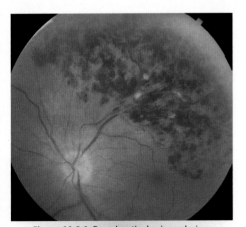

Figure 11.9.1 Branch retinal vein occlusion.

3. Dexamethasone intravitreal implant or off-label intravitreal steroid (e.g., triamcinolone 40 mg/mL, inject 1 to 4 mg). See 11.8, CENTRAL RETINAL VEIN OCCLUSION.

📝 **NOTE:** There is an evolving trend, particularly in cases of severe edema, to initiate treatment with pharmacologic agents for rapid visual recovery followed by focal laser for better durability of effect. Multiple pharmacologic trials (BRAVO and CRUISE) have validated that early anti-VEGF treatment leads to better visual outcomes.

Follow Up

In general, every month initially, with gradual interval taper based on vision, presence of ME, and treatment response. At each visit, the patient should be checked for neovascularization and ME.

REFERENCES

Campochiaro PA, Heier JS, Feiner L, et al. Ranibizumab for macular edema following branch retinal vein occlusion: six-month primary end point results of a phase III study. *Ophthalmology.* 2010;117(6):1102-1112.

Varma R, Bressler NM, Suñer I, et al. Improved vision-related function after ranibizumab for macular edema after retinal vein occlusion: results from the BRAVO and CRUISE trials. *Ophthalmology.* 2012;119(10):2108-2118.

11.10 Hypertensive Retinopathy

Symptoms

Usually asymptomatic, although may have decreased vision.

Signs

(See Figure 11.10.1.)

Critical. Generalized or localized retinal arteriolar narrowing, almost always bilateral.

Other
• Chronic HTN: Arteriovenous crossing changes ("AV nicking"), retinal arteriolar sclerosis

("copper" or "silver" wiring), CWSs, flame-shaped hemorrhages, arterial macroaneurysms, central or branch occlusion of an artery or vein. Rarely, neovascular complications can develop.
• Acute ("malignant") HTN or accelerated HTN: Hard exudates often in a "macular star" configuration, retinal edema, CWSs, flame-shaped hemorrhages, optic nerve head edema. Rarely serous RD or VH. Areas of focal chorioretinal atrophy (from previous choroidal infarcts [Elschnig spots]) are a sign of past episodes of acute HTN.
  (See Figure 11.10.2.)

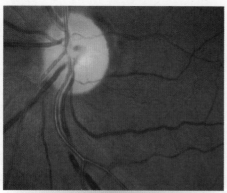

Figure 11.10.1 Chronic hypertensive retinopathy with arteriolar narrowing and arteriovenous nicking.

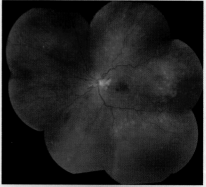

Figure 11.10.2 Acute ("malignant") hypertensive retinopathy.

NOTE: When unilateral, suspect carotid artery obstruction on the side of the normal-appearing eye, sparing the retina from the effects of the HTN.

Differential Diagnosis

- Diabetic retinopathy: Hemorrhages are usually dot-blot and microaneurysms are common; vessel attenuation is less common. See 11.12, DIABETIC RETINOPATHY.
- Collagen vascular disease: May show multiple CWSs, but few to no other fundus findings characteristic of HTN.
- Anemia: Mainly hemorrhage without marked arterial changes.
- Radiation retinopathy: History of irradiation. Most commonly occurs within a few years, but can develop at any time.
- CRVO or BRVO: Unilateral, multiple hemorrhages, venous dilation, and tortuosity. May be the result of HTN. See 11.8, CENTRAL RETINAL VEIN OCCLUSION or 11.9, BRANCH RETINAL VEIN OCCLUSION.

Etiology

- Primary HTN: No known underlying cause.
- Secondary HTN: Typically the result of preeclampsia/eclampsia, pheochromocytoma, kidney disease, adrenal disease, aortic coarctation, others.

Workup

1. History: Known HTN, diabetes, or adnexal radiation?
2. Check blood pressure.
3. Complete ocular examination, particularly dilated fundus examination.
4. Refer patient to a medical internist or an emergency department. The urgency depends on the blood pressure reading and whether the patient is symptomatic. A systolic blood pressure ≥180 mm Hg, a diastolic blood pressure ≥110 mm Hg or the presence of chest pain, difficulty breathing, headache, change in mental status, or blurred vision with optic disc swelling requires immediate medical attention.
5. Patients may need workup for secondary causes of hypertension such as those listed above.

Treatment

Control the HTN, as per the internist.

Follow Up

Every 2 to 3 months at first and then every 6 to 12 months.

11

11.11 Ocular Ischemic Syndrome/Carotid Occlusive Disease

Symptoms

Decreased vision, ocular or periorbital pain, afterimages or prolonged recovery of vision after exposure to bright light, may have a history of transient monocular visual loss (amaurosis fugax). Usually unilateral, although up to 20% of cases can be bilateral. Typically occurs in patients aged 50 to 80 years. Men outnumber women 2:1.

Signs

Critical. Although retinal veins are dilated and irregular in caliber, they are typically not tortuous. The retinal arterioles are narrowed. Associated findings include midperipheral retinal hemorrhages (80%), iris neovascularization (66%), neovascularization of the disc (35%), and neovascularization of the retina (8%).

Other. External collateral vessels on the forehead, episcleral injection, corneal edema, mild anterior uveitis, neovascular glaucoma, iris atrophy, cataract, retinal microaneurysms, CWSs, spontaneous pulsations of the central retinal artery, and cherry-red spot. CRAO may occur.

Differential Diagnosis

- CRVO: Diffuse retinal hemorrhages. Dilated and tortuous retinal veins. Decreased vision after exposure to light and orbital pain are not typically found. Ophthalmodynamometry and IVFA may aid in differentiating OIS from

CRVO. See 11.8, CENTRAL RETINAL VEIN OCCLUSION.

- Diabetic retinopathy: Bilateral, usually symmetric. Hard exudates are often present. See 11.12, DIABETIC RETINOPATHY.
- Aortic arch disease: Caused by atherosclerosis, syphilis, or Takayasu arteritis. Produces a clinical picture identical to OIS, but usually bilateral. Examination reveals absent arm and neck pulses, cold hands, and arm muscle spasms with exercise.

Etiology

- Ipsilateral carotid artery disease: Usually ≥90% stenosis.
- Ipsilateral ophthalmic artery disease: Less common.
- Ipsilateral central retinal artery obstruction: Rare.
- Giant cell arteritis: Rare.

Workup

1. History: Previous episodes of transient monocular visual loss? Cold hands or arm muscle spasms with exercise?
2. Complete ocular examination: Search carefully for anterior chamber flare, asymmetric cataract, and NVI/NVA/NVD/NVE.
3. Medical examination: Evaluate for HTN, diabetes, and atherosclerotic disease. Check pulses. Cardiac and carotid auscultation.

4. Laboratory workup for GCA in the appropriate settings. See 10.17, GIANT CELL ARTERITIS.
5. Consider IVFA for diagnostic purposes.
6. Noninvasive carotid artery evaluation: Duplex Doppler US, oculoplethysmography, magnetic resonance angiography, others.
7. Consider orbital color Doppler US.
8. Consider ophthalmodynamometry if CRVO diagnosis cannot be excluded.
9. Carotid arteriography is reserved for patients in whom surgery is to be performed.
10. Consider cardiology consultation, given the high association with cardiac disease.

Treatment

1. Carotid endarterectomy for significant stenosis. Refer to neurovascular surgeon.
2. Consider PRP and anti-VEGF agents in the presence of neovascularization.
3. Manage glaucoma if present. See 9.14, NEOVASCULAR GLAUCOMA.
4. Control HTN, diabetes, and cholesterol. Refer to internist.
5. Lifestyle modification (e.g., smoking cessation).

Follow Up

Depends on the age, general health of the patient, and the symptoms and signs of disease. Surgical candidates should be evaluated urgently.

11.12 Diabetic Retinopathy

Diabetic Retinopathy Disease Severity Scale

- No apparent retinopathy.
- Mild nonproliferative diabetic retinopathy (NPDR): Microaneurysms only.
- Moderate NPDR: More than mild NPDR, but less than severe NPDR (see Figure 11.12.1). May have CWSs and venous beading.
- Severe NPDR: Any of the following in the absence of PDR: Diffuse (traditionally >20) intraretinal hemorrhages in all four quadrants, two quadrants of venous beading, or one quadrant of prominent intraretinal microvascular abnormalities (see Figure 11.12.2).

- PDR: Neovascularization of one or more of the following: iris, angle, optic disc, or elsewhere in retina; or vitreous/preretinal hemorrhage (see Figures 11.12.3 and 11.12.4).
- Diabetic macular edema (DME): May be present in any of the stages listed above. DME affecting or threatening the fovea is an indication for treatment (see Figures 11.12.5 and 11.12.6).

Differential Diagnosis for Nonproliferative Diabetic Retinopathy

- CRVO: Optic disc swelling, veins are more dilated and tortuous, hard exudates and microaneurysms usually not found,

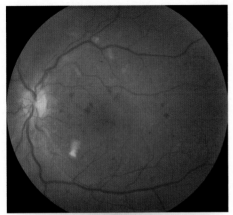

Figure 11.12.1 Moderate nonproliferative diabetic retinopathy with microaneurysms and cotton–wool spots.

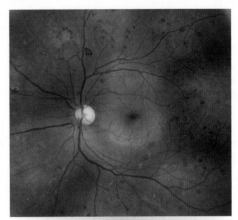

Figure 11.12.3 Proliferative diabetic retinopathy with neovascularization and scattered microaneurysms.

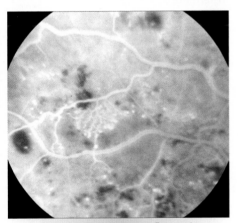

Figure 11.12.2 Intravenous fluorescein angiography of intraretinal microvascular abnormality.

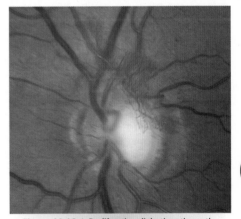

Figure 11.12.4 Proliferative diabetic retinopathy with neovascularization of the optic disc.

hemorrhages are nearly always in the NFL ("splinter hemorrhages"). CRVO is generally unilateral and of more sudden onset. See 11.8, CENTRAL RETINAL VEIN OCCLUSION.

- BRVO: Hemorrhages are distributed along a vein and do not cross the horizontal raphe (midline). See 11.9, BRANCH RETINAL VEIN OCCLUSION.
- OIS: Hemorrhages mostly in the midperiphery and larger; exudates are absent. Usually accompanied by pain; mild anterior chamber reaction; corneal edema; episcleral vascular

congestion; a mid-dilated, poorly reactive pupil; iris neovascularization. See 11.11, OCULAR ISCHEMIC SYNDROME/CAROTID OCCLUSIVE DISEASE.

- Hypertensive retinopathy: Hemorrhages fewer and typically flame-shaped, microaneurysms rare, and arteriolar narrowing present often with arteriovenous crossing changes ("AV nicking"). See 11.10, HYPERTENSIVE RETINOPATHY.
- Radiation retinopathy: Usually develops within a few years of radiation. Microaneurysms are rarely present. See 11.5, COTTON–WOOL SPOT.

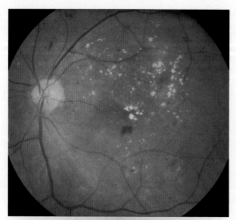

Figure 11.12.5 Nonproliferative diabetic retinopathy with clinically significant macular edema.

Differential Diagnosis for Proliferative Diabetic Retinopathy

- Neovascular complications of CRAO, CRVO, or BRVO: See specific sections.
- Sickle cell retinopathy: Peripheral retinal neovascularization. "Sea fans" of neovascularization present. See 11.20, SICKLE CELL RETINOPATHY (INCLUDING SICKLE CELL DISEASE, ANEMIA, AND TRAIT).
- Embolization from intravenous drug abuse (talc retinopathy): Peripheral retinal neovascularization in patient with history of intravenous drug abuse. Typically see talc particles in retinal vessels. See 11.33, CRYSTALLINE RETINOPATHY.
- Sarcoidosis: May have uveitis, exudates around veins ("candle-wax drippings"), NVE, or systemic findings. See 12.6, SARCOIDOSIS.
- Other inflammatory syndromes (e.g., systemic lupus erythematosus).
- OIS: See 11.11, OCULAR ISCHEMIC SYNDROME/CAROTID OCCLUSIVE DISEASE.
- Radiation retinopathy: See above.
- Hypercoagulable states (e.g., antiphospholipid syndrome).

Workup

1. Slit lamp examination using gonioscopy with careful attention for NVI and NVA, preferably before pharmacologic dilation.

2. Dilated fundus examination by using a 90- or 60-diopter or fundus contact lens with a slit lamp to rule out neovascularization and ME. Use indirect ophthalmoscopy to examine the retinal periphery.
3. Check fasting blood sugar, hemoglobin A1c, and lipid panel.
4. Check blood pressure.
5. Consider IVFA to determine areas of perfusion abnormalities, foveal ischemia, microaneurysms, and subclinical neovascularization, especially if considering focal macular laser therapy.
6. Consider OCT to evaluate for presence and extent of DME. OCT angiography (OCTA) can be useful to check for presence of significant central macular ischemia.

Treatment

Diabetic Macular Edema

1. Anti-VEGF agents (FDA-approved ranibizumab and aflibercept, as well as off-label bevacizumab) are first-line therapy for center-involving DME.
2. Those patients who have a suboptimal response to these anti-VEGF agents or require ongoing, frequent anti-VEGF therapy can consider intravitreal corticosteroid therapy with FDA-approved dexamethasone or long-acting fluocinolone acetonide injectable implants. Off-label intravitreal corticosteroid (e.g., triamcinolone 40 mg/mL, injecting 1 to 4 mg) can also be considered. Complications include cataract formation and elevated IOP.
3. Focal macular laser treatment can be considered in patients with extrafoveal microaneurysms causing significant edema. Macular laser can also be considered in patients for whom anti-VEGF and intravitreal steroid injections are contraindicated. Most practitioners avoid using anti-VEGF agents in pregnant patients, though no study has definitively shown adverse fetal side effects.

Proliferative Diabetic Retinopathy

1. PRP is indicated for any one of the following high-risk characteristics **(see Figure 11.12.7)**:
   - NVD greater than one-fourth to one-third of the disc area in size.

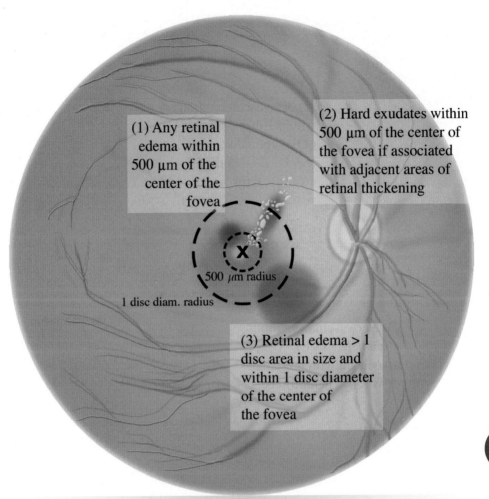

(1) Any retinal edema within 500 μm of the center of the fovea

(2) Hard exudates within 500 μm of the center of the fovea if associated with adjacent areas of retinal thickening

500 μm radius

1 disc diam. radius

X

(3) Retinal edema > 1 disc area in size and within 1 disc diameter of the center of the fovea

Figure 11.12.6 Clinically significant macular edema.

- Any degree of NVD when associated with preretinal hemorrhage or VH.
- NVE greater than one-half of the disc area in size when associated with preretinal hemorrhage or VH.
- Any NVI or NVA.

2. Anti-VEGF therapy can be utilized for PDR as an alternative to PRP and is the preferred initial therapy in the presence of DME or if the view to the peripheral retina is limited by VH. Anti-VEGF therapy without PRP should be utilized cautiously, as patients lost

to follow up have been shown to have worse anatomic and visual outcomes.

 NOTE: Some physicians treat NVE or any degree of NVD without preretinal hemorrhage or VH, especially in unreliable patients.

Indications for Vitrectomy

Vitrectomy may be indicated for any one of the following conditions:

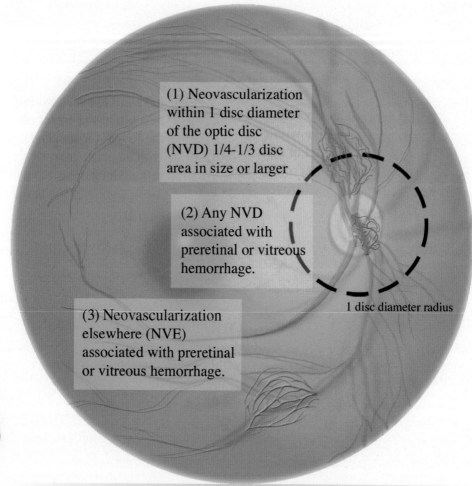

(1) Neovascularization within 1 disc diameter of the optic disc (NVD) 1/4-1/3 disc area in size or larger

(2) Any NVD associated with preretinal or vitreous hemorrhage.

(3) Neovascularization elsewhere (NVE) associated with preretinal or vitreous hemorrhage.

1 disc diameter radius

Figure 11.12.7 High-risk characteristics for diabetic retinopathy.

1. Dense, nonclearing or recurrent VH causing significant decreased vision.
2. Traction RD involving and progressing within the macula.
3. Macular epiretinal membranes (ERMs) or vitreomacular traction causing significant visual symptoms.
4. Dense premacular hemorrhage.
5. Chronic DME not responsive to other treatment.
6. Severe retinal neovascularization and fibrous proliferation that is unresponsive to laser photocoagulation or anti-VEGF therapy.

NOTE: Young patients with type 1 diabetes are known to have more aggressive PDR and therefore may benefit from earlier vitrectomy, laser photocoagulation, or anti-VEGF therapy. B-scan US may be required to rule out tractional detachment of the macula in eyes with dense VH obscuring a fundus view.

Follow Up

1. Diabetes without retinopathy. Annual dilated examination.
2. Mild NPDR. Dilated examination every 6 to 9 months.

TABLE 11.12.1 Recommendations Based on the Baseline Diabetic Retinopathy in Pregnancy

Baseline Diabetic Retinopathy	Gestational Diabetes	None or Minimal Nonproliferative Diabetic Retinopathy (NPDR)	Mild-to-Moderate NPDR	High-Risk NPDR	Proliferative Diabetic Retinopathy (PDR)
Gestational course	No risk of retinopathy	No progression in vast majority. Of those who progress, only a few have visual impairment.	Progression in up to 50%. Postpartum regression in many.	Progression in up to 50%. Postpartum regression in some.	Tends to progress rapidly.
Eye examinations	None	First and third trimester	Every trimester	Monthly	Monthly
Treatment	None	None	None, unless high-risk proliferative retinopathy develops.	None, unless high-risk proliferative retinopathy develops.	Treat PDR with panretinal photocoagulation. Observe diabetic macular edema (high rate of spontaneous postpartum regression).

3. Moderate to severe NPDR. Dilated examination every 4 to 6 months.

4. PDR (not meeting high-risk criteria). Dilated examination every 2 to 3 months.

5. Diabetes and pregnancy. Changes that occur during pregnancy have a high likelihood of postpartum regression. See **Table 11.12.1** for follow-up recommendations.

NOTE: The Diabetes Control and Complications Trial showed that strict control of blood sugar with insulin (in type 1 diabetes) decreases the progression of diabetic retinopathy, as well as nephropathy and neuropathy.

REFERENCES

Wilkinson CP, Ferris FL III, Klein RE, et al. Proposed international clinical diabetic retinopathy and diabetic macular edema disease severity scales. *Ophthalmology.* 2003;110:1677-1682.

Mitchell P, Bandello F, Schmidt-Erfurth U, et al. The RESTORE Study ranibizumab monotherapy or combined with laser versus laser monotherapy for diabetic macular edema. *Ophthalmology.* 2011;118:615-625.

Korobelnik JF, Do DV, Schmidt-Erfurth U, et al. Intravitreal aflibercept for diabetic macular edema. *Ophthalmology.* 2014;121(11):2247-2254.

Boyer DS, Yoon YH, Belfort R Jr, et al. Three-year, randomized, sham-controlled trial of dexamethasone intravitreal implant in patients with diabetic macular edema. *Ophthalmology.* 2014;121(10):1904-1914.

Cunha-Vaz J, Ashton P, Iezzi R, et al. Sustained delivery fluocinolone acetonide vitreous implants: long-term benefit in patients with chronic diabetic macular edema. *Ophthalmology.* 2014;121(10):1892-1903.

Diabetic Retinopathy Clinical Research Network. Panretinal photocoagulation vs intravitreous ranibizumab for proliferative diabetic retinopathy: a randomized trial. *J Am Med Assoc.* 2015;314(20):2137-2146.

Obeid A, Su D, Patel SN, et al. Outcomes of eyes lost to follow-up with proliferative diabetic retinopathy that received panretinal photocoagulation versus intravitreal anti-vascular endothelial growth factor. *Ophthalmology.* 2019;126(3):407-413.

11

11.13 Vitreous Hemorrhage

Symptoms

Sudden, painless loss of vision or sudden appearance of black spots, cobwebs, or haze in the vision.

Signs

(See Figure 11.13.1.)

Critical. In severe VH, the red fundus reflex may be absent, and there may be limited or no view to the fundus. Red blood cells may be seen in the anterior vitreous (or anterior chamber). In mild VH, there may be a partially obscured view to the fundus. Chronic VH has a yellow ocher appearance from hemoglobin breakdown.

Other. A mild RAPD is possible in the setting of dense hemorrhage. Depending on the etiology, there may be other fundus abnormalities.

Differential Diagnosis

- Vitritis (white blood cells in the vitreous): Usually not sudden onset; anterior or posterior uveitis may also be present. No red blood cells are seen in the vitreous. See 12.3, POSTERIOR UVEITIS.
- RD: May occur without a VH, but the symptoms may be similar. In VH due to RD, the peripheral retina may be obscured on

indirect ophthalmoscopy requiring B-scan US to detect the detachment. See 11.3, RETINAL DETACHMENT.

Etiology

- Diabetic retinopathy: Usually history of diabetes with diabetic retinopathy. Diabetic retinopathy is usually evident in the contralateral eye. In VH due to PDR, the peripheral retina is often visible on indirect ophthalmoscopy. See 11.12, DIABETIC RETINOPATHY.
- PVD: Common in middle-aged or elderly patients. Usually patients note floaters and flashing lights. See 11.1, POSTERIOR VITREOUS DETACHMENT.
- Retinal break: Commonly superior in cases of dense VH. This may be demonstrated by scleral depression and, if poor view, B-scan US. See 11.2, RETINAL BREAK.
- RD: May be diagnosed by B-scan US if the retina cannot be viewed on clinical examination. See 11.3, RETINAL DETACHMENT.
- Retinal vein occlusion (usually a BRVO): Commonly occurs in older patients with a history of high blood pressure. See 11.9, BRANCH RETINAL VEIN OCCLUSION.
- Exudative age-related macular degeneration (AMD): Usually with advanced CNV. Poor vision before the VH as a result of the underlying macular disease. Macular drusen and/or other findings of AMD are found in the contralateral eye. B-scan US may aid in the diagnosis. See 11.17, NEOVASCULAR OR EXUDATIVE (WET) AGE-RELATED MACULAR DEGENERATION.
- Sickle cell disease: May have peripheral retinal neovascularization in the contralateral eye, typically in a "sea fan" configuration and salmon color. See 11.20, SICKLE CELL RETINOPATHY (INCLUDING SICKLE CELL DISEASE, ANEMIA, AND TRAIT).
- Trauma: By history.
- Valsalva: By history.
- Intraocular tumor: May be visible on ophthalmoscopy or B-scan US. See 5.13, MALIGNANT MELANOMA OF THE IRIS and 11.36, CHOROIDAL NEVUS AND MALIGNANT MELANOMA OF THE CHOROID.

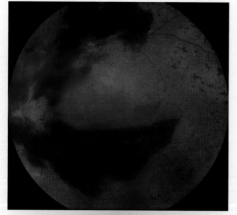

Figure 11.13.1 Vitreous and preretinal hemorrhage due to proliferative diabetic retinopathy.

- Subarachnoid or subdural hemorrhage (Terson syndrome): Frequently bilateral preretinal or VHs may occur. A severe headache usually precedes the fundus findings. Coma may occur.
- Others: Ruptured arterial macroaneurysm, Eales Disease, Coats disease, retinopathy of prematurity, retinal capillary angiomas of von Hippel–Lindau syndrome, congenital prepapillary vascular loop, retinal cavernous hemangioma, HTN, radiation retinopathy, anterior segment hemorrhage because of an intraocular lens, bleeding diathesis, hematologic malignancy, etc. See specific sections.

NOTE: In infancy and childhood, consider birth trauma, child abuse (e.g., shaken baby syndrome), congenital X-linked retinoschisis, pars planitis, bleeding dyscrasias, and hematologic malignancies.

Workup

1. History: Any ocular or systemic diseases? Trauma?
2. Complete ocular examination, including slit lamp examination with undilated pupils to check for iris neovascularization, IOP measurement, and dilated fundus examination of both eyes by using indirect ophthalmoscopy. In cases of spontaneous VH, scleral depression is performed if a retinal view can be obtained.
3. When no retinal view can be obtained, B-scan US is performed to detect an associated RD or intraocular tumor. Flap RTs may be detected with scleral depression and may be seen on B-scan US (elevated flap).
4. IVFA may aid in defining the etiology, although the quality of the angiogram depends on the density of the hemorrhage. Additionally, it may be useful to highlight abnormalities in the contralateral eye.

Treatment

1. If the etiology of VH is not known and a retinal break or an RD or both cannot be ruled out (i.e., there is no known history of one of the diseases mentioned previously, there are no changes in the contralateral eye, and the fundus is obscured by a total VH), close observation versus vitrectomy are options.
2. Observation:
   - No heavy lifting, no straining, no bending. Keep head of bed elevated. This reduces the chance of recurrent bleeding and allows blood to settle inferiorly, permitting a view of the superior peripheral fundus, a common site for possible retinal breaks.
   - Eliminate aspirin, nonsteroidal anti-inflammatory drugs (NSAIDs), and other anticlotting agents unless medically necessary.
   - The underlying etiology is treated as soon as possible (e.g., retinal breaks are sealed with cryotherapy or laser photocoagulation, detached retinas are repaired, and proliferative retinal vascular diseases are treated with anti-VEGF therapy or laser photocoagulation).
3. Vitrectomy:
   - VH accompanied by RD or RT on B-scan US.
   - Nonclearing VH. Because two-thirds of patients with an idiopathic, fundus-obscuring hemorrhage will have RTs or an RD, early vitrectomy should be considered.
   - VH with neovascularization of the iris.
   - Hemolytic or ghost cell glaucoma.

Follow Up

If observation is elected, the patient is evaluated daily for the first 2 to 3 days. If a total, dense VH persists, and the etiology remains unknown, vitrectomy should be considered.

11.14 Cystoid Macular Edema

Symptoms

Decreased vision.

Signs

(See Figures 11.14.1 to 11.14.3.)

Critical. Irregularity and blunting of the foveal light reflex, macular thickening with or without small intraretinal cysts in the foveal region.

Other. Vitreous cells, optic nerve swelling, and dot hemorrhages may be observed depending upon etiology of CME.

Etiology

- Postoperative, following any ocular surgery, including laser photocoagulation and cryotherapy. The peak incidence of post cataract extraction CME, or Irvine–Gass, is approximately 6 to 10 weeks; the incidence increases with cataract surgical complications including vitreous loss, vitreous to the corneoscleral wound, iris prolapse, or uveal incarceration.
- Diabetic retinopathy: See 11.12, DIABETIC RETINOPATHY.
- CRVO and BRVO: See 11.8, CENTRAL RETINAL VEIN OCCLUSION and 11.9, BRANCH RETINAL VEIN OCCLUSION.
- Uveitis: Particularly pars planitis; see 12.2, INTERMEDIATE UVEITIS.

- Retinitis pigmentosa (RP): See 11.28, RETINITIS PIGMENTOSA AND INHERITED CHORIORETINAL DYSTROPHIES.
- Topical drops: Epinephrine, dipivefrin, and prostaglandin analogs, especially in patients who have undergone cataract surgery.
- Retinal vasculitis: Eales disease, Behçet syndrome, sarcoidosis, necrotizing angiitis, multiple sclerosis, cytomegalovirus retinitis, others.
- Retinal telangiectasias: Coats disease, idiopathic macular telangiectasia, others.
- AMD: See 11.16, NONEXUDATIVE (DRY) AGE-RELATED MACULAR DEGENERATION and 11.17, NEOVASCULAR OR EXUDATIVE (WET) AGE-RELATED MACULAR DEGENERATION.
- ERM: See 11.26, EPIRETINAL MEMBRANE (MACULAR PUCKER, SURFACE-WRINKLING RETINOPATHY, CELLOPHANE MACULOPATHY).
- Associated with other ocular conditions: RD, subfoveal CNV, intraocular tumors, others.
- Others: Systemic HTN, collagen vascular disease, autosomal dominant CME, others.
- Pseudo-CME (no leakage on IVFA): Nicotinic acid maculopathy (typically seen only with relatively high doses of nicotinic acid), taxane drugs, X-linked retinoschisis (can see leakage with ICGA), myopic foveal schisis, Goldmann–Favre disease (and other NR2E3-related retinopathies), pseudohole from an ERM.

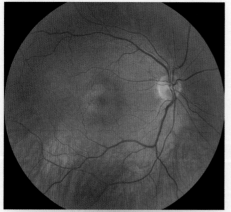

Figure 11.14.1 Cystoid macular edema.

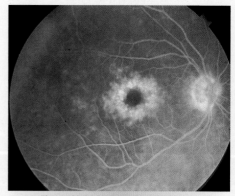

Figure 11.14.2 Intravenous fluorescein angiography of cystoid macular edema.

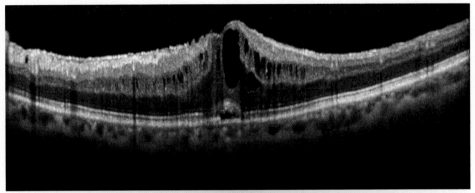

Figure 11.14.3 Optical coherence tomography of cystoid macular edema.

Workup

1. History: Recent intraocular surgery? Diabetes? Previous uveitis or ocular inflammation? Night blindness or family history of eye disease? Medications, including topical epinephrine, dipivefrin, or prostaglandin analogs?

2. Complete ocular examination, including gonioscopy to rule out the presence of retained lens fragments following cataract surgery and haptic malposition of implanted anterior chamber intraocular lens. Thorough peripheral fundus evaluation (scleral depression inferiorly may be required to detect pars planitis). Macular examination is best performed with a slit lamp and a 60- or 90-diopter lens, fundus contact lens, or a Hruby lens.

3. IVFA shows early leakage of perifoveal capillaries and late macular staining, classically in a petaloid or spoke-wheel pattern. Optic nerve head leakage is sometimes observed (Irvine–Gass syndrome). Fluorescein leakage does not occur in select cases of pseudo-CME (see above).

4. OCT can be utilized to document the presence of CME and demonstrate the efficacy of therapy. OCT outlines the loss of foveal contour resulting from enlarged cystic spaces within the retina and thickening of the macula.

5. Other diagnostic tests when indicated: Fasting blood sugar and hemoglobin A1c, ERG, others.

> **NOTE:** Subclinical CME commonly develops after cataract extraction and is noted on IVFA (angiographic CME). OCT shows no CME and these cases are not treated.

Treatment

Treat the underlying disorder if possible. For CME related to specific etiologies (e.g., diabetes, retinal vein occlusion, intermediate uveitis, etc.), see specific sections.

1. Topical NSAID (e.g., ketorolac 0.5% q.i.d., bromfenac 0.09%, or nepafenac 0.3% daily) often in conjunction with topical steroids (e.g., prednisolone acetate 1% q.i.d.).

2. Discontinue topical epinephrine, dipivefrin, or prostaglandin analog drops and medications containing nicotinic acid.

3. Other forms of therapy are often used to treat CME depending upon etiology:

   • Subtenon steroid (e.g., triamcinolone 40 mg/mL, inject 0.5 to 1.0 mL).

   • Intravitreal steroid (e.g., triamcinolone 40 mg/mL, inject 1 to 4 mg).

   • Intravitreal anti-VEGF therapy (e.g., bevacizumab 1.25 mg in 0.05 mL).

   • Systemic steroids (e.g., prednisone 40 mg p.o. daily for 5 days and then taper over 2 weeks).

   • Systemic NSAIDs (e.g., indomethacin 25 mg p.o. t.i.d. for 6 weeks).

   • Topical or systemic carbonic anhydrase inhibitors (e.g., dorzolamide 2% t.i.d. or acetazolamide 500 mg p.o. daily starting dose) in cases of RP-associated CME.

   • CME with or without vitreous incarceration in a surgical wound may be improved by vitrectomy or YAG laser lysis of the vitreous strand.

11

Follow Up

Postsurgical CME patients should be started on a topical NSAID and a topical steroid with follow up in 4 to 6 weeks to determine response to topical drop therapy. Other forms of CME should be followed in a similar time frame to monitor response to initial therapy.

11.15 Central Serous Chorioretinopathy

Symptoms

Central scotoma, blurred or dim vision, objects may appear distorted (metamorphopsia) and miniaturized (micropsia), colors may appear faded. Usually unilateral, but can be bilateral (more likely in older patients, may not be symptomatic at the same time). May be asymptomatic.

Signs

(See Figure 11.15.1.)

Critical. Localized serous detachment of the neurosensory retina in the macula without subretinal blood or lipid exudates. The margins of the detachment are sloping and merge gradually into the attached retina.

Other. Visual acuity usually ranges from 20/20 to 20/200. Amsler grid testing reveals relative scotoma and distortion of straight lines. May have a small RAPD, serous RPE detachment, or deposition of subretinal fibrin. Focal RPE changes may indicate sites of previous episodes.

Differential Diagnosis

These entities may produce a serous detachment of the neurosensory retina in the macula

- AMD: Patient usually ≥50 years old, drusen, pigment epithelial alterations, may have choroidal (subretinal) neovascularization, often bilateral. See 11.16, NONEXUDATIVE (DRY) AGE-RELATED MACULAR DEGENERATION and 11.17, NEOVASCULAR OR EXUDATIVE (WET) AGE-RELATED MACULAR DEGENERATION.

- Optic pit: The optic disc has a small defect (a pit) in the nerve tissue. A serous RD may be present, contiguous with the optic disc. See 11.34, OPTIC PIT.

- Macular detachment as a result of an RRD or macular hole: In RRD, a hole in the retina can be found. See 11.3, RETINAL DETACHMENT and 11.25, VITREOMACULAR ADHESION (VMA)/VITREOMACULAR TRACTION (VMT)/ MACULAR HOLE.

- Choroidal tumor, particularly choroidal hemangioma: See 11.36, CHOROIDAL NEVUS AND MALIGNANT MELANOMA OF THE CHOROID.

- Hypertension: See 11.10, HYPERTENSIVE RETINOPATHY.

- Pigment epithelial detachment (PED): The margins of a PED are more distinct than those of CSCR, and the RPE is elevated. Occasionally, PED may accompany CSCR or AMD.

- Others: Idiopathic choroidal effusion, inflammatory choroidal disorders, and chronic renal failure.

Etiology

- Idiopathic: Most common in young adult to middle-aged men. In women, CSCR has an association with pregnancy. Increased incidence in patients with lupus.

- Increased endogenous cortisol: This might explain a possible association with psychological or physiologic stress (type A personality). Rare cases exist with cortisol producing adrenal adenomas or Cushing syndrome.

- Exogenous cortisol: Corticosteroid use, including nasal corticosteroid sprays and topical creams.

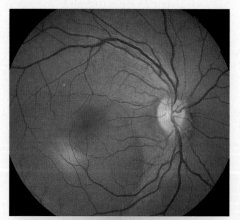

Figure 11.15.1 Central serous chorioretinopathy.

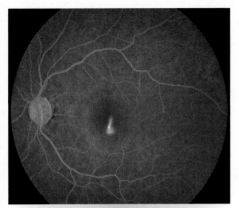

Figure 11.15.2 Intravenous fluorescein angiography of central serous chorioretinopathy showing "smoke-stack" pattern of dye leakage.

Workup

1. Amsler grid test to document the area of field involved. See Appendix 4, AMSLER GRID.
2. Slit lamp examination of the macula with a fundus contact, Hruby, or 60- or 90-diopter lens to rule out concomitant CNV. In addition, search for an optic pit of the disc.
3. Dilated fundus examination with indirect ophthalmoscopy to rule out a choroidal tumor or RRD.
4. OCT is helpful in demonstrating subretinal fluid or PEDs and for monitoring purposes. Enhanced-depth imaging OCT often demonstrates choroidal thickening and may be a useful adjunct in diagnosis **(see Figures 11.15.2** and **11.15.3)**.
5. IVFA and ICGA if the diagnosis is uncertain or presentation atypical, CNV is suspected, or laser treatment is to be considered. IVFA shows the nearly pathognomonic "smoke-stack" pattern of dye leakage in 10% to 20% of cases. ICGA shows choroidal artery and choriocapillaris filling delays and characteristic multifocal hyperfluorescent patches in the early phase.
6. In cases of chronic CSCR, a systemic workup including cortisol levels and renal function should be considered.

Treatment

1. Observation: Acute CSCR is usually self-limited with good visual prognosis. Worse prognosis for patients with recurrent disease, multiple areas of detachment, or prolonged course.
2. Stop corticosteroids, if possible, including topical skin and nasal spray preparations.
3. Laser photocoagulation: May accelerate visual recovery, but long-term benefit and safety are unclear. May increase risk of CNV formation. Given the CNV risk, use low laser intensity. Consider laser for:
   - Persistence of a serous detachment for several months.
   - Recurrence of the condition in an eye that sustained a permanent visual deficit from a previous episode.

11

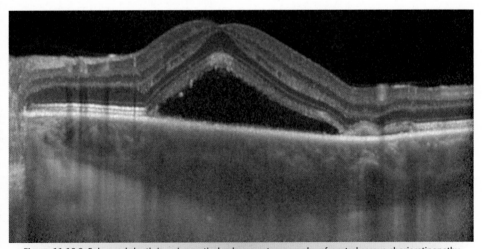

Figure 11.15.3 Enhanced-depth imaging optical coherence tomography of central serous chorioretinopathy showing subretinal fluid and choroidal thickening.

- Occurrence in the contralateral eye after a permanent visual deficit resulted from a previous episode.
- Patient requires prompt restoration of vision (e.g., occupational necessity).

4. Photodynamic therapy (PDT): May be helpful for chronic CSCR. Half-dose PDT may be considered for rapid SRF resolution in patients with acute CSCR.

5. Mineralocorticoid receptor antagonists: Eplerenone and spironolactone have been associated with improved anatomic and visual outcomes in chronic CSCR.
6. If CNV develops, consider anti-VEGF therapy.

Follow Up

1. Examine patients every 6 to 8 weeks until resolution.

11.16 Nonexudative (Dry) Age-Related Macular Degeneration

Symptoms

Gradual loss of central vision, Amsler grid changes; may be asymptomatic.

Signs

(See Figures 11.16.1 and 11.16.2.)

Critical. Macular drusen, clumps of pigment in the outer retina, and RPE atrophy, almost always in both eyes.

Other. Confluent retinal and choriocapillaris atrophy (e.g., geographic atrophy), dystrophic calcification.

Differential Diagnosis

- Peripheral drusen: Drusen only located outside of the macular area.

- Myopic degeneration: Characteristic peripapillary changes and macular changes without drusen. See 11.22, HIGH MYOPIA.
- CSCR: Serous retinal elevation, RPE detachments, and mottled RPE, without drusen, hemorrhage, or exudate, usually in patients <50 years of age. See 11.15, CENTRAL SEROUS CHORIORETINOPATHY.
- Inherited central retinal dystrophies: Stargardt disease, pattern dystrophy, Best disease, others. Variable macular pigmentary changes, atrophy, or accumulation of lipofuscin or a combination of these. Usually <50 years, without drusen, familial occurrence. See specific entities.
- Toxic retinopathies (e.g., chloroquine toxicity): Mottled hypopigmentation with ring of hyperpigmentation (bull's eye maculopathy) without drusen. Possible history of drug ingestion or exposure.

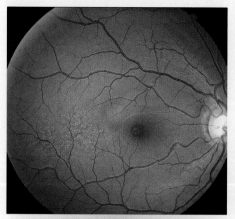

Figure 11.16.1 Dry AMD with fine drusen.

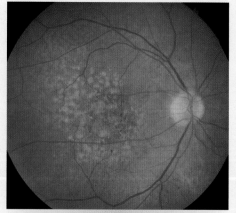

Figure 11.16.2 Dry AMD with soft drusen.

- Inflammatory maculopathies: Multifocal choroiditis, rubella, serpiginous choroidopathy, and others. Variable chorioretinal atrophy, often with vitreous cells and without drusen. See specific entities.

Workup

1. History: Presence of risk factors (e.g., family history, smoking)? See risk factors for loss of vision, 11.17, NEOVASCULAR OR EXUDATIVE (WET) AGE-RELATED MACULAR DEGENERATION.
2. Amsler grid or preferential hyperacuity perimetry (PHP) testing at home to detect central or paracentral scotoma potentially indicative of neovascular transformation. See Appendix 4, AMSLER GRID.
3. Macular examination with a 60- or 90-diopter or a fundus contact lens: Look for risk factors for conversion to the exudative form, such as soft drusen or pigment clumping. Look for geographic atrophy. Look for signs of the exudative form such as edema, SRF, lipid exudation, or hemorrhage (disappearance of drusen may herald the development of CNV).
4. Baseline and periodic FAF may be useful to monitor for progression, particularly geographic atrophy.
5. IVFA or OCT when exudative AMD is suspected based on subjective or objective change in vision or examination findings. Drusen and RPE atrophy are often more visible on IVFA and FAF. OCTA is also a potentially useful diagnostic test as a noninvasive substitute for IVFA or if IVFA is inconclusive, especially with masquerade conditions such as pattern dystrophy or CSCR.

Treatment

Patients with intermediate dry AMD (one large druse [125 microns] and/or ≥20 medium drusen [63 to 125 microns]), or advanced dry or exudative AMD in one eye but not the other eye, are at high risk for development of advanced stages of AMD. The original Age-Related Eye Disease Study (AREDS) report demonstrated that treatment with a vitamin/mineral formula consisting of vitamin C (500 mg), vitamin E (400 IU), beta-carotene (15 mg), zinc (80 mg), and cupric oxide (5 mg) reduces the risk of progression to advanced AMD by approximately 25% over 5 years and reduces the risk of vision loss caused by advanced AMD by approximately 19% by 5 years. A second study (AREDS2) evaluated the role of increased intake of different carotenoids (lutein and zeaxanthin) as well as two specific omega-3 long-chain polyunsaturated fatty acids (docosahexaenoic acid [DHA] + eicosapentaenoic acid [EPA]). The addition of lutein + zeaxanthin, DHA + EPA, or both to the original AREDS formulation did not further reduce risk of progression to advanced AMD but was found to be equally effective.

NOTE: Beta-carotene (in the original AREDS formula) should be withheld in past or present smokers because of increased risk of lung cancer. The AREDS2 formulation (with lutein + zeaxanthin) is preferred as it does not contain beta-carotene.

In addition, recommend consumption of green leafy vegetables if approved by a primary care physician (intake of vitamin K decreases effectiveness of warfarin) and foods containing high levels of omega-3 fatty acids such as cold water fish and nuts.

1. Low-vision aids may benefit some patients with bilateral loss of macular function.
2. Refer to an internist for management of presumed risk factors: HTN, hypercholesterolemia, smoking cessation, etc.
3. Those at high risk for progressing to exudative AMD may benefit from home monitoring technology for earlier detection such as the PHP ForseeHome device. Early detection of CNV increases the likelihood of better visual acuity results after intravitreal anti-VEGF therapy is initiated.
4. Certain genetic mutations confer an increased risk for AMD (e.g., polymorphisms of complement factor H and ARMS2 genes). This may or may not influence response to treatment and so, at this time, genetic screening in AMD patients is not routinely performed.

Follow Up

Every 6 to 12 months, watching for signs of the exudative form. Daily use of Amsler grid or PHP device with instructions to return promptly if a change is noted.

REFERENCES

Age-Related Eye Disease Study Research Group. A randomized, placebo-controlled, clinical trial of high-dose supplementation with vitamins C and E, beta-carotene, and zinc for age-related macular degeneration and vision loss: AREDS report no. 8. *Arch Ophthalmol.* 2001;119:1417-1436.

The Age-Related Eye Disease Study 2 (AREDS2) Research Group. Lutein + zeaxanthin and omega-3 fatty acids for age-related macular degeneration: The age-related eye disease study 2 (AREDS2) randomized clinical trial. *J Am Med Assoc.* 2013;309(19):2005-2015.

AREDS2-HOME Study Research Group; Chew EY, Clemons TE, et al. Randomized trial of a home monitoring system for early detection of choroidal neovascularization home monitoring of the Eye (HOME) study. AREDS2-HOME Study. *Ophthalmology.* 2014;121(2):535-544.

11.17 Neovascular or Exudative (Wet) Age-Related Macular Degeneration

Symptoms

Variable onset of central visual loss, central or paracentral scotoma, metamorphopsia, photopsias in the central visual field.

Signs

(See Figures 11.17.1 and 11.17.2.)

Critical. Drusen and SRF, ME or RPE detachment associated with CNV.

Other. Subretinal or intraretinal blood. Retinal exudates, subretinal fibrosis (disciform scar). Retinal angiomatous proliferation (RAP) is an intraretinal variant of neovascular AMD and is characterized by focal telangiectatic retinal vessels with an adjacent superficial retinal hemorrhage and associated intraretinal edema and RPE detachment. Some neovascular AMD patients may present with VH.

Risk Factors for Loss of Vision

Advanced age, hyperopia, blue eyes, family history, soft (large) drusen, focal subretinal pigment clumping, RPE detachments, systemic HTN, and smoking. Note that patients with wet AMD in one eye have a 10% to 12% risk per year of developing CNV in the fellow eye. The risk increases for eyes with multiple or confluent soft drusen with RPE clumping.

Differential Diagnosis

- Ocular histoplasmosis syndrome: Small white-yellow chorioretinal scars and peripapillary atrophy. May also present with CNV. See 11.24, OCULAR HISTOPLASMOSIS.
- Angioid streaks: Bilateral subretinal red-brown or gray irregular bands often radiating from the optic disc. See 11.23, ANGIOID STREAKS.

11

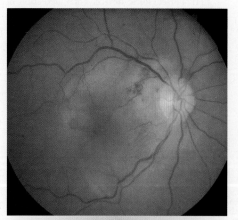

Figure 11.17.1 Exudative AMD.

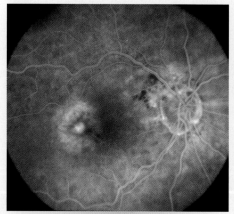

Figure 11.17.2 Intravenous fluorescein angiography of exudative AMD.

- High myopia: Significant myopic refractive error, lacquer cracks, tilted disc. See 11.22, HIGH MYOPIA.
- Idiopathic polypoidal choroidal vasculopathy (IPCV): Multiple serosanguineous macular and RPE detachments. ICGA highlights characteristic choroidal polyp-like aneurysmal dilations most often located in the peripapillary region. This is considered a variant of neovascular AMD and is more common in those of Asian and African descent. See 11.18, IDIOPATHIC POLYPOIDAL CHOROIDAL VASCULOPATHY (POSTERIOR UVEAL BLEEDING SYNDROME).
- Other CNV-predisposing conditions include drusen of the optic nerve, choroidal rupture, choroidal tumors, photocoagulation scars, inflammatory focal chorioretinal spots, and idiopathic causes.

Types of Neovascular AMD Lesions

- Occult CNV (Type 1): Ill-defined, stippled, flat, or elevated subtle late leakage on IVFA and located in the sub-RPE location by OCT.
- Classic CNV (Type 2): Early-phase IVFA demonstrates a well-delineated area of lacy hyperfluorescence with prominent leakage in later phases and located in the subneurosensory retinal location by OCT.
- RAP (Type 3): Focal intraretinal hyperfluorescence on IVFA and ICGA. High-speed ICGA is particularly sensitive and may show characteristic "hair pin loop" with retinal feeder and draining vessels. OCTA shows this focal form of neovascularization to be intraretinal.

Workup

1. Slit lamp biomicroscopy with a 60-, 90-diopter, or fundus contact lens to detect CNV and associated exudation. Must examine both eyes.
2. Perform IVFA or OCTA if CNV is suspected. IVFA is useful to confirm neovascular AMD size, type, and location. OCTA is useful as a noninvasive alternative to IVFA or when IVFA is inconclusive such as in pattern dystrophy or central CSCR. OCTA is also useful if there is an allergy to fluorescein dye or in pregnancy when it is best to avoid dye use.

3. OCT is helpful in determining retinal thickness, CNV thickness, location, and extent of ME, SRF, and RPE detachment. OCT is the primary modality for following response to treatment.
4. ICGA may help delineate the borders of certain obscured occult CNV, particularly with subretinal blood or exudation. It also shows RAP and IPCV lesions better than IVFA.

Treatment

- Ranibizumab: Anti-VEGF antibody fragment injected intravitreally that is FDA-approved for all CNV subtypes. In the original phase 3 efficacy trials (MARINA and ANCHOR), ranibizumab was given monthly to patients, with close to 40% of patients in both studies gaining three or more lines of visual acuity at 1 year. While the best visual results may occur with monthly dosing, PRN or treat-and-extend (TAE) individualized dosing regimens may yield similar visual results with less frequent injections.
- Aflibercept: Anti-VEGF fusion protein that binds all isoforms of VEGF-A and placental growth factor. FDA-approved as intravitreal injection for the treatment of neovascular AMD. Phase 3 VIEW studies showed similar efficacy at 1 year to monthly intravitreal ranibizumab with aflibercept dosed q8 weeks after a 12-week monthly induction phase.
- Bevacizumab: Full-length anti-VEGF antibody. Originally FDA-approved for systemic administration to treat colon cancer. Off-label use as intravitreal injection at a dose of 1.25 mg is effective in treating neovascular AMD. It is cost-effective and commonly used in clinical practice. The Comparison of Age-Related Macular Degeneration Treatments Trial (CATT) study demonstrated the noninferiority of bevacizumab as compared to ranibizumab at 1 year.
- Brolicizumab: Single-chain humanized anti-VEGF antibody fragment that binds all isoforms of VEGF-A. FDA-approved as intravitreal injection for the treatment of neovascular AMD. Phase 3 studies when dosed at q8 or q12 week intervals based on disease activity demonstrated the noninferiority of brolicizumab as compared to aflibercept dosed at q8 week intervals at 1 year after a

11

12-week monthly induction phase (HAWK and HARRIER).

- PDT: FDA-approved intravenous infusion of photosensitizing dye (verteporfin) followed by nondestructive (cold) laser application to activate the dye within the CNV. PDT can be performed as often as every 3 months for 1 to 2 years. Small, classic subfoveal CNV responds best, but small occult or minimally classic subfoveal CNV may also respond. PDT decreases vision loss but does not improve vision as monotherapy. Now rarely used.

- Thermal laser photocoagulation: Results are best for extrafoveal CNV (≥200 mm from fovea) or peripapillary CNV. Laser photocoagulation treatment is complicated by high CNV recurrence rates. Uncommonly used.

Follow Up

Depends on the treatment algorithm used, but typically monthly follow up until the CNV lesion is inactive with resolution of exudative signs based on examination and OCT. Patients receiving anti-VEGF therapy need indefinite follow up, though the follow-up frequency depends on treatment response and treatment algorithm, for example, as needed (PRN) versus TAE. Patients receiving intravitreal injections should be given warning symptoms for endophthalmitis and RD.

REFERENCES

Rosenfeld PJ, Brown DM, Heier JS, et al. Ranibizumab for neovascular age-related macular degeneration. *N Engl J Med.* 2006;355:1419-1431.

Lalwani GA, Rosenfeld PJ, Fung AE, et al. A variable-dosing regimen with intravitreal ranibizumab for neovascular age-related macular degeneration: year 2 of the PrONTO Study. *Am J Ophthalmol.* 2009;148(1):43-58.

The CATT Research Group. Ranibizumab and bevacizumab for neovascular age-related macular degeneration. *N Engl J Med.* 2011;364:1897-1908.

Heier JS, Brown DM, Chong V. Intravitreal aflibercept (VEGF trap-eye) in wet age-related macular degeneration. *Ophthalmology.* 2012;119:2537-2548.

Dugel, PU, Koh A, Ogura Y, et al. HAWK and HARRIER: phase 3, multicenter, randomized, double-masked trials of brolucizumab for neovascular age-related macular degeneration. *Ophthalmology.* 2020;127(1):72-84.

11.18 Idiopathic Polypoidal Choroidal Vasculopathy

Symptoms

Decreased central vision; may be sudden or gradual.

Signs

Critical. Subretinal red-orange, polyp-like lesions of the choroidal vasculature. Can be macular (more symptomatic) or peripapillary **(see Figure 11.18.1)**.

Other. Bilateral subretinal and/or sub-RPE blood, VH, circinate subretinal exudates, subretinal fibrosis (disciform scar), SRF, atypical CNV, and multiple serous PEDs.

Risk Factors

More common in females, individuals of African or Asian descent, and in patients with HTN. Can occur at a younger age compared to neovascular AMD, but usually without significant drusen or geographic atrophy.

Differential Diagnosis

- See 11.17, NEOVASCULAR OR EXUDATIVE (WET) AGE-RELATED MACULAR DEGENERATION.

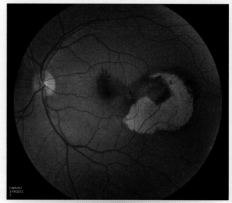

Figure 11.18.1 Polypoidal choroidal vasculopathy OS.

- See 11.19, RETINAL ARTERIAL MACROANEURYSM.
- Peripheral exudative hemorrhagic chorioretinopathy (PEHCR [peripheral CNV]): Occurs in the peripheral retina and presents with subretinal fluid, subretinal blood, exudation, RPE detachment, and/or subretinal fibrosis.

Workup

1. Slit lamp biomicroscopy with a 60-, 90-diopter, or fundus contact lens to detect signs of exudation.
2. ICGA is the gold standard for diagnosis. ICGA is used to confirm the presence of a branching network of vessels arising from the inner choroidal circulation with terminal aneurysmal dilations (popcorn lesions). Unlike occult CNV, the IPCV lesions do not stain late unless active leakage is present.
3. IVFA is performed to evaluate for other causes of CNV.
4. OCT is used to assess for ME, SRF, and PEDs and can detect polyps in some eyes.

Treatment

Asymptomatic lesions may be observed and may resolve spontaneously. IPCV with exudation and/or hemorrhagic complications has been treated with anti-VEGF monotherapy, PDT, or a combination. The EVEREST-II and PLANET studies demonstrated level I evidence that anti-VEGF monotherapy as well as combination therapy give excellent functional visual outcomes in patients presenting with symptomatic IPCV. Thermal laser photocoagulation, feeder vessel treatment, and pneumatic displacement of large submacular hemorrhage have also been used with varying success.

Follow Up

The prognosis of IPCV is generally better than for neovascular AMD. Symptomatic or macular IPCV is followed every 1 to 2 months with periodic OCT, IVFA, and ICGA as needed for disease progression. Consider treatment, or retreatment, if symptomatic, persistent, or new leakage occurs.

REFERENCES

Cheung CMG, Lai TYY, Ruamviboonsuk P, et al. Polypoidal choroidal vasculopathy: definition, pathogenesis, diagnosis, and management. *Ophthalmology*. 2018;125(5):708-724.

Koh A, Lai TYY, Takahashi K, et al. Efficacy and safety of ranibizumab with or without verteporfin photodynamic therapy for polypoidal choroidal vasculopathy: a randomized clinical trial. *JAMA Ophthalmol*. 2017;135:1206-1213.

11.19 Retinal Arterial Macroaneurysm

11

Symptoms

Decreased vision; history of systemic HTN. Usually unilateral, but 10% bilateral.

Signs

(See Figures 11.19.1 and 11.19.2.)

Critical. Acute hemorrhages in multiple layers of the retina (subretinal, intraretinal, preretinal) possibly with VH; often with a white or yellow spot in the middle of the retinal arterial macroaneurysm (RAM). Chronic leakage may cause a ring of hard exudates and retinal edema around the aneurysm resulting in decreased vision if the macula is involved.

Other. ME, arteriolar emboli, capillary telangiectasia, arterial or venous occlusions distal to macroaneurysm.

Differential Diagnosis

- Coats disease: Unilateral retinal vascular telangiectasias. Extensive yellow intraretinal and subretinal exudates. Hemorrhages not typical. See 8.1, LEUKOCORIA.
- Idiopathic retinal vasculitis, aneurysms, and neuroretinitis: A syndrome characterized by retinal vasculitis, multiple arterial macroaneurysms, neuroretinitis, and peripheral capillary nonperfusion.
- Diabetic retinopathy: Hemorrhages are not subretinal. See 11.12, DIABETIC RETINOPATHY.
- Valsalva retinopathy: No associated hard exudates. See 11.21, VALSALVA RETINOPATHY.
- Retinal telangiectasias: Juxtafoveal or parafoveal retinal telangiectasias can cause hard exudates in a circinate pattern usually temporal to macula. Association with diabetes.

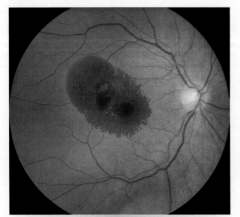

Figure 11.19.1 Retinal artery macroaneurysm on presentation.

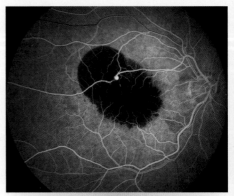

Figure 11.19.2 Intravenous fluorescein angiography of a retinal artery macroaneurysm.

- Others: Retinal capillary hemangioma (hemangioblastoma), retinal cavernous hemangioma, choroidal melanoma, hemorrhagic RPE detachment seen in AMD, IPCV, etc.

Etiology

Acquired vascular dilation of retinal artery or arteriole usually at the site of arteriolar bifurcation or arteriovenous crossing. Usually related to systemic HTN and general atherosclerotic disease.

Workup

1. History: Systemic disease, particularly HTN or diabetes?
2. Complete ocular examination with dilated retinal examination with a 60- or 90-diopter lens and indirect ophthalmoscopy. Look for concurrent retinal venous obstruction (present in one-third of cases) and signs of hypertensive retinopathy (visible in fellow eye as well).
3. Check blood pressure.

4. Consider checking lipid panel as well as fasting or random blood sugar and hemoglobin A1c.
5. IVFA may demonstrate early hyperfluorescence if there is no blockage from hemorrhage. Late frames may show leakage or staining of vessel wall.
6. OCT is helpful in demonstrating and following any ME.

Treatment

Consider laser treatment if edema and/or exudate threatens central vision. Caution must be taken when treating arterioles that supply the central macula since distal thrombosis and obstruction with resultant ischemia can occur. Laser can also cause aneurysmal rupture resulting in retinal and vitreous hemorrhage. Anti-VEGF agents may be beneficial in patients with macroaneurysm-associated ME. Dense or nonclearing vitreous hemorrhage, sub–internal limiting membrane (ILM) hemorrhage, or thick submacular hemorrhage may benefit from vitrectomy.

Follow Up

Frequency based on the amount and location of exudate and hemorrhage.

11.20 Sickle Cell Retinopathy (Including Sickle Cell Disease, Anemia, and Trait)

Symptoms

Usually without ocular symptoms. Floaters, flashing lights, or loss of vision with advanced disease.

Systemically, patients often have painful crises with severe abdominal or musculoskeletal pain. Patients are typically of African or Mediterranean descent.

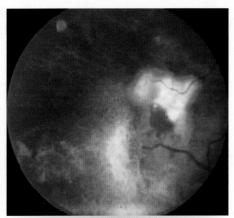

Figure 11.20.1 Sickle cell retinopathy neovascular sea fan with associated vitreous hemorrhage.

Signs

(See Figure 11.20.1.)

Critical. Peripheral retinal neovascularization in the shape of a fan ("sea fan sign"), sclerosed peripheral retinal vessels, or a dull gray peripheral fundus background color as a result of peripheral arteriolar occlusions and ischemia.

Other. Venous tortuosity, midperipheral fundus pigmented lesions with spiculated borders (black sunbursts), superficial intraretinal hemorrhages (salmon patch), refractile (iridescent) intraretinal deposits following hemorrhage resorption, angioid streaks, comma-shaped capillaries of the conjunctiva (especially along the inferior fornix). VH and traction bands, RD, CRAO, macular arteriolar occlusions, and enlargement of the foveal avascular zone occasionally develop.

Staging

- Stage 1: Peripheral arteriolar occlusions.
- Stage 2: Peripheral arteriovenous anastomoses.
- Stage 3: Neovascular proliferation.
- Stage 4: VH.
- Stage 5: RD.

Differential Diagnosis of Peripheral Retinal Neovascularization

- Sarcoidosis: Peripheral sea fan neovascularization often associated with uveitis. Increased frequency in young patients of African descent. See 12.6, SARCOIDOSIS.

- Diabetic retinopathy: Posterior pathology more prominent. Associated dot-blot hemorrhages. See 11.12, DIABETIC RETINOPATHY.
- Embolic (e.g., talc) retinopathy: History of intravenous drug abuse. May see refractile talc particles in macular arterioles. See 11.33, CRYSTALLINE RETINOPATHY.
- Eales disease: Peripheral retinal vascular occlusion of unknown etiology; diagnosis of exclusion.
- Others: Retinopathy of prematurity, FEVR, chronic myelogenous leukemia, radiation retinopathy, pars planitis, carotid–cavernous fistula, OIS, collagen vascular disease, hypercoagulable state. See specific sections.

Workup

1. Medical history and family history: Sickle cell disease, diabetes, or known medical problems? Intravenous drug abuse?
2. Dilated fundus examination using indirect ophthalmoscopy.
3. Sickledex, sickle cell preparation, and hemoglobin electrophoresis.

NOTE: Patients with sickle cell trait (i.e., HbSC), as well as hemoglobin C disease, may have a negative Sickledex preparation. Retinopathy is most common with HbSC (most severe) and HbS-Thal and less common with HbSS (sickle cell disease).

1. Consider IVFA (particularly widefield) to aid in diagnostic and therapeutic considerations.

Treatment

There are no well-established indications or guidelines for treatment. Isolated retinal neovascularization itself does not require treatment, as there may be a high probability of autoinfarction. Neovascularization with associated VH should receive PRP to the avascular area (anterior to the neovascularization). RD and VH may be best treated with vitrectomy. Anti-VEGF agents may be beneficial, but caution should be used in cases with significant traction.

Follow Up

1. No retinopathy: Annual dilated fundus examinations.
2. Retinopathy present: Repeat dilated fundus examination every 3 to 6 months, depending on severity.

11

11.21 Valsalva Retinopathy

Symptoms

Decreased vision or asymptomatic. History of Valsalva maneuver (forceful exhalation against a closed glottis), which may occur during heavy lifting, coughing, vomiting, or straining during bowel movement. Sometimes, no history of Valsalva can be elicited.

Signs

(See Figure 11.21.1.)

Critical. Single or multiple hemorrhages under the ILM in the area of the macula. Can be unilateral or bilateral. Blood may turn yellow after a few days.

Other. Vitreous, intraretinal, subretinal, and subconjunctival hemorrhage can occur.

Differential Diagnosis

- PVD: Can cause VH acutely as well as peripheral retinal and disc margin hemorrhages. However, sub-ILM hemorrhage is rare. See 11.1, POSTERIOR VITREOUS DETACHMENT.
- RAM: Hemorrhages in multiple layers of the retina and vitreous. Can also have a circinate ring of hard exudates around a macroaneurysm. See 11.19, RETINAL ARTERIAL MACROANEURYSM.
- Diabetic retinopathy: Microaneurysms, dot-blot hemorrhages, and hard exudates bilaterally. No isolated sub-ILM hemorrhage.

Can also cause VH. See 11.12, DIABETIC RETINOPATHY.

- CRVO or BRVO: Unilateral, multiple intra-retinal hemorrhages, venous dilation, and tortuosity. See 11.8, CENTRAL RETINAL VEIN OCCLUSION and 11.9, BRANCH RETINAL VEIN OCCLUSION.
- Anemia or leukemia: May have multiple, bilateral flame and dot-blot hemorrhages as well as CWSs. Can also present with sub-ILM hemorrhage.
- RT: Can be surrounded by hemorrhage obscuring the tear. Tears rarely occur in the macula.

Etiology

Valsalva causes sudden increase in intraocular venous pressure leading to rupture of superficial capillaries in macula or elsewhere in the retina. May be associated with anticoagulant therapy.

Workup

1. History: History of Valsalva including any recent heavy lifting, straining during bowel movement, coughing, sneezing, vomiting, etc.? The patient may not remember the incident.
2. Complete ocular examination, including dilated retinal examination with a slit lamp and a 60- or 90-diopter lens, and indirect ophthalmoscopy. Look for findings suggestive of a different etiology including microaneurysms, dot-blot hemorrhages, CWSs, RT, PVD.
3. If dense VH is present, perform a B-scan US to rule out RT or RD.
4. IVFA may be helpful to rule out other causes including RAM or diabetic retinopathy.

Treatment

Prognosis is excellent. Most patients are observed, as sub-ILM hemorrhage usually resolves after a few days to weeks. Occasionally laser is used to permit the blood to drain into the vitreous cavity, thereby uncovering the macula. Vitrectomy rarely considered, typically only for nonclearing VH.

Follow Up

May follow up every 2 weeks for the initial visits to monitor for resolution, then follow up routinely.

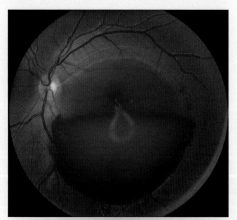
Figure 11.21.1 Valsalva retinopathy.

11

11.22 Pathologic/Degenerative Myopia

Symptoms

Decreased vision. Usually asymptomatic until middle adulthood.

Signs

(See Figure 11.22.1.)

Critical. Myopic crescent (a crescent-shaped area of white sclera or choroidal vessels adjacent to the disc, separated from the normal-appearing fundus by a hyperpigmented line); an oblique (tilted) insertion of the optic disc, with or without vertical elongation. Macular pigmentary abnormalities; hyperpigmented spots in the macula (Fuchs spots). Typically, a refractive correction of more than −6.00 diopters, axial length ≥26.5 mm.

Other. Risk for CNV or RRD. Temporal optic disc pallor, posterior staphyloma, entrance of the retinal vessels into the nasal part of the optic cup. The retina and choroid may be seen to extend over the nasal border of the optic disc. Well-circumscribed areas of atrophy, spots of subretinal hemorrhage, choroidal sclerosis, yellow subretinal streaks (lacquer cracks), peripheral retinal thinning, and lattice degeneration may occur. Visual field defects may be present.

Differential Diagnosis

- AMD: May develop CNV and a similar macular appearance, but typically are drusen present, and myopic disc features are absent. See 11.16, NONEXUDATIVE (DRY) AGE-RELATED MACULAR DEGENERATION and 11.17, NEOVASCULAR OR EXUDATIVE (WET) AGE-RELATED MACULAR DEGENERATION.

- Ocular histoplasmosis: Peripapillary atrophy with risk for CNV. A pigmented ring may separate the disc from the peripapillary atrophy, as opposed to a pigmented ring separating the atrophic area from the adjacent retina. Round choroidal scars (punched-out lesions) are scattered throughout the fundus. See 11.24, OCULAR HISTOPLASMOSIS.

- Tilted discs: Anomalous discs with a scleral crescent, most often inferonasally, an irregular vascular pattern as the vessels emerge from the disc (situs inversus), and an area of fundus ectasia in the direction of the tilt (inferonasally). Many patients have myopia and astigmatism but no chorioretinal degeneration or lacquer cracks. Visual field defects corresponding to the areas of fundus ectasia are often seen. Most cases are bilateral.

- Gyrate atrophy: Rare. Multiple, well-demarcated areas of chorioretinal atrophy that in childhood start in the midperiphery and then coalesce to involve a large portion of the fundus. Increased blood levels of ornithine. Patients are often highly myopic. See 11.28, RETINITIS PIGMENTOSA AND INHERITED CHORIORETINAL DYSTROPHIES.

- Toxoplasmosis: Well-circumscribed chorioretinal scar that does not typically develop CNV. Active disease shows retinitis and vitritis. See 12.5, TOXOPLASMOSIS.

Workup

1. Manifest and/or cycloplegic refraction.
2. IOP measurement by applanation tonometry (Schiøtz or Tono-pen tonometry may underestimate IOP in highly myopic eyes).
3. Dilated retinal examination with indirect ophthalmoscopy to search for retinal breaks or detachment. Scleral depression may be helpful but should be performed with care over a staphyloma.
4. Slit lamp biomicroscopy with a 60-, 90-diopter, or fundus contact lens to examine macula and search for CNV (gray or green

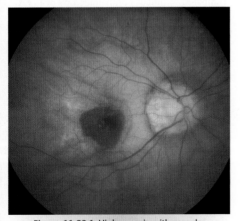

Figure 11.22.1 High myopia with macular hemorrhage.

11

lesion beneath the retina, subretinal blood or exudate, or SRF).

5. IVFA for suspected CNV.

6. OCT can reveal CNV as well as macular detachment over a staphyloma. Additionally, OCT can be useful in identifying foveal schisis, a possible cause of vision loss in patients with high myopia.

Treatment

1. Symptomatic retinal breaks are treated with laser photocoagulation, cryotherapy, or scleral buckling surgery. Treatment of asymptomatic retinal breaks may be considered when there is no surrounding pigmentation or demarcation line.

2. Anti-VEGF agents are used for CNV due to high myopia. Laser photocoagulation therapy may be considered for extrafoveal or juxtafoveal CNV within several days of obtaining an IVFA, but is seldom performed. See 11.17, Neovascular or Exudative (Wet) Age-Related Macular Degeneration.

3. For glaucoma suspects, a single visual field often cannot distinguish myopic visual field loss from early glaucoma. Progression of visual field loss in the absence of progressive myopia, however, suggests the presence of glaucoma and the need for therapy. See 9.1, Primary Open Angle Glaucoma.

4. Recommend one-piece polycarbonate safety goggles for sports because of increased risk of choroidal rupture from minor trauma.

Follow Up

In the absence of complications, reexamine every 6 to 12 months, watching for the related disorders discussed above.

11.23 | Angioid Streaks

Symptoms

Usually asymptomatic. Decreased vision may result from CNV.

Signs

(See Figure 11.23.1.)

Critical. Bilateral reddish-brown or gray bands located deep to the retina, due to breaks within Bruch membrane, usually radiating in an irregular or spoke-like pattern from the optic disc. CNV may occur.

Other. Mottled fundus appearance with an orange hue (peau d'orange), most common in the temporal midperiphery. Subretinal hemorrhages after mild blunt trauma. Reticular pigmentary changes in the macula; small, white, pinpoint chorioretinal scars (histo-like spots) in the midperiphery; crystalline bodies within the macula. Drusen of the optic disc (especially with pseudoxanthoma elasticum [PXE]). Granular pattern of hyperfluorescent lines on IVFA. Widespread RPE damage is more evident on FAF compared to fundus ophthalmoscopy or IVFA.

Differential Diagnosis

• Lacquer cracks of myopic chorioretinal degeneration: High myopia present. See 11.22, High Myopia.

• Choroidal rupture: Subretinal streaks are usually concentric to the optic disc, yellow-white in color. See 3.18, Traumatic Choroidal Rupture.

Etiology

Fifty percent of cases are associated with systemic diseases; the rest are idiopathic.

• PXE: Most common. Loose skin folds in the neck, axillae, and on flexor aspects of joints; cardiovascular complications; increased risk of gastrointestinal bleeds.

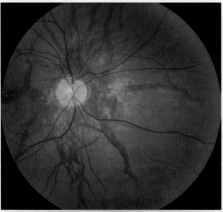
Figure 11.23.1 Angioid streaks.

- Ehlers–Danlos syndrome: Hyperelasticity of skin, loose joints.
- Paget disease of bone: Enlarged skull, bone pain, history of bone fractures, hearing loss, possible cardiovascular complications. May be asymptomatic but may develop visual loss due to optic nerve compression by enlarging bone. Increased serum alkaline phosphatase and urine calcium. Ten percent develop late angioid streaks.
- Sickle cell disease: May be asymptomatic or have decreased vision from fundus abnormalities. May have a history of recurrent infections and painless or painful crises. See 11.20, SICKLE CELL RETINOPATHY (INCLUDING SICKLE CELL DISEASE, ANEMIA, SICKLE AND TRAIT).
- Less common: Thalassemia, acromegaly, senile elastosis, lead poisoning, Marfan syndrome, hemolytic anemia, and others.

Workup

1. History: Any known systemic disorders? Previous ocular trauma?
2. Complete ocular examination: Look carefully at the macula with a slit lamp using a 60-, 90-diopter, or fundus contact lens to detect CNV.
3. FAF if diagnosis uncertain or IVFA or OCTA if CNV suspected.

4. Physical examination: Look for clinical signs of etiologic diseases.
5. Serum alkaline phosphatase and urine calcium levels if Paget disease of bone is suspected.
6. Sickle cell preparation and hemoglobin electrophoresis in patients of African descent.
7. Skin or scar biopsy if PXE is suspected.
8. CBC if hematologic etiology suspected.

Treatment

1. Anti-VEGF therapy is now used for angioid streak-associated CNV, as focal laser photocoagulation and PDT have discouraging outcomes. See 11.17, NEOVASCULAR OR EXUDATIVE (WET) AGE-RELATED MACULAR DEGENERATION.
2. Management of any underlying systemic disease by an internist.
3. Recommend wearing one-piece polycarbonate safety glasses for sports due to an increased risk of subretinal hemorrhage and choroidal rupture from minor trauma.

Follow Up

1. Fundus examination every 6 months, monitoring for CNV.
2. Instruct patient to check Amsler grid daily and return immediately if changes are noted. See Appendix 4, AMSLER GRID.

11

11.24 Ocular Histoplasmosis

Symptoms

Most often asymptomatic; can present with decreased or distorted vision, especially when CNV develops. Patients often have lived in or visited the Ohio–Mississippi River Valley or areas where histoplasmosis is endemic. Usually in the 20- to 50-year age range.

Signs

(See Figure 11.24.1.)

Critical. Classic triad. Need two of the three to make the diagnosis:

1. Yellow-white, punched-out round spots, chorioretinal scars, usually <1 mm in diameter in any fundus location (histo-spots). Pigment clumps in or at the margin of the spots may be seen.

2. A macular CNV appearing as a gray-green patch beneath the retina, associated with retinal edema, SRF, subretinal blood or exudate, or a pigment ring evolving into a disciform scar.
3. Peripapillary atrophy or scarring, sometimes with nodules or hemorrhage. There may be a rim of pigment separating the disc from the area of atrophy or scarring.

Other. Curvilinear rows of small histo-spots in the peripheral fundus. No vitreous or aqueous cells.

Differential Diagnosis

- Multifocal choroiditis with panuveitis: Similar clinical findings, except anterior or vitreous inflammatory cells or both, are also present. See 12.3, POSTERIOR UVEITIS.

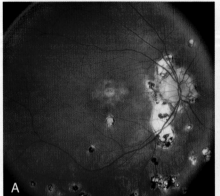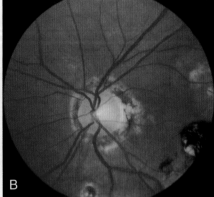

Figure 11.24.1 **A** and **B**: Ocular histoplasmosis.

- High myopia: May have atrophic spots in the posterior pole and a myopic crescent on the temporal side of the disc with a rim of pigment on the outer (not inner) edge, separating the crescent from the retina. Atrophic spots are whiter than histo-spots. See 11.22, HIGH MYOPIA.

- AMD: Macular changes may appear similar, but typically there are macular drusen and patients are ≥50 years of age. RPE more diffusely abnormal. There are no atrophic round spots similar to histoplasmosis and no scarring or atrophy around the disc. See 11.16, NONEXUDATIVE (DRY) AGE-RELATED MACULAR DEGENERATION and 11.17, NEOVASCULAR OR EXUDATIVE (WET) AGE-RELATED MACULAR DEGENERATION.

- Old toxoplasmosis: Pigmented chorioretinal lesion with fibrosis and overlying vitreous condensations. See 12.5, TOXOPLASMOSIS.

- Angioid streaks: Histo-like spots in the midperiphery and macular degeneration may occur. Jagged red, brown, or gray lines deep to the retinal vessels and radiating from the optic disc. See 11.23, ANGIOID STREAKS.

Etiology

Fungal infection caused by *Histoplasma capsulatum*. Once acquired by inhalation, the organisms can pass to the choroid through the bloodstream. Importantly, ocular histoplasmosis is *not* thought to represent active infection and antifungal therapy is not indicated.

Workup

1. History: Time spent in the Ohio–Mississippi River Valley or endemic area? Prior exposure to fowl?

2. Amsler grid test (see Appendix 4, AMSLER GRID) to evaluate the central visual field of each eye.

3. Slit lamp examination: Anterior chamber or vitreous cells and flare should not be present.

4. Dilated fundus examination: Concentrate on the macular area with a slit lamp and 60-, 90-diopter, or fundus contact lens. Look for signs of CNV and vitreous cells.

5. IVFA and OCT to help detect CNV and monitor response to treatment.

Treatment

1. Antifungal treatment is not helpful.

2. Intravitreal anti-VEGF therapy for CNV is the mainstay of treatment. PDT for subfoveal CNV and focal laser photocoagulation for extrafoveal CNV may rarely be used as well.

Follow Up

1. Instruct all patients to use an Amsler grid daily and to return immediately if any sudden visual change is noted.

2. Patients treated with anti-VEGF injections are seen every 4 to 6 weeks, depending on clinical response to therapy. Generally, a more complete treatment response is achieved with

fewer injections than in AMD. Patients are often able to stop injections rather than undergoing lifelong treatment. Patients treated with PDT or focal laser are typically seen at 2 to 3 weeks, 4 to 6 weeks, 3 months, and 6 months after treatment, and then every 6 months thereafter.

3. A careful macular examination and OCT is performed at each visit. IVFA may be repeated whenever renewed neovascular activity is suspected.

4. Patients without CNV are seen every 6 months when macular changes are present in one or both eyes and yearly when no macular disease is present in either eye.

11.25 Vitreomacular Adhesion/Vitreomacular Traction/Macular Hole

Symptoms

Variable decreased vision (typically around 20/200 level for a full-thickness hole, better for a partial-thickness hole), metamorphopsia, or central scotoma. Three times more likely in women; usually occurs in sixth to eighth decade. 10% bilateral.

Signs

(See Figures 11.25.1 and 11.25.2.)

Critical. A full-thickness macular hole appears as a round, red spot in the center of the macula, usually from one-third to two-thirds of a disc diameter in size; may be surrounded by a gray halo/cuff of SRF. Vitreomacular traction (VMT) demonstrates loss of the normal foveolar depression and often a yellow spot or ring in the center of the macula.

Other. Small, yellow precipitates deep to the retina in the hole or surrounding retina; retinal cysts at the margin of the hole or a small operculum above the hole, anterior to the retina (Gass stage 3 or 4); or both.

Gass Staging of Macular Hole

- Stage 1: An impending hole, yellow spot, or ring in fovea.
- Stage 2: Small full-thickness hole.
- Stage 3: Full-thickness hole with cuff of SRF, no PVD.
- Stage 4: Full-thickness hole with cuff of SRF, with complete PVD.

NOTE: A new classification system using OCT has been developed. It is based on size of the full-thickness hole, presence of VMT, and underlying etiology (e.g., primary VMT versus secondary trauma).

11

Differential Diagnosis

May be difficult to distinguish a macular hole from a pseudohole (no loss of foveal tissue) or a lamellar macular hole (partial-thickness).

- Macular pucker with a pseudohole: An ERM (surface-wrinkling) on the surface of the retina may simulate a macular hole. See 11.26, EPIRETINAL MEMBRANE (MACULAR PUCKER, SURFACE-WRINKLING RETINOPATHY, CELLOPHANE MACULOPATHY). Look for a sheen from ILM changes or ERM.
- Lamellar hole: Not as red as a full-thickness hole, and a surrounding gray halo is usually not present.

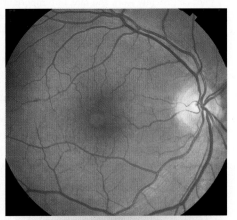
Figure 11.25.1 Macular hole.

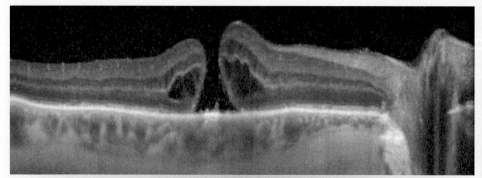

Figure 11.25.2 Optical coherence tomography of macular hole.

- Intraretinal cysts (e.g., chronic CME with prominent central cyst).
- Solar retinopathy: Small, round, red or yellow lesion at the center of the fovea, with surrounding fine gray pigment in a sun gazer or eclipse watcher. See 11.35, SOLAR RETINOPATHY.

Etiology

May be caused by vitreous or ERM traction on the macula, trauma, or CME. In early stages of vitreomacular adhesion (VMA)/VMT, the vitreous cortex is attached to the fovea but detached from the perifoveal region, exerting anteroposterior traction on the fovea. Increased tractional forces can allow for eventual progression to full-thickness macular hole.

Workup

1. History: Previous trauma? Previous eye surgery? Sun gazer?
2. Complete ocular examination, including a macular examination with a slit lamp and 60-, 90-diopter, or fundus contact lens. If a PVD is present, careful examination of the peripheral fundus to rule out peripheral breaks is important.
3. A true macular hole can be differentiated from a pseudo- or lamellar hole by directing a thin, vertical slit beam across the area in question using a 60- or 90-diopter lens with the slit lamp biomicroscope. The patient with a true hole will report a break in the line (Watzke–Allen test). A pseudohole or lamellar hole may cause distortion of the line, but it should not be broken.

4. IVFA may be helpful in identifying exudative retinal vascular disease (i.e., diabetic retinopathy, vein occlusion, pseudophakic CME) in cases which also have VMA/VMT.
5. OCT is critical for evaluating the vitreoretinal interface and determining the degree of traction from vitreous or ERMs. It is also useful in staging macular holes, differentiating from pseudo- or lamellar holes, and evaluating for progression (see Figure 11.25.3).

Treatment

1. Stage 1 macular holes can be observed, as 50% resolve spontaneously.
2. Ocriplasmin is a recombinant protease with activity against components of the vitreoretinal interface (fibronectin and laminin). It is FDA-approved for the treatment of symptomatic VMA, VMT, and macular hole. It does not consistently work and rare, but important side effects such as ERG changes, lens subluxation, and dyschromatopsias have limited acceptance of this drug.
3. For symptomatic macular holes, pars plana vitrectomy with ILM peel and gas tamponade remains the gold standard for treatment. It is preferable to operate within the first 6 months of onset for highest chance of visual recovery. Serious complications are rare, but cataract progression in phakic patients is almost universal.

Follow Up

1. Follow-up intervals vary depending on symptoms, examination, and surgical management.
2. Patients with high myopia are usually seen at least twice a year.

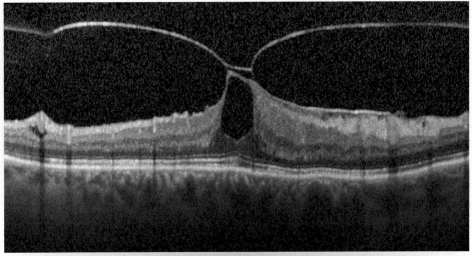

Figure 11.25.3 Optical coherence tomography of vitreomacular traction.

3. All patients are seen promptly if RD symptoms develop.

4. Because there is a small risk that the condition may develop in the contralateral eye, patients are given an Amsler grid for periodic home monitoring.

REFERENCE

Duker JS, Kaiser PK, Binder S, et al. The International Vitreomacular Traction Study Group classification of vitreomacular adhesion, traction, and macular hole. *Ophthalmology.* 2013;120(12):2611-2619.

11.26 Epiretinal Membrane (Macular Pucker, Surface-Wrinkling Retinopathy, Cellophane Maculopathy)

11

Symptoms

Most are asymptomatic; can have decreased or distorted vision or both. Incidence increases with age. Twenty percent bilateral, though often asymmetric.

Signs

(See Figure 11.26.1.)

Critical. Spectrum ranges from a fine, glistening membrane (cellophane maculopathy) to a thick, gray-white membrane (macular pucker) present on the surface of the retina in the macular area.

Other. Retinal folds radiating out from the membrane; displacement, straightening, or tortuosity of the macular retinal vessels; ME or macular detachment. A ring-shaped condensation of the ERM around the fovea may simulate a macular hole (pseudohole).

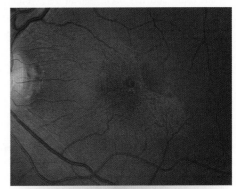

Figure 11.26.1 Epiretinal membrane with pseudohole.

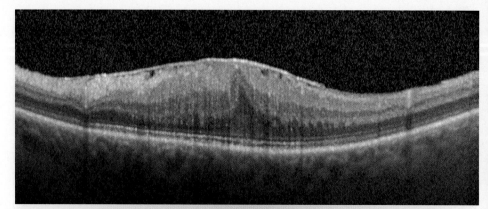

Figure 11.26.2 Optical coherence tomography of epiretinal membrane.

Differential Diagnosis

- Diabetic retinopathy: May produce preretinal fibrovascular tissue, which may displace retinal vessels or detach the macula. ME may be present. See 11.12, DIABETIC RETINOPATHY.
- CME. See 11.14, CYSTOID MACULAR EDEMA.

Etiology

- PVD. See 11.1, POSTERIOR VITREOUS DETACHMENT.
- Retinal break, RRD. A higher risk of ERM for PVD patients who also have a tear or RRD versus PVD alone. See 11.2, RETINAL BREAK and 11.3, RETINAL DETACHMENT.
- Idiopathic. ERM can occur without obvious cause and has been seen in very young children.
- After retinal cryotherapy or photocoagulation.
- After intraocular surgery, trauma, or vitreous hemorrhage.
- Uveitis.See Chapter 12, UVEITIS.
- Other retinal vascular disease (diabetic retinopathy, vein occlusion, etc.).

Workup

1. History: Previous eye surgery or eye disease? Diabetes?
2. Complete ocular examination, particularly a thorough dilated fundus evaluation and careful macula evaluation with a slit lamp and a 60- or 90-diopter, Hruby, or fundus contact lens. A careful peripheral examination should be performed to rule out a retinal break.
3. OCT is helpful in evaluating ERMs (see Figure 11.26.2).

Treatment

1. Treat the underlying disorder.
2. Examine the periphery to rule out a retinal break.
3. Surgical peeling of the membrane can be considered when it significantly reduces the vision.

Follow Up

This is not an emergent condition, and treatment may be instituted at any time. Often does not progress over time. A small percentage of ERMs recur after surgical removal.

11.27 Choroidal Effusion/Detachment

Symptoms

Decreased vision or asymptomatic in a serous choroidal detachment. Decreased vision may occur if the choroidal detachments extend posteriorly with a shadow or involve the macula. Moderate-to-severe pain and red eye may also occur with a hemorrhagic choroidal detachment.

Signs

(See Figure 11.27.1.)

Critical. Smooth, bullous, orange-brown elevation of the retina and choroid that usually extends 360 degrees around the periphery in a lobular configuration. The ora serrata can be seen without scleral depression.

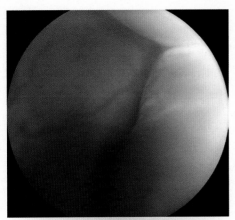

Figure 11.27.1 Choroidal detachment.

Other. *Serous choroidal detachment:* Low IOP (often <6 mm Hg), shallow anterior chamber with mild cell and flare, positive transillumination.

Hemorrhagic choroidal detachment: High IOP (if detachment is large), shallow anterior chamber with mild cell and flare, no transillumination.

Differential Diagnosis

- Melanoma of the ciliary body: Not typically multilobular or symmetric in each quadrant of the globe. Pigmented melanomas do not transilluminate. B-scan US usually helps to differentiate between the two. See 11.36, CHOROIDAL NEVUS AND MALIGNANT MELANOMA OF THE CHOROID.
- RRD: Appears white and undulates with eye movements. A break is usually seen in the retina, and pigment cells are often present in the vitreous. Serous choroidal detachment can occur as the result of chronic RRD. See 11.3, RETINAL DETACHMENT.

Etiology

Serous

- Intraoperative or postoperative: Wound leak, perforation of the sclera from a superior rectus bridle suture, iritis, cyclodialysis cleft, leakage or excess filtration from a filtering bleb, after RD repair by scleral buckling or vitrectomy, or after laser photocoagulation or cryotherapy.
- Traumatic: Often associated with a ruptured globe.
- Uveitis: posterior uveitis or scleritis.

- Other: Nanophthalmos, uveal effusion syndrome, carotid–cavernous fistula, primary or metastatic tumor, etc. See specific sections.

Hemorrhagic

- Intraoperative or postoperative: From anterior displacement of the ocular contents and rupture of the short posterior ciliary arteries.
- Spontaneous (e.g., after perforation of a corneal ulcer). May have no inciting event, especially if on anticoagulants.

Workup

1. History: Recent ocular surgery or trauma? Known eye or medical problem?
2. Slit lamp examination: Check for presence of a filtering bleb and perform Seidel test to rule out a wound leak. See Appendix 5, SEIDEL TEST TO DETECT A WOUND LEAK.
3. Gonioscopy of the anterior chamber angle: Look for a cyclodialysis cleft.
4. Dilated retinal examination: Determine whether there is SRF, indicating a concomitant RD, and whether an underlying choroidal disease or tumor is present. Examination of the contralateral eye may be helpful in diagnosis.
5. In cases suggestive of melanoma, B-scan US and transillumination of the globe are helpful in making a diagnosis. B-scan US is also useful in distinguishing between serous and hemorrhagic choroidal detachment and in determining if hemorrhage is mobile or coagulated.

Treatment

General Treatment

1. Cycloplegic (e.g., atropine 1% t.i.d.).
2. Topical steroid (e.g., prednisolone acetate 1% four to six times per day).
3. Consider oral steroids.
4. Surgical drainage of the suprachoroidal fluid may be indicated for a flat or progressively shallow anterior chamber, particularly in the presence of inflammation (because of the risk of peripheral anterior synechiae), or corneal decompensation resulting from lens–cornea touch. "Kissing" choroidals (apposition of two lobules of detached choroid) can usually be tolerated as long as there is not intractable pain or IOP elevation.

11

Specific Treatment: Repair the Underlying Problem

1. Serous:
   - Wound or filtering bleb leak: Patch for 24 hours, decrease steroids and add aqueous suppressants, suture the site, use cyanoacrylate glue, place a bandage contact lens on the eye, or a combination of these.
   - Cyclodialysis cleft: Laser therapy, diathermy, cryotherapy, or suture the cleft to close it.
   - Uveitis: Topical cycloplegic and steroid as discussed previously.

- Inflammatory disease: See the specific entity.
- RD: Surgical repair. Proliferative vitreoretinopathy after repair is common.

2. Hemorrhagic: Drainage of the choroidal detachment using intraocular infusion with or without vitrectomy is performed for severe cases. More successful if hemorrhage is liquefied, which occurs 7 to 10 days after the initial event. Otherwise use general treatment.

Follow Up

In accordance with the underlying problem.

11.28 | Retinitis Pigmentosa and Inherited Chorioretinal Dystrophies

RETINITIS PIGMENTOSA

Symptoms

Decreased night vision (often night blindness) and loss of peripheral vision. Decrease in central vision can occur early or late in the disease process depending on whether rod or cone involvement is predominant. The same is true for color vision.

Signs

(See Figure 11.28.1.)

Critical. Classically, vitreous cells (most consistent sign), clumps of pigment dispersed throughout the peripheral retina in a perivascular pattern, often assuming a "bone spicule" arrangement (though bone spicules may be absent), areas of RPE depigmentation or atrophy, arteriolar narrowing, and, later, waxy optic disc pallor. Progressive visual field loss, usually a ring scotoma, which progresses to a small central field. ERG usually moderately to markedly reduced.

Other. Focal or sectoral pigment clumping, CME, ERM, posterior subcapsular cataract.

Inheritance Patterns

- Autosomal recessive (most common): Diminished vision (severe) and night blindness occur early in life.
- Autosomal dominant (least severe): More gradual onset of RP, typically in adult life, variable penetrance, late onset of cataract. Visual loss less severe.
- X-linked recessive (rarest and most severe): Onset similar to autosomal recessive. Female carriers often have salt-and-pepper fundus. Visual loss is severe.
- Sporadic.

Treatment

Some evidence supports that diets high in vitamin A (15,000 IU/d) and lutein (12 mg/d) may help slow midperipheral visual field loss in nonsmokers with RP, but the literature remains inconclusive. If high-dose vitamin A therapy is initiated, monitor liver function tests and vitamin A levels. Both epiretinal and subretinal microchip implants have been used with some success to

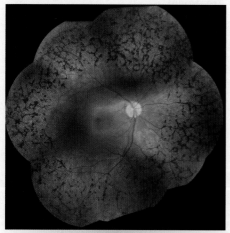

Figure 11.28.1 Retinitis pigmentosa.

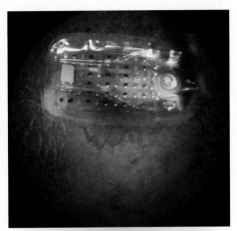

Figure 11.28.2 Epiretinal microchip implant in patient with advanced retinal pigment epithelium.

improve vision in patients with very advanced RP (see **Figure 11.28.2**). Clinical trials are ongoing with a variety of designs to determine the safety and efficacy of retinal implant technology. In addition, research in gene therapy for specific types of RP is underway.

SYSTEMIC DISEASES ASSOCIATED WITH HEREDITARY RETINAL DEGENERATION

Refsum Disease (Phytanoyl-CoA Hydroxylase Deficiency)

Autosomal recessive RP (often without bone spicules) with increased serum phytanic acid level. May have cerebellar ataxia, peripheral neuropathy, deafness, dry skin, anosmia, liver disease, and cardiac abnormalities. Treat with low-phytanic acid, low-phytol diet (minimize the amount of milk products, animal fats, and green leafy vegetables). Check serum phytanic acid levels every 6 months.

Hereditary Abetalipoproteinemia (Bassen–Kornzweig Syndrome)

Autosomal recessive RP (usually without bone spicules) with fat intolerance, diarrhea, crenated erythrocytes (acanthocytes), ataxia, progressive restriction of ocular motility, and other neurologic symptoms as a result of deficiency in lipoproteins and malabsorption of the fat-soluble vitamins (A, D, E, and K). Diagnosis based on serum apolipoprotein-B deficiency.

Treatment

1. Water-miscible vitamin A, 10,000 to 15,000 IU p.o. daily.
2. Vitamin E, 200 to 300 IU/kg p.o. daily.
3. Vitamin K, 5 mg p.o. weekly.
4. Restrict dietary fat to 15% of caloric intake.
5. Biannual serum levels of vitamins A and E; yearly ERG, and dark adaptometry.
6. Consider supplementing the patient's diet with zinc.

Leber Congenital Amaurosis

Group of autosomal recessive retinal dystrophies that represent the most common genetic cause of congenital blindness in children. Fundus appearance is variable but typically shows a pigmentary retinopathy. Moderate-to-severe vision loss identified at or within a few months of birth, infantile nystagmus, poor and/or paradoxic pupillary response, photophobia, oculodigital sign (eye poking), and markedly reduced or flat ERG. Associated with keratoconus. Voretigene neparvovec (Luxturna) is the first FDA-approved gene therapy for any inherited retinal degeneration. Treatment involves subretinal injection of an AAV2 viral vector carrying RPE65 DNA.

Usher Syndrome

Multiple subtypes exist, all autosomal recessive. Associated with congenital sensorineural hearing loss which is usually stable throughout adult life. Genes involved code a protein complex present in inner ear hair cells and retinal photoreceptor cells. Molecular testing for certain subtypes is available.

Bardet–Biedl Complex

Mainly autosomal recessive group of different diseases with similar findings including pigmentary retinopathy, hypogonadism, obesity, polydactyly, mental retardation, and others. Lawrence–Moon syndrome is a related but separate entity associated with spastic paraplegia, but without the polydactyly and obesity.

Kearns–Sayre Syndrome

Salt-and-pepper pigmentary degeneration of the retina with normal arterioles. Progressive limitation of ocular movement without diplopia, ptosis, short stature, and/or cardiac conduction defects.

11

Ocular signs usually appear before age 20 years. Mitochondrial inheritance. Refer the patient to a cardiologist. Patients may need a pacemaker. See 10.12, CHRONIC PROGRESSIVE EXTERNAL OPHTHALMOPLEGIA.

Other RP Syndromes

- Spielmeyer–Vogt–Batten–Mayou syndrome: Associated with seizures, dementia, and ataxia.
- Alström, Cockayne, and Alport syndromes: Associated with hearing loss.
- Zellweger syndrome: Associated with hypotonia, hypertelorism, and hepatomegaly.
- Others: Incontinentia pigmenti, Jansky–Bielschowsky, etc.

Differential Diagnosis

- **Phenothiazine toxicity**
  - Thioridazine: Pigment clumps between the posterior pole and the equator, areas of retinal depigmentation, retinal edema, visual field abnormalities (central scotoma and general constriction), depressed or extinguished ERG. Symptoms and signs may occur within weeks of starting phenothiazine therapy, particularly if very large doses (≥2,000 mg/d) are taken. Usually, more than 800 mg/d chronically needed for toxicity. Discontinue if toxicity develops. Follow every 6 months.
  - Chlorpromazine: Abnormal pigmentation of the eyelids, cornea, conjunctiva (especially within the palpebral fissure), and anterior lens capsule; anterior and posterior subcapsular cataract; rarely, a pigmentary retinopathy with visual field and ERG changes similar to that described for thioridazine. Usually, 1,200 to 2,400 mg/d for longer than 12 months needed for toxicity. Discontinue if toxicity develops. Follow every 6 months.
- **Syphilis:** Positive bloodwork, asymmetric visual fields, abnormal fundus appearance, may have a history of recurrent uveitis. No family history of RP. The ERG is usually preserved to some degree.
- **Congenital rubella:** A salt-and-pepper fundus appearance may be accompanied by microphthalmos, cataract, deafness, a congenital heart abnormality, or another systemic abnormality. The ERG is usually normal.

- **Bietti crystalline dystrophy:** Autosomal recessive condition characterized by crystals of unknown composition in the peripheral corneal stroma and in the retina at different layers. Can cause choroidal atrophy, decreased night vision, decreased visual acuity, and a flat ERG.
- **After resolution of a serous RD:** The history is diagnostic (e.g., toxemia of pregnancy, Harada disease).
- **Pigmented paravenous retinochoroidal atrophy:** Paravenous localization of RPE degeneration and pigment deposition. No definite hereditary pattern. Variable visual fields and ERG (usually normal).
- **After severe blunt trauma:** Usually due to spontaneous resolution of RD.
- **After ophthalmic artery occlusion.**
- **Carriers of ocular albinism:** See 13.8, ALBINISM.

NOTE: The pigment abnormalities are at the level of the RPE with phenothiazine toxicity, syphilis, and congenital rubella. With resolved RD, the pigment is intraretinal.

Workup

1. Medical and ocular history pertaining to the diseases discussed previously.
2. Drug history.
3. Family history with pedigree and genetic testing for diagnostic and counseling purposes (see above).
4. Ophthalmoscopic examination.
5. Formal visual field testing (e.g., Humphrey).
6. Dark-adaption studies and ERG: May help distinguish stationary rod dysfunction (congenital stationary night blindness) from RP (a progressive disease).
7. Fundus photographs.
8. Consider syphilis testing (RPR or VDRL and FTA-ABS or treponemal-specific assay).
9. If the patient is male and inheritance pattern is unknown, examine his mother and perform an ERG on her. Women carriers of X-linked disease often have abnormal pigmentation in the midperiphery and abnormal results on dark-adapted ERGs.
10. If neurologic abnormalities such as ataxia, polyneuropathy, deafness, or anosmia are present, obtain a fasting (at least 14 hours) serum phytanic acid level to rule out Refsum disease.

11. If hereditary abetalipoproteinemia is suspected, obtain serum cholesterol and triglyceride levels (levels are low), a serum protein and lipoprotein electrophoresis (lipoprotein deficiency is detected), and peripheral blood smears (acanthocytosis is seen).

12. If Kearns–Sayre syndrome is suspected, the patient must be examined by a cardiologist with sequential EKGs; patients can die of complete heart block. All family members should be evaluated.

Treatment

For syphilis, see 12.12, SYPHILIS. For vitamin A deficiency, see 13.7, VITAMIN A DEFICIENCY.

No definitive treatment for RP is currently known. See above, RETINITIS PIGMENTOSA.

Cataract surgery may improve central visual acuity. Topical or oral carbonic anhydrase inhibitors (e.g., acetazolamide 500 mg/d) may be effective for CME.

All patients benefit from genetic counseling and instruction on how to deal with their visual handicaps. Tinted lenses may provide comfort outdoors and may provide better contrast enhancement. In advanced cases, low-vision aids and vocational rehabilitation are helpful.

HEREDITARY CHORIORETINAL DYSTROPHIES AND OTHER CAUSES OF NYCTALOPIA (NIGHT BLINDNESS)

- Gyrate atrophy: Nyctalopia and decreased peripheral vision usually presenting in the first decade of life, followed by progressive constriction of visual field. Scalloped RPE and choriocapillaris atrophy in the midperiphery during childhood that coalesces to involve the entire fundus, posterior subcapsular cataract, high myopia with astigmatism. Constriction of visual fields and abnormal to nonrecordable ERG. Plasma ornithine level is 10 to 20 times normal; lysine is decreased. Consider ERG and IVFA if the ornithine level is not markedly increased. Autosomal recessive.

Treatment

1. Reduce dietary protein consumption and substitute artificially flavored solutions of essential amino acids without arginine (e.g., arginine-restricted diet). Monitor serum ammonia levels.

2. Supplemental vitamin B6 (pyridoxine). The dose is not currently established; consider 20 mg/d p.o. initially and increase up to 500 mg/d p.o. if there is no response. Follow serum ornithine levels to determine the amount of supplemental vitamin B6 and the degree to which dietary protein needs to be restricted. Serum ornithine levels between 0.15 and 0.2 mmol/L are optimal.

 NOTE: Only a small percentage of patients are vitamin B6 responders.

- Choroideremia: Males present in the first to second decade of life with nyctalopia, followed by insidious loss of peripheral vision. Decreased central vision occurs late. In males, early findings include dispersed pigment granules in the periphery with focal areas of RPE atrophy. Late findings include total absence of RPE and choriocapillaris. No bone spicules. Retinal arteriolar narrowing and optic atrophy can occur late in the process. Constriction of visual fields, normal color vision, markedly reduced ERG. Female carriers have small, scattered, square intraretinal pigment granules overlying choroidal atrophy, most marked in the midperiphery. No effective treatment for this condition is currently available. Darkly tinted sunglasses may ameliorate symptoms. X-linked recessive. Consider genetic counseling.

- Vitamin A deficiency: Marked night blindness. Numerous small, yellow-white, well-demarcated spots deep in the retina seen peripherally. Dry eye and/or Bitôt spots (white keratinized lesions) on the conjunctiva. See 13.7, VITAMIN A DEFICIENCY.

- Zinc deficiency: May cause abnormal dark adaptation (zinc is needed for vitamin A metabolism).

- Congenital stationary night blindness: Night blindness from birth, normal visual fields; may have a normal or abnormal fundus, not progressive. Paradoxic pupillary response. One variant is Oguchi disease—the fundus has a tapetum appearance in the light-adapted state but appears normally colored when dark-adapted (may take up to 12 hours) (see Figures 11.28.3 and 11.28.4).

- Undercorrected myopia: The most common cause of poor night vision.

11

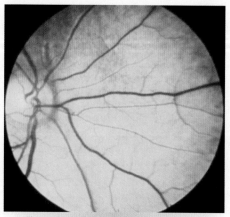

Figure 11.28.3 Oguchi disease with fundus exhibiting tapetum appearance in a light-adapted state.

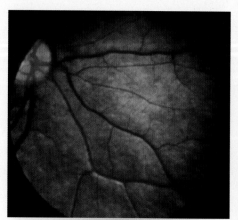

Figure 11.28.4 Oguchi disease exhibiting Mizuo phenomenon, with a normally colored fundus in dark-adapted state.

11.29 Cone Dystrophies

Symptoms

Slowly progressive visual loss, photophobia, and poor color vision, with onset during the first 3 decades of life. Vision is worse in bright than dim light.

Signs

Critical

- Early: Essentially normal fundus examination, even with poor visual acuity. Abnormal cone function on ERG (e.g., a reduced single-flash photopic response and a reduced flicker response).
- Late: Bull's eye macular appearance or central geographic atrophy of the RPE and choriocapillaris.

Other. Nystagmus, temporal pallor of the optic disc, spotty pigment clumping in the macular area, tapetal-like retinal sheen. Rarely rod degeneration may ensue, leading to an RP-like picture (e.g., a cone–rod degeneration, which may have an autosomal dominant inheritance pattern).

Inheritance

Usually sporadic. Hereditary forms are usually autosomal dominant or less often X-linked.

Differential Diagnosis

- Stargardt disease: Especially in early stage when yellowish lesions are absent and ERG is usually normal. See 11.30, STARGARDT DISEASE (FUNDUS FLAVIMACULATUS).
- Chloroquine/hydroxychloroquine maculopathy: May produce a bull's eye macular appearance and poor color vision. History of medication use, no family history of cone degeneration, no nystagmus. See 11.32, CHLOROQUINE/HYDROXYCHLOROQUINE TOXICITY.
- Central areolar choroidal dystrophy: Geographic atrophy of the RPE with normal photopic ERG.
- AMD: Can have geographic atrophy of the RPE, but with normal color vision and photopic ERG. See 11.16, NONEXUDATIVE (DRY) AGE-RELATED MACULAR DEGENERATION and 11.17, NEOVASCULAR OR EXUDATIVE (WET) AGE-RELATED MACULAR DEGENERATION.
- Congenital color deficiency: Normal visual acuity, onset at birth, not progressive.
- RP: Night blindness and peripheral visual field loss. Often with peripheral retinal bone spicules. Can be distinguished by dark-adaptation testing and ERG. See 11.28, RETINITIS PIGMENTOSA AND INHERITED CHORIORETINAL DYSTROPHIES.

- Optic neuropathy or atrophy: Decreased acuity, impaired color vision, temporal or diffuse optic disc pallor, or both. See 10.17, ARTERITIC ISCHEMIC OPTIC NEUROPATHY (GIANT CELL ARTERITIS), 10.18, NONARTERITIC ISCHEMIC OPTIC NEUROPATHY, and 10.20, MISCELLANEOUS OPTIC NEUROPATHIES.
- Nonphysiologic visual loss: Normal results on ophthalmoscopic examination, IVFA, OCT, ERG, and electrooculogram (EOG). Patients can often be tricked into seeing better by special testing. See 10.25, NONPHYSIOLOGIC VISUAL LOSS.

Workup

1. Family history.
2. Complete ophthalmic examination, including formal assessment for dyschromatopsia (e.g., Farnsworth–Munsell 100-hue test).
3. Formal visual field test.
4. Full-field ERG: abnormal photopic response with normal rod-isolated response.

5. OCT can show disruption of outer retinal layers but may be normal even in patients with electrophysical abnormalities.
6. FAF can be useful in the diagnosis (particularly sensitive to disturbances in the RPE), as well as for monitoring these diseases.

Treatment

There is no proven cure for cone dystrophy. The following measures may be palliative:

1. Heavily tinted glasses or contact lenses may help maximize vision.
2. Miotic drops (e.g., pilocarpine 0.5% to 1% q.i.d.) are occasionally tried to improve vision and reduce photophobia.
3. Genetic counseling.
4. Low-vision aids as needed.

Follow Up

Yearly.

11.30 Stargardt Disease (Fundus Flavimaculatus)

Symptoms

Decreased vision in childhood or young adulthood. Early in the disease, the decrease in vision is often out of proportion to the clinical ophthalmoscopic appearance; therefore, care must be taken not to label the child a malingerer.

Signs

(See Figures 11.30.1 to 11.30.3.)

Critical. Any of the following may be present.
- A relatively normal-appearing fundus except for slight granularity in the foveola.
- Yellow or yellow-white, fleck-like deposits at the level of the RPE, often in a pisciform (fishtail) configuration.
- Atrophic macular degeneration: May have a bull's eye appearance as a result of atrophy of the RPE around a normal central core of RPE, a "beaten-metal" appearance, pigment clumping, or marked geographic atrophy.

 NOTE: In early stages, vision declines **before** visible macular changes develop.

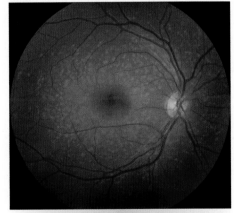

Figure 11.30.1 Stargardt disease.

Other. Atrophy of the RPE just outside of the macula or in the midperipheral fundus, normal peripheral visual fields in most cases, and rarely an accompanying cone or rod dystrophy. The ERG is typically normal in the early stages but may become abnormal late in the disease. The EOG can be subnormal.

11

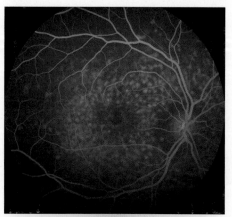

Figure 11.30.2 Intravenous fluorescein angiography of Stargardt disease exhibiting silent choroid.

Inheritance

Usually autosomal recessive, but occasionally autosomal dominant (dominant cases may be asymptomatic into middle age).

Differential Diagnosis

- Fundus albipunctatus: Diffuse, small, white, discrete dots, most prominent in the midperipheral fundus and rarely present in the fovea; congenital stationary night blindness variant; no atrophic macular degeneration or pigmentary changes. Visual acuity and visual fields remain normal. Prolonged dark-adaptation time with normal ERG.

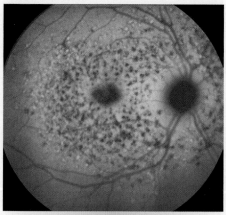

Figure 11.30.3 Fundus autofluorescence in Stargardt disease.

- Retinitis punctata albescens: Similar clinical appearance to fundus albipunctatus, but visual acuity, visual field, and night blindness progressively worsen. A markedly abnormal ERG develops. Variant of RP.
- Drusen: Small, yellow-white spots deep to the retina, sometimes calcified, usually developing later in life. IVFA may be helpful (all drusen exhibit hyperfluorescence, whereas fundus flavimaculatus lesions show variable hyperfluorescence and some areas without flecks show hyperfluorescence).
- Cone or cone–rod dystrophy: May have normal fundus in early stages. May have bull's eye maculopathy, but have significant color vision deficit and a characteristic ERG. See 11.29, CONE DYSTROPHIES.
- Batten disease and Spielmeyer–Vogt syndrome: Autosomal recessive lysosomal storage disease characterized by progressive dementia and seizures. May have bull's eye maculopathy, variable degree of optic atrophy, attenuation of retinal vasculature, and peripheral RPE changes. Shows characteristic curvilinear or fingerprint inclusions on electron microscopy of peripheral blood or conjunctival biopsy. Variants of RP.
- Chloroquine/hydroxychloroquine maculopathy: History of medication use. See 11.32, CHLOROQUINE/HYDROXYCHLOROQUINE TOXICITY.
- Nonphysiologic visual loss: Normal ophthalmoscopic examination, IVFA, OCT, ERG, and EOG. Patients can often be tricked into seeing better by special testing. See 10.25, NONPHYSIOLOGIC VISUAL LOSS.

Workup

Indicated when the diagnosis is uncertain or must be confirmed.

1. History: Age at onset, medications, family history?
2. Dilated fundus examination.
3. OCT may show photoreceptor disorganization, outer retinal atrophy, and RPE changes, which may appear early even with a normal fundus examination.
4. IVFA often shows blockage of choroidal fluorescence producing a "silent choroid" or "midnight fundus" as a result of increased lipofuscin in RPE cells.

5. FAF can be helpful in diagnosis and in monitoring disease progression.
6. ERG and EOG.
7. Formal visual field examination (e.g., Octopus, Humphrey).
8. Consider genetic testing: Sequencing of the ABCA4 gene (found to be abnormal in many cases of Stargardt disease and other related maculopathies).

Treatment

Avoid vitamin A supplementation. Ultraviolet light-blocking glasses when outdoors may be beneficial. Low-vision aids, services dedicated to helping the visually handicapped, and genetic counseling are helpful.

11.31 Best Disease (Vitelliform Macular Dystrophy)

Symptoms

Decreased vision, scotoma, metamorphopsia, or asymptomatic.

Signs

(See Figure 11.31.1.)

Critical. Yellow, round, subretinal lesion(s) likened to an egg yolk (lipofuscin) or in some cases to a pseudohypopyon. Typically bilateral and located in the fovea, measuring approximately one to two disc areas in size. Likely present at birth, though may not be detected until examination is performed. Ten percent of lesions are multiple and extrafoveal. ERG is typically normal, while EOG is abnormal, showing severe loss of the light response.

Other. The lesions may degenerate, and patients may develop macular CNV (20% of patients), hemorrhage, and atrophic scarring. In the scar

stage, it may be indistinguishable from AMD. Hyperopia is common due to shortened axial length along with angle closure glaucoma; may also have esophoria or esotropia.

Inheritance

Autosomal dominant with variable penetrance and expression. Due to mutation of the *BEST1* gene. Carriers may have normal fundi but an abnormal EOG.

Differential Diagnosis

• Pattern dystrophy: A type of pattern dystrophy, adult-onset foveomacular dystrophy, can mimic Best disease. The egg yolk lesions are usually smaller, appearing from ages 30 to 50 years. The condition is dominantly inherited, and the EOG may or may not be abnormal. Typically due to mutation of the *PRPH2* gene, rather than *BEST1*. Visual acuity is usually normal or slightly decreased until the sixth decade of life, when central vision may be compromised by geographic atrophy. There is no effective treatment for this entity, unless CNV develops and thus anti-VEGF injections may be used to treat CNV.

• AMD: See above and 11.16, NONEXUDATIVE (DRY) AGE-RELATED MACULAR DEGENERATION.

Workup

1. Family history. It is often helpful to examine family members.
2. Complete ocular examination, including a dilated retinal examination, carefully inspecting the macula with a slit lamp and a fundus contact, or handheld (60-, 90-diopter) lens.

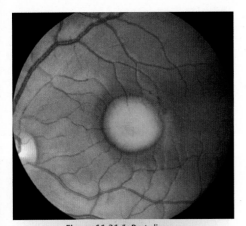
Figure 11.31.1 Best disease.

11

3. EOG is highly specific and can be used to confirm the diagnosis or to detect the carrier state of the disease.
4. Genetic testing to confirm mutation of *BEST1* gene.
5. Consider IVFA and OCT to detect the presence of or to delineate CNV.

Treatment

There is no effective treatment for the underlying disease. Treatment for CNV is controversial because it may heal without devastating visual loss. In the era of intravitreal anti-VEGF agents, these are now typically first-line agents for CNV, but PDT and focal laser may also play a potential role. Additionally, due to development of subretinal hemorrhage with mild trauma, polycarbonate lenses are recommended at all times and especially while playing sports. See 11.17, NEOVASCULAR OR EXUDATIVE (WET) AGE-RELATED MACULAR DEGENERATION, for detailed treatment options for CNV.

Follow Up

Patients with CNV should be treated promptly. Otherwise, there is no urgency in seeing patients with this disease. Patients are given an Amsler grid (see Appendix 4, AMSLER GRID), instructed on its use, and told to return immediately if a change is noted.

11.32 Chloroquine/Hydroxychloroquine Toxicity

Symptoms

Often asymptomatic early, then decreased vision, abnormal color vision, reduced dark adaptation.

Signs

Critical. Bull's eye macula (ring of depigmentation surrounded by a ring of increased pigmentation), loss of foveal reflex.

Other. Increased pigmentation in the macula, arteriolar narrowing, vascular sheathing, peripheral pigmentation, decreased color vision, CME, visual field abnormalities (central, paracentral, or peripheral scotoma), abnormal ERG and EOG, and abnormal dark adaptation. Whorl-like corneal changes may also be observed.

Major Risk Factors

- Chloroquine daily dosage: >2.3 mg/kg real weight
- Hydroxychloroquine daily dosage: >5.0 mg/kg real weight
- Duration of use: >5 years, assuming no other risk factors
- Renal disease, tamoxifen use, comorbid macular disease

Differential Diagnosis of Bull's Eye Maculopathy

- Cone dystrophy: Family history, usually <30 years of age, severe photophobia, abnormal to nonrecordable photopic ERG. See 11.29, CONE DYSTROPHIES.
- Stargardt disease: Family history, usually <25 years of age, may have white-yellow flecks in the posterior pole and midperiphery. See 11.30, STARGARDT DISEASE (FUNDUS FLAVIMACULATUS).
- AMD: Drusen; pigment clumping, atrophy, and exudative changes in the neovascular form. See 11.16, NONEXUDATIVE (DRY) AGE-RELATED MACULAR DEGENERATION and 11.17, NEOVASCULAR OR EXUDATIVE (WET) AGE-RELATED MACULAR DEGENERATION.
- Batten disease and Spielmeyer–Vogt syndrome: Pigmentary retinopathy, seizures, ataxia, and progressive dementia. See 11.30, STARGARDT DISEASE (FUNDUS FLAVIMACULATUS).

Treatment

Discontinue the medication in conjunction with the prescribing physician if signs of toxicity develop.

Baseline Workup

Baseline evaluation should be performed within the first year of starting the medication.

1. Best corrected visual acuity.
2. Ophthalmoscopic examination, including dilated fundus examination with particular attention to any pigmentary alterations.
3. Consider posterior pole fundus photographs.
4. Consider visual fields and OCT if maculopathy is present.

Follow Up

After 5 years of medication use (sooner in presence of major risk factors), begin annual screening:

1. Automated visual fields: Preferably white SITA testing and 10-2 pattern for non-Asians. 24-2 or 30-2 pattern recommended for Asian patients in whom toxicity often manifests in the more peripheral macula.

2. Spectral domain OCT: Parafoveal photoreceptor layer thinning and/or disruption of outer retinal layers ("flying saucer sign"), RPE atrophy, loss of foveal contour. Consider wide angle scans including vascular arcades in Asian patients.

3. Additional tools that may be used as available or in suspect cases include multifocal ERG and FAF **(see Figure 11.32.1)**

NOTE: Once ocular toxicity develops, it usually does not regress even if the drug is withdrawn. In fact, new toxic effects may develop, and old ones may progress even after the chloroquine/hydroxychloroquine has been discontinued.

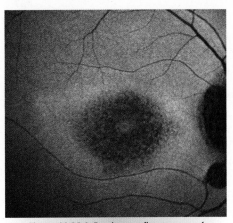

Figure 11.32.1 Fundus autofluorescence of hydroxychloroquine toxicity.

REFERENCE

Marmor MF, Kellner U, Lai TY, et al; American Academy of Ophthalmology. Recommendations on screening for chloroquine and hydroxychloroquine retinopathy (2016 Revision). *Ophthalmology.* 2016;123(6):1386-1394.

11.33 Crystalline Retinopathy

Symptoms

Decreased vision or asymptomatic.

Signs

Critical. Intraretinal refractile bodies.

Other. If crystals are intravascular and cause capillary nonperfusion, peripheral neovascularization as well as neovascularization of the optic nerve can develop (most commonly with talc). ME, macular pucker, and VH may also occur. Skin may reveal evidence of intravenous drug abuse.

Differential Diagnosis

• Hard exudates: Intraretinal lipid exudates as can be seen in multiple conditions (e.g., diabetic retinopathy, CRVO/BRVO, Coats disease, retinal telangiectasia, RAM). Hard exudates are not seen within retinal vessels.

• Calcific drusen: Seen in dry AMD. Drusen are subretinal, not intravascular.

Etiology

• Canthaxanthin toxicity: Oral tanning agent causing ring-shaped deposits in the superficial retina. Generally asymptomatic and usually resolves over many years when the drug is stopped. Usually requires a total of 19 g over 2 years. Crystals appear more prominent in eyes with preexisting retinal disease and patients taking beta-carotene.

• Tamoxifen: Used in patients with hormone receptor-positive breast cancer. Toxicity usually requires 7.7 g total. Crystals appear in the inner retina usually around the macula and may cause ME. Vision may improve with discontinuation of drug, but crystals remain. Asymptomatic patients taking tamoxifen do not need to be screened. Consider medication change if evidence of toxicity in consultation with patient's oncologist.

• Retinal arterial emboli: Seen within vessel. See 11.6, CENTRAL RETINAL ARTERY OCCLUSION and 11.7, BRANCH RETINAL ARTERY OCCLUSION.

11

- Talc: Red-yellow refractile particles seen intravascularly in intravenous drug users. Usually requires chronic IV drug use over several months to years before retinopathy develops.
- Methoxyflurane: An inhalational anesthetic agent. Calcium oxalate crystals deposited throughout the body can lead to irreversible renal failure. Crystals seen in both the RPE and inner retina.
- Bietti crystalline dystrophy: Crystals of unknown composition in the peripheral corneal stroma and in the retina at different layers. See 11.28, RETINITIS PIGMENTOSA AND INHERITED CHORIORETINAL DYSTROPHIES.
- Idiopathic juxtafoveal/parafoveal telangiectasis: Telangiectasis of juxtafoveal or parafoveal retinal capillaries leading to exudation and deposition of crystals on the ILM which may be Mueller foot plates or calcium or cholesterol deposits. Patients can develop ME and/or CNV. Vascular damage is very similar to that seen in diabetic retinopathy, and some patients with this condition are later found to have insulin resistance.
- Other: Nitrofurantoin toxicity, Sjögren–Larsson syndrome, West-African crystalline maculopathy, chronic RD, and others.

Workup

1. Complete past medical and medication history: Intravenous drug use? Cardiovascular risk factors such as HTN, elevated cholesterol? Breast cancer? Use of oral tanning agents? History of anesthesia in patient with renal failure?
2. Complete ocular examination, including dilated retinal evaluation using a slit lamp and 60- or 90-diopter lens along with indirect ophthalmoscopy. Carefully assess the location, depth, color, and morphology of crystals as well as the potential presence of ME, neovascularization of the disc and peripheral retina, or retinal infarction. Examine the cornea for crystals.
3. Consider carotid Doppler US and echocardiography in older patients and those with cardiovascular risk factors.
4. Examine patient for evidence of intravenous drug abuse.
5. Consider testing for diabetes if idiopathic juxtafoveal/parafoveal telangiectasis suspected.
6. IVFA may be helpful to demonstrate areas of nonperfusion distal to an intravascular crystal. OCT may be helpful to determine depth.

Treatment

1. Stop tamoxifen or canthaxanthin use if responsible for toxicity.
2. Stop intravenous drug use.
3. If cholesterol, calcium, or fibrin-platelet emboli, see 10.22, TRANSIENT VISUAL LOSS/ AMAUROSIS FUGAX, 11.6, CENTRAL RETINAL ARTERY OCCLUSION, and 11.7, BRANCH RETINAL ARTERY OCCLUSION.
4. If there is peripheral nonperfusion or neovascularization, consider PRP or anti-VEGF agents. Visual loss may be permanent if there has been vascular nonperfusion in the macula secondary to blockage from intraretinal crystals.

Follow Up

Depends on the underlying etiology.

11.34 | Optic Pit

Symptoms

Asymptomatic if isolated. May notice distortion of straight lines or edges, blurred vision, a blind spot, or micropsia if macular fluid develops.

Signs

(See Figure 11.34.1.)

Critical. Small, round depression (usually gray, yellow, or black in appearance) in the nerve tissue of the optic disc. Most are temporal, approximately one-third are central, but may be present anywhere on the nerve head.

Other. Peripapillary atrophy, white or gray membrane overlying pit, rarely RAPD, various visual field defects. May develop localized detachment of the sensory retina and/or retinoschisis extending from the disc to the macula, usually unilateral.

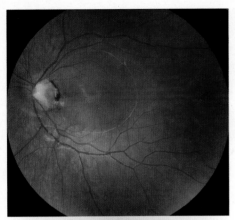

Figure 11.34.1 Optic pit with associated serous macular detachment.

Differential Diagnosis

- Acquired pit (pseudopit): Sometimes seen in patients with low-tension glaucoma or primary open-angle glaucoma. See 9.1, PRIMARY OPEN-ANGLE GLAUCOMA.
- Other causes of cyst, fluid, or hole in the macula. OCT is key. See 11.15, CENTRAL SEROUS CHORIORETINOPATHY.

Workup

- Complete ophthalmologic examination including slit lamp examination of the optic nerve and macula with a 60-, 90-diopter, or fundus contact lens to evaluate for macular fluid.
- Measure IOP.
- Obtain baseline automated visual field testing.
- If macular fluid is present, consider OCT to characterize precisely and IVFA to rule out CSCR or CNV.

Treatment

1. Isolated optic pit: No treatment required.
2. Optic pit with macular fluid causing vision loss: Watchful waiting or vitrectomy and intravitreal gas are most commonly used. Laser photocoagulation to the temporal margin of the optic disc and macular buckling have also been described.

Follow Up

1. Isolated optic pits: Yearly examination including IOP check, dilated fundus examination, and visual field testing if indicated; sooner if symptomatic. Patients should be given an Amsler grid. See Appendix 4, AMSLER GRID. Monitor for and treat amblyopia if present.
2. Optic pits with serous macular detachment or retinoschisis: Refer for retinal evaluation.

11.35 Solar or Photic Retinopathy

Symptoms

Decreased visual acuity, central/paracentral scotomata, dyschromatopsia, metamorphopsia. Typically bilateral.

Signs

(See Figure 11.35.1.)

Critical. Acute findings include a yellow-white spot in the fovea with or without surrounding granular gray pigmentation. Classic late finding is a red, sharply demarcated lesion in the fovea.

Other. Visual acuity usually ranges from 20/25 to 20/100. Amsler grid testing may reveal

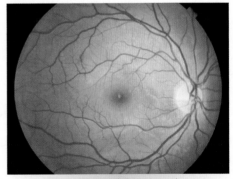

Figure 11.35.1 Solar retinopathy.

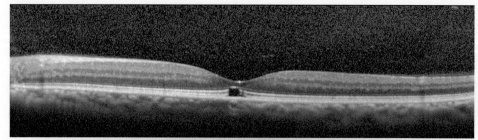

Figure 11.35.2 Optical coherence tomography of solar retinopathy.

central or paracentral scotoma. Resolution of acute findings within several weeks may leave a variable appearance to the fovea (e.g., pigmentary disturbance, lamellar hole, normal appearance, etc). Eyes with better initial visual acuities are more likely to have unremarkable fundoscopic examinations at follow up.

Differential Diagnosis

- Macular hole or vitreomacular traction: See 11.25, VITREOMACULAR ADHESION (VMA)/ VITREOMACULAR TRACTION (VMT)/MACULAR HOLE.
- Idiopathic macular telangiectasia type 2: May have OCT findings similar to those seen in chronic solar retinopathy, although on IVFA juxtafoveal capillary telangiectasis is seen with leakage. May be complicated by CNV.
- Intraretinal cysts, as for example in chronic CME, but this can be differentiated by OCT.
- Pattern dystrophy: Adult-onset foveomacular dystrophy. See 11.31, BEST DISEASE (VITELLIFORM MACULAR DYSTROPHY).

Etiology

Unprotected solar eclipse viewing, sungazing (e.g., related to religious rituals, psychiatric illnesses, hallucinogenic drugs), sunbathing, vocational exposure (e.g., aviation, military service, astronomy, arc welding)

Workup

- History: Eclipse viewing or sungazing? Work exposure? Photosensitizing medications?
- Complete ocular examination, including a dilated fundus examination and careful inspection of the macula with a slit lamp using a 60-, 90-diopter, or fundus contact lens.
- Amsler grid testing may identify central or paracentral scotomata.
- IVFA typically shows a window defect late in the disease course.
- OCT findings in the acute setting include hyporeflectivity at the level of the RPE and occasional hyperreflectivity of the injured neurosensory retina. In the chronic stage, a central hyporeflective defect at the level of the photoreceptor inner segment–outer segment junction is seen (see Figure 11.35.2).

Treatment

1. Observation. Eyes with better visual acuities on initial examination tend to recover more vision. Long-term significant reduction in visual acuity is rare. However, central or paracentral scotomata may persist despite improvement in visual acuity.

11.36 Choroidal Nevus and Malignant Melanoma of the Choroid

CHOROIDAL NEVUS

Symptoms

Usually asymptomatic. Rare symptoms include flashes of light (if SRF present) or decreased visual acuity (if directly subfoveal).

Signs

(See Figure 11.36.1.)

Critical. Flat or minimally elevated pigmented or nonpigmented choroidal lesion.

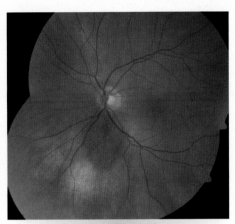

Figure 11.36.1 Choroidal nevus.

Other. Usually <2 mm thick with gradual elevation from the choroid. Overlying drusen become more prominent with age and can appear as hard cuticular drusen or soft drusen. RPE atrophy, hyperplasia, and detachment can occur. Rarely, overlying orange pigment (lipofuscin) or SRF is detected. Minimal growth of <1 mm over many years can be found. If >1 mm growth is observed over shorter period (1 year), transformation into melanoma should be considered.

Risk Factors for Malignant Transformation

These are remembered by the mnemonic "to find small ocular melanoma doing imaging" whereby the first letter of each word (TFSOM-DIM) represents a risk factor found using multimodal imaging.

- T: Thickness >2 mm (US).
- F: Fluid subretinal (OCT).
- S: Symptoms (vision loss, <20/50 on Snellen visual acuity).
- O: Orange pigment hyperautofluorescence (autofluorescence).
- M: Melanoma hollow (US).
- DIM: Diameter >5 mm (photography).

> **NOTE:** If four or more factors are present, the lesion has a >50% chance to show growth and is likely to be a small choroidal melanoma.

Differential Diagnosis

See below for differential diagnosis of pigmented/nonpigmented choroidal lesions.

Workup

1. Complete ophthalmologic examination including dilated fundus examination with evaluation of the lesion using a 20-diopter lens.
2. Detailed clinical drawing of the lesion with careful attention to location and size.
3. Baseline color photos of the lesion to assist in diameter assessment and in documenting growth.
4. OCT to document the overlying retinal features, SRF, and the lesion itself using enhanced-depth imaging.
5. Autofluorescence to document the presence of lipofuscin or RPE disturbance.
6. US for tumor thickness measurement and internal acoustic qualities.

Treatment

Observation. First examination should be in 3 to 4 months to confirm stability and then one to two times yearly to document lack of change.

Follow Up

Low-risk lesions can be followed with annual dilated fundus examination. High-risk lesions should be followed every 3 to 6 months.

MALIGNANT MELANOMA OF THE CHOROID

Symptoms

Decreased vision, visual field defect, floaters, light flashes, rarely pain; often asymptomatic.

Signs

(See Figure 11.36.2.)

Critical. Gray-green or brown (melanotic) or yellow (amelanotic) choroidal mass that exhibits one or more of the following:

- Presence of SRF.
- Thickness ≥2 mm, especially with an abrupt elevation from the choroid.

11

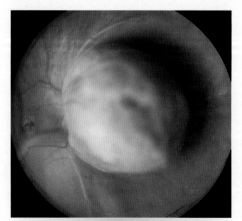

Figure 11.36.2 Choroidal melanoma.

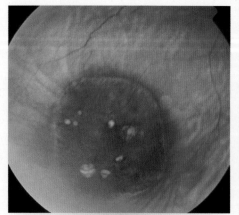

Figure 11.36.3 Congenital hypertrophy of the retinal pigment epithelium.

- Ill-defined, large areas of geographic orange pigment over the lesion.
- A dome, mushroom, or plateau shape with congested blood vessels in the apex of the tumor.
- Break in Bruch membrane with subretinal hemorrhage.
- Growth.

NOTE: A diffuse choroidal melanoma can appear as a minimally thickened dark choroidal lesion without a prominently elevated mass and can simulate a nevus.

Other. Overlying cystoid retinal degeneration, VH or vitreous pigmented cells, drusen on the tumor surface, CNV, proptosis (from orbital invasion). Choroidal melanoma rarely occurs in darker pigmented individuals and more commonly occurs in light-skinned, blue- or green-eyed individuals.

Differential Diagnosis of Pigmented Lesions

- Choroidal nevus: See above.
- Congenital hypertrophy of the RPE: Flat black lesions that have crisp margins and often occur in the peripheral fundus. The margins are often well delineated with a surrounding depigmented and pigmented halo. Depigmented lacunae within the lesion appear as the lesion ages. Asymptomatic **(see Figure 11.36.3)**.

- Reactive hyperplasia of the RPE: Related to previous trauma or inflammation. Lesions are black, flat, have irregular margins, and may have associated white gliosis. Often multifocal.
- Subretinal blood: From any cause can simulate a melanoma, including AMD, IPCV, PEHCR, others. IVFA and ICGA may aid in differentiation. See specific sections.
- Melanocytoma of the optic nerve: A black optic nerve lesion with fibrillated margins. It can grow slowly in approximately 15% cases. IVFA may allow differentiation.
- Choroidal detachment: Follows ocular surgery, trauma, or hypotony of another etiology. Dark peripheral multilobular fundus mass. The ora serrata is often visible without scleral depression. Localized suprachoroidal hemorrhage can be very difficult to differentiate from melanoma based on appearance alone. Transillumination may help distinguish a serous choroidal detachment (but not hemorrhagic) from melanoma. In these situations, IVFA is the study of choice, usually allowing differentiation between the two entities. See 11.27, CHOROIDAL EFFUSION/DETACHMENT.

Differential Diagnosis of Nonpigmented Lesions

- Choroidal hemangioma: Red-orange, may be elevated, not mushroom shaped.
- Metastatic carcinoma: Cream or light brown, flat or slightly elevated, extensive SRF, may be multifocal or bilateral. Patient may have

a history of cancer (especially breast or lung cancer).

- Choroidal osteoma: Yellow-orange, usually close to the optic disc, pseudopod-like projections of the margin; often bilateral; typically occurs in young women in their teens or twenties. US may show a minimally elevated, calcified plaque-like lesion.

- Posterior scleritis: Patients may have choroidal folds, pain, proptosis, uveitis, or anterior scleritis associated with an amelanotic mass. Look for the T-sign on US. See 5.7, SCLERITIS.

- Lymphoma: Yellow-orange infiltration; can be unilateral or bilateral; often there is associated orbital or conjunctival lymphoma.

- Sclerochoroidal calcification: Asymptomatic, yellow-white, sub-RPE, and subchoroidal plaques. Typically bilateral and commonly postequatorial and superotemporal. May be elevated. May be the result of calcification of the insertion of the oblique muscles. B-scan US shows an elevated, calcified lesion. Typically idiopathic and seen in elderly patients. Can be associated with abnormalities of calcium-phosphorus metabolism and cases of renal tubular hypokalemic metabolic alkalosis (e.g., Gitelman and Bartter syndromes). Renal function, parathyroid hormone, and serum electrolytes including calcium and magnesium should be checked.

Workup

1. History: Ocular surgery or trauma, cancer, anorexia, weight loss, or systemic illness?

2. Dilated fundus examination using indirect ophthalmoscopy.

3. IVFA: Can rule out lesions that simulate melanoma, but may not differentiate melanoma from large nevus, metastases, or hemangioma.

4. A-scan and B-scan US: Documents thickness and confirms clinical impression. With choroidal melanoma, US usually shows low-to-moderate reflectivity with choroidal excavation. Thickness is often >2 mm. May show a mushroom appearance.

5. OCT: Often documents fresh SRF.

6. Autofluorescence: Often shows prominent overlying lipofuscin (orange pigment).

7. ICGA: Can show double circulation with prominent blood vessels within the melanoma.

8. Consider fine-needle aspiration biopsy for genetic analysis of the tumor for prognostication and in selected cases for cytologic confirmation.

9. Consider CT scan or MRI of the orbit and brain (useful in patients with opaque media):

   - If melanoma is confirmed, systemic follow up is done according to the risk level for metastatic disease. Blood work: Lactate dehydrogenase, gamma-glutamyl transferase, aspartate and alanine aminotransferases, and alkaline phosphatase twice yearly. If liver enzymes are elevated, consider an MRI or liver scan to rule out liver metastases.
   - Annual chest x-ray.
   - Annual MRI of the liver.
   - Annual complete physical examination by a medical internist or oncologist.

10. Referral to an internist or oncologist for breast examination, full skin examination, chest CT, and possibly a carcinoembryonic antigen assay if choroidal metastases are suspected.

Treatment

Depending on the results of the metastatic workup, the tumor characteristics, the status of the contralateral eye, and the age and general health of the patient, melanoma of the choroid may be managed by observation, photocoagulation, transpupillary thermotherapy, radiation therapy, local resection, enucleation, or exenteration. Most cases are managed with plaque radiotherapy. Anti-VEGF injections every 4 months for the first 2 years have been shown to minimize ultimate vision loss from radiation retinopathy. In some cases, sector photocoagulation is added.

REFERENCES

Shields CL, Dalvin LA, Ancona-Lezama D, et al. Choroidal nevus imaging features in 3,806 cases and risk factors for transformation into melanoma in 2,355 cases: the 2020 Taylor R. Smith and Victor T. Curtin lecture. *Retina.* 2019;39(10):1840-1851.

Shields CL, Dalvin LA, Chang M, et al. Visual outcome at 4 years following iodine-125 plaque radiotherapy and prophylactic intravitreal bevacizumab (every 4 months for 2 years) for uveal melanoma in 1131 patients. *JAMA Ophthalmol.* 2019;138(2):136-146. doi:10.1001/jamaophthalmol.2019.5132

11

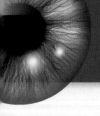

Chapter 12

Uveitis

APPROACH TO UVEITIS

Uveitis is not a single disease but a collection of 30 to 40 different disorders that may be characterized by clinical symptoms, anatomic location, morphology, presence or absence of key anatomic findings (such as ciliary flush, keratic precipitates [KP], iris nodules, synechiae, snowballs, snowbanks, retinal vasculitis, macular edema, and optic neuropathy), and response to treatment. A thorough history and review of systems with a complete examination will typically narrow the differential diagnosis to a much more manageable number of possibilities on which the workup should be based. There is no one "uveitis workup." The use of a "shotgun" approach to diagnostic testing is not only not cost-effective but will often lead to incorrect diagnoses and treatment based on a misunderstanding of the sensitivity, specificity, and positive and negative predictive values of a given test.

The Standardization of Uveitis Nomenclature Working Group has emphasized the clinical presentation of the disease, laterality, and the anatomic location of inflammation in the evaluation of patients with uveitis.

- The history defines the course of the disease.
  - Onset (sudden versus insidious)
  - Duration
    - Limited (<3 months) versus persistent (>3 months).
  - Course
    - Acute (sudden onset and limited duration).
    - Recurrent (flare-ups occurring >3 months after stopping therapy).
    - Chronic (persistent or flaring up <3 months after stopping therapy).
    - Note that by these criteria, the term "acute or chronic" has no meaning, and uveitis controlled with medication should be considered "suppressed" and not "in remission."

- Laterality
  - Unilateral.
  - Unilateral/alternating (bilateral and nonsimultaneous).
  - Bilateral and simultaneous.
- Anatomic location
  - Anterior: cells limited to the anterior chamber (iritis) or with some anterior vitreous involvement (iridocyclitis)
    - Anterior chamber cells must be greater than vitreous cells.
    - Isolated anterior uveitis should NEVER be diagnosed without assessment of the retina.
  - Intermediate uveitis: Cells in the vitreous cavity (vitritis) without chorioretinal involvement; may have anterior chamber cells
    - Vitreous cells must be greater than anterior chamber cells.
  - Posterior: isolated retinitis, choroiditis, or both
    - Retinochoroiditis: primarily retinal with secondary choroidal involvement.
    - Chorioretinitis: primarily choroidal with secondary retinal involvement.
    - There may be posterior vitreous cells.
    - Optic disc edema and hyperemia may be present.
    - Neuroretinitis.
    - Retinal vasculitis
      - Venous.
      - Arterial.
      - Mixed venous/arterial.
    - Lesions in posterior uveitis should be characterized by:
      - Color
        - White lesions are usually retinal.
        - Yellow lesions are usually choroidal.
        - Pigmented lesions usually indicate long-standing disease.

- Presence or absence of hemorrhage
- Presence or absence of retinal vasculitis
- Border appearance: creamy versus granular versus sharply defined
- Pattern
  - Focal or paucifocal.
  - Multifocal.
- Morphology
  - Placoid.
  - Punched-out.
  - Serpiginous.
  - Amoeboid.
  - Ovoid.
  - Punctate.
- Panuveitis: concurrent anterior, intermediate, and posterior uveitis.

> 📝 **NOTE:** Macular edema and peripheral retinal vasculitis do not by themselves define posterior uveitis (e.g., pars planitis may have cystoid macular edema [CME], peripheral vascular sheathing and leakage, and optic disc edema but it is still an intermediate uveitis).

Hypopyon (layering of white blood cells in the anterior chamber)
- Usually white, flat-topped.
- Bloody hypopyon often suggests herpetic uveitis.
- Shifting hypopyon (changes with head position) suggests Behçet disease.

Consider different causes of or predisposing factors to uveitis (recognizing there may be substantial overlap)
- Infectious.
- Systemic inflammatory disease.

- Vascular disorders.
- Host immune status.
- Genetic.
- Drug-induced.
- Trauma.
- Environmental.

The principles of the uveitis workup should be as follows:

1. Distinguish infectious from noninfectious uveitis.
2. Distinguish purely ocular disease from uveitis associated with systemic conditions.
3. Consider masquerade syndromes (e.g., retained intraocular foreign body, tumors, chronic retinal detachment, etc.).
4. Obtain additional testing only if the results will influence the differential diagnosis, medical or surgical management, prognosis, or referral patterns.
5. Recognize that up to 40% of uveitis is undifferentiated (the term preferred to "idiopathic," since nearly all noninfectious uveitis has no known cause) and explain this to patients.
6. Imaging, like laboratory testing, should be based on the disease and not used indiscriminately. Testing may include:
   - Optical coherence tomography (OCT).
   - Intravenous fluorescein angiography (IVFA).
   - Indocyanine green angiography (ICGA).
   - Fundus autofluorescence (FAF).
   - OCT angiography.
   - Visual field testing.
   - Electrophysiology.

12

12.1 Anterior Uveitis (Iritis/Iridocyclitis)

Symptoms

- Acute: Pain, redness, photophobia, consensual photophobia (pain in the affected eye when a light is shone in the fellow eye), excessive tearing, and decreased vision.
- Chronic: Decreased vision (from cataract, vitreous debris, CME, or epiretinal membrane [ERM]) and floaters. May have periods of exacerbations and remissions with few acute symptoms (e.g., juvenile idiopathic arthritis [JIA]).

Signs

Critical
- Cells and flare in the anterior chamber (see **Tables 12.1.1** and **12.1.2**) and ciliary flush.

Keratic Precipitates
- Fine KP: Herpes simplex or varicella zoster virus, cytomegalovirus (CMV), Fuchs heterochromic iridocyclitis (FHIC).
- Small, nongranulomatous KP (NGKP): HLA-B27-associated, trauma, masquerade

TABLE 12.1.1 Grading of Anterior Chamber Cells

Grade	Cells in 1 × 1 mm Field
0	<1
0.5+	1 to 5
1+	6 to 15
2+	16 to 25
3+	26 to 50
4+	>50

syndromes, JIA, Posner–Schlossman syndrome (glaucomatocyclitic crisis), drug-induced. Granulomatous uveitides such as sarcoidosis can present with NGKP; the reverse rarely occurs.
- Granulomatous KP (large, greasy, "mutton-fat"; mostly on the inferior cornea): Sarcoidosis, syphilis, tuberculosis (TB), JIA-associated, sympathetic ophthalmia, lens-induced, Vogt–Koyanagi–Harada (VKH) syndrome, and others.
- CMV uveitis often has characteristic "coin-shaped" KP not found in other herpetic uveitides.
- The location of KP can be helpful diagnostically.
  - Diffuse KP are characteristic of FHIC and herpetic uveitides.
  - KP underneath areas of stroma opacification suggest herpes simplex or, less often, varicella zoster keratouveitis.
  - Granulomatous KP in an inferior peripheral crescent underneath areas of stromal haze (often with fine, deep stromal vascularization) are highly suggestive of sarcoidosis.

TABLE 12.1.2 Grading of Anterior Chamber Flare

Grade	Description
0	None
1+	Faint
2+	Moderate (iris/lens details clear)
3+	Marked (iris/lens details hazy)
4+	Intense (fibrin/plastic aqueous)

- Granulomatous KP in Arlt triangle (apex near central cornea, base at inferior limbus) are nonspecific.
- "Crenated" KP are translucent and discrete, usually medium-large lesions characteristic of regressed granulomatous anterior uveitis.

Other. Low intraocular pressure (IOP) more commonly seen (secondary to ciliary body hyposecretion), elevated IOP can occur (e.g., herpetic, lens-induced, FHIC, Posner–Schlossman syndrome), fibrin (e.g., HLA-B27 or endophthalmitis), hypopyon (e.g., HLA-B27, Behçet disease, infectious endophthalmitis, rifabutin-induced, tumor), iris nodules (e.g., sarcoidosis, syphilis, TB), iris atrophy (e.g., herpetic, oral fourth-generation fluoroquinolones), iris heterochromia (e.g., FHIC), iris synechiae (especially HLA-B27, sarcoidosis), band keratopathy (especially JIA in younger patients, any chronic uveitis in older patients), uveitis in a "quiet eye" (consider JIA, FHIC, and masquerade syndromes), and CME **(see Figure 12.1.1)**.

Differential Diagnosis

- Intermediate or panuveitis with spillover into the anterior chamber: Mainly floaters and decreased vision, positive fundoscopic findings (see 12.3, POSTERIOR UVEITIS).
- Traumatic iritis. See 3.5, TRAUMATIC IRITIS.
- Posner–Schlossman syndrome: Recurrent episodes of very high IOP and minimal inflammation. Many cases are caused by herpetic uveitis (herpes simplex virus [HSV], varicella

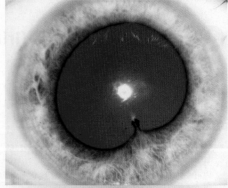

Figure 12.1.1 Anterior uveitis with posterior synechiae.

zoster virus [VZV], and CMV). See 9.8, GLAUCOMATOCYCLITIC CRISIS/POSNER–SCHLOSSMAN SYNDROME.

- Drug-induced uveitis (e.g., rifabutin, cidofovir, sulfonamides, pamidronate, systemic fluoroquinolones [especially moxifloxacin], biologic drugs, cancer immunotherapy [checkpoint inhibitors], and some chemotherapeutic drugs).
- Sclerouveitis: Uveitis secondary to scleritis; typically presents with profound pain and tenderness to palpation. See 5.7, SCLERITIS.
- Contact lens-associated red eye (CLARE): Red eye, corneal edema, epithelial defects, iritis with or without hypopyon, hypoxic subepithelial or stromal infiltrates (often multiple) may be present.
- Infectious keratouveitis: Corneal infiltrate is present. See 4.11, BACTERIAL KERATITIS.
- Infectious endophthalmitis: History of recent ocular surgery (including intravitreal injections), penetrating trauma, systemic infections (e.g., urinary tract infections), recent bowel or dental surgery, and skin wounds. Signs and symptoms include pain, hypopyon, fibrinous anterior chamber reaction, vitritis, decreased vision, and red eye; may have an endogenous source with fever, elevated white blood cell count. See 12.13 to 12.16, ENDOPHTHALMITIS SECTIONS.
- Schwartz–Matsuo syndrome: Pigment released from a chronic retinal detachment clogs the trabecular meshwork, resulting in elevated IOP.
- Tumor: Retinoblastoma and juvenile xanthogranuloma in children, primary intraocular lymphoma in elderly, metastatic disease in all ages, and others.
- Pseudouveitis from pigment dispersion syndrome. Other findings include Krukenburg spindle and iris transillumination defects. Pigment cells in the anterior chamber are smaller than white blood cells and may disappear when viewed with a red-free light.

Etiology

- Undifferentiated (idiopathic) (30% to 50% of anterior uveitis has no identifiable cause or disease association).
- HLA-B27-associated uveitis: Systemic associations include ankylosing spondylitis, reactive arthritis (Reiter syndrome), psoriatic arthritis, and inflammatory bowel disease.

> **NOTE:** Bilateral acute recurrent alternating anterior uveitis is very characteristic of HLA-B27 uveitis.

- Lens-induced uveitis: Immune reaction to the lens material, often secondary to incomplete cataract extraction, trauma with lens capsule damage, or hypermature cataract. See 9.12, LENS-RELATED GLAUCOMA.
- Postoperative iritis: Anterior chamber inflammation following intraocular surgery. Rule out acute endophthalmitis, retained lens fragments, iris chafing, or recurrence of preexisting anterior uveitis (e.g., HLA B27-associated uveitis). A small percentage of patients (especially African-Americans) with well-positioned posterior chamber intraocular lenses (IOL) may have a low-grade, steroid-responsive anterior uveitis that recurs when low-dose topical steroids are tapered off. Endophthalmitis must be considered if severe inflammation and pain are present. See 12.14, CHRONIC POSTOPERATIVE UVEITIS.
- Uveitis–glaucoma–hyphema (UGH) syndrome: Usually secondary to irritation from an IOL (particularly a closed-loop anterior chamber lens or single-piece IOL in ciliary sulcus). A milder variant with iris chafing but no hyphema can occur (look for iris transillumination defects in an undilated pupil). See 9.16, POSTOPERATIVE GLAUCOMA.
- Behçet disease: Young adults, acute simultaneous bilateral shifting hypopyon and iritis, aphthous ulcers, genital ulcerations, erythema nodosum, retinal vasculitis (arteries and/or veins), and hemorrhages, may have recurrent episodes.
- VKH disease: acute unilateral or bilateral anterior uveitis occurs in chronic VKH disease.
- Lyme disease: May have a history of a tick bite and rash. See 13.3, LYME DISEASE.
- Anterior segment ischemia: Unilateral. Flare out of proportion to a cellular reaction. Corneal edema is common. Pain. Secondary to carotid insufficiency, tight scleral buckle, or previous extraocular muscle surgeries.
- Tubulointerstitial nephritis and uveitis (TINU) syndrome: Uncommon but frequently underdiagnosed; usually bilateral nongranulomatous uveitis in children and young adults, female predilection. May be precipitated by oral

12

nonsteroidal anti-inflammatory drug (NSAID) therapy. Systemic symptoms include abdominal pain, fatigue, and malaise. Urinary beta-2 microglobulin, urinary casts, and increased serum creatinine helpful diagnostically.

- Toxoplasmosis: granulomatous unilateral anterior uveitis, posterior synechiae, and mutton-fat KP in Arlt triangle typically present. Occurs only with concurrent toxoplasmic retinitis.

- Other rare infectious etiologies of anterior uveitis: Mumps, influenza, adenovirus, measles, chlamydia, leptospirosis, Kawasaki disease, rickettsial disease, chikungunya virus, and others. Ask about recent travel history.

Chronic

- JIA: Usually occurs in young girls with pauciarticular arthritis (≤4 joints involved); may be painless and asymptomatic with minimal injection. Usually bilateral. Iritis may precede typical arthritis. Positive antinuclear antibody (ANA), negative rheumatoid factor, and increased erythrocyte sedimentation rate (ESR) are most commonly seen. Associated with glaucoma, cataracts, band keratopathy, and CME. Uveitis less commonly occurs in polyarticular and rarely in systemic JIA (Still disease).

- Chronic iridocyclitis of children: Usually occurs in young girls; it is similar to JIA in signs and symptoms but lacks arthritis.

- FHIC: Floaters with or without blurred vision and glare, but few other symptoms, diffuse iris stromal atrophy often causing a lighter-colored iris with transillumination defects and blunting of the iris architecture. Gonioscopy may reveal fine vessels that cross the trabecular meshwork. Fine, stellate KP over the entire corneal endothelium, and mild anterior chamber reaction. Vitreous opacities, glaucoma, and cataracts are common, but macular edema and posterior synechiae are absent. Topical corticosteroids not helpful. Cataract surgery may cause anterior chamber hemorrhage from rupture of fine angle vessels, but outcomes are usually excellent.

- Sarcoidosis: More common in African-Americans and Scandinavians. Usually bilateral; can have extensive posterior synechiae and conjunctival or iris nodules. See 12.6, SARCOIDOSIS.

- HSV/VZV/CMV: May be chronic or acute and recurrent. Diffuse KP, increased IOP, and iris atrophy (transillumination defects). History of a unilateral recurrent red eye, occasionally history of skin vesicles, or history of shingles. Corneal scars associated with decreased corneal sensation may be present. HSV and VZV anterior uveitis usually require long-term oral acyclovir, valacyclovir, or famciclovir; CMV anterior uveitis usually requires oral valganciclovir. All three types usually require chronic low-dose topical corticosteroids for suppression.

- Syphilis: Anterior and intermediate uveitis are most common. May have a maculopapular rash, iris roseola (vascular papules on the iris), and interstitial keratitis with ghost vessels in late stages. Inflammation of any ocular structure may occur. Placoid chorioretinitis is virtually pathognomonic. Neurosyphilis can cause meningismus. See 12.12, SYPHILIS.

- TB: "Sticky" uveitis with extensive posterior synechiae, usually bilateral. Positive protein derivative of tuberculin (PPD) and/or interferon-gamma release assay (IGRA) (e.g., QuantiFERON-TB Gold), typical chest radiograph findings (helpful but not necessary for diagnosis; most TB uveitis occurs in patients without pulmonary TB), occasionally phlyctenular or interstitial keratitis, and sometimes signs of posterior uveitis. See 12.3, POSTERIOR UVEITIS.

- Others: Leprosy, brucellosis, and other infectious causes.

Workup

1. Obtain a thorough history and review of systems. Specifically ask about fevers, chills, fatigue, malaise, cough, shortness of breath, joint pain/swelling/stiffness, diarrhea, blood in urine/stool, skin rashes, and oral or genital ulcers.

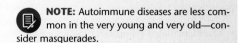 **NOTE:** Autoimmune diseases are less common in the very young and very old—consider masquerades.

2. Complete ocular examination, including an IOP check, gonioscopy, and a dilated fundus examination. The vitreous should be evaluated for cells.

3. A laboratory workup may be unnecessary in certain situations:

   • First episode of a mild, unilateral, nongranulomatous uveitis with a history and examination that is not suggestive of systemic disease or herpetic uveitis.

   • Uveitis in the setting of known systemic disease such as sarcoidosis or the use of medicines known to cause uveitis (e.g., rifabutin).

   • Clinical findings are classic for a particular diagnosis (e.g., herpetic keratouveitis, FHIC, and toxoplasmosis).

4. In all other situations requiring laboratory or diagnostic testing, a targeted workup is recommended. If too many tests are ordered unnecessarily, a portion of them may come back false-positive and confuse the diagnosis. See **Table 12.1.3**. However, if a patient presents with bilateral, granulomatous, or recurrent uveitis without a suspected diagnosis, our practice is to at least evaluate for sarcoidosis,

TABLE 12.1.3 Suggested Diagnostic Workup for Anterior Uveitis

Ankylosing spondylitis	HLA B27, SI joint films, rheumatology consult
Reactive arthritis	HLA B27, SI joint films (if symptomatic), swab for *Chlamydia*
Psoriatic arthritis	HLA B27, rheumatology and/or dermatology consult
Lyme disease	Lyme antibody immunofluorescent assay (e.g., ELISA)
Juvenile idiopathic arthritis or any suspect uveitis in children	Rheumatoid factor, antinuclear antibodies, HLA-B27, radiographs of affected joints, urinalysis and renal function tests, rheumatology consult
Sarcoidosis	Chest radiograph and/or chest CT, PPD or IGRA, ACE, lysozyme
Syphilis	RPR or VDRL, FTA-ABS or treponemal-specific assay; HIV testing if positive
Ocular ischemic syndrome	Intravenous fluorescein angiography, carotid Doppler studies

syphilis, and TB (in at-risk patients). Consider additional workup as needed based on history and examination.

• Syphilis testing (see 12.12 Syphilis).

• PPD and/or IGRA. Limit use of TB testing to patients:

   • At risk of TB (e.g., immigrants from high-risk areas such as India, human immunodeficiency virus [HIV]-positive patients), homeless patients, or prisoners).

   • If immunosuppressive therapy (especially biologics) are being considered.

   • If anti-inflammatory therapy is not working.

• Chest radiograph or chest CT to rule out sarcoidosis and pulmonary tuberculosis.

• Angiotensin-converting enzyme (ACE) ± lysozyme (questionable utility).

• Lyme antibody (consider in endemic areas).

• HLA-B27 (in acute unilateral or bilateral alternating anterior uveitis; especially if hypopyon is present; ask about symptoms of a seronegative spondyloarthropathy).

• Anterior chamber paracentesis for polymerase chain reaction (PCR) testing for suspected herpes virus-associated anterior uveitis (HSV, VZV, and CMV) and toxoplasmosis.

   • Serologic tests for infectious diseases have a low positive predictive value due to high seroprevalence in the general population, but negative tests (e.g., IgM and IgG for *Toxoplasma gondii*) may help to rule out the disease.

12

📝 **NOTE:** In children with uveitis, sarcoidosis and syphilis are much less common and no lab test should be ordered routinely except as indicated by the history and findings. Evaluation for systemic disease by a pediatric rheumatologist may be warranted (e.g., JIA and TINU).

Treatment

1. Cycloplegic (e.g., cyclopentolate 1% t.i.d. for mild to moderate inflammation; atropine 1% b.i.d. to q.i.d. for severe inflammation).

2. Topical steroid (e.g., prednisolone acetate 1%) q1–6h, depending on the severity of

inflammation. Most cases of moderate to severe acute uveitis require q1–2h dosing initially. Difluprednate 0.05% may allow less frequent dosing than prednisolone acetate. Consider a loading dose (prednisolone acetate 1% one drop every minute for 5 minutes at bedtime and awakening) or fluorometholone 0.1% ophthalmic ointment at night. If the anterior uveitis is severe, unilateral, and is not responding to topical steroids, then consider periocular repository steroids (e.g., 0.5 to 1.0 mL subtenon injection of triamcinolone 40 mg/mL). See Appendix 10, TECHNIQUE FOR RETROBULBAR/SUBTENON/SUBCONJUNCTIVAL INJECTIONS.

> **NOTE:** The periocular use of triamcinolone is off-label and must be discussed with patients. A trial of topical steroids at full strength for several weeks may help identify patients at risk of a significant IOP increase from steroids. Additionally, periocular depot steroids should be used with extreme caution in patients with scleritis because of possible scleral melting.

3. If there is no improvement on maximal topical and repository steroids, or if the uveitis is bilateral and severe, consider systemic steroids, or immunosuppressive therapy. Consider referral to a uveitis specialist and rheumatologist.

> **NOTE:** Prior to giving periocular depot steroids, it is important to rule out infectious causes; oral steroids in such cases may be helpful starting 1 to 2 days after initiation of treatment for the underlying infection.

4. Treat secondary glaucoma with aqueous suppressants. Avoid pilocarpine. Glaucoma may result from:
   - Cellular blockage of the trabecular meshwork. See 9.7, INFLAMMATORY OPEN ANGLE GLAUCOMA.
   - Secondary angle closure from synechiae formation. See 9.4, ACUTE ANGLE CLOSURE GLAUCOMA.
   - Neovascularization of the iris and angle. See 9.14, NEOVASCULAR GLAUCOMA.
   - Steroid-response. See 9.9, STEROID-RESPONSE GLAUCOMA.

   - Although topical prostaglandins may rarely cause uveitis, they should be tried if other medical management is ineffective before considering glaucoma surgery.

5. If an exact etiology for the anterior uveitis is determined, then additional ocular and/or systemic management may be indicated.
   - Ankylosing spondylitis: Often requires systemic anti-inflammatory agents (e.g., NSAIDs such as naproxen). Consider consulting rheumatology, physical therapy, and cardiology (increased incidence of cardiomegaly, conduction defects, and aortic insufficiency).
   - Inflammatory bowel disease (IBD): Often benefits from systemic steroids, sulfadiazine, or other immunosuppressive agents. Obtain a medical or gastrointestinal consult.
   - Reactive arthritis (previously known as Reiter syndrome): If urethritis is present, then the patient and sexual partners are treated for chlamydia (e.g., single-dose azithromycin 1 g p.o.). Obtain medical and/or rheumatology or urology consult.
   - Psoriatic arthritis: Consider a rheumatology and/or dermatology consult.
   - Glaucomatocyclitic crisis: See 9.8, GLAUCOMATOCYCLITIC CRISIS/POSNER-SCHLOSSMAN SYNDROME.
   - Lens-induced uveitis: Usually requires removal of the lens material. See 9.12, LENS-RELATED GLAUCOMA.
   - Herpetic uveitis: Herpes simplex typically requires topical or oral antivirals and steroid drops for nonepithelial corneal disease. Herpetic iridocyclitis benefits from topical steroids and systemic antiviral medications (e.g., acyclovir, valacyclovir, or famciclovir); topical antivirals are usually ineffective for uveitis due to poor intraocular penetration. See 4.15, HERPES SIMPLEX VIRUS and 4.16, HERPES ZOSTER OPHTHALMICUS/VARICELLA ZOSTER VIRUS.
   - UGH syndrome: See 9.16, POSTOPERATIVE GLAUCOMA.
   - Behçet disease: See 12.7, BEHÇET DISEASE.
   - Lyme disease: See 13.3, LYME DISEASE.
   - JIA: Topical steroids can be useful acutely for reducing cells and flare, but should be minimized for long-term therapy to reduce the risk of cataract and glaucoma, both of which

are more common in children. Systemic steroid therapy in children may cause growth suppression and should be avoided if possible. Prolonged cycloplegic therapy may be required and necessitate appropriate refractive correction. Consultation with rheumatology, pediatrics, and/or a uveitis specialist is useful as immunomodulatory therapy (e.g., methotrexate, adalimumab, and infliximab) is often needed. Regular follow up is essential, as flares may be asymptomatic; recurrent or chronic disease can lead to irreversible damage and various sequelae including synechiae, glaucoma (or hypotony), CME, epiretinal membrane, and cataract formation.

> **NOTE:** Cataract surgery in patients with JIA-associated uveitis has a high complication rate. Avoid cataract surgery if possible until the patient is inflammation-free for at least 3 months. An IOL may be placed in select circumstances and is preferable to aphakia in well-controlled disease.

- Chronic iridocyclitis of children: Same as JIA.
- FHIC: Usually does not respond to or require steroids (a trial of steroids may be attempted, but they should be tapered quickly if there is no response); cycloplegics are not necessary.

> **NOTE:** Patients with FHIC usually do well with cataract surgery; however, they may develop a hyphema.

- Sarcoidosis: See 12.6, SARCOIDOSIS.
- Syphilis: See 12.12, SYPHILIS.
- Tuberculosis: Refer the patient to an internist, infectious disease specialist, or public health officer for consideration of systemic treatment. Patients with ocular TB frequently have no pulmonary disease but still require systemic four-drug antituberculous therapy. Concomitant oral steroids or methotrexate may be necessary.

Follow Up

1. Every 1 to 7 days in the acute phase, depending on the severity; every 1 to 3 months when stable.
2. At each visit, the anterior chamber reaction and IOP should be evaluated.
3. A vitreous and fundus examination should be performed for all flare-ups, when vision is affected, or every 3 to 6 months. Macular edema is a frequent cause of decreased vision even after the uveitis is controlled; OCT can be very useful.
4. If the anterior chamber reaction has resolved, then the steroid drops can be slowly tapered with intermittent examinations to ensure that the inflammation does not return during the taper (usually one drop per day every 3 to 7 days [e.g., q.i.d. for 1 week, then t.i.d. for 1 week, then b.i.d. for 1 week, etc.]). Steroids are usually discontinued following the taper when the anterior chamber is quiet. Occasionally, long-term, low-dose steroids every day or every other day are required to keep the inflammation from recurring. Punctal occlusion techniques may increase the potency of the drug and decrease systemic absorption. The cycloplegic agents also can be tapered off as the anterior chamber reaction improves and no new posterior synechiae are noted.

> **NOTE:** Topical steroids should be tapered slowly to prevent severe rebound inflammation. If oral steroids are used, consider concurrent calcium 600 mg with vitamin D 400 units twice a day to reduce the risk of osteoporosis. In patients with very severe disease, note that doses of prednisone >60 mg/d increase the risk of ischemic necrosis of bone, and a three-day course of intravenous methylprednisolone 1 g/d for 3 days should be considered instead. Regular monitoring of glucose, blood pressure, lipids, and bone density should be done by a primary care doctor or rheumatologist if long-term oral steroid therapy is necessary.

12

12.2 Intermediate Uveitis

Symptoms

Painless floaters and decreased vision. Minimal photophobia or external inflammation. Most often bilateral and classically affects patients aged 15 to 40 years.

Signs

(See Figure 12.2.1.)

Critical. Vitreous cells and cellular aggregates floating predominantly in the inferior vitreous (snowballs). Younger patients may present with vitreous hemorrhage. White exudative material over the inferior ora serrata and pars plana (snowbank) is suggestive of pars planitis.

NOTE: Snowbanking is typically in the inferior vitreous and can often be seen only with indirect ophthalmoscopy and scleral depression.

Other. Peripheral retinal vascular sheathing, peripheral neovascularization, mild anterior chamber inflammation, CME, posterior subcapsular cataract, band keratopathy, secondary glaucoma, ERM, and exudative retinal detachment. Posterior synechiae in pars planitis are uncommon and, if present, usually occur early in the course of the disease. Choroidal neovascularization is rare.

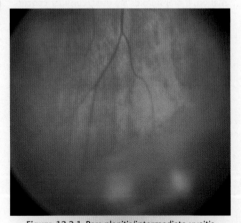

Figure 12.2.1 Pars planitis/intermediate uveitis with snowballs.

Etiology

- Pars planitis (>70%). Autoimmune disease of unknown cause in teenagers and young adults; insidious onset; bilateral but may be asymmetric; no clear gender predilection. CME most common cause of vision loss; vitreous hemorrhage may cause acute vision loss.
- Sarcoidosis. See 12.6, SARCOIDOSIS.
- Multiple sclerosis. See 10.14, OPTIC NEURITIS.
- Lyme disease. See 13.3, LYME DISEASE.
- Syphilis. See 12.12, SYPHILIS.
- TINU: Rare cause of uveitis, mostly in young females but wide age distribution. Ocular disease usually follows renal disease but occasionally precedes or is concurrent. More commonly presents as anterior uveitis. Requires co-management with a nephrologist; eye disease may linger long after resolution of nephritis.
- Primary intraocular lymphoma: intermediate uveitis may be the initial manifestation. Ask about neurologic symptoms in older patients; low threshold for CNS imaging. Referral to a retina specialist or an ocular oncologist for diagnostic pars plana vitrectomy and send the undiluted specimen to an experienced ocular cytopathologist; consider testing for interleukin-10 and MYD88 mutation. Oral steroids prior to biopsy may decrease the yield.
- Toxocariasis. See 12.3, POSTERIOR UVEITIS and 8.1, LEUKOCORIA.
- Others: IBD, Bartonellosis (cat-scratch disease), Whipple syndrome, primary Sjögren syndrome, etc.
- Masquerade syndromes include retinoblastoma in children, old vitreous hemorrhage, and asteroid hyalosis.

Workup

1. Complete ocular examination. Includes gonioscopy to evaluate for possible neovascularization.
2. Appropriate workup may include chest radiograph and/or chest CT, PPD and/or IGRA, ACE ± lysozyme, RPR or VDRL, and FTA-ABS or treponemal-specific assay. Obtain urinary beta-2 microglobulin, hemoglobin, creatinine, and urinalysis if TINU is suspected.

3. Consider IVFA and/or OCT to document CME or retinal vasculitis.

4. Consider lab testing for Lyme disease, toxoplasmosis, and cat-scratch disease in the appropriate clinical context. In older individuals, consider workup for malignancy/lymphoma.

5. Consider magnetic resonance imaging (MRI) of the brain ± orbits with gadolinium to evaluate for demyelinating lesions if the review of systems is positive for current or previous focal neurologic deficits. Refer to a neurologist for multiple sclerosis workup if necessary.

Treatment

Treat all vision-threatening complications (e.g., CME and vitritis) in symptomatic patients with active disease. Mild vitreous cell in the absence of symptoms, CME, or vision loss may be observed in cases of noninfectious intermediate uveitis.

1. Topical prednisolone acetate 1% or difluprednate 0.05% q1–2h. Consider subtenon steroid (e.g., 0.5 to 1.0 mL injection of triamcinolone 40 mg/mL). May repeat the injections every 6 to 8 weeks until the vision and CME have stabilized. Slowly taper the frequency of injections. Subtenon steroid injections must be used with caution in patients with steroid-induced glaucoma. See Appendix 10, TECHNIQUE FOR RETROBULBAR/SUBTENON/ SUBCONJUNCTIVAL INJECTIONS.

2. If there is minimal improvement after three subtenon steroid injections 1 to 2 months apart, consider systemic steroids (e.g., prednisone 40 to 60 mg p.o. daily for 4 to 6 weeks), tapering gradually according to the patient's response. High-dose systemic steroid therapy should last no longer than 2 to 3 months, followed by a taper to no more than 5 to 10 mg/d. Other options include sustained-release steroid implants (e.g., dexamethasone 0.7 mg intravitreal implant; fluocinolone acetonide 0.19 or 0.59 mg intravitreal implant) and immunomodulatory therapy (e.g., antimetabolites, calcineurin inhibitors, and anti-tumor necrosis factor agents), usually in conjunction with rheumatology.

NOTE: In bilateral cases, systemic steroid therapy may be preferred to periocular injections. However, in children and adolescents, growth suppression (in addition to the usual complications of long-term systemic steroids) is a major concern.

3. Transscleral cryotherapy to the area of snowbanking should be considered in patients who fail to respond to either oral or subtenon corticosteroids and who have neovascularization.

4. Pars plana vitrectomy may be useful in cases refractory to systemic steroids or to treat vitreous opacification, tractional retinal detachment, ERM, and other complications. Additionally, vitreous biopsy through a pars plana vitrectomy may be indicated in cases of suspected masquerade syndromes, especially intraocular lymphoma.

 NOTE

1. Some physicians delay steroid injections for several weeks to observe whether the IOP increases on topical steroids (steroid response). If a marked steroid response is found, depot injections should be avoided.

2. Intravitreal preservative-free triamcinolone acetonide and the dexamethasone or fluocinolone acetonide implants are more effective for uveitic macular edema than periocular triamcinolone.

3. Intravitreal anti-VEGF drugs (e.g., ranibizumab, bevacizumab, and aflibercept) are effective in the treatment of uveitic CME but only if the uveitis itself is suppressed.

4. Oral acetazolamide 250 mg two to four times a day can reduce CME but is often not well tolerated due to nausea, diarrhea, fatigue, malaise, anorexia, or hypokalemia.

5. Topical NSAIDs are usually not effective in patients with uveitic CME.

6. Cataracts are a frequent complication of intermediate uveitis. If cataract extraction is performed, the patient should ideally be free of inflammation for 3 months preceding the operation. Consider starting the patient on oral prednisone 60 mg daily 2 to 5 days prior to surgery and tapering the prednisone over the next 1 to 4 weeks. Aggressive perioperative use of topical NSAIDS (e.g., ketorolac 0.5% q.i.d.) and topical steroids (e.g., prednisolone acetate 1% q2h or difluprednate 0.05% six times a day) starting 2 to 5 days preoperatively and continued for at least 4 to 6 weeks postoperatively may reduce the risk of pseudophakic CME and recurrent uveitis. Consider a combined pars plana vitrectomy at the time of cataract surgery if significant vitreous opacification is present.

12

Follow Up

1. In the acute phase, patients are re-evaluated every 1 to 4 weeks, depending on the severity of the condition.
2. In the chronic phase, re-examination is performed every 3 to 6 months. Monitor for neovascularization, CME, ERM, glaucoma, and cataract.

Other Causes of Vitreous Cells

- Ocular ischemia.
- Spillover from anterior uveitis.
- Masquerade syndromes: Always consider these in the very old or very young patients.
  - Large cell lymphoma: Persistent vitreous cells in patients >50 years old, which usually do not respond completely to systemic steroids. Yellow-white subretinal infiltrates, retinal edema and hemorrhage, anterior chamber inflammation, or neurologic signs may be present.
  - Malignant melanoma: A retinal detachment and associated vitritis may obscure the underlying tumor. See 11.36, CHOROIDAL NEVUS AND MALIGNANT MELANOMA OF THE CHOROID.
  - Retinitis pigmentosa: Vitreous cells and macular edema may accompany waxy pallor of the optic disc, "bone-spicule" pigmentary changes, and attenuated retinal vessels. See 11.28, RETINITIS PIGMENTOSA AND INHERITED CHORIORETINAL DYSTROPHIES.
  - Rhegmatogenous retinal detachment (RRD): A small number of pigmented anterior vitreous and anterior chamber cells frequently accompany an RRD. Uveitis due to chronic retinal detachment (Schwartz–Matsuo syndrome) is one of the masquerade syndromes. See 11.3, RETINAL DETACHMENT.
  - Retained intraocular foreign body (IOFB): Persistent inflammation after a penetrating ocular injury. May have iris heterochromia. Diagnosed by indirect ophthalmoscopy, gonioscopy, B-scan ultrasonography (US), US biomicroscopy (UBM), or computed tomography (CT) scan of the globe. See 3.15, INTRAOCULAR FOREIGN BODY.
  - Retinoblastoma: Almost always occurs in young children. May also present with a pseudohypopyon and vitreous cells. One or more elevated white retinal lesions are usually, but not always, present. See 8.1, LEUKOCORIA.
  - Leukemia: Unilateral retinitis and vitritis may occur in patients already known to have leukemia. Prompt laboratory testing (complete blood count [CBC] with differential) and anterior chamber paracenteses (if there is anterior uveitis) for histology and immunostaining usually diagnostic.
  - Amyloidosis: Retrolenticular footplate-like deposits, vitreous globules, or vitreous membranes without any signs of anterior segment inflammation. Serum protein electrophoresis and diagnostic vitrectomy confirm the diagnosis. Rare.
  - Asteroid hyalosis: Small, white, refractile particles (calcium soaps) adherent to collagen fibers and floating in the vitreous. Usually asymptomatic and of no clinical significance.

Workup

1. Complete history and review of systems: Ask about systemic disease or infection, skin rash, tattoos, intravenous drug abuse, indwelling catheter, risk factors for AIDS, recent eye trauma or surgery, travel (particularly to Ohio-Mississippi River Valley, Southwestern United States, New England, or Middle Atlantic area), and exposures (e.g., tick bite).
2. Complete ocular examination, including IOP measurement and careful ophthalmoscopic examination. Indirect ophthalmoscopy with scleral depression of the ora serrata.
3. Consider IVFA for diagnosis or therapeutic planning.
4. Blood tests (any of the following may be obtained, depending on the suspected diagnosis, but a "shotgun" approach is inappropriate): *Toxoplasma* titer, ACE level, serum lysozyme, RPR or VDRL, FTA-ABS or treponemal-specific assay, ESR, ANA, ANCA, HLA-B51 (Behçet disease), HLA-A29 (birdshot retinochoroidopathy), *Toxocara* titer, IGRA ± PPD, and/or Lyme antibody. In neonates or immunocompromised patients, consider checking titers for HSV, VZV, CMV, and rubella virus. Cultures of blood and i.v. sites may be helpful when infectious etiologies are suspected. PCR techniques are available for HSV, VZV, CMV, and *Toxoplasma*.

5. Chest radiograph or CT.

6. CT/MRI of the brain and lumbar puncture when either lymphoma is suspected or there is any potential for central nervous system (CNS) involvement from an HIV-associated opportunistic infection.

7. Diagnostic vitrectomy when appropriate (see individual sections).

8. See individual sections for more specific guidelines on workup and treatment.

12.3 Posterior and Panuveitis

Symptoms

Blurred vision and floaters. Scotomas and metamorphopsia are common. Photopsias are often present in posterior uveitis. Pain, redness, and photophobia are often present due to anterior chamber inflammation.

NOTE: Panuveitis describes a pattern of severe, diffuse inflammation of both anterior and posterior segments. Often bilateral. Endophthalmitis or posterior scleritis should be considered in patients with posterior uveitis and significant pain.

Signs

Critical. Cells in the posterior vitreous, vitreous haze, retinal or choroidal inflammatory lesions, and retinal vasculitis (sheathing and exudates around vessels).

Other. Anterior and intermediate uveitis (indicative of panuveitis), retinal neovascularization, CME, ERM, and choroidal neovascular membranes.

Differential Diagnosis

Panuveitis

Possible etiologies are listed below:

- Sarcoidosis: See 12.6, SARCOIDOSIS.
- Syphilis: See 12.12, SYPHILIS.
- VKH syndrome: See 12.11, VOGT–KOYANAGI–HARADA SYNDROME.
- Behçet disease: See 12.1, ANTERIOR UVEITIS (IRITIS/IRIDOCYCLITIS) and 12.7, BEHÇET DISEASE.
- Lens-induced uveitis: See 9.12, LENS-RELATED GLAUCOMA.
- Sympathetic ophthalmia: See 12.18, SYMPATHETIC OPHTHALMIA.

- Tuberculosis: Produces varied clinical manifestations. The diagnosis is usually made by ancillary laboratory tests and response to antituberculosis therapy. Miliary tuberculosis may produce multifocal, small, yellow-white choroidal lesions. Most patients have concomitant anterior granulomatous or nongranulomatous uveitis.

- Tattoo-associated uveitis: Anterior, intermediate, or panuveitis mimicking sarcoidosis; associated with induration and itching of tattooed but not adjacent skin. Posterior synechiae and resistance to steroid therapy are common. Often requires immunosuppressive therapy. Removal of preexisting tattoos not usually effective and often not feasible.

White Dot Syndromes

- Acute posterior multifocal placoid pigment epitheliopathy (APMPPE): Acute visual loss in young adults, often after a viral illness. Multiple, creamy yellow–white or gray, plaque-like subretinal lesions in both eyes **(see Figure 12.3.1A and B)**. Lesions block early and stain late on IVFA. Usually spontaneously improves over weeks to months without treatment. May be associated with a cerebral vasculitis (consider MRA if the patient has a headache or other neurologic symptoms), in which case, systemic steroids are indicated.

- Multiple evanescent white dot syndrome (MEWDS): Photopsias and acute unilateral visual loss, often after a viral illness and usually in young women. May have a shimmering scotoma. Uncommonly bilateral, sequential, or recurrent. Characterized by multiple, small white lesions deep in the retina or at the level of the retinal pigment epithelium with foveal granularity and occasionally vitreous cells. Fluorescein angiography may show a classic perifoveal "wreath-like" pattern. There is often an enlarged blind spot on formal visual field

12

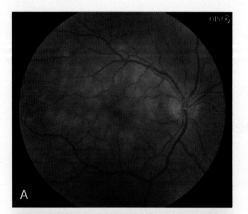

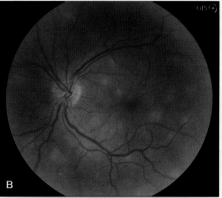

Figure 12.3.1 Fundus photographs of right (A) and left (B) eye showing creamy yellow subretinal lesions in APMPPE. Note a pigmented choroidal nevus along the inferotemporal arcade in the left eye.

testing. Vision typically returns to normal within 6 to 8 weeks without treatment.

- Birdshot retinochoroidopathy: Usually middle-aged patients with multiple bilateral, oval, creamy-yellow spots deep to the retina, approximately 1 mm in diameter, scattered throughout the fundus but most prominent in inferior quadrants. A mild to moderate vitritis is present. Retinal vasculitis, CME, and optic nerve edema may be present. ICG angiography shows characteristic hypofluorescent spots but fluorescein angiography often shows only retinal vasculitis, CME, and "quenching" of dye. Positive HLA-A29 in 95% to 100% of patients. Early systemic immunosuppression is often recommended.

- Multifocal choroiditis with panuveitis: Visual loss in young myopic women more often than men, typically bilateral. Multiple, small, round, and pale inflammatory lesions (similar to histoplasmosis) are located at the level of the pigment epithelium and choriocapillaris. Unlike histoplasmosis, vitritis occurs in 98% of patients. The lesions can occur in the macula and midperiphery and frequently respond to oral or periocular steroids, but typically recur with tapering, so that immunosuppressive therapy is often necessary. Choroidal neovascularization (CNV) occurs in about 1/3 of patients, and so patients should return for urgent evaluation if they have decreased vision or metamorphopsia.

- Punctate inner choroidopathy: Blurred vision, paracentral scotoma, and/or photopsias, usually in young myopic women. Multiple, small round yellow-white spots predominantly in posterior pole with minimal intraocular inflammation. Lesions become well-demarcated atrophic scars within weeks. CNV may develop in up to 40% of patients. Systemic immunosuppression is usually indicated.

- Serpiginous choroidopathy: Typically bilateral, recurrent chorioretinitis characterized by acute lesions (yellow-white subretinal patches with indistinct margins) bordering old atrophic scars. The chorioretinal changes usually extend from the optic disc outward; however, one-third may begin in the macula. Patients are typically aged 30 to 60 years. CNV may develop. Systemic immunosuppression is usually indicated. Must be distinguished from the "serpiginous" pattern of tuberculous chorioretinitis.

- Toxocariasis: Typically unilateral. Usually occurs in children. The most common presentations are a macular granuloma (elevated white retinal/subretinal lesion) with poor vision, unilateral intermediate uveitis with peripheral granuloma, or endophthalmitis. A peripheral lesion may be associated with a fibrous band extending to the optic disc, sometimes resulting in macular vessel dragging. A severe vitritis and anterior uveitis may be present. A negative undiluted *Toxocara* titer in an immunocompetent host usually rules out this disease. See 8.1, LEUKOCORIA.

- Presumed ocular histoplasmosis syndrome: Punched-out chorioretinal scars, peripapillary atrophy, CNV is common. Vitreous cells are absent. See 11.24, OCULAR HISTOPLASMOSIS.

Retinitis

- CMV retinitis: White patches of necrotic retina with granular borders, often mixed with retinal hemorrhage. Vascular sheathing (secondary frosted branch angiitis) in about 20% of eyes. Vitritis and anterior uveitis are usually mild. Seen in immunocompromised patients (most commonly in advanced HIV/AIDS, but also inherited or iatrogenic disorders of the immune system; rarely after periocular or intravitreal steroid injections) and congenitally infected neonates. See 12.9, CYTOMEGALOVIRUS RETINITIS.
- Acute retinal necrosis (ARN): Unilateral or bilateral peripheral white patches of thickened necrotic retina with vascular sheathing that progress rapidly. Marked vitritis and anterior uveitis are typically present. See 12.8, ACUTE RETINAL NECROSIS.
- Progressive outer retinal necrosis (PORN): Clinically similar to ARN, but may not have vitreous cells. Involves the posterior pole or optic nerve early, and classically spares the vessels. Occurs exclusively in severely immunocompromised patients, especially advanced HIV/AIDS, with rapid progression over several days. See 12.8, ACUTE RETINAL NECROSIS.
- Toxoplasmosis: Unilateral retinal lesion may or may not be associated with an adjacent pigmented chorioretinal scar or clumps of scars. Focal dense vitritis over an area of white retinitis constitutes the "headlight in a fog" morphology. See 12.5, TOXOPLASMOSIS.
- Candida: Early discrete drusen-like choroidal lesions progressing to yellow-white, fluffy retinal, or preretinal lesions. See 12.17, CANDIDA RETINITIS/UVEITIS/ENDOPHTHALMITIS.

Vasculitis

Retinal sheathing around vessels. Branch retinal vein and branch retinal artery occlusions may occur.

- Periphlebitis (predominantly veins)
  - Sarcoidosis: Yellow "candlewax" exudates around veins.
  - Syphilis.
  - Pars planitis: Most prominent in the inferior periphery, neovascularization may be present.

- Eales disease: Peripheral neovascularization and/or avascular retina.
  - Multiple sclerosis.
  - Birdshot retinochoroidopathy.
- Arteritis (predominantly arteries)
  - Giant cell arteritis.
  - Polyarteritis nodosum.
  - Frosted branch angiitis.
  - Churg–Strauss disease.
  - ARN.
  - Idiopathic retinal vasculitis, aneurysms, and neuroretinitis (IRVAN).
  - Susac syndrome.
- Both arteries and veins
  - Systemic lupus erythematosus.
  - Granulomatosis with polyangiitis (GPA, formerly Wegener granulomatosis).
  - Behçet disease.
  - HLA-B27-associated (rare).

Postsurgical/Trauma

See 12.13, POSTOPERATIVE ENDOPHTHALMITIS; 12.14, CHRONIC POSTOPERATIVE UVEITIS; 12.15, TRAUMATIC ENDOPHTHALMITIS; and 12.18, SYMPATHETIC OPHTHALMIA.

Other Infectious Causes of Posterior Uveitis

- Cat-scratch disease: Unilateral stellate macular exudates, optic nerve swelling, vitreous cells, and positive Bartonella serology. See 5.3, PARINAUD OCULOGLANDULAR CONJUNCTIVITIS.
- Diffuse unilateral subacute neuroretinitis: Unilateral visual loss in children and young adults, caused by a nematode. Optic nerve swelling, vitreous cells, and deep gray-white retinal lesions are present initially, but may be subtle. Later, optic atrophy, narrowing of retinal vessels, and atrophic pigment epithelial changes develop. Vision, visual fields, and ERG deteriorate with time. Treatment is to laser nematode.
- Lyme disease: Produces varied forms of posterior uveitis. See 13.3, LYME DISEASE.
- *Nocardia*, *Coccidioides* species, *Aspergillus* species, *Cryptococcus* species, meningococcus, ophthalmomyiasis, onchocerciasis, and cysticercosis (seen more commonly in Africa and Central and South America).

12

12.4 Human Leukocyte Antigen–B27–Associated Uveitis

Symptoms

Acute pain, blurred vision, and photophobia. Associated systemic complaints may include lower back, cervical, or heel pain (typically worse on awakening), arthritis, oral ulcers, pain with urination, gastrointestinal complaints, and rashes.

Signs

Critical. Recurrent, unilateral (or alternating bilateral) nongranulomatous anterior uveitis.

Other. Severe anterior chamber reaction with cell, flare, and fibrin. Most common cause of unilateral hypopyon. Tendency to form posterior synechiae early. Ciliary flush. More common in men than women.

Differential Diagnosis

- Other hypopyon uveitides: Behçet disease (posterior involvement more common than in HLA-B27), infectious endophthalmitis, retinoblastoma, metastatic tumors, drug-induced (e.g., rifabutin), sarcoidosis, and masquerade syndromes.
- Idiopathic anterior uveitis.

Types of HLA-B27 Disease

- HLA-B27-associated uveitis without systemic disease.
- Ankylosing spondylitis: Young adult men, often with lower back pain or stiffness, abnormalities on sacroiliac spine radiographs, increased ESR, positive HLA-B27, and negative rheumatoid factor (seronegative spondyloarthropathy).
- IBD: Crohn disease and ulcerative colitis. Chronic diarrhea, bloody stool, and crampy abdominal pain. Patients who have IBD and are HLA B27-negative may be more likely

to get sclerokeratitis or peripheral ulcerative keratitis than uveitis.

- Reactive arthritis (Reiter syndrome): Young adult men, conjunctivitis, urethritis, polyarthritis, occasionally keratitis, increased ESR, and positive HLA-B27. May have recurrent episodes. Arthritis tends to involve the lower extremities.
- Psoriatic arthritis: Characteristic skin findings with arthritis typically involving the upper extremities.

NOTE: Over half of patients presenting with HLA-B27-positive acute anterior uveitis have an underlying seronegative spondyloarthropathy, and of those, over half are diagnosed only after the onset of uveitis.

Workup

1. HLA-B27 to confirm the diagnosis.
2. Ankylosing spondylitis: Sacroiliac spine radiographs or CT scan show sclerosis and narrowing of the joint spaces; ESR often elevated but nonspecific.
3. IBD: A medicine or gastroenterology consult.
4. Reactive arthritis: Conjunctival and urethral swabs for chlamydia if indicated. Consult medicine or rheumatology.
5. Psoriatic arthritis: A rheumatology or dermatology consult.

Treatment

See 12.1, ANTERIOR UVEITIS (IRITIS/IRIDOCYCLITIS). Patients with HLA-B27 uveitis often suffer multiple recurrences. For particularly severe relapsing cases, consider longer-term steroid-sparing immunomodulatory therapy, often in conjunction with rheumatology.

12.5 Toxoplasmosis

Symptoms

Blurred vision and floaters. May have redness and photophobia. Pain depends on the severity of associated iridocyclitis.

Signs

(See Figure 12.5.1.)

Critical. New, unilateral white retinal lesion often associated with an old pigmented chorioretinal scar. There is a moderate to severe focal vitreous inflammatory reaction directly over the lesion. Scar may be absent in cases of newly acquired toxoplasmosis.

Other

- Anterior: Mild anterior chamber spillover may be present, increased IOP in 10% to 20%.
- Posterior: Vitreous debris, optic disc swelling due to peripapillary lesions often with edema extending into the retina, neuroretinitis with/without macular star, optic neuritis with significant vitritis, retinal vasculitis, rarely retinal artery or vein occlusion in the area of the inflammation. Kyrieleis arteritis is periarterial exudate accumulation, which may occur near the retinitis or elsewhere in the retina; IVFA does not show vascular occlusion. Chorioretinal scars are occasionally found in the uninvolved eye. CME may be present.

NOTE: Toxoplasmosis is the most common cause of posterior uveitis and accounts for approximately 90% of focal necrotizing retinitis.

Toxoplasmosis can also develop in the deep retina (punctate outer retinal toxoplasmosis) with few to no vitreous cells present. More common in HIV-infected patients. See SPECIAL CONSIDERATION IN IMMUNOCOMPROMISED PATIENTS at the end of this section.

Differential Diagnosis

See 12.3, POSTERIOR UVEITIS, for a complete list. The following rarely may closely simulate toxoplasmosis.

- Syphilis (See 12.12, SYPHILIS) and tuberculosis.
- Toxocariasis: Usually affects children. Chorioretinal scars are not typically seen. See 12.3, POSTERIOR UVEITIS and 8.1, LEUKOCORIA.
- ARN. See 12.8, ACUTE RETINAL NECROSIS (see **Table 12.8.1**).
- PORN. See 12.8, ACUTE RETINAL NECROSIS (see **Table 12.8.1**).

Workup

See 12.3, POSTERIOR UVEITIS, for work-up recommendations when the diagnosis is in doubt.

1. History: risk factors include handling or eating raw meat (e.g., venison), exposure to cats or especially kittens (sources of acquired infection), and hunters who dress their own game. Inquire about risk factors for HIV in atypical cases (e.g., multifocal retinitis). Water- and airborne outbreaks of toxoplasmosis reported.
2. Complete ocular examination, including a dilated fundus evaluation.
3. Serum anti-*Toxoplasma* antibody titer to indicate remote (IgG) or recent (IgM) infection (usually not necessary). IgM is found approximately 2 weeks to 6 months after initial infection, after which only IgG remains positive.
4. PCR testing from aqueous or vitreous specimens for *Toxoplasma gondii* is more specific than serologic testing.

The high population seropositivity reduces the positive predictive value of a positive titer, but a negative titer makes the diagnosis unlikely.

12

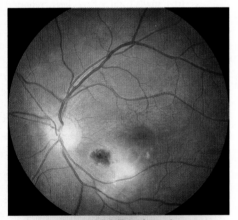

Figure 12.5.1 Toxoplasmosis.

NOTE: Request a 1:1 dilution because any titer of serum antibodies is significant in the setting of classic fundus findings.

5. *Toxoplasma* antibody titers and PCR may be performed on anterior chamber taps or through diagnostic vitrectomy in equivocal cases.
6. Consider RPR or VDRL, FTA-ABS or treponemal-specific assay, PPD or IGRA, chest radiograph or CT, and a *Toxocara* ELISA when the diagnosis is uncertain.
7. Consider HIV testing in atypical cases or high-risk patients. See below.

Treatment

1. Mild peripheral retinochoroiditis.
   - Self-limited in immunocompetent patients. May consider observation only for peripheral lesions.
   - Treat elevated IOP with antiglaucoma medications and anterior uveitis with topical cycloplegic (e.g., cyclopentolate 1% to 2% t.i.d.) with or without topical steroid (e.g., prednisolone acetate 1% q2h).
2. Treatment usually recommended for lesions in the macula, within 2 to 3 mm of the disc, threatening a large retinal vessel, associated with severe vitritis causing decreased vision, or disease in an immunocompromised patient. Immunocompromised patients may require extended treatment.
   - Classic first-line triple therapy (for 4 to 6 weeks):
     - Pyrimethamine, 200 mg p.o. load (or two 100 mg doses p.o. 12 hours apart), and then 25 to 50 mg p.o. daily. Do not give pyrimethamine to pregnant or breastfeeding women (spiramycin 1 g p.o. t.i.d. for women who seroconvert in pregnancy).
     - Folinic acid 10 mg p.o. every other day (to minimize bone marrow toxicity of pyrimethamine).
     - Sulfadiazine 2 g p.o. load and then 1 g p.o. q.i.d. Expensive and difficult to obtain; trimethoprim/sulfamethoxazole 160 mg/800 mg twice daily may be substituted as described below.
     - Prednisone may be added 20 to 60 mg p.o. daily beginning at least 24 hours after initiating antimicrobial therapy

and tapered 10 days before stopping antibiotics. Periocular steroids should not be given.

Systemic steroids should only rarely be used in immunocompromised patients. Before systemic steroid use, evaluation of fasting blood sugar/hemoglobin A1C and studies to rule out tuberculosis are prudent.

NOTE: Due to potential bone marrow suppression, a CBC must be obtained once per week while a patient is taking pyrimethamine. If the platelet count decreases below 100,000, then reduce the dosage of pyrimethamine and increase the folinic acid. Patients taking pyrimethamine should not take vitamins that contain folic acid. The medication should be given with meals to reduce anorexia.

- Alternate regimens:
  - Clindamycin 150 to 450 mg p.o. t.i.d. to q.i.d. (maximum 1.8 g/d) may be used alone, with pyrimethamine as the alternative therapy (if the patient is sulfa allergic), or as an adjunct (quadruple therapy). Patients on clindamycin should be warned about pseudomembranous colitis, and the medication should be stopped if diarrhea develops. Intravitreal injection of clindamycin (0.1 mg/0.1 mL) can be effective for macular-threatening cases, or when the patient is intolerant to systemic medication. Combined intravitreal clindamycin (0.1 mg/0.1 mL) and dexamethasone (0.4 mg/0.1 mL) have been reported helpful.
  - Atovaquone 750 mg p.o. q.i.d., used as an alternative similar to clindamycin.
  - Trimethoprim/sulfamethoxazole (160 mg/800 mg) one tablet p.o. b.i.d., with or without clindamycin and prednisone.
  - Azithromycin loading dose 1 g (day 1) and then 250 to 500 mg daily. May be used alone or in combination with pyrimethamine (50 mg daily).
  - Spiramycin 400 mg p.o. t.i.d. may be considered in cases of pregnancy, but must be obtained from CDC.
  - Anterior segment inflammation is treated as above.

3. Vitrectomy has been used for nonclearing dense vitritis or other complications.
4. Maintenance therapy (if the patient is immunosuppressed)
   - Trimethoprim/sulfamethoxazole 160 mg/800 mg one tablet p.o. three times a week.

   or

   - If sulfa-allergic (common in HIV-infected patients), may use clindamycin 300 mg p.o. q.i.d.
5. Prophylaxis: In a patient with a history of toxoplasmosis undergoing cataract or refractive surgery, consider using trimethoprim/sulfamethoxazole b.i.d. during the perioperative period.

Follow Up

In 3 to 7 days for blood tests and/or ocular assessment, and then every 1 to 2 weeks on therapy.

SPECIAL CONSIDERATION IN IMMUNOCOMPROMISED PATIENTS

Vitritis usually much less prominent. Adjacent retinochoroidal scars may not be present. The lesions may be single or multifocal, discrete or diffuse, and unilateral or bilateral. CNS imaging is essential because of high association with CNS disease (e.g., toxoplasmic encephalopathy in HIV patients). Diagnostic vitrectomy may be necessary because of the multiple simulating entities and the variability of laboratory diagnostic tests. Systemic steroids for ocular toxoplasmosis should be used very cautiously in patients with AIDS.

12.6 Sarcoidosis

Symptoms

Unilateral or bilateral ocular pain, photophobia, and decreased vision. May have an insidious onset, especially in older patients with chronic disease. Systemic findings may include shortness of breath, parotid enlargement, fever, arthralgias, and rarely neurologic symptoms including cranial nerve palsy. Most common in the 20- to 50-year age group. Most common in African Americans and Scandinavians.

Signs

Critical. Iris nodules, large mutton-fat KP (especially in Arlt triangle), and sheathing along peripheral retinal veins (candlewax drippings).

Other. Conjunctival nodules, enlargement of the lacrimal gland, dry eyes, posterior synechiae, glaucoma, cataract, intermediate uveitis, CME, vitritis, round and pale choroidal lesions that may simulate multifocal choroiditis or birdshot retinochoroidopathy, chorioretinitis, optic nerve granuloma, optic disc or peripheral retinal neovascularization **(see Figure 12.6.1)**.

Systemic. Tachypnea, facial nerve palsy, enlargement of salivary or lacrimal glands, bilateral symmetric hilar adenopathy on chest radiograph or CT, erythema nodosum (erythematous, tender nodules beneath the skin, often found on the shins), lupus pernio (a dusky purple rash on nose and cheeks), arthritis, lymphadenopathy, hepatosplenomegaly.

NOTE: Uveitis, secondary glaucoma, cataracts, and CME are the most common vision-threatening complications of ocular sarcoidosis.

Differential Diagnosis

- Other causes of mutton-fat KP and iris nodules include syphilis, tuberculosis, sympathetic ophthalmia, tattoo-associated uveitis, and lens-related uveitis. See 12.1, ANTERIOR UVEITIS (IRITIS/IRIDOCYCLITIS).

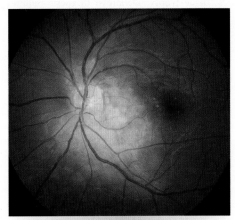

Figure 12.6.1 Sarcoid choroidal granuloma.

12

- Intermediate uveitis may be idiopathic or secondary to sarcoid, multiple sclerosis, Lyme disease, and others. See 12.2, INTERMEDIATE UVEITIS.
- Posterior uveitis with multiple chorioretinal lesions may be from birdshot retinochoroidopathy, intraocular lymphoma, syphilis, sympathetic ophthalmia, multifocal choroiditis, VKH syndrome, and others. See 12.3, POSTERIOR UVEITIS.

Workup

The following are the tests that are obtained when sarcoidosis is suspected clinically. See 12.1, ANTERIOR UVEITIS (IRITIS/IRIDOCYCLITIS) and 12.3, POSTERIOR UVEITIS, for other uveitis workup.

1. Chest radiography: May reveal bilateral and symmetric hilar adenopathy and/or infiltrates indicative of pulmonary fibrosis, but may be normal in many patients and a negative result does not rule out sarcoidosis. Chest CT is more sensitive but more expensive. In cases of unilateral or atypical lung disease, consider malignancy.

2. Serum ACE: Elevated in 60% to 90% of patients with active sarcoidosis. Similar to chest radiography, a normal level does not rule out sarcoidosis, and elevation is not specific. HIV, tuberculosis, histoplasmosis, and leprosy may also present with elevated ACE. Patients with underlying lung disease (e.g., COPD) or patients on oral steroids and/or ACE inhibitors may have falsely low ACE levels. ACE levels in children are less helpful in diagnosis.

3. Tissue biopsy: Definitive diagnosis requires demonstration of noncaseating granulomatous inflammation. Obtain biopsy of accessible affected lesions, including lymph nodes or edges of skin plaques or nodules. Sarcoid granulomas are not present in erythema nodosum and these lesions should not be sampled. An acid-fast stain and a methenamine–silver stain may be performed to rule out tuberculosis and fungal infection. A nondirected conjunctival biopsy in the absence of visible lesions has a low yield and is not recommended. Indurated areas of tattooed skin with concurrent uveitis may suggest tattoo-associated uveitis; skin biopsy may show noncaseating granulomas while the chest X-ray (CXR) is normal.

4. PPD or IGRA: Useful for differentiating tuberculosis from sarcoidosis when pulmonary findings are present. Up to 50% of sarcoidosis patients are anergic and have no response to PPD or controls.

5. Other: Some authors recommend serum and urine calcium levels, liver function tests, and a serum lysozyme. A positive result on one of these tests in the absence of chest radiographic or other findings is usually not helpful in diagnosis. A serum lysozyme may be useful in children, in whom ACE levels are often normal.

If laboratory and chest radiographic studies suggest sarcoidosis or in the setting of a negative workup but a high clinical suspicion of the disease, the following tests should be considered:

1. Chest CT is more sensitive than CXR.

2. Whole-body gallium scan is sensitive for sarcoidosis. A "panda sign" indicates involvement of lacrimal, parotid, and submandibular glands. A "lambda sign" indicates involvement of bilateral hilar and right paratracheal lymph nodes. A positive gallium scan and an elevated ACE level are 73% sensitive and 100% specific for sarcoidosis. Cost and inconvenience are drawbacks.

3. Referral to a pulmonologist for pulmonary function tests and transbronchial lung biopsy.

4. The risks of an invasive diagnostic test or radiation exposure must be weighed against the impact the results will have on treatment.

Treatment

Refer patients to an internist or pulmonologist for systemic evaluation and medical management. Consider early referral to a uveitis specialist in complicated cases. A poor visual outcome has been reported with posterior uveitis, glaucoma, delay in definitive treatment, or presence of macula-threatening conditions such as CME.

1. Anterior uveitis:
   - Cycloplegic (e.g., cyclopentolate 1% t.i.d. or atropine 1% b.i.d.).
   - Topical steroid (e.g., prednisolone acetate 1% q1–6h).

2. Posterior uveitis:
   - Supplement calcium with vitamin D (e.g., 600 mg with 400 iU) once or twice daily and consider a histamine type 2 receptor (H2) blocker (e.g., ranitidine 150 mg p.o. b.i.d.) or proton pump inhibitor (e.g., pantoprazole 40 mg daily).

- Periocular steroids (e.g., 0.5 to 1.0 mL injection of triamcinolone 40 mg/mL) may be considered instead of systemic steroids, especially in unilateral or asymmetric cases. Can repeat injection every 3 to 4 weeks. See Appendix 10, TECHNIQUE FOR RETROBULBAR/SUBTENON/SUBCONJUNCTIVAL INJECTIONS.

3. Immunosuppressives (e.g., methotrexate, azathioprine, mycophenolate mofetil, cyclosporine, cyclophosphamide, and infliximab) have been used effectively as steroid-sparing agents. Decisions regarding therapy should be individualized given known side effect profiles of each regimen.

> **NOTE:** Topical steroids alone are inadequate for the treatment of posterior uveitis.

4. CME: See 11.14, CYSTOID MACULAR EDEMA.
5. Glaucoma: See 9.7, INFLAMMATORY OPEN ANGLE GLAUCOMA; 9.9, STEROID-RESPONSE GLAUCOMA; 9.4, ACUTE ANGLE CLOSURE GLAUCOMA; or 9.14, NEOVASCULAR GLAUCOMA, depending on the etiology of the glaucoma.
6. Retinal neovascularization: May require panretinal photocoagulation.
7. Orbital disease is managed with systemic steroids as described previously.
8. Optic nerve granulomas require consultation with a neuro-ophthalmologist and treatment with systemic steroids.
9. Pulmonary disease, facial nerve palsy, CNS disease, and renal disease require systemic steroids and management by an internist or neurologist.

Follow Up

1. Patients are re-examined in 1 to 7 days, depending on the severity of inflammation. The steroid dosages are adjusted in accordance with the treatment response. Slowly taper the steroids and cycloplegic agent as the inflammation subsides. Monitor IOP and re-evaluate the fundus at each visit.
2. Patients with quiescent disease are seen every 3 to 6 months.
3. Patients being treated with steroids or systemic immunosuppression are monitored every 2 to 6 weeks, pending clinical response.
4. Poor response to steroid treatment should prompt a workup for other causes of uveitis or referral to a subspecialist.

12.7 Behçet Disease

Symptoms

Sudden onset of bilateral decreased vision, floaters, and photophobia. Pain is usually mild or moderate.

Signs

Critical. Painful oral aphthous ulcers (well-defined borders with a white yellow necrotic center, often with surrounding erythema, found in 98% to 100% of patients) at least three times per year and two of the following: genital ulcers, skin lesions, positive Behçetine (pathergy) test (formation of a local pustule that appears 48 hours after skin puncture with a needle), and eye lesions. May have other skin findings including erythema nodosum, pseudofolliculitis, palpable purpura, superficial thrombophlebitis, or dermographism.

Other. Other systemic manifestations include arthritis, hemoptysis from pulmonary artery involvement, renal involvement, gastrointestinal disease with bowel ulceration, epididymitis, and neuro-Behçet (e.g., vasculitis, encephalitis, cerebral venous thrombosis, neuropsychiatric symptoms).

Ocular Signs

- Anterior: Bilateral hypopyon and anterior chamber reaction; scleritis occasionally reported.

> **NOTE:** Patients with Behçet disease almost never have fibrin even if the anterior chamber reaction is severe, thus the hypopyon appears mobile ("shifting") in contrast to HLA-B27-associated uveitis.

- Posterior: Vitritis, retinal vasculitis affecting both arteries and veins, venous obstruction, arterial attenuation, retinal neovascularization, focal necrotizing retinitis, waxy optic nerve pallor, and retinal detachment.

12

Epidemiology

Age 20 to 40 years; especially Japanese, Turkish, or Middle Eastern descent.

Differential Diagnosis

- Sarcoidosis: May occasionally present with oral ulcers. See 12.6, SARCOIDOSIS.
- HLA-B27: Usually unilateral or bilateral alternating uveitis. Severe fibrinous uveitis. Oral ulcers are less painful and severe. See 12.4, HUMAN LEUKOCYTE ANTIGEN–B27–ASSOCIATED UVEITIS.
- ARN: Confluent retinal whitening in the periphery. More pain than Behçet disease. See 12.8, ACUTE RETINAL NECROSIS.
- GPA: Nephritis, orbital inflammation, sinus, and pulmonary inflammation.
- Syphilis. See 12.12, SYPHILIS.
- Systemic lupus erythematosus and other collagen vascular diseases.

Workup

- Chest radiograph or CT, ACE level, PPD or IGRA, RPR or VDRL, and FTA-ABS or treponemal-specific assay.
- Consider HLA-B27 in young men with a positive review of systems suggesting seronegative spondyloarthropathy.
- Granular-staining cytoplasmic antineutrophil cytoplasmic antibody (c-ANCA) if GPA is suspected.
- Consider HLA-B51 and HLA-DR5 testing for Behçet disease (positive and negative predictive values are uncertain).
- Consider Behçetine (pathergy) test. The test is considered positive if there is development of a papule of 2 mm or more in size 48 hours after 5-mm deep skin prick with a 20-gauge needle.

Treatment

If untreated, bilateral blindness often develops within 3 to 4 years. Death may result from CNS involvement. Proper referral for immunosuppressive therapy is critical.

1. Topical corticosteroids (e.g., prednisolone acetate 1% q1–6h depending on severity of inflammation) and cycloplegics (e.g., atropine 1% b.i.d.) for anterior inflammation.
2. Systemic corticosteroids should be started (prednisone 1 mg/kg p.o. daily or intravenous methylprednisolone sodium succinate 1 g daily for 3 days, followed by prednisone). Steroids delay the onset of blindness but do not alter the long-term outcome. Prior to systemic immunosuppressive therapy, it is important to rule out syphilis, tuberculosis, and hepatitis.
3. All patients with Behçet disease and posterior uveitis should be referred to a specialist for initiation of immunosuppressive therapy. TNF-antagonists such as infliximab or adalimumab are now considered first-line therapy for Behçet disease. Calcineurin inhibitors (tacrolimus and cyclosporine) and antimetabolites (e.g., mycophenolate mofetil, methotrexate, and azathioprine) can be used, but take 1 to 2 months to achieve the full effect.

Follow Up

Daily during acute episodes to monitor inflammation and IOP. Refer to a uveitis specialist for further follow up.

12.8 Acute Retinal Necrosis

Symptoms

Blurred vision, floaters, ocular pain, and photophobia. Affected patients are usually immunocompetent.

Signs

(See Figure 12.8.1.)

Critical. The American Uveitis Society criteria include one or more foci of retinal necrosis with discrete borders in the peripheral retina, rapid progression of disease in the absence of antiviral therapy, circumferential spread, evidence of occlusive vasculopathy with arterial involvement, and prominent inflammatory reaction in the anterior chamber and vitreous. If untreated, the circumferential progression of necrosis may become confluent and spread posteriorly. The macula is typically spared early in the disease course.

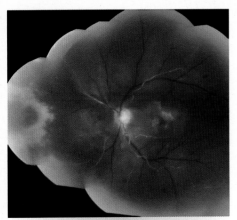

Figure 12.8.1 Acute retinal necrosis.

Other. Anterior chamber reaction; KP; conjunctival injection; episcleritis or scleritis; increased IOP; sheathed retinal arterioles and sometimes venules, especially in the periphery; retinal hemorrhages (minor finding); optic disc edema; delayed RRD occurs in approximately 70% of patients secondary to large irregular posterior breaks. Usually begins unilaterally but may involve the second eye in one-third of cases within weeks to months. An optic neuropathy with disc edema or pallor sometimes develops.

Etiology

ARN is a clinical syndrome caused by the herpes virus family: VZV (older patients), HSV (younger patients), or rarely, CMV or Epstein-Barr virus (EBV).

Differential Diagnosis

See 12.3, POSTERIOR UVEITIS.
- CMV retinitis (**Table 12.8.1**).
- PORN: Rapidly progressive retinitis characterized by clear vitreous and sheet-like opacification deep to normal-looking retinal vessels, and occasional spontaneous vitreous hemorrhage. PORN is usually found in immunocompromised individuals and frequently leads to rapid bilateral blindness due either to the infection itself or to secondary retinal detachment, making prompt diagnosis and treatment essential. Unlike ARN, pain and vitritis are minimal and macular involvement occurs early.
- Syphilis.
- *Toxoplasma* chorioretinitis.
- Behçet disease.
- Sarcoidosis.
- Fungal or bacterial endophthalmitis.
- Large cell lymphoma. Consider in patients >50 years of age with refractory unilateral vitritis, yellow-white subretinal infiltrates, and absence of pain.

Workup

See 12.3, POSTERIOR UVEITIS, for a nonspecific uveitis workup.

1. History: Risk factors for AIDS or other immunocompromised states (iatrogenic, autoimmune, malignancy, or genetic)? If yes, the differential diagnosis includes CMV retinitis and PORN. Ask about history of shingles (especially zoster ophthalmicus) or herpes

12

TABLE 12.8.1 Cytomegalovirus (CMV) Retinitis Versus Acute Retinal Necrosis (ARN) Versus Progressive Outer Retinal Necrosis (PORN) Versus Toxoplasmosis

	CMV	ARN	PORN	Toxoplasmosis
Retinal hemorrhages	Common	Uncommon	Uncommon	Usually absent
Vitritis	Minimal	Significant	Absent	Significant
Pain	Absent	Significant	Absent	Moderate
Immune status	Immunocompromised	Usually healthy	Immunocompromised	Either
Appearance	"Brushfire" border with the leading edge of active retinitis and necrotic retina and mottled retinal pigment epithelium in its wake	Sharply demarcated lesions with a nearly homogeneous appearance	Multifocal patches of deep retinal necrosis, rapid progression with the involvement of the macula	"Headlight in the fog" with dense vitritis and smooth edges

simplex infections. Head trauma (including neurosurgery) and ocular surgery may precipitate ARN. Rarely, ARN can follow periocular or intravitreal corticosteroid injections. Most patients have no identifiable precipitating factors.

2. Complete ocular examination: Evaluate the anterior chamber and vitreous for cells, measure IOP, and perform a dilated retinal examination using indirect ophthalmoscopy; gentle scleral depression as necrotic retina has an increased risk of retinal detachment.

3. Consider a CBC with differential, RPR or VDRL, FTA-ABS or treponemal-specific assay, ESR, *Toxoplasma* titers, PPD or IGRA, and chest radiograph or CT to rule out other etiologies.

4. Consider HIV testing.

5. Anterior chamber paracentesis for herpes virus and *Toxoplasma* PCR to confirm the causative virus is highly specific but sensitivity may vary. See Appendix 13, ANTERIOR CHAMBER PARACENTESIS.

6. Consider IVFA to identify retinal vasculitis and areas of ischemia.

7. MRI of the brain and orbits in cases of suspected optic nerve dysfunction.

8. CT or MRI of the brain and lumbar puncture if large cell lymphoma, tertiary syphilis, or encephalitis is suspected.

Treatment

NOTE: All patients with ARN should be referred to a specialist.

1. Prompt inpatient or outpatient treatment. The goal is to decrease the incidence of disease in the fellow eye. Treatment does not reduce the rate of retinal detachment in the first eye.

2. Oral antivirals (valacyclovir 1 to 2 g t.i.d. or famciclovir 500 mg t.i.d. preferred; acyclovir 800 mg five times per day second-line option as it achieves lower intravitreal levels) with supplemental intravitreal injections with foscarnet (2.4 mg/0.1 mL) or ganciclovir (2 mg/0.1 mL) given one to two times per week. Alternative therapy includes intravenous acyclovir 10 mg/kg t.i.d. for 5 to 14 days (requires dose adjustment for renal

insufficiency) with supplemental intravitreal injections as noted above, followed by oral valacyclovir 1 g t.i.d. or acyclovir 400 to 800 mg five times per day. Either of these regimens is maintained for up to 14 weeks from the onset of infection. Involvement of the second eye typically starts within 6 weeks of initial infection. Published literature suggests that primary treatment with oral antivirals in conjunction with the above intravitreal injections has similar efficacy as intravenous therapy. Stabilization and early regression of retinitis are usually seen within 4 days. The lesions may progress during the first 48 hours of treatment. The ideal duration of oral antiviral therapy remains unproven, but since replicating virus in the anterior chamber can be found up to 2 months after the onset of disease, a minimum of 2 months of therapy is recommended, and some experts recommend lifetime therapy to reduce the risk of second-eye involvement (especially if the first eye becomes nonfunctional).

3. Topical cycloplegic (e.g., atropine 1% t.i.d.) and topical steroid (e.g., prednisolone acetate 1% q2–6h) in the presence of anterior segment inflammation.

4. The benefits of antiplatelet therapy (e.g., aspirin 81 to 650 mg daily) to minimize vascular thrombosis and help prevent further retinal ischemia remain unproven.

5. Systemic steroids may be considered, particularly when the optic nerve is thought to be involved. Steroids are usually delayed at least 24 hours after the initiation of antiviral therapy, or when regression of retinal necrosis is evident. A typical oral corticosteroid regimen is prednisone 60 to 80 mg/d for 1 to 2 weeks followed by a taper over 2 to 6 weeks. Subtenon injection of triamcinolone (40 mg/1 mL) can be considered after adequate loading of antiviral therapy but may interfere with the clearance of virus by the eye.

6. See 9.7, INFLAMMATORY OPEN ANGLE GLAUCOMA, for increased IOP.

7. Consider prophylactic barrier laser photocoagulation posterior to active retinitis to wall off or prevent subsequent RRD (efficacy unclear).

8. Pars plana vitrectomy, with long-acting gas or silicone oil, is the best way to repair the associated complex RRD. Proliferative vitreoretinopathy is common.

12

Follow Up

1. Patients are seen daily initially and are examined every few weeks to months for the following year; examination of both eyes is essential.
2. A careful fundus evaluation is performed at each visit to rule out retinal holes that may lead to a detachment. If barrier laser demarcation has been done and the retinitis subsequently crosses the posterior margin, consider applying additional laser therapy.
3. Pupillary evaluation should be performed, and optic neuropathy should be considered if the retinopathy does not explain the amount of visual loss.

12.9 | Cytomegalovirus Retinitis

CMV is the most frequent ocular opportunistic infection in patients with AIDS, but is 80% to 90% less common in the era of combination antiretroviral therapy (cART). CMV is almost never seen unless the CD4+ count is <100 cells/mm³. Because active retinitis is often asymptomatic, patients with CD4+ counts <100 cells/mm³ should be seen at least every 3 to 6 months. May also be seen in other immunocompromised states (e.g., leukemia and post-transplant). Local ocular immunosuppression (regional steroid injections) may precipitate CMV retinitis in otherwise healthy patients.

Symptoms

Scotoma or decreased vision in one or both eyes, floaters, or photopsias. Pain and photophobia are uncommon. Often asymptomatic.

Signs

Critical
- Indolent form: Peripheral granular opacities with or without hemorrhage. The absence of hemorrhage does not rule out CMV retinitis.
- Fulminant form: Confluent areas of necrosis with prominent hemorrhage, starting along the major retinal vascular arcades. Progressive retinal atrophy may also indicate active CMV (see Figure 12.9.1).

Other. Anterior uveitis with nongranulomatous, stellate KP almost always present but mild. Vitritis is usually mild. Retinal pigment epithelial (RPE) atrophy and pigment clumping result once the active process resolves. RRD occurs in approximately one-third of patients with CMV retinitis with increased risk when >25% of the retina is involved.

Workup

1. History and complete ocular examination.
2. Consider anterior chamber paracentesis with viral PCR in equivocal cases. See Appendix 13, ANTERIOR CHAMBER PARACENTESIS.
3. Refer the patient to an internist or an infectious disease specialist for systemic evaluation and treatment.

Treatment

See **Table 12.9.1** for treatment details.

1. Oral therapy with valganciclovir 900 mg p.o. b.i.d. for induction (21 days), followed by 900 mg p.o. daily for maintenance. Alternatively, intravenous ganciclovir 5 mg/kg b.i.d. or foscarnet 90 mg/kg b.i.d. (adjusting for renal function) may be used, followed by oral therapy valganciclovir (900 mg p.o. b.i.d. to complete 3-week induction, then 900 mg p.o. daily). Patients with progression of retinitis

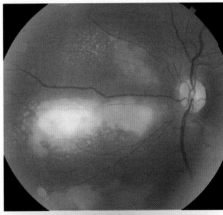

Figure 12.9.1 CMV retinitis.

12

TABLE 12.9.1 Therapy for CMV Retinitis

Drug	Dosing	Toxicities	Contraindications
Ganciclovir[a]	Induction: 5 mg/kg i.v. b.i.d. for 14 days Maintenance: 5 mg/kg i.v. daily	Neutropenia,[b] thrombocytopenia, anemia; Discontinue nursing	Absolute neutrophil count <500/mm³, platelets <25,000/mm³; Potentially embryotoxic
Valganciclovir	Induction: 900 mg p.o. b.i.d. for 21 days Maintenance: 900 mg p.o. daily	Neutropenia,[b] thrombocytopenia, and anemia; Discontinue nursing	Absolute neutrophil count <500/mm³, platelets <25,000/mm³; Potentially embryotoxic
Foscarnet	Induction: 90 mg/kg i.v. b.i.d. twice/wk Maintenance: 90 to 120 mg/kg i.v. daily[c] (monitor creatinine and electrolytes; adjust dosing as needed)	Renal impairment neutropenia, anemia, and electrolyte imbalances	Use caution with renal impairment or electrolyte imbalances
Cidofovir	Induction: 5 mg/kg i.v. weekly for 3 wks maintenance: 3 to 5 mg/kg i.v. every 2 wks	Dose- and schedule-dependent nephrotoxicity, hypotony (necessitates discontinuation), iritis (steroid responsive); Must be given with probenecid	Recurrent uveitis, moderate to severe kidney disease, intolerance to probenecid

[a]Compared with intravitreal therapy alone, there is a decreased risk of mortality (50%), systemic disease (90%), and fellow eye involvement (80%) in patients treated with systemic anti-CMV therapy. Moreover, the risk of retinitis progression is significantly greater in eyes treated with intravitreal therapy alone.
[b]Compared with i.v. ganciclovir, there is an increased risk of systemic disease (30%) and fellow eye involvement (50%) after 6 months. However, the relapse-free interval is greatly increased.
[c]During the induction phase, 500 mL of normal saline is used for each dose. During maintenance, 1000 mL of saline should be used.

despite induction or who have disease that threatens the macula may benefit from intravitreal antiviral injections, but systemic therapy is still necessary to prevent the involvement of the fellow eye. The goal of treatment is quiescent retinitis (nonprogressive areas of RPE atrophy with a stable opacified border).

2. Under the direction of an internist or infectious disease specialist, HAART should be initiated or optimized; immune recovery with sustained CD4+ counts >200 cells/mm³ results in decreased risk of retinal detachment, second-eye involvement, antiviral resistance, and mortality. Also, monitor for toxicity of anti-CMV therapy (valganciclovir and ganciclovir cause bone marrow toxicity; foscarnet is nephrotoxic and can cause electrolyte abnormalities and seizures; intravenous ganciclovir and foscarnet require placement of an indwelling catheter, which may cause line infection and sepsis).

3. Small, macula-sparing RRDs may be treated with laser demarcation, but multiple retinal breaks are typical and may be missed; pars plana vitrectomy with silicone oil is indicated for most detachments, especially those involving the macula.

4. Primary prophylaxis (prevention of CMV retinitis) with oral valganciclovir in high-risk patients is usually not recommended because of potential toxicity except in transplant patients.

Follow Up

1. Ganciclovir resistance (reflected by positive blood or urine CMV cultures) may occur with prolonged treatment.

2. All currently available anti-CMV therapy is virostatic, not virocidal, and almost all patients eventually relapse if not treated with HAART. Serial fundus photographs helpful for comparison.

3. Relapse is defined as recurrent or new retinitis, movement of opacified border, or expansion of the atrophic zone.

4. Relapse can occur from resistance or subtherapeutic intraocular drug levels. Reinduction with the same medication is the first line of treatment.

5. Clinical resistance is defined as persistent or progressive retinitis despite induction level medication for 6 weeks. Laboratory

confirmation is possible for low-grade UL97 (viral phosphotransferase) or high-grade UL54 (viral DNA polymerase) mutations.

6. If resistance is recognized, a change in therapy from one antiviral to the other is indicated. Consider intravenous cidofovir 5 mg/kg once weekly for 2 weeks and then 3 to 5 mg/kg every 2 weeks. Cidofovir itself may cause uveitis and renal impairment and must be given with probenecid to reduce the nephrotoxicity. Intravitreal cidofovir is contraindicated because of the high risk of uveitis and hypotony. Cross-resistance can occur since all three anti-CMV drugs are CMV DNA polymerase inhibitors.

7. Discontinuation of anti-CMV maintenance therapy may be considered in select patients receiving HAART who have CD4+ counts >100 cells/mm³ for greater than 6 months and completely quiescent CMV retinitis. In these patients, whose immune system can control CMV, stopping maintenance therapy may prevent drug toxicity and drug-resistant organisms. In iatrogenically immunosuppressed patients, cessation or reduction in dosage of immunosuppressive drugs may be required for long-term control of CMV retinitis.

8. Immune recovery uveitis (IRU): Occurs in previously immunocompromised patients (HIV/iatrogenic) with CMV after the CD4+ count or immune system reconstitutes. In the presence of a functioning immune system, the CMV antigens elicit an inflammatory response that is predominantly posterior (e.g., vitritis, papillitis, CME, and ERM). Treatment may require topical, periocular, or intraocular steroids. Antivirals should be continued to avoid reactivation of CMV in cases of borderline CD4+ counts.

12.10 Noninfectious Retinal Microvasculopathy/HIV Retinopathy

Noninfectious retinopathy is the most common ocular manifestation of HIV/AIDS. About 50% to 70% of patients with AIDS have this condition.

Symptoms

Rarely symptomatic (focal scotomata and decreased contrast).

Signs

Cotton–wool spots, intraretinal hemorrhages, and microaneurysms. An ischemic maculopathy may occur with significant visual loss in 3% of affected patients.

Workup

HIV retinopathy is a marker of low CD4+ counts. Look for concomitant opportunistic infections (see 12.9, CYTOMEGALOVIRUS RETINITIS). Rule out the other causes for unexplained cotton–wool spots (see 11.5, COTTON–WOOL SPOT).

Treatment

No specific ocular treatment is necessary, but the retinopathy resolves with cART and increased CD4+ counts.

Follow Up

Patients with CD4+ counts <50 should be examined every 3 to 4 months.

12.11 Vogt–Koyanagi–Harada Syndrome

Autoimmune disease featuring inflammation of melanocyte-containing tissues.

Symptoms

Decreased vision, photophobia, pain, and red eyes; accompanied or preceded by a headache, stiff neck, nausea, vomiting, fever, and malaise. Hearing loss, noise causing ear pain, and tinnitus frequently occur. Typically bilateral.

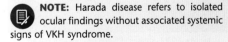 **NOTE:** Harada disease refers to isolated ocular findings without associated systemic signs of VKH syndrome.

Signs

Diagnostic criteria include the following:

* (1) no history of ocular trauma, (2) no evidence of other disease processes, (3) bilateral anterior or panuveitis, (4) neurologic/auditory findings (usually occur before ocular disease), and (5) dermatologic findings (usually occur after ocular disease).
* Complete VKH includes criteria 1 to 5, incomplete VKH includes criteria 1 to 3 and either 4 or 5, and probable VKH (isolated ocular disease) includes criteria 1 to 3.
   (See Figure 12.11.1.)

Critical

* Anterior: Anterior chamber flare and cells, granulomatous (mutton-fat) KP, perilimbal vitiligo (e.g., depigmentation around the limbus).
* Posterior: Bilateral serous retinal detachments with underlying choroidal thickening, vitreous cells, opacities, and optic disc edema.
* Systemic (four phases):
  * Prodromal: loss of high-frequency hearing, tinnitus, meningismus, encephalopathy, and hypersensitivity of the skin to touch.
  * Uveitic: acute ocular findings (see preceding bullets).
  * Convalescent: alopecia, vitiligo, poliosis, "sunset glow" fundus (yellow-orange appearance of the fundus due to depigmentation of the RPE and choroid).
  * Chronic recurrent: recurrence of anterior uveitis, subretinal fibrosis, neovascularization, glaucoma, and cataract.

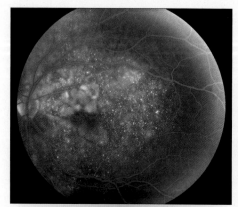

Figure 12.11.2 IVFA of VKH.

* IVFA: Multiple pinpoint leaking areas of hyperfluorescence at the level of the retinal pigment epithelium **(see Figure 12.11.2)**.

Other

* Anterior: Iris nodules, peripheral anterior or posterior synechiae, scleritis, hypotony, or increased IOP from the forward rotation of ciliary processes.
* Posterior: Sunset glow fundus (mottling and atrophy of the retinal pigment epithelium after the serous retinal detachment resolves), retinal vasculitis, choroidal neovascularization, and chorioretinal scars.
* Systemic: Neurologic signs, including loss of consciousness, paralysis, and seizures.

Epidemiology

Typically, patients are aged 20 to 50 years, female (77%), and have pigmented skin (especially Asian, Middle Eastern, Hispanic, or Native American).

Differential Diagnosis

See **Table 12.11.1** for the differential of serous retinal detachments and 12.3, POSTERIOR UVEITIS. In particular, consider the following:

* Sympathetic ophthalmia: History of trauma or surgery (especially repeated vitreoretinal procedures) in the contralateral eye. Usually no systemic signs. See 12.18, SYMPATHETIC OPHTHALMIA.
* APMPPE: Ophthalmoscopic and IVFA features may be very similar, but there is less vitreous inflammation and no anterior segment involvement. See 12.3, POSTERIOR UVEITIS.

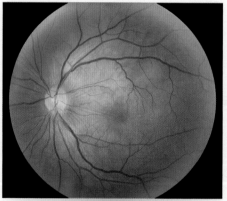

Figure 12.11.1 Vogt–Koyanagi–Harada (VKH) disease.

12

TABLE 12.11.1 Differential Diagnosis of Serous Retinal Detachments

Harada Disease
Malignant hypertension
Toxemia of pregnancy
Disseminated intravascular coagulopathy
Idiopathic uveal effusion syndrome
Sympathetic ophthalmia
Posterior scleritis
Central serous chorioretinopathy
Choroidal tumors (including metastases)
Choroidal neovascularization
Congenital optic disc pit
Nanophthalmos

- Posterior scleritis: Typically unilateral, not typically associated with neurologic or dermatologic findings. Associated with an ultrasonographic "T" sign.
- Systemic arterial hypertension and pregnancy-related hypertension: Acute elevation in blood pressure can produce multifocal serous retinal detachments.
- Other granulomatous panuveitides (e.g., syphilis, sarcoidosis, and tuberculosis).

Workup

See 12.3, POSTERIOR UVEITIS, for a nonspecific uveitis workup.

1. History: Neurologic symptoms, hearing loss, or hair loss? Previous eye surgery or trauma?
2. Complete ocular examination, including a dilated retinal evaluation.
3. CBC, RPR or VDRL, FTA-ABS or treponemal-specific assay, ACE, PPD or IGRA, blood pressure, and possibly chest radiograph or CT to rule out similar-appearing disorders.
4. Consider B-scan ultrasonography to rule out posterior scleritis.

5. Consider a CT or MRI of the brain with or without contrast in the presence of neurologic signs to rule out a CNS disorder.
6. Lumbar puncture during attacks with meningeal symptoms for cell count and differential, protein, glucose, VDRL, Gram and methenamine–silver stains, and culture. CSF pleocytosis is often seen in VKH and APMPPE.
7. Consider IVFA to evaluate for pinpoint leaking areas of hyperfluorescence at the level of the retinal pigment epithelium.

Treatment

Inflammation is initially controlled with steroids; the dose depends on the severity of the inflammation. In moderate to severe cases, the following regimen can be used. Steroids are tapered very slowly as the condition improves.

1. Topical steroids (e.g., prednisolone acetate 1% q1h).
2. Systemic steroids (e.g., prednisone 60-80 mg p.o. daily or intravenous methylprednisolone sodium succinate 1 g daily for 3 days followed by oral therapy) with concurrent calcium/vitamin D supplementation and antiulcer prophylaxis.
3. Topical cycloplegic (e.g., cyclopentolate 1% t.i.d. or atropine 1% b.i.d.).
4. Treatment of any specific neurologic disorders (e.g., seizures or coma).
5. For patients who cannot tolerate or are unresponsive to long-term oral steroids, consider immunosuppressive agents (e.g., antimetabolites, calcineurin inhibitors, cytotoxic agents, and TNF-alpha inhibitors).

Follow Up

1. Initial management may require hospitalization if intravenous corticosteroids are initiated.
2. Weekly, then monthly re-examination is performed, watching for recurrent inflammation and increased IOP.
3. Steroids are tapered very slowly, and most patients should be transitioned to steroid-sparing immunosuppressants for long-term management. Inflammation may recur up to 9 months after the steroids have been discontinued. If this occurs, steroids should be reinstituted.

12

12.12 Syphilis

ACQUIRED SYPHILIS

Signs

Systemic. Most patients with syphilis will never develop ocular involvement. A history of sexually transmitted disease, HIV, or high-risk sexual activity should be elucidated. Men who have sex with men are at an increased risk.

- Primary: Chancre (ulcerated, painless lesion), regional lymphadenopathy.
- Secondary: Skin or mucous membrane lesions, generalized lymphadenopathy, constitutional symptoms (e.g., sore throat, fever), and symptomatic or asymptomatic meningitis.
- Latent: No clinical manifestations.
- Tertiary: Cardiovascular disease (e.g., aortitis), CNS disease (e.g., meningovascular disease, general paresis, and tabes dorsalis).

Ocular

- Primary: A chancre may occur on the eyelid or conjunctiva, madarosis (loss of lashes or eyebrows).
- Secondary: Uveitis (posterior and panuveitis more common than anterior), optic neuritis, chorioretinitis, serous retinal detachments, retinitis, retinal vasculitis, conjunctivitis, dacryoadenitis, dacryocystitis, episcleritis, scleritis, interstitial keratitis, and others. See **Figure 12.12.1A** and **B**.
- Tertiary: Optic atrophy, old chorioretinitis, interstitial keratitis, chronic anterior uveitis, Argyll Robertson pupil (see 10.3, ARGYLL ROBERTSON PUPIL), in addition to signs seen in secondary disease.

> 📝 **NOTE:** Presentations strongly suggestive of syphilis include the following: patchy hyperemia of the iris with fleshy, pink nodules near the iris sphincter; acute posterior placoid chorioretinitis (multifocal white placoid lesions in the posterior pole); and punctate inner retinitis (superficial punctate creamy white lesions).

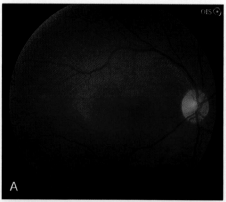

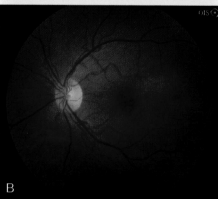

Figure 12.12.1 Fundus photographs of the right (A) and left (B) eye showing placoid retinopathy in secondary syphilis.

Differential Diagnosis

See 12.1, ANTERIOR UVEITIS (IRITIS/IRIDOCYCLITIS) and 12.3, POSTERIOR UVEITIS.

Workup

See 12.1, ANTERIOR UVEITIS (IRITIS/IRIDOCYCLITIS) and 12.3, POSTERIOR UVEITIS, for general uveitis workup recommendations.

1. Complete ophthalmic examination, including pupillary and dilated fundus examination. Palmar skin lesions are common and easily assessed in the clinic.

2. The "reverse algorithm" should be used, with treponemal testing done first to confirm the disease, and (if reactive) then nontreponemal testing to allow for assessment of treatment response. Treponemal testing with enzyme immunoassay (EIA), chemiluminescent immunoassays (CIA), FTA-ABS, or *Treponema pallidum* microhemagglutination assay (MHA-TP) tests are highly sensitive and specific in all but the primary stage of syphilis, during which ocular involvement is very rare. Quantitative nontreponemal tests such as RPR or VDRL are then done to assess the activity of the infection and are then repeated periodically after treatment to confirm resolution of infection. Once reactive, treponemal tests do not normalize and cannot be used to assess the patient's response to treatment.

3. VDRL and RPR should not be used for screening as false-negative results can occur in early primary, latent, or late syphilis due to low sensitivity. False-negatives are also possible due to interference from excessively high titers (prozone reaction). False-positive results can occur due to viral illnesses, pregnancy, and test cross-reactivity with autoimmune or collagen vascular diseases. RPR and VDRL titers are used to follow treatment response.

4. In a patient with findings consistent with syphilis but no documented history of treatment, a positive treponemal test with a negative nontreponemal test still mandates treatment.

5. HIV testing is indicated in any patient with syphilis because of the relatively aggressive course in HIV-infected individuals as well as the high frequency of co-infection.

6. Patients should be evaluated for concomitant sexually transmitted diseases, with notification sent to the local health department when indicated.

7. Lumbar puncture with VDRL or FTA testing, protein, and cell count with differential should be performed in all cases of confirmed syphilitic uveitis, which should be considered consistent with neurosyphilis. Persistently stable or elevated CSF VDRL titers are concerning for incomplete treatment or reinfection.

Treatment Indications

In the presence of uveitis consistent with syphilis:

1. Treponemal testing negative: Syphilis unlikely, consider re-testing if there is high suspicion and/or evaluating for other causes of uveitis.

2. Treponemal testing positive and nontreponemal testing negative:
   - If appropriate past treatment cannot be documented, treatment for syphilis is indicated.
   - If appropriate past treatment can be documented, treatment for syphilis is not indicated if another cause is identified and the patient responds to therapy for that condition.

3. Treponemal testing positive and nontreponemal testing positive: Treat for syphilis.

NOTE: Patients with concurrent HIV and active syphilis may have negative serologies (both treponemal and nontreponemal) because of their immunocompromised state. These patients manifest aggressive, recalcitrant syphilis and should be treated with neurosyphilis dosages over longer treatment periods. Consultation with infectious disease is recommended. Treatment of their comorbid HIV infection is paramount.

Treatment

1. Syphilitic uveitis represents a breakdown of the blood–brain (ocular) barrier and should be treated as neurosyphilis: Aqueous crystalline penicillin G 3 to 4 million units q4h for 10 to 14 days, followed by benzathine penicillin 2.4 million units intramuscularly (i.m.) weekly for 3 weeks.

2. If anterior segment inflammation is present, treatment with a cycloplegic (e.g., cyclopentolate 1% b.i.d.) and topical steroid (e.g., prednisolone acetate 1% q2h) should be started.

3. Oral steroids may be started 24 to 48 hours after induction of penicillin therapy and may speed visual recovery, but ultimately, have not been shown to affect final visual outcomes. Oral steroids may also help prevent systemic inflammatory complications associated with the Jarisch–Herxheimer reaction.

12

NOTE

- Incomplete response to i.m. penicillin is possible, while a full course of i.v. therapy is virtually always effective; therefore, i.v. therapy is considered definitive therapy.
- Treatment for chlamydial infection with a single dose of azithromycin 1 g p.o. is typically indicated.
- Therapy for penicillin-allergic patients should be done in consultation with an infectious disease specialist. The CDC recommends admission and penicillin desensitization for patients who have a serious penicillin allergy and have neurosyphilis. Alternative regimens include ceftriaxone 2 g i.v./i.m. daily for 10 to 14 days or doxycycline 200 mg p.o. b.i.d. for 21 to 28 days. Notably, cephalosporins have a small risk for cross-reactivity in patients with a penicillin allergy.

Follow Up

1. Uveitis (negative CSF VDRL): Repeat serum VDRL/RPR testing q3 months after treatment. If a titer of 1:8 or more does not decline fourfold within 6 months, the titer increases fourfold, or clinical symptoms or signs of syphilis persist or recur, then repeat lumbar puncture checking VDRL and retreatment may be indicated. If a pretreatment VDRL/RPR titer is <1:8, retreatment is indicated only when the titer increases or when signs of syphilis recur.

2. Uveitis and neurosyphilis (positive CSF VDRL): Requires follow up with an infectious disease specialist. Repeat lumbar puncture should be performed every 6 months for 2 years, less frequently if the cell count returns to normal sooner. The cell count should decrease to a normal level within this period, and the CSF VDRL titer should decrease fourfold within 6 to 12 months. A significantly elevated CSF protein decreases more slowly. Failure of these indices to improve is concerning for incomplete treatment or reinfection.

CONGENITAL SYPHILIS

Ocular signs include bilateral interstitial keratitis, secondary cataracts, salt-and-pepper chorioretinitis, and chronic anterior uveitis. Hutchinson triad of congenital syphilis includes peg-shaped widely spaced incisors, interstitial keratitis, and deafness. Serologic testing is similar to acquired syphilis above. Standard treatment is with penicillin G, but dosing should be managed by a pediatrician or an infectious disease specialist.

12.13 Postoperative Endophthalmitis

ACUTE (DAY[S] AFTER SURGERY)

Symptoms

Sudden onset of decreased vision and increasing eye pain after surgical procedure.

Signs

(See Figure 12.13.1.)

Critical. Hypopyon, fibrin, severe anterior chamber reaction, vitreous cells and haze, and decreased red reflex.

Other. Eyelid edema, corneal edema, intense conjunctival injection, chemosis (all are highly variable).

Organisms

- Postcataract extraction:
  - Most common: *Staphylococcus epidermidis.*
  - Common: *Staphylococcus aureus,* Streptococcal species (except Pneumococcus).
  - Less common: Gram-negative bacteria (species including *Pseudomonas, Aerobacter, Proteus, Klebsiella, Bacillus, Enterobacter, Haemophilus influenzae, Escherichia coli*) and anaerobes.
- Bleb associated: *Streptococcus* or Gram-negative infections.
- Postvitrectomy: *S. epidermidis.*
- Postintravitreal injection: *S. epidermidis* and oral flora (notably streptococcal species).

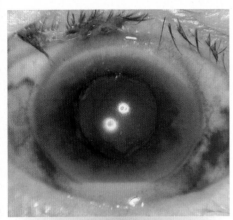

Figure 12.13.1 Postoperative endophthalmitis with hypopyon.

Differential Diagnosis

- Toxic anterior segment syndrome (TASS): Occurs 6 to 24 hours after cataract surgery. Diffuse corneal edema with KP. Due to endotoxin from surgical instruments or fluids. Usually responds to intensive topical steroid and cycloplegic therapy but may require endothelial keratoplasty or penetrating keratoplasty for persistent corneal edema.
- Acute noninfectious uveitis flare: Ask about history of previous uveitis; HLA-B27-associated anterior uveitis may be precipitated by trauma, including surgery.
- Sterile (noninfectious) endophthalmitis (e.g., following intravitreal triamcinolone acetonide or anti-VEGF injection).
- Lens-particle uveitis (retained lens fragment in the angle or vitreous or retained lens cortex in the capsular bag).
- See 12.14, CHRONIC POSTOPERATIVE UVEITIS.

Workup

1. Complete ocular history and examination. Look for wound/bleb leak, exposed suture, vitreous to wound, blepharitis, or other predisposing factors for endophthalmitis.
2. Consider B-scan US if there is limited view to the posterior segment, which may confirm marked vitritis and/or membrane formation and establishes a baseline against which the success of therapy can be measured.

3. If vision is light perception postcataract extraction, a diagnostic (and therapeutic) vitrectomy is often indicated. Cultures (blood, chocolate, Sabouraud, and thioglycolate) and smears (Gram and Giemsa stains) should be obtained and intravitreal antibiotics are given. If vision is hand motion or better, vitreous aspiration or an anterior chamber paracentesis if the vitreous specimen cannot be obtained of 0.2 mL is performed and variably sent for culture. See Appendix 13, ANTERIOR CHAMBER PARACENTESIS.

Treatment

1. Prevention: Preparation of the conjunctiva with 5% povidone-iodine in all cases and the eyelids for incisional eye surgery prior to surgery has been proven to reduce the risk of endophthalmitis. Intraoperative (e.g., intracameral) antibiotics have also been shown to reduce endophthalmitis risk. While perioperative use of topical broad-spectrum antibiotics may decrease bacterial load, it has not been proven to lower the rates of endophthalmitis and may promote antibiotic resistance.
2. Anterior chamber or vitreous tap for Gram stain, culture, and sensitivities along with timely intravitreal injections using broad-spectrum antibiotics (often vancomycin and ceftazidime, amikacin if penicillin allergic). See Appendix 11, INTRAVITREAL TAP AND INJECT and Appendix 12, INTRAVITREAL ANTIBIOTICS. Consider intravitreal steroids (e.g., dexamethasone 0.4 mg/0.1 mL) in select cases with severe vitreous inflammation.
3. Consider admission to hospital for observation.
4. Consider intensive topical steroids (e.g., prednisolone acetate 1% q1h around the clock) for control of anterior segment inflammation.
5. Consider intensive topical fortified antibiotics (e.g., vancomycin and tobramycin, q1h around the clock for 24-48 hours) in the setting of filtering blebs, wound leaks, or exposed sutures. See Appendix 9, FORTIFIED TOPICAL ANTIBIOTICS/ANTIFUNGALS.
6. Atropine 1% b.i.d. to t.i.d.
7. For postcataract extraction endophthalmitis, immediate pars plana vitrectomy is beneficial if visual acuity on presentation is light perception. Vitrectomy for other causes of

12

endophthalmitis (bleb-related, posttraumatic, or endogenous) may be beneficial in select cases.

8. Systemic antibiotics may be considered. Intravenous antibiotics are not routinely used. Consider i.v. fluoroquinolones (e.g., moxifloxacin) in special circumstances (e.g., bleb-related endophthalmitis or trauma). Some oral antibiotics (e.g., moxifloxacin 400 mg p.o. daily) may reach therapeutic vitreous levels and could be considered as alternatives to intravenous antibiotics.

9. Subconjunctival antibiotics (vancomycin and ceftazidime) were used in the Endophthalmitis Vitrectomy Study; however, their use has become less common.

Follow Up

1. Monitor the clinical course q12–24h early on.
2. Relief of pain is a useful early sign of response to therapy.
3. Early prednisone 60 mg p.o. daily for 5 days was part of the Endophthalmitis Vitrectomy Study protocol. However, its use depends on the causative organism, the patient's comorbidities (e.g., diabetic), as well as the severity and duration of the disease. Once the infection is sterilized, postendophthalmitis inflammation may be significant and should be treated with aggressive topical and occasionally oral steroids.
4. After 48 hours, patients should show clinical improvement (e.g., relief of pain, decreased inflammation, and decreased hypopyon). Consider reinjecting antibiotics if there is no improvement or if Gram stain shows an unusual organism. Consider vitrectomy if the patient is deteriorating.
5. The antibiotic regimen is refined according to the treatment response, culture results, and culture sensitivity.
6. If the patient is responding well, topical antibiotics and steroids may be slowly tapered. Close outpatient follow up is warranted.

SUBACUTE (WEEKS TO MONTHS AFTER SURGERY)

Symptoms

Variable. Insidious decreased vision, increasing redness, and pain.

Signs

Critical. Anterior chamber and vitreous inflammation, lens capsular plaque, hypopyon; clumps of fibrinous exudate in the anterior chamber, on the iris surface, or along the pupillary border; vitreous abscesses; and vitritis.

Other. Variable conjunctival injection, KP, corneal edema, and blebitis.

Organisms

- *S. epidermidis* or other common bacteria (e.g., streptococci with a filtering bleb).

    Cutibacterium acnes (formerly *Propionibacterium acnes*), or other rare, indolent bacteria: Recurrent, anterior uveitis, may have a hypopyon and granulomatous KP, but with minimal conjunctival injection and pain. A white plaque or opacities on the lens capsule may be evident. Only a transient response to steroids.
- Fungi (*Aspergillus, Candida, Cephalosporium, Penicillium* species, and others).

Differential Diagnosis

- Lens-particle uveitis: Perform gonioscopy and dilated exam to look for retained lens fragment(s) in angle or vitreous.
- IOL-induced uveitis (iris chafing): Look for iris transillumination and IOL decentration. Most common with one-piece acrylic IOL (thick, square-edge haptics) in the sulcus and with any lens that impinges on the iris or ciliary body.
- See 12.14, CHRONIC POSTOPERATIVE UVEITIS.

Workup

1. Complete ocular history and examination.
2. Aspiration of vitreous for smears (Gram, Giemsa, and methenamine–silver) and cultures (blood, chocolate, Sabouraud, thioglycolate, and a solid medium for anaerobic culture).

See Appendix 11, INTRAVITREAL TAP AND INJECT. Intravitreal antibiotics are given as described previously. See Appendix 12, INTRAVITREAL ANTIBIOTICS.

NOTE: C. acnes will be missed unless proper anaerobic cultures are obtained and held for extended culture (14 days).

Treatment

1. Initially treat as acute postoperative endophthalmitis, as described previously, but do not start steroids.
2. Immediate pars plana vitrectomy is beneficial if visual acuity on presentation is light perception within 6 weeks after cataract surgery. Prompt vitrectomy for endophthalmitis due to other procedures has not been studied in a large randomized trial.
3. If a fungal infection is suspected, administer intravitreal amphotericin B (5 to 10 µg/0.1 mL) or intravitreal voriconazole (100 µg/0.1 mL).
4. Removal of the intraocular lens and capsular remnants may be required for diagnosis and treatment of C. acnes endophthalmitis, which may be sensitive to intravitreal penicillin, cefoxitin, clindamycin, or vancomycin.

5. If S. epidermidis is isolated, intraocular vancomycin (including irrigation of the capsular bag) alone may be sufficient.
6. Antimicrobial therapy should be modified in accordance with culture results, sensitivity testing, clinical course, and tolerance of therapeutic agents.
7. A vitrectomy with limited capsulectomy of the capsular plaque may be considered if vitreous aspiration cultures are negative or if the clinical response is incomplete. In cases with an incomplete response, removal of the entire capsule and IOL, along with intravitreal antibiotics, should be considered.

Follow Up

1. Dependent on the organism.
2. In general, follow up is as described previously for acute postoperative endophthalmitis.

12.14 | Chronic Postoperative Uveitis

Routine postoperative inflammation is typically mild, responds promptly to steroids, and usually resolves within 6 weeks. Consider the following etiologies when postoperative inflammation is atypical.

Etiology

- Severe intraocular inflammation in the early postoperative course:
  - Infectious endophthalmitis: Deteriorating vision, pain, fibrin, or hypopyon in the anterior chamber, vitritis. See 12.13, POSTOPERATIVE ENDOPHTHALMITIS.
  - Retained lens material: A severe granulomatous inflammation with mutton-fat KP, resulting from an hypersensitivity reaction to lens protein exposed during surgery and may result in elevated IOP. See 9.12, LENS-RELATED GLAUCOMA.
  - Aseptic (sterile) endophthalmitis: A severe noninfectious postoperative uveitis caused by intraoperative injections (e.g., triamcinolone acetonide) or excess tissue manipulation, especially of vitreous manipulation, during surgery. A hypopyon and a mild vitreous cellular reaction may develop.

Usually not characterized by profound or progressive pain or visual loss. A fibrinoid reaction is typically absent. Eyelid swelling and chemosis are atypical. Conjunctival injection is often absent. Usually resolves with topical steroid therapy.

- TASS: An acute, sterile inflammation following uneventful surgery that develops rapidly within 6 to 24 hours. Characterized by anterior chamber cell and flare, possibly with fibrin or hypopyon, and severe corneal edema in excess of what would be expected following surgery. IOP may be increased. May be caused by any material placed in the eye during surgery including irrigating or injected solutions (e.g., due to the presence of a preservative or incorrect pH or concentration of a solution) or improperly cleaned instruments.
- Acute iridocyclitis flare: HLA-B27-associated and herpetic uveitis flares can be triggered by surgical trauma.
- Persistent postoperative inflammation (e.g., beyond 6 weeks):
  - Poor compliance with topical steroids.
  - Steroid drops tapered too rapidly.

12

- Retained lens material.
- Iris or vitreous incarceration in the wound.
- UGH syndrome: Irritation of the iris or ciliary body by an IOL. Increased IOP and red blood cells in the anterior chamber accompany the anterior segment inflammation. See 9.16, POSTOPERATIVE GLAUCOMA.
- Retinal detachment: Often produces a low-grade anterior chamber reaction. See 11.3, RETINAL DETACHMENT.
- Sub-acute endophthalmitis (e.g., *C. acnes* and other indolent bacteria, fungal, or partially treated bacterial endophthalmitis).
- Epithelial downgrowth: Corneal or conjunctival epithelium grows into the eye through a corneal wound and may be seen on the posterior corneal surface and iris. The iris may appear flattened with loss of detail because of the spread of the membrane across the anterior chamber angle onto the iris. Large cells may be seen in the anterior chamber, and glaucoma may be present. The diagnosis of epithelial downgrowth can be confirmed by observing the immediate appearance of white spots after medium-power argon laser treatment to the areas of iris covered by the membrane. An anterior chamber tap may also reveal many epithelial cells.
- Preexisting chronic uveitis: See 12.1, ANTERIOR UVEITIS (IRITIS/IRIDOCYCLITIS).
- Sympathetic ophthalmia: Diffuse granulomatous inflammation in both eyes, after penetrating trauma or surgery. See 12.18, SYMPATHETIC OPHTHALMIA.

Workup and Treatment

1. History: Is the patient taking the steroid drops properly? Did the patient stop the steroid drops abruptly? Was there a postoperative wound leak allowing epithelial downgrowth? Previous history of uveitis?
2. Complete ocular examination of both eyes, including a slit lamp assessment of the anterior chamber reaction, a determination of whether vitreous or residual lens material

is present in the anterior chamber, and an inspection of the lens capsule looking for capsular opacities (e.g., *C. acnes* capsular plaque). Perform gonioscopy (to evaluate for iris or vitreous to the wound or small retained lens fragments), an IOP measurement, vitreous evaluation for inflammatory cells, and a dilated posterior and peripheral fundus examination (to rule out retained lens material in the inferior pars plana, retinal detachment, or signs of chorioretinitis).

3. Obtain B-scan US when the fundus view is obscured. Consider UBM to assess the IOL position, for iris-IOL contact, and to evaluate for retained lens material.
4. When concerned for subacute postoperative endophthalmitis: A vitreous tap should be performed (see Appendix 11, INTRAVITREAL TAP AND INJECT) with anaerobic cultures, using both solid media and broth to isolate atypical organisms such as *C. acnes* (routine cultures also are obtained; see 12.13, POSTOPERATIVE ENDOPHTHALMITIS). The anaerobic cultures should be incubated in an anaerobic environment as rapidly as possible and held for an extended incubation period (14 days).
5. Consider an anterior chamber paracentesis for diagnostic smears and cultures. See Appendix 13, ANTERIOR CHAMBER PARACENTESIS.
6. Consider diagnostic medium-power argon laser treatment to areas of iris with suspected epithelial downgrowth.

In the setting of a capsular plaque, transient improvement in inflammation with steroids, and a negative work up, surgery may be required to diagnose and treat subacute endophthalmitis such as *C. acnes*. Initially, a vitrectomy with limited capsulectomy of the capsular plaque and injection of intravitreal antibiotics should be considered. Removal of the entire capsule and IOL may be required if there is an incomplete response as it usually successfully eradicates the infection.

See 12.1, ANTERIOR UVEITIS (IRITIS/IRIDOCYCLITIS); 12.3, POSTERIOR UVEITIS; 12.13, POSTOPERATIVE ENDOPHTHALMITIS; and 12.18, SYMPATHETIC OPHTHALMIA for more specific information on diagnosis and treatment.

12

12.15 Traumatic Endophthalmitis

This condition constitutes an emergency requiring prompt attention.

Symptoms and Signs

Similar to 12.13, POSTOPERATIVE ENDOPHTHALMITIS. An occult or missed IOFB must be ruled out. See 3.15, INTRAOCULAR FOREIGN BODY.

NOTE: Patients with *Bacillus* endophthalmitis may have a high fever, leukocytosis, proptosis, a corneal ring ulcer, and rapid visual deterioration.

Organisms

Staphylococcus species, *Streptococcus* species, Gram-negative species, fungi, *Bacillus* species, and others. Mixed flora may be present. Understanding the mechanism of injury is helpful in predicting the type of infecting organism (e.g., penetrating trauma from organic matter increases the risk of fungal infection).

Differential Diagnosis

- Phacoanaphylactic inflammation: A sterile hypersensitivity reaction as a result of exposed lens protein associated with anterior chamber reaction, KP, and sometimes elevated IOP. See 9.12, LENS-RELATED GLAUCOMA.
- Lens cortex: Fluffed up and hydrated cortical lens material, especially in younger patients with soft nuclei after violation of the lens capsule, associated with large anterior chamber lens particles, but no KP.
- Sterile inflammatory response from a retained IOFB, blood in the vitreous, retinal detachment, or as a result of surgical manipulation.

Workup

Same as for 12.13, POSTOPERATIVE ENDOPHTHALMITIS, in addition to an orbital CT scan (axial, coronal, and parasagittal views) with thin 1-mm cuts and B-scan US to evaluate for IOFB.

Treatment

1. Consider hospitalization.
2. Management for a ruptured globe or penetrating ocular injury if present. See 3.14, RUPTURED GLOBE AND PENETRATING OCULAR INJURY.
3. Removal of an intraocular foreign body in traumatic endophthalmitis is paramount in controlling the infection. See 3.15, INTRAOCULAR FOREIGN BODY.
4. Intravitreal antibiotics (e.g., ceftazidime 2.2 mg in 0.1 mL and vancomycin 1 mg in 0.1 mL; clindamycin 1 mg in 0.1 mL or amikacin 0.4 mg in 0.1 mL may also be considered for anaerobic coverage, especially if high concern for *Bacillus*, intraocular foreign body, or when there is a penicillin allergy). Intravitreal aminoglycosides should be used with caution, given their potential risk of macular infarction. These medications may be repeated every 48 to 72 hours as needed. See Appendix 12, INTRAVITREAL ANTIBIOTICS.
5. Systemic antibiotics (e.g., ciprofloxacin 400 mg i.v. q12h or moxifloxacin 400 mg p.o. or i.v. daily; and cefazolin 1 g i.v. q8h). Consider an infectious disease consult for guidance in specific cases. May need to adjust dose for renal insufficiency and for children.
6. The benefit of pars plana vitrectomy is unknown for traumatic endophthalmitis without IOFB. However, pars plana vitrectomy reduces the overall infectious and inflammatory burden and provides sufficient material for diagnostic culture and pathologic investigation.
7. Give tetanus toxoid 0.5 mL intramuscularly if immunization is not up-to-date. See Appendix 2, TETANUS PROPHYLAXIS.
8. Steroids are typically not used until fungal organisms are ruled out, although recent reports have demonstrated that topical steroids may not be as deleterious as previously thought. Topical and oral steroids may be used at the discretion of the physician to control postinfection inflammation once the infection is sterilized.

Follow Up

Same as for 12.13, POSTOPERATIVE ENDOPHTHALMITIS.

12

12.16 Endogenous Bacterial Endophthalmitis

Symptoms

Decreased vision in an acutely ill (e.g., septic) or recently hospitalized patient, the immunocompromised, a patient with an indwelling catheter, an intravenous drug user, or in a patient with a history of a recent systemic procedure (e.g., heart valve replacement or repair). No history of recent intraocular surgery.

Signs

Critical. Chorioretinitis, vitreous cells and debris, anterior chamber cell and flare, and/or a hypopyon.

Other. Iris microabscesses, absent red reflex, retinal inflammatory infiltrates, flame-shaped retinal hemorrhages with or without white centers, retinal/subretinal/choroidal abscesses, corneal edema, eyelid edema, chemosis, conjunctival injection, and panophthalmitis with orbital involvement (proptosis, restricted ocular motility). May be bilateral.

Organisms

Bacillus cereus (especially in i.v. drug users), streptococci, *Neisseria meningitidis*, *S. aureus*, *H. influenzae*, Klebsiella in East Asia, and others.

Differential Diagnosis

- Endogenous fungal endophthalmitis: May see fluffy, white vitreous opacities. Organisms include *Aspergillus* and *Candida*. See 12.17, CANDIDA RETINITIS/UVEITIS/ENDOPHTHALMITIS.
- Viral retinitis: one or more foci of retinal whitening with variable levels of vitreous inflammation. See 12.8 ACUTE RETINAL NECROSIS.
- Retinochoroidal infection (e.g., toxoplasmosis and toxocariasis): Yellow or white retinochoroidal lesions.
- Noninfectious posterior or intermediate uveitis (e.g., sarcoidosis and pars planitis). Unlikely to get the first episode coincidentally during sepsis.
- Neoplastic conditions (e.g., large cell lymphoma and retinoblastoma).

Workup

1. History: Duration of symptoms? Systemic symptoms of underlying disease or infection? Indwelling catheter? Intravenous drug use? Immunocompromised? Recent medical procedures?
2. Complete ocular examination, including a dilated fundus evaluation.
3. B-scan US if there is no view to the fundus to assess for vitritis, abscesses.
4. Complete medical workup by an infectious disease specialist.
5. Chest X-ray; cultures of blood, urine, all indwelling catheters, and i.v. lines; Gram stain of any discharge. Consider a transesophageal or transthoracic echocardiogram to rule out endocarditis. A lumbar puncture is indicated when meningeal signs are present.

Treatment

All treatment should be coordinated with an internal medicine physician.

1. Hospitalize the patient.
2. Broad-spectrum (i.v. and/or oral) antibiotics are started after appropriate smears and cultures are obtained. Antibiotic choices vary according to the suspected source of septic infection (e.g., gastrointestinal tract, genitourinary tract, and cardiac) and are determined in consultation with an infectious disease specialist. Dosages recommended for meningitis and severe infections are used. If oral antibiotics are used, confirm that the regimen includes antibiotics with good vitreous penetration.

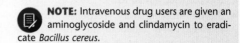 **NOTE:** Intravenous drug users are given an aminoglycoside and clindamycin to eradicate *Bacillus cereus*.

3. Topical cycloplegic (e.g., atropine 1% b.i.d. to t.i.d.).
4. Topical steroid (e.g., prednisolone acetate 1% q1–6h titrated to the degree of anterior segment inflammation).

12

5. Consider intravitreal antibiotics if there is significant or worsening vitreous involvement (e.g., ceftazidime 2.2 mg in 0.1 mL and vancomycin 1 mg in 0.1 mL; clindamycin 1 mg in 0.1 mL, or amikacin 0.4 mg in 0.1 mL may also be considered for anaerobic coverage, especially if there is high concern for *Bacillus*, intraocular foreign body, or when there is a penicillin allergy). Intravitreal aminoglycosides, including amikacin, may cause macular infarction. The timing of intravitreal antibiotics is controversial although they offer higher intraocular concentrations. Consider intravitreal antifungal agents, if clinically suspicious. See Appendix 11, INTRAVITREAL TAP AND INJECT, and Appendix 12, INTRAVITREAL ANTIBIOTICS.

6. Consider pars plana vitrectomy if severe or nonresponsive to initial therapy. Vitrectomy offers the benefits of reducing infective and inflammatory load and providing sufficient material for diagnostic culture and pathologic study. Additionally, intravitreal antibiotics may be administered at the time of surgery.

7. Periocular antibiotics (e.g., subconjunctival or subtenon injections) are sometimes used. See Appendix 10, TECHNIQUE FOR RETROBULBAR/ SUBTENON/SUBCONJUNCTIVAL INJECTIONS.

Follow Up

1. Daily in the hospital.

2. Peak and trough levels for many antibiotic agents are obtained every few days. Renal function needs monitoring during aminoglycoside therapy. The antibiotic regimen is guided by the culture and sensitivity results, as well as the patient's clinical response to treatment. Intravenous antibiotics are maintained for at least 2 weeks (pending identification of clinical source and response to treatment).

12.17 Candida Retinitis/Endophthalmitis

Symptoms

Decreased vision, floaters, and pain that is often bilateral. Patients typically have a history of recent hospitalization, recent abdominal surgery, being immunocompromised, possessing a long-term indwelling line or catheter (e.g., for hyperalimentation, hemodialysis, or antibiotics), or using intravenous drugs.

Signs

(See Figure 12.17.1.)

Critical. Discrete, multifocal, yellow-white, choroidal to chorioretinal fluffy lesions from one to several disc diameters in size. With time, the lesions increase in size, break into the vitreous, and appear as "cotton balls" or a "string of pearls".

Other. Vitreous cell and haze, vitreous abscesses, retinal hemorrhages with or without pale centers, anterior chamber cells, and hypopyon. A retinal detachment may develop.

Differential Diagnosis

The following should be considered in immunocompromised patients.

- CMV retinitis: Multifocal areas of granular retinal whitening with a minimal to mild vitreous reaction, more likely to be associated with retinal hemorrhage. See 12.9, CYTOMEGALOVIRUS RETINITIS.

- Toxoplasmosis: Yellow-white retinal lesions often with an adjacent chorioretinal scar. See 12.5, TOXOPLASMOSIS.

- Pneumocystis choroidopathy: Rare manifestation of widely disseminated *Pneumocystis*

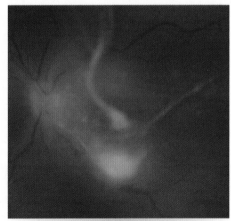

Figure 12.17.1 Candida chorioretinitis with vitreous involvement.

12

carinii infection. Usually in AIDS patients. Often asymptomatic. History of *P. carinii* and treatment with aerosolized pentamidine. Multifocal, yellow, round, deep choroidal lesions approximately one-half to two-disc diameters in size, located in the posterior pole. No vitritis. Patients are often cachectic. Treatment is with i.v. trimethoprim/sulfamethoxazole or i.v. pentamidine in conjunction with an infectious disease specialist.

- Others: Herpes viral retinitis; *Nocardia*, *Aspergillus*, and *Cryptococcus* species; Atypical *Mycobacterium*, coccidioidomycosis, and others.

Workup

1. History: History of bacteremia or fungemia? Underlying medical conditions? Medications? Indwelling catheter? Intravenous drug use? Other risk factors for immunocompromised state?
2. Skin examination for signs of intravenous drug injection.
3. Most clinicians recommend that all patients with candidemia have a complete, dilated fundoscopic examination (ideally within 72 hours), as ocular involvement may be asymptomatic. A repeat fundoscopic examination is recommended 2 weeks after the initial negative examination.
4. Blood, urine, and catheter tip fungal cultures; these often need to be repeated several times and may be negative despite ocular candidiasis. Blood cultures may need to be held a full 7 days and may take 3 to 4 days to become positive for *Candida* species.
5. Consider vitrectomy to obtain a specimen and remove opacified vitreous. Cultures and smears can confirm the diagnosis. Amphotericin B 5 to 10 μg in 0.1 mL or voriconazole 50 to 100 μg in 0.1 mL is injected into the vitreous cavity after the procedure.
6. Baseline CBC, renal function tests, and liver function tests.

Treatment

1. Suspected fungal endophthalmitis without a clear source should be considered evidence of a disseminated infection and requires further systemic evaluation and workup.
2. Hospitalize all unreliable patients, systemically ill patients, or those with moderate to severe vitreous involvement.
3. An infectious disease specialist should be consulted for systemic workup to evaluate for a source and other sites of involvement.
4. Typically, chorioretinitis without vitreous involvement can be successfully treated with systemic therapy alone with one of the following regimens: Fluconazole 800 mg p.o. loading dose followed by 400 to 800 mg p.o. daily. Alternatively, voriconazole 400 mg i.v. b.i.d. daily for 2 doses followed by 300 mg i.v. or p.o. b.i.d. may also be considered in fluconazole-resistant species. For fluconazole- and voriconazole-resistant species, liposomal amphotericin B (3 to 5 mg/kg i.v. daily) is recommended. Therapy should be guided by cultures and sensitivities. Other agents that may be used include caspofungin, itraconazole, and micafungin.
5. Intravitreal injection of antifungal agents as above (voriconazole or amphotericin B) if there is vitreous involvement. Depending on the response and location of retinal involvement (anterior versus posterior), injections may be repeated.
6. Topical cycloplegic agent (e.g., atropine 1% b.i.d. to t.i.d.).
7. See 9.7, INFLAMMATORY OPEN ANGLE GLAUCOMA, for IOP control.

Follow Up

1. Patients are seen daily early on. Visual acuity, IOP, and the degree of anterior chamber and vitreous inflammation are assessed.
2. Patients receiving azole antifungals require liver function tests every 1 to 2 weeks and as clinically indicated. Patients receiving amphotericin require monitoring of electrolytes, kidney function, and CBC as directed by an infectious disease specialist.

12.18 Sympathetic Ophthalmia

Symptoms

Bilateral eye pain, photophobia, decreased vision, and red eyes. A history of penetrating trauma or intraocular surgery (most commonly vitreoretinal surgery) to one eye (usually 4 to 8 weeks before, but ranges from days to decades, with 90% occurring within 1 year). Sympathetic ophthalmia is rare (the literature estimates an annual incidence of 0.03/100,000 people).

Signs

Critical. Suspect anytime there is inflammation in the uninvolved eye after unilateral ocular trauma or surgery. Bilateral severe anterior chamber reaction with large mutton-fat KP; may have asymmetric involvement with typically more reaction in uninjured eye. Posterior segment findings include small depigmented nodules at the level of the retinal pigment epithelium (corresponding to Dalen–Fuchs nodules histopathologically) and diffuse thickening of the choroid. Signs of previous injury or surgery in one eye are usually present. In developed countries, repeated vitreoretinal procedures following ocular trauma are the most common risk factors.

Other. Nodular infiltration of the iris, peripheral anterior synechiae, neovascularization of the iris, occlusion, and seclusion of the pupil, cataract, exudative retinal detachment, and papillitis. The earliest sign may be loss of accommodation, or a mild anterior or posterior uveitis in the uninjured eye.

Differential Diagnosis

- VKH syndrome: Similar signs, but no history of ocular trauma or surgery. Other systemic symptoms. See 12.11, VOGT–KOYANAGI–HARADA SYNDROME.
- Phacoantigenic (formerly phacoanaphylaxis) endophthalmitis: Severe anterior chamber reaction from injury to the lens capsule. The contralateral eye is uninvolved. See 9.12, LENS-RELATED GLAUCOMA.
- Sarcoidosis: Often associated systemic symptoms involving the lungs or skin, elevated ACE level, or characteristic pulmonary changes on chest CT. May cause a bilateral granulomatous panuveitis. See 12.6, SARCOIDOSIS.

- Syphilis: Positive treponemal and reflex non-treponemal testing. May cause bilateral granulomatous panuveitis. See 12.12, SYPHILIS.
- Tuberculosis: Positive PPD or IGRA with possible characteristic findings on CXR or chest CT. May cause bilateral granulomatous panuveitis.
- Multifocal choroiditis with panuveitis: Usually bilateral, with no history of trauma.

Workup

1. History: Any prior eye surgery or injury? History of sexually transmitted disease or high-risk sexual activity? Difficulty breathing?
2. Complete ophthalmic examination, including a dilated retinal examination.
3. Assess for any systemic findings to rule out VKH (e.g., neurologic, skin, or auditory changes).
4. CBC, EIA, or another treponemal testing followed by reflex, nontreponemal testing if positive.
5. Chest radiograph and/or CT chest to evaluate for tuberculosis and sarcoidosis.
6. IVFA or B-scan ultrasound, or both, to help confirm the diagnosis.

Treatment

1. Prevention: Historically enucleation of a blind, traumatized eye within 14 days of the trauma has been recommended to reduce the risk of sympathetic ophthalmia. However, this has limited support in the literature and should only be performed if the eye has been deemed unsalvageable. Once sympathetic ophthalmia develops, enucleation of the sympathizing eye appears to have no benefit.
2. Initial treatment with high dose oral steroids (e.g. prednisone 1 mg/kg p.o. daily) with calcium/vitamin D supplementation and gastric ulcer prophylaxis may be used initially to control ocular inflammation.
3. However long-term local or systemic immunosuppression is essential in most cases. Local control can be achieved with intravitreal steroid implants (e.g., dexamethasone 0.7 mg

12

intravitreal implant or the fluocinolone acetonide 0.19 or 0.59 mg intravitreal implants). Inflammatory control can also be achieved with steroid-sparing systemic immunosuppression. The choice of specific local or systemic immune suppression should be made in conjunction with a uveitis specialist and individualized for each patient.

4. Cycloplegic (e.g., cyclopentolate 1% b.i.d.) for active anterior chamber inflammation.

5. Topical steroids for active anterior chamber inflammation (e.g., prednisolone acetate 1% q1–2h or difluprednate 0.05% q2h), which are tapered slowly as the inflammation improves.

6. Periocular or intravitreal steroids (e.g., subconjunctival triamcinolone acetate 40 mg in 1 mL) may be used to aid in local control prior to pursuing long-term options. See Appendix 10, TECHNIQUE FOR RETROBULBAR/SUBTENON/SUBCONJUNCTIVAL INJECTIONS.

Follow Up

1. Every 1 to 7 days initially, to monitor the effectiveness of therapy and IOP.

2. As the condition improves, the follow-up interval may be extended to every 3 to 4 weeks.

3. Oral steroids may be used initially to quell inflammation with rapid, sequential initiation of long-term local or steroid-sparing systemic immunosuppression to allow for tapering of oral steroids. The goal should be to slowly taper oral prednisone to 5 mg or less by 3 months to avoid the adverse effects of systemic steroids. Because of the possibility of recurrence, periodic checkups are important.

4. The long-term prognosis in patients treated with immunosuppressive therapy can be good, with 81% of eyes seeing ≥20/40 at the final follow up.

Chapter 13

General Ophthalmic Problems

13.1 Acquired Cataract

Symptoms

Slowly progressive visual loss or blurring, usually over months to years, affecting one or both eyes. Glare, especially in bright sun or from oncoming headlights while driving at night, and altered color perception may occur, but not to the same degree as in optic neuropathies. Characteristics of the cataract determine specific symptoms.

Signs

(See Figure 13.1.1.)

Critical. Opacification or discoloration of the normally clear crystalline lens.

Other. Blurred view of the retina with dimming or disruption of the red reflex on retinoscopy. Myopic shift from nuclear sclerosis may cause increased near vision—so-called "second sight." Cataract alone does not cause a relative afferent pupillary defect (RAPD).

Etiology

- Age-related: Most common. Advanced forms include mature, hypermature, and Morgagnian.
- Trauma: Penetrating, concussion (Vossius ring), and electric shock.
- Toxic: Steroids in any form (including intravitreal injections), miotics, antipsychotics (e.g., phenothiazines), and others.
- Secondary.
  - Chronic anterior uveitis. See 12.1, ANTERIOR UVEITIS (IRITIS/IRIDOCYCLITIS).
  - History of vitrectomy.
  - Repeated intravitreal injections (if trauma to lens occurs during a procedure).
  - Ionizing radiation.
  - Tumor (ciliary body).

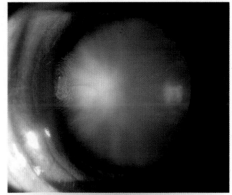

Figure 13.1.1 Cataract with early cortical changes and nuclear sclerosis.

- Acute angle closure glaucoma: May have glaukomflecken. See 9.4, ACUTE ANGLE CLOSURE GLAUCOMA.
- Degenerative ocular disease: Retinitis pigmentosa, Leber congenital amaurosis, gyrate atrophy, Wagner and Stickler syndromes associated with posterior subcapsular cataracts, and others.
- Endocrine/metabolic/chromosomal.
  - Diabetes: Juvenile form characterized by rapidly progressing white "snowflake" opacities in the anterior and posterior subcapsular locations. Age-related cataracts form earlier than in nondiabetics.
  - Hypocalcemia: Small, white, iridescent cortical changes, usually seen in the presence of tetany.
  - Wilson disease: Red-brown pigment deposition in the cortex beneath the anterior capsule (a "sunflower" cataract). See 13.9, WILSON DISEASE.

- Myotonic dystrophy: Multicolored bire-fringent opacities, "Christmas-tree" cataract behind the anterior capsule.
- Others: Down syndrome, neurofibromatosis type 2 (posterior subcapsular cataract), atopic dermatitis (anterior subcapsular), etc.

Types

1. Nuclear: Yellow or brown discoloration of the central lens. Typically blurs distance vision more than near (myopic shift).
2. Posterior subcapsular: Plaque-like opacity near the posterior aspect of the lens. Best seen with retroillumination as a dark shadow against the red reflex. Glare and difficulty reading are common complaints. Symptoms may improve postdilation. Associated with ocular inflammation, steroid use, diabetes, trauma, radiation, or excessive alcohol use. Classically occurs in patients <50 years of age. Typically more rapid onset.
3. Cortical: Vacuoles and radial or spoke-like opacities in the periphery that expand to involve the anterior and posterior lens. Glare is the most common complaint. Often asymptomatic until central changes develop.

NOTE: Traditionally, a mature cataract is defined as lenticular changes sufficiently dense to totally obscure the view of the posterior lens and posterior segment of the eye. No iris shadow is seen on oblique illumination at the pupillary margin. Rarely, the cortex may liquefy and the nucleus becomes free floating within the capsule; this is known as a hypermature or Morgagnian cataract. If the liquefied cortex leaks through the intact capsule, wrinkling of the lens capsule may be seen and phacolytic glaucoma may develop. See 9.12.1, PHACOLYTIC GLAUCOMA. A visually significant cataract is one which subjectively causes bothersome visual symptoms.

Workup

Determine the etiology, whether the cataract is responsible for the decreased vision, and whether surgical removal would improve vision.

1. History: Medications (e.g., tamsulosin and other drugs used for urinary retention [alpha-1 antagonists] strongly associated with intraoperative floppy iris syndrome)? Systemic diseases? Trauma? Ocular disease or poor vision before the cataract?
2. Complete ocular examination, including distance and near vision, pupillary examination, and refraction. When best corrected acuity is 20/30 or better, glare testing is helpful to demonstrate decreased vision. A dilated slit lamp examination using both direct and retroillumination techniques is required to view the cataract properly. Fundus examination, concentrating on the macula, is essential in ruling out other causes of decreased vision.
3. For preoperative planning, note the degree of pupil dilation, density of the cataract, and presence or absence of pseudoexfoliation, phacodonesis (quivering of the lens indicating zonular damage or weakness), or corneal guttae.
4. B-scan ultrasonography (US) if the fundus is not visible to rule out detectable posterior segment disease.
5. The potential acuity meter (PAM) or laser interferometry can be used to estimate the visual potential when cataract extraction is considered in an eye with posterior segment disease.

NOTE: PAM and laser interferometry often overestimate the eye's visual potential in the presence of macular holes or macular pigment epithelial detachments. Interferometry also overestimates visual potential in cases of amblyopia. Near vision is often the most accurate manner of evaluating macular function if the cataract is not too dense. Nonetheless, both PAM and laser interferometry are useful clinical tools.

6. Keratometry readings and measurement of axial length are required for determining the power of the desired intraocular lens (IOL). Corneal pachymetry or endothelial cell count is occasionally helpful if corneal guttae are present.

Treatment

1. Cataract surgery may be performed for the following reasons:
   - To improve visual function in patients with symptomatic visual disability.
   - As surgical therapy for ocular disease (e.g., lens-related glaucoma or uveitis).

13

- To facilitate management of ocular disease (e.g., to allow a fundus view to monitor or treat diabetic retinopathy or glaucoma).
2. Correct any refractive error (e.g., prescription of corrective lenses) if the patient declines cataract surgery.
3. A trial of mydriasis (e.g., cyclopentolate 1% b.i.d. to t.i.d.) may be used successfully in some patients who desire nonsurgical treatment. The benefits of this therapy are only temporary. Most useful for posterior subcapsular cataracts.

Follow Up

Unless there is a secondary complication from the cataract (e.g., glaucoma), a cataract itself does not require urgent action. If a patient requires bilateral cataract extraction, surgery is typically first performed on the more advanced cataract. Patients who decline surgical removal are reexamined annually or sooner if symptoms worsen.

If congenital, see 8.8, PEDIATRIC CATARACT.

13.2 Subluxed or Dislocated Crystalline Lens

Definition

- Subluxation: Partial disruption of the zonular fibers. Lens is decentered but remains partially visible through the pupil.
- Dislocation: Complete disruption of the zonular fibers. Lens is fully displaced out of the pupillary aperture.

Symptoms

Decreased vision, double vision that persists when covering one eye (monocular diplopia).

Signs

(See Figure 13.2.1.)

Critical. Decentered or displaced lens, iridodonesis (quivering of the iris), and phacodonesis (quivering of the lens).

Other. Change in refractive error, marked astigmatism, cataract, angle closure glaucoma as a result of pupillary block, vitreous in the anterior chamber, and asymmetry of the anterior chamber depth.

Etiology

- Trauma: Most common. Results in subluxation if >~25% of the zonular fibers are ruptured. Need to rule out a predisposing condition (see other etiologies).
- Pseudoexfoliation: Flaky material seen as scrolls in a "target pattern" on anterior lens capsule; associated with glaucoma and poor pupillary dilation; higher risk of complications during cataract surgery due to weak zonular fibers (see 9.11, PSEUDOEXFOLIATION SYNDROME/EXFOLIATIVE GLAUCOMA).
- Marfan syndrome: Bilateral lens subluxation, classically superotemporally. Increased risk of retinal detachment. Autosomal dominant with cardiomyopathy, aortic aneurysm, aortic dissection, tall stature with long extremities, and kyphoscoliosis.
- Homocystinuria: Bilateral lens subluxation, classically inferonasally. Increased risk of retinal detachment. Autosomal recessive often with mental retardation, skeletal deformities, high incidence of thromboembolic events (particularly with general anesthesia). Lens subluxation may be the first manifestation in patients with mild disease.
- Weill–Marchesani syndrome: Small lens can dislocate into the anterior chamber, causing reverse pupillary block. Usually autosomal recessive with short fingers and stature, seizures, microspherophakia (small, round lens), myopia, and no mental retardation.
- Others: Acquired syphilis, congenital ectopia lentis, simple ectopia lentis, aniridia, Ehlers–Danlos syndrome, Crouzon syndrome, hyperlysinemia, sulfite oxidase deficiency, high myopia, chronic inflammation, hypermature cataract, etc.

Workup

1. History: Trauma? Family history of disorders listed above? Systemic illness (e.g., syphilis)? Neurologic symptoms (e.g., seizures)?
2. Determine whether the condition is unilateral or bilateral. Determine direction of lens

13

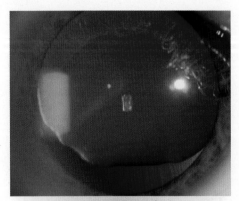

Figure 13.2.1 Ectopia lentis.

displacement and evaluate for subtle phaco-donesis by observing the lens during back and forth saccadic eye movements. Check for pseudoexfoliation. Evaluate for acute or remote signs of ocular trauma including hyphema, angle recession, iridodialysis, cyclo-dialysis, retinal tears and detachments.

3. Systemic examination: Evaluate stature, extremities, hands, and fingers; often in conjunction with an internist, including blood and urine tests to rule out homocystinuria and echocardiography to rule out aortic aneurysms in patients with possible Marfan syndrome. Consider genetic testing when appropriate and available.

4. Syphilis screening tests (rapid plasma reagin [RPR] or venereal disease research laboratory [VDRL] and fluorescent treponemal antibody absorption [FTA-ABS] or treponemal-specific assay).

Treatment

1. Lens dislocated into the anterior chamber.
   - Dilate the pupil, place the patient on his or her back, and attempt to replace the lens into the posterior chamber by head manipulation. It may be necessary to indent the cornea after topical anesthesia with a Zeiss gonioprism or cotton swab to reposition the lens. After the lens is repositioned in the posterior chamber, constrict the pupil with pilocarpine 0.5% to 1% q.i.d. and perform a peripheral laser iridotomy to prevent pupillary block.
   or
   - Surgically remove the lens and consider placing an IOL (preferred treatment if significant cataract, corneal decompensation,

prior treatment failure, recurrent dislocation, or compliance issues with pilocarpine).

2. Lens dislocated into the vitreous.
   - Lens capsule intact, patient asymptomatic, no signs of inflammation: Observation versus pars plana lensectomy and possible IOL placement.
   - Lens capsule broken with intraocular inflammation: Pars plana lensectomy with possible IOL placement.

3. Subluxation.
   - Asymptomatic or stable refractive error: Observe in adults. Timely refractive correction to prevent amblyopia in children.
   - Uncorrectable astigmatism, unstable refractive errors, or monocular diplopia: Surgical removal of the lens and possible IOL placement.
   - Symptomatic cataract: Options include surgical removal of the lens, mydriasis (e.g., atropine 1% daily) and aphakic correction (i.e., contact lens if the other eye is phakic or pseudophakic to prevent anisometropia), pupillary constriction (e.g., pilocarpine 4% gel q.h.s.) and phakic correction, or a large optical iridectomy (away from the lens) with aphakic correction.

4. Pupillary block: Treatment is identical to that for aphakic pupillary block. See 9.16, POSTOPERATIVE GLAUCOMA.

5. If Marfan syndrome suspected, refer the patient to a cardiologist for an annual echocardiogram and management of any cardiac-related abnormalities. Prophylactic systemic antibiotics may be needed if the patient undergoes surgery (or a dental procedure) to prevent endocarditis.

6. If homocystinuria is suspected: Refer to an internist. The usual therapy consists of:
   - Pyridoxine (vitamin B6) daily oral supplementation and a methionine-restricted, cysteine-supplemented diet.
   - Avoid surgery if possible because of the risk of thromboembolic complications. If surgical intervention is necessary, anticoagulant therapy is indicated in conjunction with internist.

Follow Up

Depends on the etiology, degree of subluxation or dislocation, and symptoms.

13.3 Pregnancy

ANTERIOR SEGMENT CHANGES

Transient loss of accommodation and increased corneal thickness, edema, and curvature. Refractive change results from hormonal status or a shift in fluid and tends to normalize after delivery. Defer prescribing new glasses until several weeks postpartum. Rigid contact lens wearers may experience contact lens intolerance due to corneal changes. Corneal refractive surgery is usually delayed at least 3 months after pregnancy or stopping nursing.

PREECLAMPSIA/ECLAMPSIA

A worldwide leading cause of maternal/fetal/neonatal morbidity and mortality. Occurs in 2% to 5% of pregnancies but may approach 10% in developing countries. Occurs after 20 weeks of gestation; most commonly in primigravida.

Symptoms

Headaches, blurred vision, photopsias, diplopia, and scotomas.

Signs

Systemic
• Preeclampsia or pregnancy-induced hypertension: Hypertension and proteinuria in previously normotensive women. Other signs include peripheral edema, liver failure, renal failure, and HELLP syndrome (hemolysis, elevated liver enzymes, and low platelet counts).
• Eclampsia: Preeclampsia with seizures.

Ocular. Focal retinal arteriolar spasm and narrowing, peripapillary or focal areas of retinal edema, retinal hemorrhages, exudates, nerve fiber layer infarcts, vitreous hemorrhage secondary to neovascularization, serous retinal detachments in 1% of preeclamptic and 10% of eclamptic patients, acute nonarteritic ischemic optic neuropathy, bilateral occipital lobe infarcts, and posterior cerebral edema (posterior reversible encephalopathy syndrome, or PRES). Differential diagnosis of PRES includes posterior circulation stroke, infectious cerebritis, coagulation disorder causing intracranial venous thrombosis, intracranial hemorrhage, occult tumor with secondary bleed, migraines, atypical seizure, or demyelination.

Natural History

1. Magnetic resonance imaging (MRI) abnormalities resolve 1 to 2 weeks after blood pressure control, at which time complete neurologic recovery can be expected.
2. Serous retinal detachments; often bilateral and bullous; resolve postpartum with residual pigment epithelial changes **(see Figure 13.3.1)**.
3. Retinal vascular changes also normalize postpartum.

Workup

1. Complete neuro-ophthalmologic assessment and fundus examination. Poor vision with brisk pupils without a RAPD suggests occipital lesions.
2. MRI findings in PRES include vasogenic edema in the parieto-occipital regions of both cerebral hemispheres involving subcortical white matter with possible extension into the gray-white junction, cortical surface, external capsule, and basal ganglia.
3. With typical presentation, further invasive studies are discouraged.
4. Systemic workup, including blood pressure monitoring and urinalysis, in conjunction with an obstetrics/gynecology specialist.

Treatment

1. Control blood pressure and electrolyte imbalances.
2. Prompt delivery ideal.

OCCLUSIVE VASCULAR DISORDERS

Pregnancy represents a hypercoagulable state possibly resulting in the development of retinal artery and vein occlusions, disseminated intravascular coagulopathy (DIC), and thrombotic thrombocytopenic purpura. Ocular DIC is characterized by widespread small-vessel thrombosis, particularly in the choroid, associated with hemorrhage, tissue necrosis, and serous retinal detachments.

13

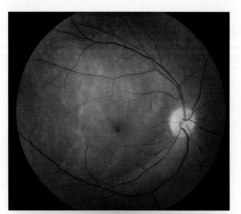

Figure 13.3.1 Serous macular detachment in a patient with preeclampsia.

MENINGIOMA OF PREGNANCY

Meningiomas may have a very aggressive growth pattern during pregnancy that is difficult to manage. They may regress postpartum but may reoccur during subsequent pregnancies.

NOTE: All pregnant women complaining of a headache should have their blood pressure, visual fields, and fundus checked (particularly looking for papilledema). MRI/MRV or lumbar puncture is often required if a hemorrhage or cortical venous thrombosis is suspected.

OTHER CONDITIONS INFLUENCED BY PREGNANCY

Multiple conditions can be impacted by pregnancy. See 3.20, PURTSCHER RETINOPATHY; 10.10, CAVERNOUS SINUS AND ASSOCIATED SYNDROMES (MULTIPLE OCULAR MOTOR NERVE PALSIES); 10.16, IDIOPATHIC INTRACRANIAL HYPERTENSION/PSEUDOTUMOR CEREBRI; 10.27, MIGRAINE; 11.12, DIABETIC RETINOPATHY; and 11.15, CENTRAL SEROUS CHORIORETINOPATHY. Remember that medications deserve special attention during pregnancy. In 2015, the Food and Drug Administration (FDA) replaced the former pregnancy risk letter categories (A, B, C, D, X) with the updated Pregnancy and Lactation Labeling Rule (PLLR). In the old system, ophthalmic drops used regularly for examination, such as proparacaine hydrochloride 0.5% for topical anesthesia and tropicamide 0.5% or 1% and phenylephrine hydrochloride 2.5% for dilation, were considered category C drugs in pregnancy. This means that their effects are unknown, as there are no adequate and well-controlled studies in humans. Many ophthalmic drops have not yet been reclassified using the new PLLR system. Physicians should familiarize themselves with the current labeling system, refer to drug package inserts, and/or consult with the patient's obstetrics and gynecology physician prior to use. If topical ophthalmic drops are utilized during pregnancy, patients should be advised to perform punctal occlusion with a finger for several minutes after drop instillation to decrease systemic absorption.

13.4 Lyme Disease

Symptoms

Ophthalmic manifestations include decreased vision, double vision, pain, photophobia, and facial weakness. Systemic complaints may include headache, malaise, fatigue, fever, chills, palpitations, or muscle/joint pains. A history of a tick bite within the previous few months may be elicited.

Signs

Ocular. Conjunctivitis (most common), episcleritis, exposure keratopathy (due to cranial nerve VII palsy), stromal keratitis, iritis, vitritis, choroiditis, optic neuritis or perineuritis, bilateral

optic nerve edema (frequently in children with disseminated disease), cranial nerve palsies, and idiopathic orbital inflammatory syndrome. See specific sections.

Critical Systemic. One or more flat, erythematous, or "bull's eye" skin lesions, which enlarge in all directions (erythema migrans); unilateral or bilateral facial nerve palsies; polyarticular migratory arthritis. May not be present at the time ocular signs develop.

Other Systemic. Meningitis, peripheral radiculoneuropathy, synovitis, joint effusions, and cardiac abnormalities.

Differential Diagnosis

- Syphilis: High-positive FTA-ABS titer may produce a low false-positive antibody titer against *Borrelia burgdorferi*. See 12.12, SYPHILIS.
- Others: Rickettsial infections, acute rheumatic fever, juvenile idiopathic arthritis, sarcoidosis, tuberculosis, herpes virus infections, etc.

Workup

1. History: Does patient live in endemic area? Prior tick bite, skin rash, facial nerve palsy, joint or muscle pains, flu-like illness? Meningeal symptoms? Prior positive Lyme antibody test?
2. Complete systemic, neurologic, and ocular examinations.
3. Two-step diagnosis with a screening assay and confirmatory Western blot for *B. burgdorferi*.

> **NOTE:** A positive interpretation is generally considered if 5 out of 10 IgG bands are positive or 2 out of 3 IgM bands are positive. IgM is helpful for acute presentation (<4 weeks). IgG antibodies may take 4 to 6 weeks to develop.

4. Serum RPR or VDRL and FTA-ABS or treponemal-specific assay. Consider serum angiotensin-converting enzyme, chest x-ray, and purified protein derivative and/or interferon-gamma release assay (e.g., QuantiFERON-TB Gold).
5. Consider lumbar puncture when meningitis is suspected or neurologic signs or symptoms are present.

Treatment

Early Lyme Disease (Including Lyme-Related Uveitis, Keratitis, or Facial Nerve Palsy)

1. Doxycycline 100 mg p.o. b.i.d. for 10 to 21 days.
2. In children, pregnant women, and others who cannot take doxycycline, substitute amoxicillin 500 mg p.o. t.i.d., cefuroxime axetil 500 mg p.o. b.i.d., clarithromycin 500 mg p.o. b.i.d., or azithromycin 500 mg p.o. daily.

Patients With Neuro-Ophthalmic Signs or Recurrent or Resistant Infection

1. Ceftriaxone 2 g i.v. daily for 2 to 3 weeks.
2. Alternatively, penicillin G, 20 million units i.v. daily for 2 to 3 weeks.

Follow Up

Every 1 to 3 days until improvement is demonstrated and then weekly until resolved.

13.5 Convergence Insufficiency

Symptoms

Eye discomfort or blurred vision from reading or near work. Most common in young adults but may be seen in older people.

Signs

Critical. An exophoria at near in the presence of poor near-fusional convergence amplitudes, a low accommodative convergence/accommodation (AC/A) ratio, and a remote near point of convergence.

Differential Diagnosis

- Uncorrected refractive error: Hyperopia or over-minused myopia.

- Accommodative insufficiency (AI): Often in prepresbyopia age range from uncorrected low hyperopia or over-minused myopia. While reading, a 4-diopter base-in prism placed in front of the eye blurs the print in AI but improves clarity in convergence insufficiency (CI). Rarely, adolescents may develop transient paresis of accommodation, requiring reading glasses or bifocals. This idiopathic condition resolves in several years.
- Convergence paralysis: Acute onset of exotropia and diplopia on near fixation only; normal adduction and accommodation. Usually results from a lesion in the corpora quadrigemina or the third cranial nerve nucleus and may be associated with Parinaud syndrome.

13

> **NOTE:** A diagnosis of convergence paralysis should prompt neuroimaging to rule out an intracranial lesion.

Etiology

- Fatigue or illness.
- Drugs (parasympatholytics).
- Uveitis.
- Glasses inducing a base-out prism effect.
- Postviral encephalitis.
- Traumatic brain injury.
- Parkinson disease.
- Idiopathic.

Workup

1. Manifest (without cycloplegia) refraction.
2. Determine the near point of convergence: Ask patient to focus on an accommodative target (e.g., a pencil eraser) and to state when double vision develops as you bring the target toward them; a normal near point of convergence is <8 cm.
3. Check for exodeviations or esodeviations at distance and near using the cover tests (see Appendix 3, COVER/UNCOVER AND ALTERNATE COVER TESTS) or the Maddox rod test.
4. Measure the patient's fusional ability at near. Have patient focus on an accommodative target at their reading distance. With a prism bar, slowly increase the amount of base-out prism in front of one eye until patient notes double vision (the break point) and then slowly reduce the amount of base-out prism until a single image is again noted (the recovery point). A low break point (10 to 15 prism diopters) or a low recovery point or both are consistent with CI.
5. Place a 4-diopter base-in prism in front of one eye while patient is reading. Determine

whether the print becomes clearer or more blurred to rule out AI.
6. Perform cycloplegic refraction after the previous tests.

> **NOTE:** These tests are performed with the patient's spectacle correction in place (if glasses are worn for near work).

Treatment

1. Correct any refractive error. Slightly undercorrect hyperopia and fully correct myopia.
2. Near-point exercises (e.g., pencil push-ups): The patient focuses on a pencil eraser while slowly moving it from arm's length toward the face. Concentrate on maintaining one image of the eraser, repeating the maneuver when diplopia manifests. Try to bring the pencil in closer each time while maintaining single vision. Repeat the exercise 15 times, five times per day.
3. Near-point exercises with base-out prisms (for patients whose near point of convergence is satisfactory or for those who have mastered pencil push-ups without a prism): The patient performs pencil push-ups as described previously, while holding a 6-diopter base-out prism in front of one eye.
4. Encourage good lighting and relaxation time between periods of close work.
5. For older patients, or those whose condition shows no improvement despite near-point exercises, reading glasses with base-in prism can be useful.
6. Consider referral to an orthoptist for vision therapy, which has been shown to be more effective in reducing symptoms and signs of CI in children than pencil push-ups.

Follow Up

Nonurgent. Patients are reexamined in 1 month.

13.6 Accommodative Spasm

Symptoms

Bilateral blurred distance vision, fluctuating vision, blurred vision when shifting gaze from near to far, headache, and eye strain while reading. Often seen in teenagers under stress. Symptoms may occur after prolonged and intense periods of near work.

Signs

Critical. Cycloplegic refraction reveals substantially less myopia (or more hyperopia) than was originally found when the refraction was performed without cycloplegia (manifest refraction). Manifest myopia may be as high as

10 diopters. Spasm of the near reflex is associated with excess accommodation, excess convergence, and miosis and is in the differential diagnosis of sixth cranial nerve palsy (see 10.8 ISOLATED SIXTH CRANIAL NERVE PALSY).

Other. Abnormally close near point of focus, miosis, and a normal amplitude of accommodation that may appear low.

Etiology

- Inability to relax the ciliary muscles. Involuntary and associated with stressful situations or functional neuroses.
- Fatigue.
- Prolonged reading may precipitate episodes.

Differential Diagnosis

- Uncorrected hyperopia: Increased plus power accepted during manifest refraction.
- Other causes of pseudomyopia: Hyperglycemia, medication induced (e.g., sulfa drugs and anticholinesterase medications), anterior displacement of the lens–iris diaphragm.
- Manifestation of iridocyclitis.

Workup

1. Complete ophthalmic examination. The manifest refraction may be highly variable, but it is important to determine the least amount of minus power or the most amount of plus power that provides clear distance vision.
2. Cycloplegic refraction.

Treatment

1. True refractive errors should be corrected. If a significant amount of esophoria at near is present, additional plus power (e.g., +2.50 diopters) in reading glasses or bifocal form may be helpful.
2. Counseling patient and parents to provide a more relaxed atmosphere and avoid stressful situations.
3. Cycloplegics have been used to break the spasm, but are rarely needed except in resistant cases.

Follow Up

Reevaluate in several weeks.

13.7 Erythema Multiforme, Stevens–Johnson Syndrome, and Toxic Epidermal Necrolysis

Erythema multiforme (EM) is distinct from Stevens–Johnson syndrome (SJS) and toxic epidermal necrolysis (TEN). SJS and TEN are considered variants along the same disease spectrum. All three conditions cause mucocutaneous lesions that can involve the eye.

Symptoms

Flu-like prodrome (fever, malaise, arthralgia, dysphagia), red eyes, eye pain/burning, and skin rash.

Signs

Systemic. Classic "target" lesions (central red macule/papule surrounded by concentric circles of a pale/white intermediate zone and outer erythematous rim), atypical "target" lesions, dusky macules, bullous lesions, tender erythematous mucocutaneous lesions involving oral (e.g., ulcerative stomatitis; hemorrhagic lip crusting), GI, respiratory, or genital tracts.

Ocular

- Acute phase: Mucopurulent or pseudomembranous conjunctivitis; episcleritis; iritis; corneal punctate erosions, epithelial defects, and ulcers; eyelid margin ulceration.
- Late complications: Severe dry eye; trichiasis; conjunctival scarring, symblepharon, and ankyloblepharon; eyelid deformities (e.g., entropion); tear deficiency; corneal neovascularization, ulceration, perforation, or scarring.

Types

1. EM minor: Mainly skin involvement; absent or mild mucosal involvement; no systemic symptoms.
2. EM major: Skin involvement with moderate-to-severe mucosal involvement; usually has systemic symptoms.

13

SJS and TEN have severe mucosal involvement and are defined by the body surface area (BSA) of skin detachment.

1. SJS: <10% BSA epidermal detachment.
2. SJS–TEN overlap: 10% to 30% BSA epidermal detachment.
3. TEN: >30% BSA epidermal detachment; most severe form with extensive vesiculobullous eruptions and epidermal sloughing. More common in children and immunosuppressed patients.

Etiology

An immune complex–mediated hypersensitivity reaction precipitated by many agents.

Erythema Multiforme

- Infectious agents (most common): herpes simplex virus, *Mycoplasma pneumoniae*, and adenovirus.
- Rarely drug exposure.

Stevens–Johnson Syndrome and Toxic Epidermal Necrolysis

- Drug exposure (most common): Antibiotics (sulfonamides, penicillins, cephalosporins), anticonvulsants (carbamazepine, phenytoin, barbiturates), NSAIDs (oxicam type), allopurinol, corticosteroids, and others. Highest risk of reaction occurs during the first 2 months of treatment.
- Allergy and autoimmune diseases.
- Genetics: HLA-B*15:02 and carbamazepine in Asian populations; HLA-B*58:01 and allopurinol.
- Radiation therapy.
- Malignancy.
- Idiopathic (50% of cases).

Workup

1. History: Attempt to determine the precipitating factor (e.g., drug exposure, recent illness).
2. Slit lamp examination, including eyelid eversion with examination of the fornices.
3. Conjunctival or corneal cultures if infection is suspected. See Appendix 8, CORNEAL CULTURE PROCEDURE.
4. Consult internal medicine for a systemic workup and dermatology for a full-body examination and possible skin biopsy which may aid in the diagnosis.

Treatment

EM: Supportive Care; Treat Underlying Infection if Identified.

SJS, TEN

1. Hospitalization, often requiring burn unit if available.
2. Remove (e.g., drug) or treat (e.g., infection) the inciting factor.
3. Supportive care is the mainstay of therapy.
4. Comanagement with internal medicine and dermatology.

Ocular

1. Ocular surface inflammation: Topical steroid drops (e.g., prednisolone acetate 1% or difluprednate 0.05% four to eight times per day).
2. Tear deficiency: Aggressive lubrication with preservative-free artificial tears, gels, and ointments. Topical cyclosporine 0.05% to 2%, punctal occlusion, moisture chambers, or tarsorrhaphy.
3. Iritis: Topical steroid drops (e.g., prednisolone acetate 1% or difluprednate 0.05% four to eight times per day) and cycloplegia (e.g., atropine 1% b.i.d.).
4. Infections: Treat as outlined in **4.11,** BACTERIAL KERATITIS.
5. Conjunctival and/or eyelid margin defects: Daily pseudomembrane peel with moistened cotton swab. Symblepharon lysis and possible amniotic membrane graft (e.g., Prokera, AmnioGraft) to minimized scarring. In severe cases, consider suturing amniotic membrane over the eyelid margin, palpebral conjunctiva, and into the fornix during the hyperacute phase (<72 hours after disease onset). When epithelial defects of the conjunctiva, eyelid margin, and/or cornea are present, prophylactic topical antibiotics should also be utilized to prevent infection.
6. Additional potential treatments:
   - Systemic or topical vitamin A.
   - Intravenous immunoglobulin.

Systemic. Manage by burn unit protocol, including hydration, wound care, and systemic antibiotics.

Follow Up

1. During hospitalization: Follow daily, with infection and IOP surveillance.
2. Outpatient: Weekly follow ups initially, watching for long-term ocular complications.
   - Topical steroids and antibiotics are maintained for 48 hours after resolution and are then tapered.
   - If there is severe conjunctival scarring, artificial tears and lubricating ointment may need to be maintained indefinitely.
3. Possible late surgical interventions.
   - Trichiasis: Repeated epilation, electrolysis, cryotherapy, or surgical repair.
   - Entropion repair with buccal mucosal grafts.

- Penetrating keratoplasty: Poor prognosis even when combined with limbal stem cell or amniotic membrane transplantation because of underlying deficiencies, such as dry eyes and limbal stem cell abnormality.
- Permanent keratoprosthesis (guarded prognosis).

Prognosis

EM is typically self-limited but can recur. SJS and TEN are potentially fatal with average reported mortality rates of 1% to 5% in SJS and up to 25% to 35% in TEN. Ocular prognosis depends on the severity of conjunctival damage. Early amniotic membrane grafting covering the palpebral and bulbar conjunctival surfaces when indicated greatly improves the prognosis.

13.8 Vitamin A Deficiency

(See **Table 13.8.1.**)

Symptoms

Night blindness (earliest and most common manifestation), dry eyes, ocular pain, and severe vision loss.

Signs

Ocular. Bitôt spots (triangular, perilimbal, gray, foamy plaques of keratinized conjunctival debris); decreased tear break-up time; bilateral conjunctival and corneal dryness; corneal epithelial defects, sterile or infectious ulceration (often peripheral with a punched-out appearance), perforation, or scarring; keratomalacia (often preceded by a gastrointestinal, respiratory, or measles infection); fundus abnormalities (yellow or white peripheral retinal dots representing focal retinal pigment epithelium [RPE] defects).

Systemic. Growth retardation in children; dry, hyperkeratotic skin; increased susceptibility to infections.

Differential Diagnosis

See 4.3, DRY EYE SYNDROME and 11.28, RETINITIS PIGMENTOSA AND INHERITED CHORIORETINAL DYSTROPHIES.

Etiology

- Primary: Dietary deficiency or chronic alcoholism (relatively uncommon in developed countries). Beyond 6 months postpartum, breast milk in vitamin A–deficient mothers is unlikely to sufficiently maintain vitamin A stores in nursing infants.
- Secondary: Lipid malabsorption (e.g., cystic fibrosis, chronic pancreatitis, inflammatory bowel disease, celiac sprue, postgastrectomy or postintestinal bypass surgery, chronic liver disease, abetalipoproteinemia [Bassen–Kornzweig syndrome]).

Workup

1. History: Malnutrition? Poor diet? Gastrointestinal or liver disease? Previous gastrointestinal surgery? Measles?
2. Complete ophthalmic examination, including careful inspection of eyelid margins and inferior fornices.
3. A positive response to treatment is a simple, cost-effective way to confirm the diagnosis.
4. Consider serum vitamin A level before treatment is initiated. Keep in mind that other vitamin deficiencies may coexist and may warrant testing.
5. Consider impression cytology of the conjunctiva, looking for decreased goblet cell density.
6. Consider dark adaptation studies and electroretinogram (may be more sensitive than the serum vitamin A level).
7. Corneal cultures if infection suspected. See Appendix 8, CORNEAL CULTURE PROCEDURE.

13

TABLE 13.8.1 World Health Organization Classification of Vitamin A Deficiency

XN	Night Blindness
X1A	Conjunctival xerosis
X1B	Bitôt spot
X2	Corneal xerosis
X3A	Corneal ulceration or keratomalacia with less than one-third corneal involvement
X3B	Corneal ulceration or keratomalacia with one-third or more corneal involvement
XS	Corneal scar
XF	Xerophthalmia fundus

Treatment

1. Immediate vitamin A replacement therapy orally (preferred) or intramuscularly in the following WHO recommended dosages for clinical xerophthalmia:
   - Children <12 months: 100,000 IU daily for 2 days, repeat in 2 weeks.
   - Adults and children >12 months: 200,000 IU daily for 2 days, repeat in 2 weeks.
   - Women of childbearing age (reduce dose due to possible teratogenic effects): Night blindness or Bitôt spots only, 10,000 IU daily for 2 weeks or 25,000 IU weekly for 4 weeks; any corneal lesions, give full adult dose as above.
2. Intensive ocular lubrication with preservative-free artificial tears every 15 to 60 minutes and preservative-free artificial tear ointment q.h.s.
3. Treat malnutrition/underlying disease if present.
4. Consider supplementing the patient's diet with zinc and vitamin A.
5. Consider corneal surgery (e.g., penetrating keratoplasty or keratoprosthesis) for corneal scars in eyes with potentially good vision.
6. Prophylaxis in endemic regions:
   - Infants: Consider 50,000 IU.
   - 6 to 12 months: 100,000 IU q4–6 months.
   - Children >12 months: 200,000 IU q4–6 months.
   - Retinyl palmitate has been used to fortify sugars in developing countries.

Follow Up

Determined by the clinical presentation and response to treatment, ranges from hospitalization to daily or weekly follow up.

13.9 Albinism

Symptoms

Decreased vision. Photosensitivity in some patients.

> **NOTE:** Patients with albinism show a wide range of visual acuities, refractive errors, nystagmus, and amblyopia.

Signs

Best corrected visual acuity ranging from 20/40 to 20/400. May have refractive error, strabismus, reduced stereopsis, nystagmus, amblyopia secondary to strabismus or anisometropia, iris transillumination defects, fundus hypopigmentation with highly visible choroidal vasculature, and foveal hypoplasia with or without failure of the retinal vessels to properly surround the fovea.

Associated Disorders

- Hermansky–Pudlak syndrome: An autosomal recessive disorder characterized by platelet dysfunction leading to easy bruising and bleeding; some individuals also have pulmonary fibrosis or colitis. More common in patients of Puerto Rican and Swiss descent. Multiple genes.

- Chédiak–Higashi syndrome: An autosomal recessive disorder affecting white blood cell function, resulting in an increased susceptibility to infections and a predisposition for lymphoma-like malignancy. *LYST* gene on chromosome 1q42.1–q42.2.
- Multiple other syndromes, some involving deafness or immunodeficiency.

Types

1. Oculocutaneous albinism: Usually autosomal recessive with hypopigmentation of the hair, skin, and eye.
   - Mutations in tyrosinase gene (OCA1): Include severe, moderate, and temperature sensitive phenotypes.
   - Mutations in the P gene (OCA2): Varying degrees of pigmentation.
2. Ocular albinism: Only ocular hypopigmentation is readily apparent. Usually X-linked recessive. Female carriers may have partial iris transillumination, patches of skin hypopigmentation, and mottling of the midperipheral and peripheral retinal pigmentation (mudsplattered fundus).

Workup

1. History: Easy bruising? Frequent nosebleeds? Prolonged bleeding after dental work? Symptoms of pulmonary fibrosis and/or colitis? Frequent infections? Difficulty hearing? Family history? Puerto Rican or Swiss descent?

2. External examination (including hair and skin color).
3. Complete ocular examination of patient and family members.
4. Check platelet aggregation studies and ultrastructure (especially preoperatively) and polymorphonuclear leukocyte function as indicated based on associated symptoms. Consult primary care or hematology as needed.
5. Ocular genetics consultation.

Treatment

There is currently no effective treatment for albinism, but the following may be helpful:

1. Treating amblyopia, strabismus, and refractive error may reduce nystagmus, if present. See 8.7, AMBLYOPIA.
2. Low vision referral when indicated.
3. Eye muscle surgery may be considered for patients with significant strabismus or an abnormal head position due to nystagmus. However, patients with albinism and strabismus rarely achieve binocularity after surgical correction. Surgery to reduce nystagmus may also have benefits.
4. Genetic counseling.
5. Advise ultraviolet sun protection.
6. Hematology consultation as indicated. Patients with Hermansky–Pudlak syndrome may require platelet transfusions before surgery.

13.10 Wilson Disease

13

Symptoms

Ocular complaints are rare. Patients experience symptoms of cirrhosis, neurologic disorders, psychiatric problems, or renal disease. Onset typically between 5 and 40 years of age.

Signs

Critical. Kayser–Fleischer ring: 1- to 3-mm, brown, yellow, green, or reddish band that represents copper deposition in the peripheral Descemet membrane **(see Figure 13.10.1).** Present in 50% to 60% of patients with isolated hepatic involvement and more than 90% of

patients with neurologic manifestations. First appears superiorly (may only be visible on gonioscopy) and eventually forms a ring involving the entire corneal periphery extending to the limbus. Anterior-segment optical coherence tomography (OCT) may be useful in detecting early Kayser–Fleischer rings that are not readily detected on slit lamp examination; appears as linear hyperreflective material on Descemet membrane.

Other. "Sunflower" cataract: Ring or stellate yellow, brown, or reddish anterior capsule opacity due to copper deposition under the lens capsule.

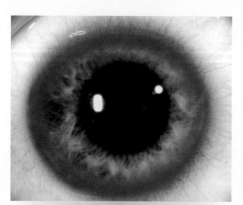

Figure 13.10.1 Kayser–Fleischer ring in Wilson disease.

Differential Diagnosis

- Kayser–Fleischer-like ring: Rarely can be seen in primary biliary cirrhosis, chronic active hepatitis, progressive intrahepatic cholestasis, and multiple myeloma. These patients usually have a normal serum ceruloplasmin level.

- Arcus senilis: White, gray, or blue ring-shaped opacification in peripheral corneal due to lipid deposition in stroma, initially appears inferiorly and superiorly before extending. A 1-mm zone of clear cornea separates the edge of the arcus from the limbus. Check a fasting lipid profile if observed in patients <40 years.

- Chalcosis: Copper deposition in basement membranes, including Descemet membrane, secondary to copper-containing intraocular foreign body. Alloys containing more than 85% copper may induce severe inflammation, while those with lower amounts may cause retinal toxicity. Corneal deposition is more diffuse.

Etiology

Autosomal recessive inborn error of copper metabolism that results in impaired copper

excretion and toxic accumulation of copper in multiple organ systems (e.g., liver, brain, cornea, kidney). *ATP7B* gene on chromosome 13.

Workup

1. Slit lamp examination: Deposition at Descemet membrane is apparent with a narrow slit beam.
2. Gonioscopy if the Kayser–Fleischer ring is not evident on slit lamp examination.
3. Check serum copper and ceruloplasmin levels, urine copper level (low serum copper and ceruloplasmin and elevated urine copper levels with ocular findings are diagnostic).
4. Referral to appropriate systemic specialists.

Treatment

1. Lifelong systemic therapy (e.g., zinc salts, D-penicillamine, trientine) is instituted by the appropriate systemic specialist. Liver transplantation may be required for fulminant hepatic failure or disease progression after medical therapy.
2. Ocular manifestations usually require no specific treatment.

Follow Up

1. Systemic therapy and monitoring.
2. Successful treatment should lead to resorption of the corneal copper deposition and clearing of the Kayser–Fleischer ring, although residual peripheral corneal changes may remain. This change can be used to monitor treatment response. Reappearance of ring may suggest noncompliance with treatment.
3. Consider referral of family members for genetic testing for early detection and prevention.

13.11 Hypotony Syndrome

Definition

Decreased visual function and other ocular symptoms related to low IOP.

Symptoms

Mild-to-severe pain, reduced vision, or may be asymptomatic. Patient with recent glaucoma filtering surgery may complain of "excessive tearing."

Signs

Critical. Low IOP, usually ≤5 mm Hg, but may occur with an IOP as high as 10 mm Hg.

Other. Corneal edema and folds, corneal decompensation, aqueous cell and flare, shallow or flat anterior chamber, retinal edema, hypotony maculopathy, chorioretinal folds, serous choroidal detachment, suprachoroidal hemorrhage, optic disc swelling, and retinal vascular tortuosity.

Etiology

- Postsurgical: Wound leak, overfiltering/bleb leak (more common with use of antimetabolites during surgery) or glaucoma drainage device, cyclodialysis cleft (disinsertion of the ciliary body from the sclera at the scleral spur), scleral perforation (e.g., from a superior rectus bridle suture or retrobulbar injection), iridocyclitis, retinal or choroidal detachment, etc.
- Posttraumatic: Same causes as postsurgical.
- Rhegmatogenous retinal detachment.
- Pharmacologic: Usually from an oral carbonic anhydrase inhibitor in combination with a topical beta-blocker. Also associated with cidofovir.
- Systemic (bilateral hypotony): Conditions that cause blood hypertonicity (e.g., dehydration, uremia, hyperglycemia), myotonic dystrophy, pregnancy, etc. Rare.
- Vascular occlusive disease (e.g., ocular ischemic syndrome, giant cell arteritis, central retinal vein or artery occlusion): Usually mild hypotony due to decreased aqueous humor production from ciliary body hypoperfusion. Rare.
- Uveitis: Secondary to ciliary body shutdown.

Workup

1. History: Recent ocular surgery or trauma? Systemic symptoms (nausea, vomiting, drowsiness, polyuria)? History of renal disease, diabetes, or myotonic dystrophy? Medications?
2. Complete ocular examination, including slit lamp evaluation of surgical or traumatic ocular wounds, IOP check, grading of anterior chamber depth, gonioscopy to rule out a cyclodialysis cleft, evaluation of the macula for folds, and indirect ophthalmoscopy to rule out retinal or choroidal detachment.
3. Seidel test (with or without gentle pressure) to rule out a wound leak. See Appendix 5, SEIDEL TEST TO DETECT A WOUND LEAK.
4. OCT of the macula to evaluate for macular folds (evidenced by rippled appearance of the RPE).

NOTE: A wound leak may drain under the conjunctiva, producing an inadvertent filtering bleb. May be seen in old extracapsular cataract extraction wounds, which are large and may not completely close. Seidel test will then be negative.

5. B-scan US when the fundus cannot be seen clinically. Consider US biomicroscopy or anterior segment OCT to aid in anterior chamber assessment, especially evaluation for cyclodialysis cleft. Macular OCT may be used for diagnosis confirmation and therapeutic monitoring.
6. Systemic workup in bilateral cases, including basic metabolic panel.

Treatment

Repair of the underlying disorder may be needed if symptoms are significant or progressive. Low IOP, even as low as 2 mm Hg, may not cause problems or symptoms and may be observed.

Wound Leak

1. Large wound leaks: Suture the wound closed.
2. Small wound leaks: Can be sutured closed or can be patched with a pressure dressing or bandage soft contact lens and an antibiotic ointment (e.g., erythromycin) for one night to allow the wound to close spontaneously. Occasionally, cyanoacrylate glue is applied to small wound leaks and covered with a bandage contact lens. Aqueous suppressants are often given concurrently to reduce aqueous flow through the wound.
3. Wound leaks under a conjunctival flap: Repair required only if vision affected or for secondary ocular complication such as a flat anterior chamber or infection.

Shallow Anterior Chamber

If the anterior chamber is very shallow or flat, start a topical cycloplegic (e.g., cyclopentolate 1% t.i.d. or atropine 1% daily) and topical steroid (e.g., prednisolone acetate 1% or difluprednate 0.05% q2h), as long as no infectious process is suspected. This will rotate the iris-lens complex posteriorly and can deepen the chamber to prevent corneal endothelial damage.

Overfiltering Bleb

Compression with a large contact lens can at times reduce bleb exuberance. Surgical repair in the operating room may be required with compression sutures (transconjunctivally or directly over the scleral flap), placement of a corneal or scleral patch graft over a shrunken scleral flap, or removal of the aqueous shunt device from the anterior chamber.

Cyclodialysis Cleft

Reattach the ciliary body to the sclera by chronic atropine therapy, diathermy, suturing, cryotherapy,

13

laser photocoagulation, or external plombage. See 3.7, IRIDODIALYSIS/CYCLODIALYSIS.

Scleral Perforation

The site may be closed by suturing or cryotherapy.

Iridocyclitis

Topical steroid (e.g., prednisolone acetate 1% or difluprednate 0.05% q1–6h) and a topical cycloplegic (e.g., cyclopentolate 1% t.i.d.). See 12.1, ANTERIOR UVEITIS (IRITIS/IRIDOCYCLITIS).

Retinal Detachment

Surgical repair. See 11.3, RETINAL DETACHMENT.

Choroidal Detachment

See 11.27, CHOROIDAL EFFUSION/DETACHMENT. Surgical drainage of the choroidal effusion along with reformation of the eye and anterior chamber is indicated for any of the following:

1. Retinal apposition ("kissing" choroidal detachments).
2. Lens–corneal touch (needs emergent attention).
3. A flat or persistently shallow anterior chamber accompanied by a failing filtering bleb or an inflamed eye.

4. Corneal decompensation.

If these findings are not present, choroidal effusion can be managed conservatively with a topical cycloplegic and topical steroids for a period of time.

Pharmacologic

Reduce or discontinue the IOP-reducing medications.

Systemic Disorder

Refer to an internist.

> **NOTE:** In myotonic dystrophy, the hypotony is rarely severe enough to produce deleterious effects, and treatment of hypotony, from an ocular standpoint, is unnecessary.

Follow Up

If vision is good, the anterior chamber is well formed, and there is no wound leak, retinal detachment, or kissing choroidal detachments, then the low IOP poses no immediate problem, and treatment and follow up are not urgent. Fixed retinal folds in the macula may develop from long-standing hypotony.

13.12 Blind, Painful Eye

Patients with a nonseeing eye and unsalvageable vision can experience mild-to-severe ocular pain for a variety of reasons.

Causes of Pain

- Corneal decompensation: Fluorescein-staining defect(s) on slit lamp examination. Pain improves with topical anesthetic.
- Uveitis: Anterior chamber or vitreous white blood cells. Corneal opacification may obscure the view of an inflammatory reaction.
- Glaucoma with elevated IOP.
- Hypotony: Ciliary body shutdown, retinal detachment, choroidal detachment, and ciliary body detachment. See 13.11, HYPOTONY SYNDROME.

Workup

1. History: Determine the etiology and duration of blindness.

2. Ocular examination: Stain the cornea with fluorescein to detect epithelial defects and measure IOP. Tonopen measurements may be required if the corneal surface is irregular. If the cornea is clear, look for neovascularization of the iris and angle by gonioscopy, and inspect the anterior chamber for cell and flare. Attempt a dilated fundus examination to rule out an intraocular tumor or retinal detachment.
3. When the fundus cannot be adequately visualized, B-scan US of the posterior segment is required to rule out an intraocular tumor, retinal, choroidal, or ciliary body detachment.

Treatment

1. Sterile corneal decompensation (if it appears infected, see 4.11, BACTERIAL KERATITIS).
   - Antibiotic or lubricating ointment (e.g., erythromycin or bacitracin–polymyxin B)

daily to q.i.d. to the eye for weeks to months (or even permanently). Can also add cycloplegic agent (e.g., atropine 1%) for additional comfort. Consider nightly taping of eyelids.

- Consider a tarsorrhaphy, amniotic membrane graft, or Gunderson conjunctival flap in refractory cases.

2. Uveitis.
   - Cycloplegia (e.g., atropine 1% b.i.d.).
   - Topical steroid (e.g., prednisolone acetate 1% q1–6h). See 12.1, ANTERIOR UVEITIS (IRITIS/IRIDOCYCLITIS).
   - Endophthalmitis should be ruled out if severe uveitis or a hypopyon is present.

3. Markedly increased IOP.
   - Topical beta-blocker (e.g., timolol 0.5% daily or b.i.d.) with or without an adrenergic agonist (e.g., brimonidine 0.1%, 0.15%, or 0.2% b.i.d. to t.i.d.). Topical carbonic anhydrase inhibitors (e.g., dorzolamide 2% t.i.d.) are effective, but potential systemic side effects may not warrant their use for pain relief; miotics and prostaglandin analogs may increase ocular irritation.
   - If the IOP remains markedly increased and is thought to be responsible for the pain, a cyclodestructive procedure (e.g., diode laser cyclophotocoagulation) may be attempted. The potential for sympathetic ophthalmia must be considered.
   - If pain persists despite the previously described treatment, a retrobulbar alcohol block may be given.

NOTE: Technique: 2 to 3 mL of lidocaine is administered in the retrobulbar region. The needle is then held in place while the syringe of lidocaine is replaced with a 1-mL syringe containing 95% to 100% alcohol (some physicians use 50% alcohol). The contents of the alcohol syringe are then injected into the retrobulbar space through the needle. The syringes are again switched, so a small amount of lidocaine can rinse out the remaining alcohol. The retrobulbar needle is then withdrawn. Patients are warned that

transient eyelid droop or swelling, limitation of eye movement, or anesthesia may result. Retrobulbar chlorpromazine (25 to 50 mg, using 25 mg/mL) or phenol can also be used. See Appendix 10, TECHNIQUE FOR RETROBULBAR/SUBTENON/SUBCONJUNCTIVAL INJECTIONS.

4. Hypotony.
   - Resolve causes of hypotony (e.g., repair wound leak, treat uveitis or ciliochoroidal detachment). If retinal detachment is found, repair may resolve hypotony.

5. Cause of pain unknown.
   - Cycloplegia (e.g., atropine 1% t.i.d.).
   - Topical steroid (e.g., prednisolone acetate 1% q1–6h).
   - Retrobulbar injections of neurolytic agents can be considered. See Appendix 10, TECHNIQUE FOR RETROBULBAR/SUBTENON/SUBCONJUNCTIVAL INJECTIONS.

6. Ocular pain refractory to topical medication therapy and/or retrobulbar injections.
   - Consider enucleation or evisceration of the eye. Evisceration should not be performed if intraocular malignancy is suspected. Enucleation does not relieve facial paresthesias.
   - Consider postinfectious or postsurgical neuralgia, in which case referral to pain management is indicated.

NOTE: Monocular patients should wear protective eye wear (e.g., polycarbonate lenses) at all times to prevent injury to the contralateral eye.

13

Follow Up

Depends on the degree of pain and clinical examination. Once the pain resolves, patients are reexamined every 6 to 12 months. B-scan US should be performed periodically (typically every 3 years) to rule out an intraocular tumor when the posterior pole cannot be visualized.

13.13 Phakomatoses

NEUROFIBROMATOSIS TYPE 1 (VON RECKLINGHAUSEN SYNDROME)

Criteria for Diagnosis

(See **Table 13.13.1.**)

> 📝 **NOTE:** Lisch nodules (light brown elevated lesions on darker iris or brown lesions on blue/hazel iris) occur at a rate of approximately age in years x 10% (e.g. 50% at 5 years old). Approximately 98% of affected individuals have Lisch nodules after puberty.

Signs

(See Figures 13.13.1 and 13.13.2.)

Ocular. Lisch nodules, visual pathway glioma (12% to 15%), prominent corneal nerves, multifocal choroidal nevi, choroidal hamartoma (detectable by near-infrared high-frequency OCT), cranial nerve lesions (e.g., superior oblique palsy), glaucoma (usually associated with plexiform neuromas of the ipsilateral upper eyelid), pulsating proptosis secondary to absence of the greater wing of the sphenoid bone, ectropion uveae, and iris melanosis.

Systemic. (See **Table 13.13.1.**)
Developmental delay, seizures, scoliosis, leukemia, juvenile xanthogranuloma, aortic and arteriovascular anomalies, and other cancers.

Inheritance

Autosomal dominant with variable expression: chromosome 17q11.2.

Workup

1. Family history. Examination of parents for Lisch nodules. If child affected, consider further systemic and ocular evaluation.
2. MRI of the brain and orbits only if indicated by a sign or symptom, including ophthalmic findings of optic nerve dysfunction, optic nerve pallor/swelling/shunt vessels, or proptosis.
3. Others: As recommended by nonophthalmic providers.

Treatment/Follow Up

Dependent upon the findings. Every year up to 6 years old when risk of visual pathway glioma diminishes. Every 2 years thereafter. More frequent follow up as needed for patients with gliomas or other signs of ophthalmic or orbital involvement, especially if risk factors for amblyopia (e.g., ptosis from plexiform neurofibroma).

NEUROFIBROMATOSIS TYPE 2

Criteria for Diagnosis

(See **Table 13.13.1.**)

TABLE 13.13.1 Diagnostic Criteria for Neurofibromatosis 1 and 2

Neurofibromatosis 1	Neurofibromatosis 2
At least two of the following:	Either A or B:

1. At least six café au lait spots
  1. 5-mm greatest diameter prepubertal or
  2. 15-mm postpubertal
2. Neurofibromas
  1. One plexiform neurofibroma or
  2. At least two of any other type
3. Axillary/groin freckling
4. Visual pathway glioma
5. At least two Lisch nodules
6. Distinctive osseous dysplasia (sphenoid wing or tibial)
7. Affected first-degree relative
	A. Bilateral acoustic neuromas (by computed tomography or magnetic resonance imaging) or
	B. Affected first-degree relative and
	  1. Unilateral acoustic neuroma or
	  2. At least two of the following:
	    Neurofibroma
	    Meningioma
	    Glioma
	    Schwannoma
	    Juvenile posterior subcapsular cataract

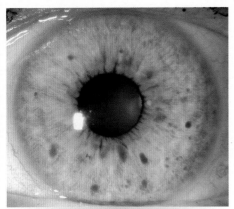

Figure 13.13.1 Lisch nodules.

Signs

Ocular. Juvenile-onset posterior subcapsular cataracts, combined hamartoma of the RPE, epiretinal membrane, optic nerve sheath meningioma, and cranial nerve palsies.

Systemic.

Inheritance

Autosomal dominant with variable expression: chromosome 22q12.2.

Workup

1. Family history. If child affected, consider further systemic and ocular evaluation.
2. Audiology and gadolinium-enhanced MRI of the brain and auditory canals should be performed.
3. OCT of epiretinal membrane.
4. Others: As indicated by symptoms and signs.

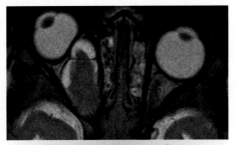

Figure 13.13.2 Optic nerve glioma.

Treatment/Follow Up

Dependent upon the findings.

STURGE–WEBER SYNDROME (LEPTOMENINGEAL ANGIOMATOSIS)

Signs

(See Figure 13.13.3.)

Ocular. Diffuse choroidal hemangioma ("tomato catsup" fundus with uniform reddish background obscuring choroidal vasculature), glaucoma (increased risk with upper eyelid or combined upper and lower eyelid port-wine birthmark or choroidal hemangioma), iris heterochromia, blood in Schlemm canal seen on gonioscopy, and secondary serous retinal detachment. Ocular signs are all ipsilateral to port-wine birthmark.

Systemic. Unilateral or bilateral (10%) port-wine birthmark (trigeminal nerve distribution patterns), developmental delay, seizures, ipsilateral facial hemihypertrophy, leptomeningeal angiomatosis, and cerebral calcifications.

Inheritance

Somatic mutation in *GNAQ*, extremely rare to transmit.

Workup

Complete general and ophthalmic examination with specific screenings for glaucoma and amblyopia. Periodic OCT macula if choroidal hemangioma present. Neuroimaging of the brain (CT or MRI).

Treatment

1. Treat glaucoma if present. Early onset (<4 years old) usually caused by goniodysgenesis (see 8.11, CONGENITAL/INFANTILE GLAUCOMA). Later onset usually caused by increased episcleral venous pressure. Presence of leptomeningeal angiomatosis is a relative contraindication to use of topical alpha-agonists.
2. Consider treating serous retinal detachment from underlying choroidal hemangioma. Laser photocoagulation success rate is low, but photodynamic therapy can be successful for smaller, circumscribed tumors. Low-dose radiotherapy using a plaque is often successful in leading to resolution of subretinal fluid.

13

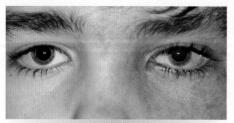

Figure 13.13.3 Nevus flammeus.

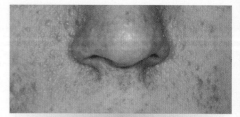

Figure 13.13.5 Adenoma sebaceum.

Follow Up

Every 6 months or sooner for glaucoma screening and yearly for retinal examination with OCT.

TUBEROUS SCLEROSIS COMPLEX (BOURNEVILLE SYNDROME)

Signs

(See Figures 13.13.4 and 13.13.5.)

Ocular. Astrocytic hamartoma of the retina or optic disc (a white, semitransparent, or mulberry-appearing tumor in the superficial retina that may undergo calcification with age; no prominent feeder vessels; no associated retinal detachment; often multifocal and bilateral) and punched-out chorioretinal depigmentation.

Systemic. Adenoma sebaceum (yellow–red angiofibromas in a butterfly distribution on the upper cheeks), seizures, periventricular hamartomas, developmental delay, subungual angiofibromas, shagreen patches, ash leaf spots (hypopigmented skin lesions that illuminate

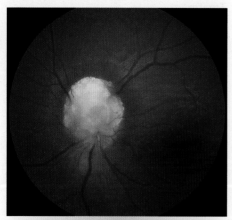

Figure 13.13.4 Retinal astrocytic hamartoma.

with Wood lamp); renal cell carcinoma or angiomyolipoma; intracardiac rhabdomyoma or lipoma; pleural cysts and possible spontaneous pneumothorax; cystic bone lesions; and hamartomas of the liver, thyroid, pancreas, or testes.

Differential Diagnosis of Astrocytic Hamartoma

Retinoblastoma. See 8.1, LEUKOCORIA.

Inheritance

Autosomal dominant with variable expression: *TSC1* gene on chromosome 9q34 or *TSC2* gene on chromosome 16p13.

Workup

1. Family history. Parents of affected child should first be evaluated by ocular and systemic examination/testing. If one parent is positive, then consider examination and testing of siblings of affected patient.
2. MRI of the brain and additional systemic testing as indicated by symptoms and signs or screening protocol.

Treatment/Follow Up

Retinal astrocytomas usually require no treatment. Ophthalmic examination every 6 months to a 1 year after lesion is identified.

VON HIPPEL–LINDAU SYNDROME

Signs

(See Figure 13.13.6.)

Ocular. Retinal capillary hemangioma/hemangioblastoma (small, round, orange–red tumor with a prominent dilated feeding artery and draining vein), sometimes associated with

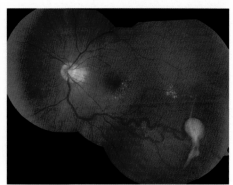

Figure 13.13.6 Retinal capillary hemangioma/ hemangioblastoma.

subretinal exudates, subretinal fluid, and total retinal detachment. Bilateral in 50%. Can produce macular traction and epiretinal membrane. Peripheral lesions often present with macular exudates.

Systemic. Central nervous system hemangioblastoma (cerebellum and spinal cord most common, 25% of cases), renal cell carcinoma, renal cysts, pheochromocytoma (possible malignant hypertension), pancreatic cysts, epididymal cystadenoma, endolymphatic sac tumor with hearing loss, and broad ligament tumors (females).

Inheritance

Autosomal dominant with variable expression: *VHL* gene on chromosome 3p26.

Differential Diagnosis of Retinal Hemangioblastoma

- Coats disease: Aneurysmal dilation of blood vessels with prominent subretinal exudate and no identifiable tumor. See 8.1, LEUKOCORIA.
- Racemose hemangiomatosis: Large, dilated, tortuous vessels form arteriovenous communications void of intervening capillary beds without exudation or subretinal fluid.
- Retinal cavernous hemangioma: Small vascular dilations (characteristic "cluster of grapes" appearance) around retinal vein without feeder vessels. Usually asymptomatic.
- Retinal vasoproliferative tumor: Vascular tumor that appears as a yellow–red retinal

mass, most commonly in the peripheral inferior retina of older patients. Visual loss usually associated with macular edema or epiretinal membrane. Feeder vessels can be slightly dilated and tortuous but not to the extent of retinal hemangioblastoma.

- Retinal macrovessel: Large, solitary, nontortuous vessel without arteriovenous connection that supplies or drains the macular area and crosses the horizontal raphe. More commonly veins than arteries.
- Congenital retinal vascular tortuosity: Tortuous retinal vessels without racemose component.
- Familial exudative vitreoretinopathy: Bilateral, temporal, peripheral exudation with retinal vascular abnormalities and traction. See 8.3, FAMILIAL EXUDATIVE VITREORETINOPATHY.

Workup

Systemic evaluation is indicated for all patients with retinal hemangioblastoma. Solitary tumors can occur without Von Hippel–Lindau disease, but multiple or bilateral tumors are diagnostic of Von Hippel–Lindau disease.

1. Family history. Begin with ocular examination of parents and consider systemic evaluation. If one parent is affected, then siblings of affected patients also need a full workup.
2. Consider periodic intravenous fluorescein angiography.
3. Young children may require examination under anesthesia to identify peripheral retinal tumors.
4. Periodic systemic evaluations for blood pressure measurements, urinary catecholamines, MRI brain, and abdominal ultrasound.
5. Other testing in response to symptoms or signs.

Treatment/Follow Up

1. If retinal hemangioblastoma is affecting or threatening vision, laser photocoagulation, cryotherapy, transpupillary thermotherapy, photodynamic therapy with verteporfin, or radiotherapy is indicated depending on size of tumor.
2. Annual dilated fundus examination or more frequently based on findings.

13

WYBURN–MASON SYNDROME (RACEMOSE HEMANGIOMATOSIS)

Signs

(See Figure 13.13.7.)

Ocular. Enormously dilated, tortuous retinal vessels with arteriovenous communications without communicating capillary beds and without mass or exudate. Rarely, proptosis from an orbital racemose hemangioma.

Systemic. Midbrain racemose hemangiomas, intracranial calcification, seizures, hemiparesis, mental changes, facial nevi, and ipsilateral pterygoid fossa, mandibular, or maxillary hemangiomas.

Inheritance

Nonheritable.

Differential Diagnosis of Racemose Hemangiomas

See Von Hippel–Lindau syndrome above.

Workup

Complete general and ophthalmic examinations. MRI of the brain.

Treatment/Follow Up

No treatment is indicated for retinal lesions. Complications include blindness and rarely intraocular hemorrhage, retinal vascular obstruction, and neovascular glaucoma. Warn of hemorrhage risk with ipsilateral dental and facial surgery. Annual follow up.

ATAXIA–TELANGIECTASIA (LOUIS–BAR SYNDROME)

Signs

Ocular. Telangiectasias of the conjunctiva, horizontal or vertical oculomotor apraxia (inability to generate saccades, but normal pursuit), and cerebellar eye movements.

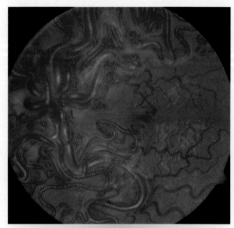

Figure 13.13.7 Racemose hemangioma.

Systemic. Progressive cerebellar ataxia with gradual deterioration of motor function. Cutaneous telangiectasias. Recurrent sinopulmonary infections. Various immunologic abnormalities (e.g., IgA deficiency and T-cell dysfunction). High incidence of malignancy (mainly leukemia or lymphoma), developmental delay and loss of motor milestones, vitiligo, premature graying of the hair, testicular or ovarian atrophy, hypoplastic or atrophic thymus, and acute radiosensitivity.

Inheritance

Autosomal recessive: *ATM* gene on chromosome 11q22.

Workup

1. Family history. Consider evaluation of siblings.
2. Consider MRI of the brain.
3. Systemic evaluations in response to signs and symptoms.

Treatment/Follow Up

No specific ocular treatment. Annual follow up. Routine dermatology monitoring and full-thickness excision of lesions as needed.

Chapter 14

Imaging Modalities in Ophthalmology

14.1 Plain Films Radiography

Description

Images of radiopaque tissues obtained by exposure of special photographic plates to ionizing radiation.

Uses in Ophthalmology

Plain films are of limited use in ophthalmology. They may be used to identify or exclude radiopaque intraorbital or intraocular foreign bodies. However, computed tomography (CT) is the study of choice to evaluate for foreign bodies, as CT has greater contrast sensitivity over conventional radiography. Plain films remain a valid screening modality before magnetic resonance imaging (MRI) if an occult metallic foreign body is suspected. Plain films should never be used in the setting of trauma or for the diagnosis of orbital fractures, as this needlessly exposes the patient to radiation without providing enough detail of orbital bone and soft tissue.

14.2 Computed Tomography

Description

CT uses ionizing radiation and computer-assisted formatting to produce multiple cross-sectional planar images. With the use of multidetector technology, CT now provides direct axial, coronal, and parasagittal images without the need for patient repositioning or data reformatting. Bone and soft tissue windows should always be reviewed in axial, coronal, and parasagittal orientations **(see Figures 14.2.1 to 14.2.3)**. Orbital studies should be obtained using the lowest radiation dose necessary for diagnosis (as low as reasonably acceptable [ALARA]—see below). This is especially important in children; for accreditation by the American College of Radiology, health care facilities must maintain specific pediatric protocols for CT. Radiopaque iodinated contrast allows for more extensive evaluation of vascular structures and areas where there is a breakdown of the normal capillary endothelial barrier (as in inflammation).

Uses in Ophthalmology

1. Excellent for defining bone abnormalities such as fractures (orbital wall or optic canal), calcification, or bony involvement of a soft tissue mass.

2. Locating suspected intraorbital or intraocular metallic foreign bodies. Glass, wood, and plastic are less radiopaque and therefore more difficult to isolate on CT.

3. Soft tissue windows are good for determining some pathologic features, including orbital cellulitis/abscess, inflammation, and tumors. May be useful in determining posterior scleral rupture when clinical examination is inconclusive, but B-scan ultrasonography is likely more sensitive. CT should never be used to definitively rule out globe rupture; clinical examination and/or surgical exploration are more sensitive modalities.

4. Excellent for imaging paranasal sinus anatomy and disease.

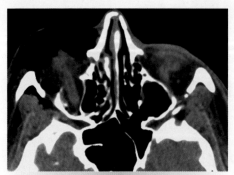

Figure 14.2.1 Axial soft tissue window of inferior orbit shows abnormality, which is difficult to assess using this window.

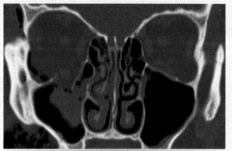

Figure 14.2.3 Coronal bone window shows the fracture again. In bone windows, the soft tissue detail fades, but bone detail is enhanced, allowing for better examination of bony anatomy.

5. Head CT is very sensitive for locating parenchymal, subarachnoid, subdural, and epidural hemorrhage in either acute or subacute settings. Although CT may show orbital hemorrhage as a nonspecific opacification within radiolucent orbital fat, it is significantly less sensitive for orbital hemorrhage than central nervous system hemorrhage.

6. Imaging modality of choice for most cases of thyroid eye disease. See 7.2.1, THYROID EYE DISEASE.

7. Loss of consciousness or unwitnessed head trauma with poor history requires CT of the brain unless otherwise recommended by a neurosurgical consultant.

8. Note that CT of the brain does not provide adequate detail of the orbital anatomy, and orbital CT does not image the entire brain. *Each site has its own specific, separate CT protocol.*

Guidelines for Ordering an Orbital Study

1. Always order a dedicated orbital study if ocular or orbital pathology is suspected. Always include views of paranasal sinuses and cavernous sinuses.

2. Order both direct axial and direct coronal views if older scanners are used. Newer, multidetector CT scanners provide excellent views in coronal and parasagittal planes with very short scan times and no patient repositioning. Multidetector CT has supplanted older technology in the vast majority of hospitals and imaging centers.

3. When evaluating traumatic optic neuropathy, request 1-mm cuts of the orbital apex and optic canal to rule out bony impingement of the optic nerve. See 3.11, TRAUMATIC OPTIC NEUROPATHY.

4. When attempting to localize ocular or orbital foreign bodies, order 1-mm cuts.

5. Intravenous contrast may be necessary for suspected infections or inflammatory conditions. Contrast is helpful in distinguishing orbital cellulitis from abscess. However, it is not mandatory to rule out orbital inflammation or postseptal involvement. Relative contraindications for contrast include renal failure, diabetes, congestive heart failure, multiple myeloma or other proteinemias, sickle cell disease, multiple severe allergies, and asthma. Check renal function and discuss

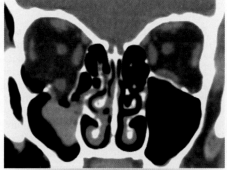

Figure 14.2.2 Coronal soft tissue window shows a large blowout fracture of the orbital floor. This finding was missed on the axial study in **Figure 14.2.1**, demonstrating the importance of reviewing both axial and coronal images.

14

the options with the radiologist for patients in whom renal insufficiency is suspected. Shellfish allergy is not a contraindication for CT contrast.

> **NOTE:** The radiologist may recommend premedication with corticosteroids and antihistamines if contrast is required and a prior allergy is suspected. Follow the protocol recommended by your radiology department.

6. Obtain a pregnancy test before obtaining CT scans in females of childbearing age.
7. CT angiography (CTA) is helpful in diagnosing intracranial vascular pathology, including aneurysms. It is available on all multidetector CT scanners and may be more sensitive than magnetic resonance angiography (MRA) in specific clinical situations. However, it requires the use of intravenous iodinated contrast. Also note that CTA requires significantly more radiation than CT. CTA should be avoided if at all possible in children; MRA is the preferred modality in the pediatric age group.

8. CT scans may be obtained in children with careful consideration of the risk of radiation exposure versus benefits of performing the scan. According to the ALARA paradigm, it is best to avoid CT if possible in children unless there is no reasonable substitute. Check with your radiologist about using a pediatric protocol to limit radiation exposure. Each CT scan exposes children to a cumulative radiation dose that may increase the risk of malignancy over their lifetime. Radiation exposure from CT scans in children is of particular concern when serial imaging is required. In these cases, MRI/MRA is often a better choice for children, although intravenous sedation or general anesthesia may be needed because of the significantly longer scanning time.

> **NOTE:** CT is an extremely valuable tool and is an acceptable imaging modality in children when necessary. Because of its easy availability, rapid scan time, excellent bone resolution, and ability to diagnose acute intracranial hemorrhage, CT is the modality of choice in head and orbital trauma in all age groups, including children.

14.3 Magnetic Resonance Imaging

Description

1. MRI uses a large magnetic field to excite protons of water molecules. The energy given off as the protons re-equilibrate to their normal state is detected by specialized receivers (coils), and that information is reconstructed into a computer image.
2. MRI obtains multiplanar images without loss of resolution.
3. The basic principles of MRI are listed in **Table 14.3.1**. **Figures 14.3.1** to **14.3.3** provide specific examples.

> **NOTE:** In general, conventional "closed" MRI scanners provide better resolution and fat suppression than open scanners, unless the open scanner contains a stronger magnet. As a rule, always try to use conventional "closed" scanners for orbital studies.

4. Contrast studies can be ordered using gadolinium, a well-tolerated, non–iodine-based paramagnetic agent.
5. Diffusion weighted imaging (DWI) is a technique that measures the Brownian motion of water within tissue. Lesions that are tightly packed by cells with a high nuclear to cytoplasmic ratio will minimize Brownian motion and "restrict diffusion." DWI is often coupled with an apparent diffusion coefficient (ADC) image. The use of DWI/ADC in the orbit is limited because of proximity of the CNS and limitations of resolution, but it can be useful in certain disorders such as lymphoma.

Uses in Ophthalmology

1. Excellent for defining the extent of orbital/central nervous system masses. Signal-specific properties of certain pathology may be helpful in diagnosis (see **Table 14.3.2**).

14

TABLE 14.3.1 Summary of Magnetic Resonance Imaging (MRI) Sequences[a]

	T1	Fat Suppression	Gadolinium	T2
Properties	Useful for intraorbital structures such as optic nerve, extraocular muscles, and orbital vessels. The strong fat signal within the orbit gives poor resolution of lacrimal gland and may also mask intraocular structures.	T1-weighted images with bright intraconal fat signal suppressed in the orbit, allowing for better anatomic detail. Essential for all orbital MRIs. Used with contrast (gadolinium).	A paramagnetic agent that distributes in the extracellular space and does not cross the intact blood–brain barrier. Gadolinium is best for T1, fat-suppressed images. The lacrimal gland, extraocular muscles, and most orbital pathology enhance with gadolinium. Essential for all orbital MRIs. Always order with fat suppression in orbital studies.	Suboptimal intraocular contrast. Demyelinating lesions (e.g., multiple sclerosis) are bright. The cerebrospinal fluid (CSF) signal may be useful in interpretation of optic nerve lesions/processes.
Interpretation	Fat is bright (high signal intensity). Vitreous and intracranial ventricles are dark.	Vitreous and fat are dark. Extraocular muscles are bright.	Most orbital masses are dark on T1 and become bright with gadolinium enhancement. Notable exceptions are listed in **Table 14.3.2.**	Fluid-containing structures such as vitreous and CSF are bright. Melanin is dark. The fluid-attenuated inversion recovery sequence on T2 suppresses the bright signal from CSF and is especially helpful in identifying the periventricular lesions of demyelinating disease.

[a]Note: High-flow areas create a dark area ("flow void"), which is helpful in identifying arterial structures (e.g., carotid siphon within the cavernous sinus).

2. Poor bone definition (e.g., fractures).

3. Excellent for diagnosing intracranial, cavernous sinus, and orbital apex lesions, many of which affect neuro-ophthalmic pathways.

4. Gadolinium is essential in defining lesion extent in suspected neurogenic tumors (meningioma, glioma).

5. All patients with clinical signs or symptoms of optic neuritis from suspected demyelinating disease should undergo brain MRI with gadolinium. Fluid-attenuated inversion recovery images are especially useful. See **Figure 14.3.4** and 10.14, OPTIC NEURITIS.

6. For orbital studies, fat suppression (also called fat saturation) should always be used in conjunction with intravenous gadolinium to enhance the visualization of the underlying pathology (e.g., optic neuritis, fat-containing lesions). Note that gadolinium without fat suppression may cause pathology to "disappear" into surrounding orbital fat.

7. DWI can help differentiate the various phases of cerebral infarction (e.g., hyperacute, acute, subacute, and chronic). DWI may also help to distinguish tightly packed, highly cellular tumors (e.g., lymphoma) from inflammation.

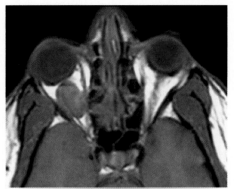

Figure 14.3.1 Axial T1-weighted image without fat suppression or gadolinium. The vitreous is dark (hypointense) relative to the bright signal from fat. A well-circumscribed mass is clearly visible in the right orbit, also hypointense. Most orbital lesions are dark in T1 prior to gadolinium injection. The notable exceptions are listed in **Table 14.3.2**.

Guidelines for Ordering the Study

1. For the vast majority of orbital studies, a head coil is indicated to provide bilateral orbital views extending to the optic chiasm.
2. Intravenous gadolinium is a useful adjunct for evaluating ocular, orbital, and perineural masses. In patients who have kidney failure, sepsis, or recent major surgery, risk of developing nephrogenic systemic fibrosis (NSF) may be a contraindication.

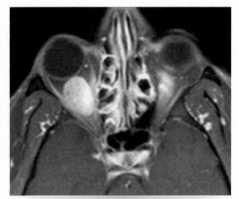

Figure 14.3.2 Axial T1 image with fat suppression and gadolinium. Note how both the vitreous and fat are dark, but the extraocular muscles become bright. The orbital mass is now clearly visible. This technique should be performed in all orbital magnetic resonance imagings.

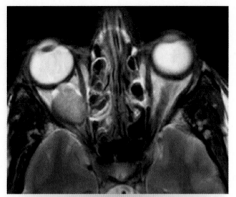

Figure 14.3.3 Axial T2-weighted image. The vitreous is hyperintense (bright) relative to the orbital fat. The lesion is also bright but in some cases may be isointense with the surrounding fat.

NSF is a rare but devastating complication of gadolinium that occurs weeks to months after administration. NSF is characterized by a scleroderma-like fibrosis of the skin, especially over extremities and trunk, which may involve the viscera. There is no known effective therapy or prophylaxis. Evaluate renal function in patients in whom renal insufficiency is suspected and discuss options with your radiology and nephrology

TABLE 14.3.2 Tissues/Lesions That Appear Bright (Hyperintense) Relative to Vitreous on T1 *Before* Gadolinium Injection[a]

Tissues/Lesions	Examples
Fat	Lipoma, liposarcoma
Mucus/ proteinaceous material	Dermoid cyst, mucocele, dacryocystocele, craniopharyngioma
Melanin	Melanoma
Subacute blood (3 to 14 days old)	Lymphangioma with blood cyst, hemorrhagic choroidal detachment, subperiosteal orbital hematoma
Certain fungal infections (iron scavengers)	*Aspergillus*

[a]Note: Most orbital lesions will become hyperintense after gadolinium infusion.

14

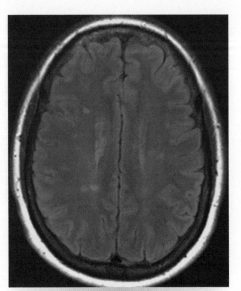

Figure 14.3.4 Magnetic resonance imaging with fluid-attenuated inversion recovery sequence of demyelinating lesions in multiple sclerosis.

departments. Recently, gadolinium deposition with specific areas of the brain has been noted in patients undergoing serial imaging. The clinical significance of this finding is unknown and is under review by the Food and Drug Administration.

3. Contraindications to MRI include severe claustrophobia, marked obesity, some cardiac pacemakers, some cardiac valves, suspected magnetic intraocular/intraorbital foreign bodies, spinal stimulators, vagal nerve stimulators, stapes implants, and specific breast and penile implants. Titanium plates and newer aneurysm clips are MRI safe, as are gold and platinum weights placed in the eyelids. When in doubt, ask the radiologist to look up the specific device in an MRI safety catalog. Any patient with a poorly documented implanted device should NOT be scanned with MRI until the issue is clarified. On occasion, specific types of pacemakers must be turned off and reset for an MRI.

14.4 Magnetic Resonance Angiography

Description

Special application of MRI technology in which signal from flowing blood is augmented while signal from stationary tissues is suppressed. MRA allows for three-dimensional rotational reconstruction. Importantly, MRA is *not* performed with gadolinium and is therefore useful in patients with a history of renal disease and other contraindications to gadolinium or CT contrast.

Uses in Ophthalmology

1. Suspected carotid stenosis, occlusion, aneurysm, or dissection.

2. Suspected intracranial and orbital arterial aneurysms (e.g., pupil-involving third cranial nerve palsy), arteriovenous malformations, and acquired arteriovenous communications.

3. Suspected orbital or intracranial vascular mass. Note that MRA is best for imaging high-flow and large-caliber lesions. Lower-flow lesions (e.g., varix) are not well seen. Both CTA and MRA have limited potential in visualizing cavernous sinus fistulas; color Doppler studies may be more sensitive in

making this diagnosis, but conventional arteriography remains the most sensitive and specific modality.

Guidelines for Ordering the Study

Conventional cerebral arteriography remains the gold standard for diagnosis of vascular lesions but carries potential morbidity and mortality in certain populations. Currently, the limit of MRA is an aneurysm larger than about 2 mm. However, the sensitivity is highly dependent on several factors: hardware, software, availability of adequate clinical history, and the experience of the neuroradiologist. Note that in one large study, the two most critical factors in missing a posterior communicating artery aneurysm (PCOM) on MRI/MRA were lack of clinical history by the referring physician and a reading by a radiologist without fellowship training in neuroradiology. Also note that most PCOM aneurysms that manifest as an oculomotor nerve paresis or palsy are at least 4 mm in diameter. Despite these potential limitations, MRA remains a safe and sensitive screening test, especially when coupled with MRI for concomitant soft tissue imaging.

14

14.5 Magnetic Resonance Venography

Magnetic resonance venography (MRV) is helpful in diagnosing central venous sinus thrombosis. MRI *and* MRV are essential parts of the workup of any patient presenting with bilateral optic disc swelling. See 10.15, PAPILLEDEMA.

14.6 Conventional Arteriography

Description

This interventional examination entails intra-arterial injection of radiopaque contrast followed by rapid-sequence x-ray imaging of the region of interest to evaluate the transit of blood through the regional vasculature. Unlike MRA or CTA, catheter arteriography allows the option of simultaneous treatment of lesions by intravascular techniques. Cerebral arteriography is the gold standard for diagnosing intracranial aneurysms, but it is being replaced as the initial imaging modality in many centers by CTA; note that, unlike catheter angiography, CTA is solely a diagnostic modality. Cerebral arteriography carries a stroke risk of 0.3% to 1.8% in patients without transient ischemic attack or previous stroke.

Uses in Ophthalmology

1. Suspected arteriovenous malformations, carotid cavernous fistulas, cavernous sinus fistula, aneurysm, and vascular masses (e.g., varix).
2. Evaluation of ocular ischemic syndrome or amaurosis fugax due to suspected atherosclerotic carotid, aortic arch, or ophthalmic artery occlusive disease. Usually carotid Doppler ultrasound, MRA, or CTA is adequate for diagnosis.

> **NOTE:** Conventional arteriography is generally contraindicated in patients with suspected carotid artery dissection (catheter placement may propagate the dissection). That said, in some centers, arteriography is used to stent areas of carotid dissection.

14.7 Nuclear Medicine

Description

Nuclear medicine imaging uses radioactive contrast (radionuclide) that emits gamma radiation, which is then gathered by a gamma-ray detector. The classic types of radionuclide scanning known to ophthalmologists include bone scanning, liver–spleen scanning, and gallium scanning. Positron emission tomography (PET) is useful in determining metabolic activity within a lesion and is usually coupled with CT for anatomic detail.

Uses in Ophthalmology

1. Scintigraphy (e.g., with technetium-99): Useful for assessing lacrimal drainage physiology in patients with inconsistent irrigation testing.
2. Systemic gallium scan: Useful for detecting extraocular sarcoidosis and Sjögren syndrome.

The use of gallium scanning for the diagnosis of sarcoidosis has been largely replaced by other testing, including serum angiotensin-converting enzyme and chest CT. See 12.6, SARCOIDOSIS.

3. Technetium-99m-tagged red blood cell study: Occasionally used to distinguish cavernous hemangioma from other solid masses in the orbit. This modality has been largely supplanted by specific MRI techniques.
4. PET/CT: The use of PET/CT for the diagnosis and management of orbital disease is still an evolving technique. Limitations in this area include the high background metabolic activity of the adjacent CNS (which may mask orbital abnormalities), the size of the orbital pathology (current PET scanners have a resolution limit of about 7 mm), and the relatively indolent nature of most orbital

14

lymphomas (decreasing the intensity of the signal on PET). PET is extremely useful in the diagnosis and surveillance of systemic pathologies, including metastases and aggressive subtypes of lymphoma. At present, the primary role of PET in the management of

orbital disease is for diagnosis, surveillance, and response to therapy of any systemic component of the pathologic process. PET is rarely obtained alone; it is typically coupled with a low-resolution CT to provide anatomic information (PET/CT).

14.8 Ophthalmic Ultrasonography

A-SCAN

Description

A-scan, or amplitude-modulated ultrasonography (US), uses ultrasonic waves (8 to 12 MHz) which travel through different tissues at different velocities in order to generate linear distance versus amplitude of reflectivity curves of the evaluated ocular and orbital tissues. A-scans are one-dimensional and used for measuring and characterizing the composition of tissues on the basis of the reflectivity curves. Not all A-scan instruments are standardized (see Figure 14.8.1).

Uses in Ophthalmology

1. Primary use in ophthalmology is measurement of axial length of the globe. This information is critical for intraocular lens (IOL) power calculations for cataract surgery. Axial length information can also be used to identify certain congenital disorders such as microphthalmia, nanophthalmos, intraocular tumor size, intrinsic tumor vascularity, and congenital glaucoma. A-scan is used to follow patients with congenital glaucoma.

2. A standardized A-scan probe calibrated on an S curve can be used for diagnostic identification of the echogenicity characteristics of masses in the globe or orbit.

3. Specialized A-mode ultrasonography can be used for corneal pachymetry (measurement of corneal thickness).

Guidelines for Ordering the Study

1. When used for IOL power calculations, make sure to check both eyes. The two eyes are usually within 0.3 mm of each other.

2. Spikes along the baseline should be sharply rising at 90 degrees.

3. If needed, keratometry readings should be obtained prior to scan or 30 minutes after the scan for accurate results.

B-SCAN   ▶

Description

(See Figure 14.8.2.)

B-scan, or brightness-modulated US, gives real-time, two-dimensional (cross-sectional) images of the eye that span from the posterior aspect of the cornea to the posterior aspect of the globe. The B-scan probe may be placed directly on the globe (after anesthetic is applied) or on the closed eyelid, which is preferred in cases of trauma or poorly cooperative patients.

Uses in Ophthalmology

1. Define ocular anatomy in the presence of media opacities (e.g., mature cataract, hyphema, corneal opacity, vitreous hemorrhage, trauma) in order to evaluate retinal and/or choroidal pathology.

2. Diagnosis of scleral rupture posterior to the muscle insertions or when media opacities prevent direct visualization.

3. Identify intraocular foreign bodies especially if made of metal or glass (spherical objects have a specific echo shadow); wood or vegetable matter has variable echogenicity; can also give a more precise location if the foreign body is next to the scleral wall.

4. Evaluation of intraocular tumor/mass consistency and vascularity, retinal detachment, choroidal detachment (serous versus hemorrhagic), and optic disc abnormalities (e.g., optic disc drusen, coloboma). Also used to monitor intraocular tumor/mass over time for response to treatment.

5. Screening of intraocular pathology (especially choroidal melanoma) in blind eyes prior to evisceration.

6. Evaluation of the posterior sclera and anterior orbit for signs of inflammation in cases of suspected posterior scleritis.

14

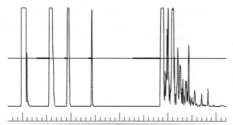

Figure 14.8.1 Normal A-scan ultrasonography.

Guidelines for Ordering the Study

1. If used in the setting of trauma to determine unknown scleral rupture, the probe is used over closed eyelids with immersion in copious amounts of sterile methylcellulose, such that no pressure is placed on the globe. The gain must be set higher to overcome the sound attenuation of the eyelids. Known ruptured globe is a relative contraindication to B-scan US.

2. When scleral integrity is not in question, B-scan US should be performed dynamically to help differentiate pathologic conditions, such as retinal detachment versus posterior vitreous detachment. To locate the exact location of retinal pathology (e.g., retinal tear, tumor), the scan should be performed directly on the globe.

3. Dense intraocular calcifications (such as those occurring in many eyes with phthisis bulbi) result in poor-quality images.

4. Silicone oil and intraocular gas in the vitreous cause distortion of the scanned image, and therefore the study should be performed in an upright patient to improve image quality.

ULTRASONOGRAPHIC BIOMICROSCOPY

Description

(See Figure 14.8.3.)

Ultrasonographic biomicroscopy uses ultrahigh frequency (50 to 100 MHz) B-mode US of the anterior one-fifth of the globe to give cross sections at near-microscopic resolution. Uses a water-bath eyelid speculum with viscous liquid in the bowl of the speculum.

Uses in Ophthalmology

1. Excellent for defining the following anatomic sites: Corneoscleral or limbal region, anterior chamber angle, iris, ciliary body, and sulcus.

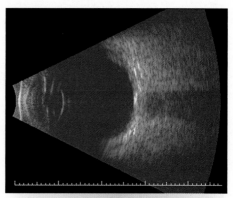

Figure 14.8.2 Normal B-scan ultrasonography.

Useful for anterior segment detail and identification of various pathologic conditions (e.g., small anterior ocular foreign bodies, ciliary body mass/cyst, plateau iris, IOL location).

2. Unexplained unilateral angle narrowing or closure.

3. Suspected cyclodialysis.

Guidelines for Ordering the Study

Known ruptured globe is a contraindication to the study.

ORBITAL ULTRASONOGRAPHY/ DOPPLER

Description

Uses B-mode US coupled with Doppler technology to visualize flow in the vessels in the orbit.

Uses in Ophthalmology

1. Superior ophthalmic vein pathology: Cavernous sinus fistula, superior ophthalmic vein thrombosis.

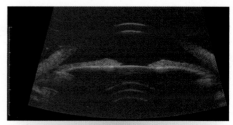

Figure 14.8.3 Normal anterior ultrasonographic biomicroscopy.

2. Orbital varix.

3. Arteriovenous malformations.

4. Vascular disease including central retinal artery occlusion, central retinal vein occlusion, ocular ischemic syndrome, and giant cell arteritis.

14.9 Photographic Studies

Description

Various methods of imaging the eye(s) or selected regions of the eye(s), using white light or various spectral wavelengths of light.

Types of Ophthalmic Photographic Imaging Studies

1. Documentary photography: Color pictures of the face, external eye, cornea, anterior segment, and fundus (white light or red-free lighting). **(See Figure 14.9.1.)**

2. Fundus autofluorescence (FAF): Imaging modality that takes advantage of the naturally and pathologically occurring fluorophores in the fundus. Provides sensitive information regarding the health of the retinal pigment epithelium (RPE) and allows early detection and monitoring of a variety of conditions such as age-related macular degeneration (AMD), macular dystrophies, and medication toxicity. Additionally, FAF is useful in the evaluation of certain ocular tumors, specifically, choroidal nevi and melanomas. **(See Figure 14.9.2.)**

3. Specular microscopy: Contact and noncontact photographic techniques used to image the corneal endothelium. The images can then be used to evaluate the quality and quantity of the endothelial cells.

4. Adaptive optics: A super high-resolution means of imaging the retina, allowing identification of rod and cone morphology, useful in delineating retinal dystrophies.

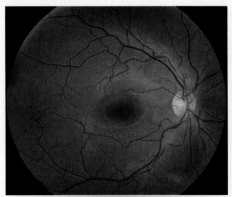

Figure 14.9.1 Normal fundus photograph.

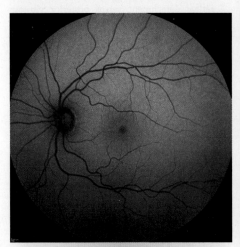

Figure 14.9.2 Normal fundus autofluorescence.

14.10 Intravenous Fluorescein Angiography

Description

(See Figure 14.10.1.)

Intravenous fluorescein angiography is a type of angiographic photography that does not rely on ionizing radiation or iodine-based contrast.

After intravenous injection of fluorescein solution (usually in a hand or arm vein), rapid-sequence photography is performed by using a camera with spectral excitation and barrier filters. Fluorescein sodium absorbs blue light, with peak absorption and excitation occurring at wavelengths of 465 to

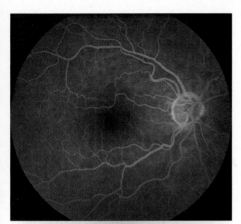

Figure 14.10.1 Normal intravenous fluorescein angiography.

490 nm. Fluorescence then occurs at the yellow-green wavelengths of 520 to 530 nm. The fluorescein molecule is 80% protein bound and does not pass through the tight junctions of a healthy blood–retinal barrier (RPE and retinal capillaries are impermeable, whereas Bruch membrane and choriocapillaris lack tight junctions and are freely permeable).

Phases of the Intravenous Fluorescein Angiography

1. Choroidal filling (background fluorescence): Begins 8 to 15 seconds after injection. Choroid is normally completely filled within 5 seconds after dye appearance within the tissue.

2. Arterial phase: Starts 1 to 2 seconds after choroidal filling.

3. Arteriovenous phase (laminar flow).

4. Venous phase: Arteriovenous transit time is the time from the first appearance of dye within the retinal arteries of the temporal arcade until the corresponding veins are completely filled, normally <11 seconds.

5. Recirculation phase: Occurs 45 to 60 seconds after arterial phase.

6. Late phase: Occurs 10 to 30 minutes post injection.

Foveal dark spot can result from xanthophyll pigment in the outer plexiform layer or tall RPE cells with increased melanin or lipofuscin. The foveal avascular zone is the central area which has no retinal capillaries (300 to 500 microns in diameter).

Describing an Abnormal Study

Hyperfluorescence

1. Leakage: Fluorescein penetrates the blood–retinal barrier and accumulates subretinally, intraretinally, or preretinally. Hyperfluorescence increases in size and brightness as study progresses (e.g., choroidal or retinal neovascularization, central serous chorioretinopathy [CSCR], cystoid macular edema [CME]).

2. Staining: Mild fluorescence appears in the late phase while its borders remain fixed (e.g., scar).

3. Pooling: Accumulation of fluorescein in fluid-filled space in retina or choroid. The margins of the space trapping fluorescein are distinct (e.g., pigment epithelial detachment [PED], CSCR).

4. Window or transmission defect: Focal area of hyperfluorescence without leakage usually due to RPE atrophy that appears early and stays stable in brightness (e.g., geographic atrophy, RPE rip, laser scar).

5. Autofluorescence: Structures that naturally fluoresce can be captured on film prior to intravenous fluorescein injection (e.g., optic nerve drusen and lipofuscin).

Hypofluorescence

1. Blockage: Due to optical density such as blood, pigment, or fibrous tissue interposed between the camera and the choriocapillaris.

2. Nonperfusion: Nonfilling vessel(s) causing relative or absolute hypofluorescence (e.g., central retinal artery occlusion). Applies to both capillaries and larger vessels.

Uses in Ophthalmology

1. Used to image retinal, choroidal, optic disc, iris vasculature, or a combination of these. It is used for diagnosis and therapeutic planning (e.g., retinal lasers).

2. Transit times between injection and appearance of dye in the choroid, retinal arteries, and veins also can be used to evaluate vascular flow. Arm to retina time is less accurate than intraretinal circulation times.

3. Suspected retinal ischemia (capillary nonperfusion) and neovascularization from various conditions (e.g., diabetes).

14

4. Suspected choroidal neovascularization (CNV) from various diseases (e.g., AMD).

Guidelines for Ordering the Study

1. Side effects of intravenous fluorescein are nausea (10%), vomiting (2%), hives, pruritus, and vasovagal response. True anaphylaxis is rare. Death may occur in 1 out of 220,000 injections. Extravasation into extracellular space at the injection site can produce local necrosis. Treat with cool compresses. Excretion in urine occurs within 24 to 36 hours. Urine will be bright yellow; remember to warn all patients about this.

2. Because it is a photographic method, moderately clear media is required for visualization.

14.11 Indocyanine Green Angiography

Description

Photographic method of ocular angiography similar to intravenous fluorescein angiography utilizing tricarbocyanine dye, an iodine-based dye. Indocyanine green (ICG) angiography differs in that fluorescence occurs in the infrared spectrum (835 nm), allowing for penetration through pigment, fluid, and blood. ICG provides better evaluation of the choroidal vasculature. ICG excitation occurs at 805 nm, with fluorescence at 835 nm. The ICG molecule is approximately 95% protein bound.

Uses in Ophthalmology

1. Suspected occult CNV.
2. Suspected recurrent CNV after prior treatment.
3. Suspected CNV with retinal PED.
4. Suspected polypoidal choroidal vasculopathy. See 11.18, IDIOPATHIC POLYPOIDAL CHOROIDAL VASCULOPATHY (POSTERIOR UVEAL BLEEDING SYNDROME).
5. Other accepted uses: Identifying feeder vessels in retinal angiomatous proliferation lesions in AMD, chronic CSCR, certain inflammatory conditions (e.g., birdshot choroidopathy), and occasionally helpful in diagnosing certain posterior segment tumors.

Guidelines for Ordering the Study

1. Contraindicated in patients with iodine or shellfish allergies.
2. Most common side effect of ICG dye administration is a vasovagal response.
3. Excreted by hepatic parenchymal cells via bile.

14.12 Optical Coherence Tomography

Description

(See Figure 14.12.1.)

Optical coherence tomography (OCT) provides noninvasive, noncontact two-dimensional or three-dimensional images by measuring optical reflections of light. In this manner, OCT is similar to US except that OCT is based on the reflection of light, not sound. The OCT scanner sends low-coherence light (~820-nm wavelength for posterior segment imaging and ~1310-nm wavelength for anterior segment imaging) emitted by a superluminescent diode to the tissue to be examined and to a reference beam. The time delays of the light reflections from retinal structures are recorded by an interferometer. Using a reference mirror, these light reflections are then translated into an imaged object with a high resolution of up to 3 microns. The most highly reflective structures are the nerve fiber layer and the RPE. Highly reflective lesions include dense pigmentation, scar tissue, subhyaloid hemorrhage, and hard exudates. Low reflectivity in pathologic conditions include intraretinal or subretinal fluid.

Spectral domain OCT has largely replaced time domain OCT due to increased image resolution, shorter acquisition time, and fewer artifacts. Enhanced depth imaging OCT is a technique used to improve the detail of the choroid. Newer modalities such as swept-source OCT and multicolor laser imaging are being evaluated. Swept-source OCT provides better resolution of retinal and choroidal structures within the same scan. Multicolor imaging complements OCT and

14

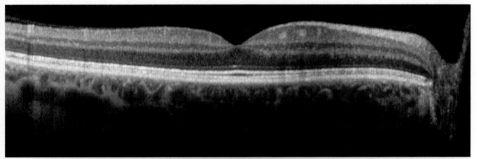

Figure 14.12.1 Normal optical coherence tomography.

uses red, green, and blue lasers to provide a topographic map of the outer, mid, and inner retina, respectively. OCT angiography (OCT-A) allows for rapid and noninvasive imaging of the retinal microvasculature and may also be applied to the anterior segment. Limitations of OCT-A include a small field of view and need for good patient cooperation.

Uses in Ophthalmology

1. Retinal diseases, including macular edema, macular atrophy, CSCR, AMD, CNV, CME, retinal detachment, PED, retinal tumors, drusen, and hard exudates.

2. Vitreoretinal interface abnormalities, including macular holes, cysts, epiretinal membranes, subhyaloid hemorrhage, and vitreoretinal strands or traction.

3. Suspected glaucoma, including quantification of the nerve fiber layer thickness, macular thickness, and optic nerve cup characteristics.

4. Suspected optic neuritis, other optic neuropathies, optic nerve drusen, disc edema, and multiple sclerosis.

5. Anterior segment pathology, such as Descemet detachment in an edematous cornea.

Guidelines for Ordering the Study

Requires patient's ability to fixate and relatively clear media.

14.13 Confocal Scanning Laser Ophthalmoscopy

Description

Confocal scanning laser ophthalmoscopy is a noninvasive imaging technique used to obtain high-resolution optical images and evaluate the topography of ocular structures. This confocal optical system provides a contour map of the desired structure in a process known as "optical sectioning." The system aims to detect reflected light from a very thin optical plane, the focal plane. A series of "focal planes" or images may be recorded and combined to create a three-dimensional image (e.g., Heidelberg retinal tomography).

Uses in Ophthalmology

1. Suspected optic nerve disease, including glaucoma and papilledema.

2. Suspected fundus elevations, including macular edema and choroidal nevi.

Guidelines for Ordering the Study

1. Requires patient's ability to fixate and relatively clear media.

2. Because the hallmark of the test is to provide comparative data, subsequent tests in the same patient need accurate alignment in the same focal plane to provide useful information.

14

14.14 Confocal Microscopy

Description

The confocal microscope optically sections the cornea to noninvasively obtain structural information of the different corneal layers.

Uses in Ophthalmology

The high level of detail available may be helpful in the detection of corneal microorganisms such as *Acanthamoeba* and fungi. It may also permit visualization of noninfectious changes such as those seen in corneal dystrophies, iridocorneal endothelial syndrome, corneal neuropathies, and epithelial downgrowth. It is excellent for imaging the corneal endothelium and obtaining endothelial cell density measurements.

14.15 Corneal Topography and Tomography

Description

Standard keratometry measures the radius of corneal curvature and then converts the radius into dioptric corneal power. Computerized corneal topography is performed using various methods, including Placido disc analysis and rasterstereography. These techniques project an image onto the cornea, most commonly a series of concentric rings, and analyze the reflection to determine corneal curvature. They can provide information on anterior corneal power and regularity. Simulated keratometry readings can be generated and the results can be represented in graphical formats, such as a variety of color maps.

Corneal tomography, the computerized reconstruction of multiple images of cornea, can give detailed information about the anterior and posterior corneal curvatures as well as corneal thickness. These techniques include scanning slit, rotating Scheimpflug photography, and anterior segment OCT-based systems. Scanning slit and rotating Scheimpflug imaging are particularly helpful in imaging posterior corneal elevation. Rotating Scheimpflug photography and anterior segment OCT can image corneal and anterior segment anatomy.

Uses in Ophthalmology

Detecting irregular astigmatism secondary to keratoconus, pellucid marginal degeneration, corneal surgery, corneal trauma, and contact lens warpage; evaluating depth of opacities in inherited corneal dystrophies and corneal scars from inflammatory or infectious etiologies. Has the ability to image normal and abnormal corneal and anterior segment structures. It may be helpful in identifying the cause of decreased vision in patients with no known cause. It is useful for refractive surgical screening and imaging the postkeratorefractive cornea. Serial imaging is critical in the evaluation of progression of corneal ectasias.

14

Appendices

A.1 Dilating Drops

MYDRIATIC AND CYCLOPLEGIC AGENTS

	Approximate Maximal Effect	Approximate Duration of Action
Mydriatic agent		
Phenylephrine, 2.5%, 10%	20 min	3 h
Cycloplegic/mydriatic agents		
Tropicamide, 0.5%, 1%	20 to 30 min	3 to 6 h
Cyclopentolate, 0.5%, 1%, 2%	20 to 45 min	24 h
Homatropine, 2%, 5%	20 to 90 min	2 to 3 d
Scopolamine, 0.25%	20 to 45 min	4 to 7 d
Atropine, 0.5%, 1%, 2%	30 to 40 min	1 to 2 wk

The usual regimen for a dilated examination is:

- Adults: Phenylephrine, 2.5% and tropicamide, 1%. Repeat these drops in 15 to 30 minutes if the eye is not dilated.
- Children (>1-year-old) and full-term infants (consider any two-agent combination from the following): Phenylephrine, 2.5%; tropicamide, 1%; and cyclopentolate, 1% to 2%. Consider repeating the drops in 30 minutes if the eye is not dilated.
- Preterm infants and neonates (consider any two-agent combination from the following): Phenylephrine, 1%; tropicamide, 1%; and

cyclopentolate, 0.2 % to 0.5%. Consider repeating the drops in 30 to 45 minutes if the eye is not dilated.

 NOTE

1. Dilating drops are contraindicated in most types of angle-closure glaucoma and in eyes with severely narrow anterior chamber angles.
2. Dilating drops tend to be less effective at the same concentration in darkly pigmented eyes.

435

A.2 Tetanus Prophylaxis

History of Tetanus Immunization (doses)	Clean Minor Wounds		All Other Wounds	
	Tetanus Toxoid*	Immune Globulin	Tetanus Toxoid	Immune Globulin
Uncertain or fewer than 2 doses	Yes	No	Yes	Yes
2	Yes	No	Yes	No[a]
3 or more	No[b]	No	No[c]	No

*Dose of tetanus toxoid is 0.5 mL intramuscularly.
[a]Unless wound is >24 hours old.
[b]Unless >10 years since the last dose.
[c]Unless >5 years since the last dose.

A.3 Cover/Uncover and Alternate Cover Tests

COVER/UNCOVER TEST

The primary purpose is to detect a tropia (a deviation when both eyes are open) and/or a phoria (a latent deviation that manifests when binocular fusion is disrupted). Ideally performed with best correction, as the patient must have adequate vision to fixate on a target.

Requirements

Full range of ocular motility, vision adequate to see the target of fixation, foveal fixation in each eye, and patient cooperation. This test should be performed before the alternate cover test (see below).

Method

1. Ask the patient to fixate on a nonaccommodative target at a distance (e.g., a letter on the vision chart).
2. Cover one of the patient's eyes while observing the uncovered eye. A refixation movement of the uncovered eye indicates the presence of a manifest deviation (tropia). Repeat the procedure, covering the opposite eye. A shift in fixation may not occur if the uncovered eye is the preferred or fixating eye. Prisms may be used to quantify the observed deviation.
3. If there is no movement of either eye, the eyes are aligned with both eyes open (no tropia).

4. Ask the patient to fixate on an accommodative target nearby. Both eyes are tested at a near distance in the manner described previously.

> **NOTE:** An esodeviation is detected by a refixation movement temporally (the eye being observed turns away from the nose). An exodeviation is detected by a refixation movement nasally (the eye being observed turns toward the nose). A hyperdeviation is detected by a refixation movement inferiorly.

ALTERNATE COVER TEST

In the absence of a tropia, the alternate cover test may be used to reveal any latent deviation that occurs with the interruption or suspension of binocular fusion (phoria). When it has been determined by the cover/uncover test that a tropia exists, the alternate cover test may be used to dissociate the two eyes and further quantify the total deviation (manifest tropia and latent phoria combined). The alternate cover test does not distinguish manifest from latent deviations.

Requirements

Same as for the cover/uncover test above.

Method

1. Ask the patient to fixate on a nonaccommodative target at a distance. To make certain that he or she is fixing on the target, ask that the letters be read or the picture described.

2. Repeatedly cover one eye and then quickly move the cover to the other eye. The eye being uncovered may be noted to swing into a position to refixate on the target, indicating the presence of a deviation. Then repeat the test at a near distance.

ALTERNATE COVER TEST WITH PRISM

Measures the size of the total deviation, regardless of whether a phoria or tropia is present.

Method

1. To measure a deviation, prisms are placed in front of one eye with the prism base placed in the direction of the eye's refixation movement. While continuing to alternately cover, as described above, increase the prism strength until eye movement ceases. The strength of the weakest prism that eliminates eye movement during alternate cover is the amount of deviation.

2. Measurements may be done for any direction of gaze by turning the patient's head away from the target while asking him or her to maintain fixation on it (e.g., the right gaze is measured by turning the patient's head toward his or her left shoulder and asking the patient to look at the target).

3. In general, measurements are taken in the straight-ahead position (both at a distance and nearby), in right gaze, left gaze, downgaze (the head is tilted up while the patient focuses on the target), upgaze (the head is tilted down while the patient focuses on the target), and with the patient's head tilted toward either shoulder. Measurements are often taken both with and without glasses in the straight-ahead position.

A.4 Amsler Grid

Used to test macular function or to detect a central or paracentral scotoma.

1. Have the patient wear his or her glasses and occlude the left eye while an Amsler grid is held approximately 12 inches in front of the right eye **(see Figure A.4.1)**.

2. The patient is asked what is in the center of the page. Failure to see the central dot may indicate a central scotoma.

3. Have the patient fixate on the central dot (or the center of the page if he or she cannot see the dot). Ask if all four corners of the diagram are visible and if any of the boxes are missing.

4. Again, while staring at the central dot, ask the patient if all of the lines are straight and continuous or if some are distorted and broken.

5. The patient is asked to outline any missing or distorted areas on the grid with a pencil.

6. Repeat the procedure, covering the right eye and testing the left.

 NOTE

1. It is very important to monitor the patient's eye for any movement away from the central dot.

2. A red Amsler grid may define more subtle defects.

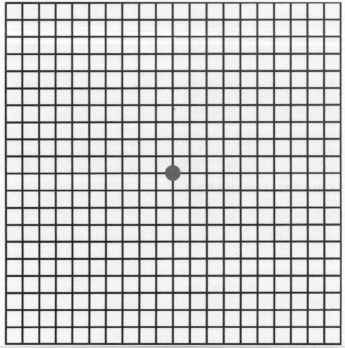

Figure A.4.1 Amsler grid.

A.5 Seidel Test to Detect a Wound Leak

Concentrated fluorescein dye (from a moistened fluorescein strip) is applied directly on the potential site of perforation while observing the site with the slit lamp **(see Figure A.5.1)**. If a perforation and leak exist, the fluorescein dye is diluted by the aqueous and appears as a green (dilute) stream within the dark orange (concentrated) dye. The stream of aqueous is best seen with the cobalt blue light of the slit lamp.

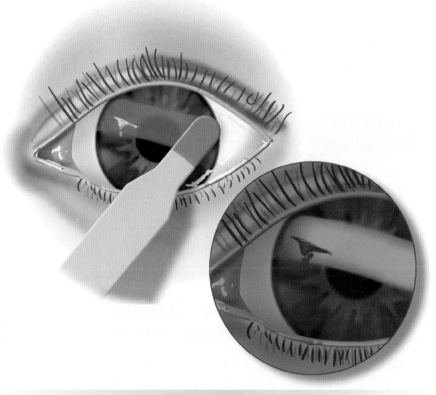

Figure A.5.1 Seidel test.

A.6 Forced Duction Test and Active Force Generation Test

Forced Duction Test

(See Figure A.6.1.)

This test distinguishes restrictive causes of decreased ocular motility from other motility disorders. One technique is the following:

1. Place a drop of topical anesthetic (e.g., proparacaine) into the eye.

2. Apply viscous lidocaine to further anesthetize the eye.

3. Use toothed forceps (e.g., Graefe fixation forceps) to firmly grasp Tenon's close to the limbus at both locations perpendicular to the desired direction of movement. Doing so helps prevent corneal abrasions should the

forceps slip. Rotate the eye in the "paretic" direction. If there is a resistance to the passive rotation of the eye, a restrictive disorder is diagnosed. This test does not require the patient to be conscious.

Active Force Generation Test

The patient is asked to look in the "paretic" direction while a sterile cotton swab is held just beneath the limbus on that same side. The amount of force generated by the "paretic" muscle is compared with that generated in the normal contralateral eye. The test can only be used in a cooperative, alert patient.

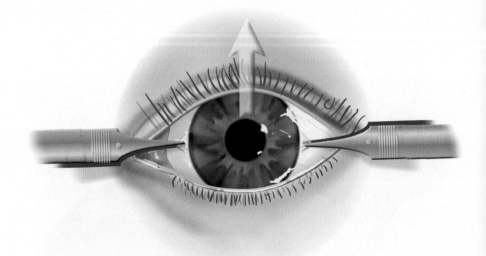

Figure A.6.1 Forced duction test.

A.7 Technique for Diagnostic Probing and Irrigation of the Lacrimal System

1. Anesthetize the eye with a drop of topical anesthetic (e.g., proparacaine) and consider holding a cotton-tipped applicator soaked in the topical anesthetic or applying viscous lidocaine on the involved punctum for several minutes for additional comfort.

2. Dilate the punctum with a punctum dilator **(see Figure A.7.1)**.

3. Gently insert a #00 Bowman probe into the punctum 2 mm vertically, and then 8 mm horizontally, toward the nose. Avoid using smaller probes, as they can create a false passage. Pull the involved eyelid laterally while slowly moving the probe horizontally to facilitate the procedure and to avoid creating a false passageway.

4. In the presence of an eyelid laceration, a torn canaliculus may be diagnosed by the appearance of the probe in the site of the eyelid laceration. See 3.8, EYELID LACERATION.

5. Irrigation of the lacrimal system is performed after removing the probe and inserting an irrigation cannula in the same manner in which the probe was inserted. Warn the patient before irrigation to expect a gag reflex. Saline (2 to 3 mL) is gently pushed into the system. Leakage through a torn eyelid also diagnoses a severed canaliculus. Resistance to the injection of the saline, ballooning of the lacrimal sac, or leakage of the saline out of either punctum may be the result of a lacrimal system obstruction. If soft-tissue edema occurs during irrigation, stop immediately—a false passage may have been created. A patent lacrimal system usually drains into the throat quite readily, and the arrival of saline may be noted by the patient. Stop irrigating as soon as the patient tastes the fluid.

NOTE: If only evaluating the patency of the lacrimal system, and not ruling out a laceration, the system can be irrigated immediately after punctum dilation.

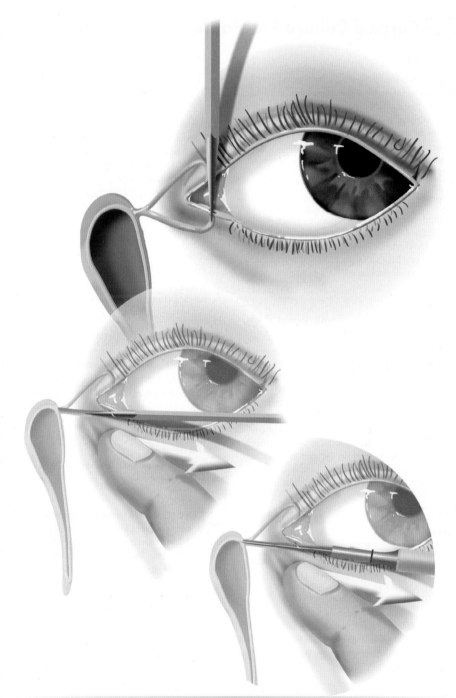

Figure A.7.1 Probing and irrigation: After anesthetizing the eye, dilate the punctum with a punctum dilator. Insert the dilator 2 mm vertically. Pull the eyelid laterally. Rotate the dilator 90 degrees and continue to advance it horizontally. Using a similar insertion technique, advance the irrigation cannula.

A.8 Corneal Culture Procedure

Indications

Small (<1 mm) infiltrates may be treated empirically with intensive commercially available broad-spectrum antibiotics without prior scraping. We routinely culture infiltrates larger than 1 to 2 mm, in the visual axis, unresponsive to initial treatment, or if we suspect an unusual organism based on history or examination. See 4.11, BACTERIAL KERATITIS.

Equipment

Slit lamp; sterile Kimura spatula, knife blade, or moistened calcium alginate swab (e.g., with nonpreserved sterile saline, or thioglycolate or trypticase soy broth); culture media; microscopy slides; and an alcohol lamp.

Procedure

1. Anesthetize the cornea with topical drops. Proparacaine is best because it appears to be less bactericidal than others.
2. At the slit lamp, scrape the ulcer base (unless significant corneal thinning has occurred) and the leading edge of the infiltrate firmly with the spatula, blade, or swab. Place the specimens on the slides first and then on the culture media. Sterilize the spatula over the flame of the alcohol lamp between each separate culture or slide. Be certain that the spatula tip temperature has returned to normal before touching the cornea again.

Media

Routine

1. Blood agar (most bacteria).
2. Sabouraud dextrose agar without cycloheximide; place at room temperature (fungi).

3. Thioglycolate broth (aerobic and anaerobic bacteria).
4. Chocolate agar; lab will place into a CO_2 jar (*Haemophilus* species, *Neisseria gonorrhoeae*).

Optional

1. Löwenstein–Jensen medium (mycobacteria, *Nocardia* species) should be included in patients with a history of LASIK or an atypical ulcer appearance.
2. Nonnutrient agar with *Escherichia coli* overlay if available (*Acanthamoeba*).

Slides

Routine

1. Gram stain (bacteria and fungi).
2. Calcofluor white; a fluorescent microscope is needed (fungi and *Acanthamoeba*).

Optional

1. Giemsa stain (bacteria, fungi, and *Acanthamoeba*).
2. Acid-fast stain (*Mycobacterium* species and *Nocardia* species).
3. Gomori methenamine silver stain and periodic acid-Schiff (PAS) stain (fungi and *Acanthamoeba*).
4. KOH wet mount (fungi, *Nocardia* species, and *Acanthamoeba*).
5. Extra slide to send to pathology at a local institution.

NOTE: When a fungal infection is suspected, deep scrapings into the base of the ulcer are essential. Sometimes a corneal biopsy is necessary to obtain diagnostic information for fungal, atypical mycobacterial, and *Acanthamoeba* infections.

A.9 Fortified Topical Antibiotics/Antifungals

📝 **NOTE:** Additional and updated information is available in the online e-book. To access, use your code from the back of the front cover at http://solution.lww.com/access

Fortified Bacitracin (10,000 U/mL)

Add enough sterile water (without preservative) to 50,000 U bacitracin dry powder to form 5 mL of solution. This provides a concentration of 10,000 U/mL. Refrigerate. Expires after 7 days.

Fortified Cefazolin (50 mg/mL)

Add enough sterile water (without preservative) to 500 mg of cefazolin dry powder to form 10 mL of solution. This provides a strength of 50 mg/mL. Refrigerate. Expires after 7 days.

Fortified Ceftazidime (50 mg/mL)

Add 10 mL of sterile water to 1 g of ceftazidime. Draw up 7.5 mL of this solution and add it to a sterile dropper bottle. Then add 7.5 mL of sterile water to the dropper bottle to produce a concentration of 50 mg/mL. Refrigerate. Expires after 7 days.

Fortified Tobramycin (or Gentamicin) (15 mg/mL)

With a syringe, inject 2 mL of tobramycin, 40 mg/mL, directly into a 5-mL bottle of tobramycin, 0.3%, ophthalmic solution. This gives a 7-mL solution of fortified tobramycin (approximately 15 mg/mL). Refrigerate. Expires after 14 days.

Fortified Vancomycin (25 mg/mL)

Add enough sterile water (without preservative) to 500 mg of vancomycin dry powder to form 10 mL of solution. This provides a strength of 50 mg/mL. To achieve a 25-mg/mL concentration, take 5 mL of 50-mg/mL solution and add 5 mL sterile water. Refrigerate. Expires after 7 days.

Fortified Voriconazole (0.5 mg/mL)

Dilute 1 mL of IV voriconazole (10 mg/mL) with 19 mL of sterile water. This provides a strength of 0.5 mg/mL. Refrigerate. Expires after 7 days. Filter the solution prior to topical administration.

A.10 Technique for Retrobulbar/Subtenon/Subconjunctival Injections

Retrobulbar Injection

1. Clean the skin of the lower eyelid and upper cheek around the area of the inferior orbital rim with an alcohol swab.

2. With the patient in primary gaze, use a 1.25-inch 25- or 27-gauge needle (preferably a short-beveled blunt retrobulbar needle) to penetrate the skin just superior to the inferior orbital rim in line with the lateral limbus.

3. Advance the needle parallel to the orbital floor. After passing parallel to the equator of the globe, redirect the needle superonasally into the muscle cone.

4. Lateral motions of the needle are made to ensure that the needle has not penetrated the sclera (at which point, the lateral motion would be inhibited).

5. Pull back on the syringe to ensure no vascular structures have been penetrated. If no aspiration occurs, slowly inject the contents of the syringe. In a successful injection, the globe may move anteriorly due to the retrobulbar pressure.

6. Withdraw the needle along the same contour as insertion. May perform orbital compression for at least 2 minutes.

Subtenon Injection

1. Apply topical anesthesia to the area to be injected (e.g., topical proparacaine or a cotton-tipped applicator soaked in proparacaine, or both, held on the area for 1 to 2 minutes). Place a drop of topical 5% povidone-iodine on the surface of the eye. If subtenon steroids are to be injected, 0.1 mL of lidocaine may

be injected in the same manner as described next, several minutes before the steroids. The inferotemporal quadrant is usually the easiest location for injection.

2. With the aperture of a 25-gauge, 5/8-inch needle facing the sclera, the bulbar conjunctiva is penetrated 2 to 3 mm from the fornix, avoiding conjunctival blood vessels.

3. As the needle is inserted, lateral motions of the needle are made to ensure that the needle has not penetrated the sclera (at which point, the lateral motion would be inhibited).

4. The curvature of the eyeball is followed, attempting to place the aperture of the needle near the posterior sclera.

5. When the needle has been pushed in to the hilt, the stopper of the syringe is withdrawn to ensure that the needle is not intravascular.

6. The contents of the syringe are injected, and the needle is removed.

Subconjunctival Injection

1. Apply topical anesthesia and antiseptic as above.

2. Forceps are used to tent the conjunctiva, allowing the tip of a 25-gauge, 5/8-inch needle to penetrate the subconjunctival space. The needle is placed several millimeters below the limbus at the 4- or 8-o'clock position, with the aperture facing the sclera and the needle pointed inferiorly toward the fornix.

3. When the entire tip of the needle is beneath the conjunctiva, the stopper of the syringe is withdrawn to ensure that the needle is not intravascular.

4. The contents of the syringe are injected, and the needle is removed.

> **NOTE:** An eyelid speculum may be helpful in keeping the eyelids open during subtenon and subconjunctival injections.

A.11 Intravitreal Tap and Inject

Supplies Needed

1. Ophthalmic proparacaine or tetracaine.
2. 5% povidone-iodine.
3. Eyelid speculum.
4. 1% or 2% lidocaine without epinephrine.
5. Alcohol wipes.
6. Cotton tip applicators as needed.
7. 1 or 3 mL syringe with an 18-gauge needle to fill a syringe with lidocaine and a 30-gauge needle (1/2 to 5/8-inch length) for subconjunctival lidocaine injection.
8. 25 or 27-gauge needle (1/2 to 5/8-inch length) on a 3 mL syringe for vitreous tap. If the patient has had a pars plana vitrectomy, a 30-gauge needle may be used.
9. 30-gauge needle (1/2 to 5/8-inch length) on a 1 mL syringe for anterior chamber tap.
10. 1 mL syringe or caliper to mark the injection site.
11. 30-gauge needle (1/2 to 5/8-inch length) on a 1 mL syringe with indicated intravitreal injection(s).
12. Specimen cap.

Procedure Steps

1. Anesthetize the eye with topical proparacaine or tetracaine.
2. Apply 1 to 2 drops of 5% povidone-iodine.
3. Insert speculum.
   a. Tips: A wire or plate speculum may be used. Plate speculum can provide more comfort if the eye is painful.
4. Using a 1 mL syringe with a 30-gauge needle, inject ~0.5 mL of lidocaine subconjunctivally (As mentioned in the video, we suggest waiting at least 5 minutes after the subconj lido before proceeding with the tap and inject. Longer may be better in very inflamed eyes. The eyelid speculum can be removed while waiting and then reinserted before the subsequent steps.). The injection should be placed in the area of the anticipated vitreous tap and injection.
   a. Tips:
      i. To optimize ocular anesthesia, wait for at least five minutes after lidocaine injection.

ii. Subconjunctival lidocaine may not yield complete ocular anesthesia with the tap, especially in very inflamed eyes. Both the physician and patient should be prepared for possible patient movement if there is any discomfort during the procedure.

5. Mark the injection site by pressing the tip of a 1 mL syringe on the surface of the eye to create an imprint. Place one edge of the syringe tip at the inferotemporal limbus. The outer edge of the tip will mark 4 mm from the limbus.

   a. Tips:

      i. The entry point of injection should be 4 mm from the limbus in phakic patients and 3.5 mm in pseudophakic patients.

      ii. Alternatively, a caliper may be used to measure the exact distance.

6. Apply another 1 to 2 drops of 5% povidone-iodine.

7. Using a 25- or 27-gauge needle on a 3-mL syringe, enter the eye at your marked site, aiming posteriorly toward the optic nerve.

   a. Tips:

      i. In phakic patients, it is crucial to remain perpendicular to the entry plane as to avoid hitting the lens.

8. Carefully pull back on the plunger to create a vacuum. The sample volume should be between 0.1 and 0.3 mL.

   a. Tips:

      i. Sample may not immediately be obtained. Several techniques can be used to optimize yield:

1. Aspirate in one location first. If there is no return of fluid, release the suction and slowly pivot the needle to a slightly different location and then try to aspirate again.

   Or

2. Carefully move the needle slowly in and out after insertion into the vitreous cavity to find a pocket of liquid vitreous.

9. If the vitreous tap is unsuccessful, convert to an anterior chamber tap. Using a 30-gauge needle on a 1-mL syringe, insert the needle and bevel up, through the clear cornea in the inferotemporal quadrant, over the iris. Gently pull back on the plunger to obtain a 0.1- to 0.2-mL sample.

   a. Tips:

      i. If the patient is phakic, it is crucial to keep the needle in the horizontal plane over the iris to avoid hitting the lens capsule. If the patient is pseudophakic, you may enter at the limbus and aim the needle more centrally while still taking care to avoid contact with the iris, intraocular lens, or corneal endothelium. A sterile cotton swab may be used to stabilize the globe by placing the tip of the swab on the nasal side of the globe to provide countertraction.

10. Place specimen cap on the syringe.

11. Prepare for intravitreal injection by applying 1 to 2 drops of 5% povidone-iodine to the surface of the eye.

12. Inject intravitreal agent(s) at the previous injection site using a 30-gauge needle on a 1-mL syringe.

13. Remove speculum.

A.12 Intravitreal Antibiotics

Intravitreal Cefazolin (2.25 mg/0.1 mL)

Reconstitute a 500-mg vial of cefazolin with 2 mL of sterile water. Draw 1 mL of the solution into a Tb syringe and inject into an empty 30-mL vial. Add 9 mL of sterile water. Mix. Withdraw 0.2 mL of the solution from the 30-mL vial into a Tb syringe. Remove the Tb syringe needle and replace it with a 30-gauge needle. Expel 0.1 mL to leave 0.1 mL of 2.25-mg/0.1-mL cefazolin solution.

Intravitreal Vancomycin (1 mg/0.1 mL)

Reconstitute a 500-mg vial of vancomycin with 10 mL of sterile water. Withdraw 1 mL of the solution and inject it into a sterile 10-mL vial. Add 4 mL of sterile water to the 10-mL vial. Mix. Withdraw 0.2 mL of vancomycin solution with a Tb syringe. Remove the Tb syringe needle and replace it with a 30-gauge needle. Expel 0.1 mL to leave 0.1 mL of 1-mg/0.1-mL vancomycin solution.

Intravitreal Amikacin (400 mcg/0.1 mL)

Withdraw 0.8 mL (40 mg) of amikacin from a 100-mg/2-mL amikacin vial. Inject into a sterile

10-mL vial. Add 9.2 mL of nonpreserved sodium chloride and mix. Withdraw 0.3 mL into a sterile Tb syringe and replace the needle with a 30-gauge needle. Expel 0.2 mL to leave 0.1 mL of 400-mcg/0.1-mL amikacin solution.

Intravitreal Ceftazidime (2 mg/0.1 mL)

Add 9.4 mL of sterile water to 1 g of ceftazidime injection (in a vial). After dissolving, vent the vial. From the ceftazidime vial, transfer 2 mL to a 10-mL sterile vial. To this sterile vial, add 8 mL of sodium chloride 0.9% nonpreserved. Withdraw 0.3 mL of the solution into a sterile Tb syringe and replace the needle with a 30-gauge needle. Expel 0.2 mL to leave 0.1 mL of a 2-mg/0.1-mL ceftazidime solution.

A.13 Anterior Chamber Paracentesis

1. Place a drop of topical anesthetic (e.g., proparacaine) on the surface of the eye.
2. Retract the eyelids with a sterile speculum.
3. Place a drop of topical 5% povidone-iodine on the surface of the eye and allow it to sit on the globe for at least 30 to 60 seconds.
4. If available, use an operating microscope or slit lamp.
5. In an eye with normal or elevated intraocular pressure, fixation forceps are not needed.
6. In eyes with intraocular pressure <8 mm Hg, fixation forceps may be necessary. Anesthetize the base of the lateral rectus muscle by holding a cotton-tipped applicator dipped in the topical anesthetic against the muscle for 1 minute. Grasp the base of the lateral rectus muscle with fixation forceps at the anesthetized site.

> **NOTE:** To best provide countertraction and minimize globe rotation, the eye is fixated at the same side of needle insertion.

7. Use a 30-gauge short needle on a syringe and remove the plunger.

8. Enter the eye at an area with a sufficiently formed anterior chamber. Keep the bevel of the needle pointing anteriorly (toward the epithelium) and away from the lens. Keep the tip of the needle over the iris (not the lens) when entering the anterior chamber **(see Figure A.13.1)**.

> **NOTE:** Make sure the plane of the needle is parallel to the plane of the iris.

9. Leave the tip of the needle in the anterior chamber for about 2 to 3 seconds. Aqueous will passively egress into the plungerless syringe.

> **NOTE:** In some instances (e.g., when an aqueous specimen is necessary), it may be necessary to withdraw aqueous. This greatly increases the risk of complication and is to be avoided if possible.

10. Withdraw the needle and place a drop of antibiotic on the eye (e.g., gatifloxacin or moxifloxacin). Consider topical antibiotics q.i.d. for 4 to 7 days.

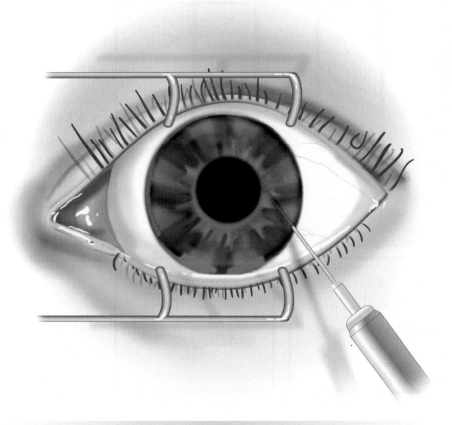

Figure A.13.1 Anterior chamber paracentesis.

A.14 Angle Classification

Proper evaluation of the configuration of the anterior chamber requires the use of at least three descriptors: the point at which the peripheral iris is adherent to the cornea or uvea, the depth of the anterior chamber, and the curvature of the peripheral iris. The Spaeth grading system of the anterior chamber angle takes into account all the three attributes.

Spaeth Grading System

(See Figure A.14.1.)

Iris Insertion

A = Anterior to the Schwalbe line (SL)

B = Between SL and scleral spur

C = Scleral spur visible (common in blacks and Asians)

D = Deep: ciliary body visible (common in whites)

E = Extremely deep: >1 mm of the ciliary body is visible

Indentation gonioscopy may be necessary to differentiate false opposition of the iris against the structures in the iridocorneal angle from

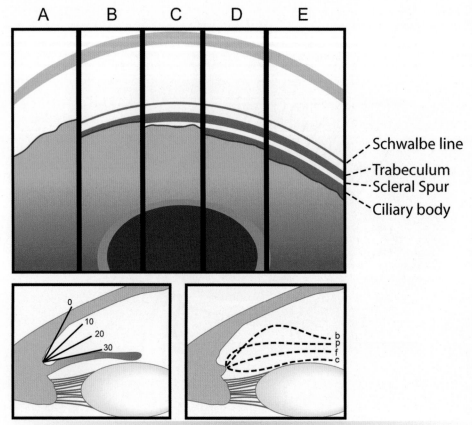

A B C D E

Schwalbe line
Trabeculum
Scleral Spur
Ciliary body

0
10
20
30

b
p
f
c

Figure A.14.1 Spaeth angle classification.

the true iris insertion. First, make note of the most posterior portion of the inner wall of the eye that can be seen without indentation. The iris is then displaced posteriorly by compressing the cornea. This allows for the determination of the true iris insertion. When the true iris insertion is different from the preindentation appearance, the preindentation appearance is placed in parentheses. For example, a (B)D grade means that without indentation, it is not possible to see any of the scleral spur or ciliary body, but with indentation, the ciliary body can be seen.

Angle of the Anterior Chamber

The angular width that is measured is the angle between a line parallel to the corneal endothelium at the Schwalbe line and a line parallel to the anterior surface of the iris.

Curvature of Iris

b = bowing anteriorly
p = plateau configuration
f = flat
c = concave posterior bowing

Pigmentation of the Posterior Trabecular Meshwork (PTM)

Viewing at 12 o'clock in the angle with the mirror at 6 o'clock position, pigmentation graded on a scale of 0 (no PTM pigment seen) to 4 + (intense PTM pigment).

General Guidelines

1. Occludable angles would include the following:
   - Any angle narrower than 10 degrees.
   - Any *p* angle configuration.

2. Potentially occludable angles include:
   - Any angle narrower than 20 degrees.
   - Any B insertion.
3. Abnormal iris insertions include:
   - Any A insertion.
   - Any B insertion.
   - C attachment in certain populations.
4. Iris bow >1+ usually indicates pupillary block.
5. Pigmentation >2+ is usually pathologic though can occur naturally in patients with heavy skin pigmentation.

Examples of the Spaeth Grading System

1. C15b 2+ ptm = Open but narrow occludable angle.
2. A40f = closed angle.
3. (B)D30p 0 ptm = open, atypical narrow angle, occludable with dilation.

4. D40c 4+ ptm = open-angle characteristic of patients with myopia or iris pigment dispersion syndrome.

Shaffer Classification

(See Figure A.14.2.)

Grade 0: The angle is closed.

Grade 1: Extremely narrow angle (10 degrees). Only the Schwalbe line, and perhaps also the top of the trabecula, can be visualized. Angle closure is probable.

Grade 2: Moderately narrow angle (20 degrees). Only the trabecular meshwork can be seen. Angle closure is possible.

Grade 3: Moderately open angle (20 to 35 degrees). The scleral spur can be seen. Angle closure is not possible.

Grade 4: Angle wide open (35 to 45 degrees). The ciliary body can be visualized with ease. Angle closure is not possible.

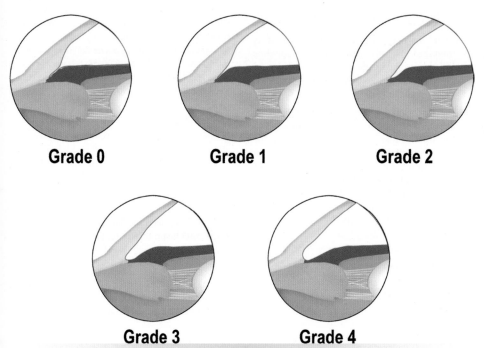

Figure A.14.2 Shaffer angle classification.

Van Herick Angle Depth Estimation

> **NOTE:** The Van Herick slit-lamp method of evaluation only allows an estimation of the anterior chamber depth and is not a substitute for formal gonioscopy. For Van Herick grading, bring the temporal aspect of the cornea into focus using a thin, bright slit beam that is offset approximately 60 degrees temporal to the oculars. The thickness of the cornea is compared to the depth of the peripheral anterior chamber.

Grade 1: Chamber depth <1/4 corneal thickness. Suggests narrow angle at increased risk for closure.

Grade 2: Chamber depth 1/4 corneal thickness. Suggests angle closure is possible.

Grade 3: Chamber depth 1/4 to 1/2 corneal thickness. Suggests low probability of angle closure.

Grade 4: Chamber depth ≥ corneal thickness. Suggests open angle without the risk of closure.

A.15 YAG Laser Peripheral Iridotomy

Also see 9.4, ACUTE ANGLE CLOSURE GLAUCOMA.

1. Perform prelaser peripheral iridotomy (LPI) gonioscopy to assess the baseline angle.

2. Inform the patient that they may experience ghost imaging after LPI due to the newly created iris defect. Preference for creation of the LPI at 3 and 9 o'clock to avoid the eyelid margin and prismatic tear film effect theorized to cause ghost images. Superior LPI discouraged even if completely covered by upper eyelid due to high rate of postoperative dysphotopsias.

3. Pretreat the eye with one drop each of apraclonidine 1% and pilocarpine (1% for lightly pigmented irides and 2% for darkly pigmented). As an alternative to pilocarpine, some ophthalmologists prefer to shine a bright light into the fellow eye immediately before engaging the laser or to employ bright ambient light. This allows for physiologic constriction of the operative pupil.

4. Recommended laser settings:
   - Power: 4 to 7 mJ (usually for a total of 12 to 21 mJ).
   - Spot size: 10 to 70 mm.
   - Shots/pulse: 3.

> **NOTE:** Darker irides usually require more total power. Always start with a lower power and titrate up as needed for each individual patient. Pretreatment with an argon laser prior to YAG laser therapy is an option for patients with darker, thicker irides or concern for intraoperative bleeding. The argon laser coagulates the tissue to reduce bleeding and thins the iris, thus encouraging easier YAG laser penetration with less applied energy. Utilize spot size 50 um with an escalating power beginning at 300 mJ, 50 laser applications to 600 mJ, 50 laser applications, and finally 900 mJ, 50 laser applications with YAG laser to follow (as below).

5. Anesthetize the eye (e.g., proparacaine).

6. Place an Abraham YAG iridotomy contact lens cushioned with 2.5% hydroxypropyl methyl cellulose or lidocaine gel, positioning the magnification button above the anticipated site of iris penetration.

> **NOTE:** Keep the lens perpendicular to the YAG beam to ensure good focus and laser concentration.

7. Focus the YAG beam on the predetermined iris location (see #2, above). Focus within an iris crypt if possible **(see Figure A.15.1)**.

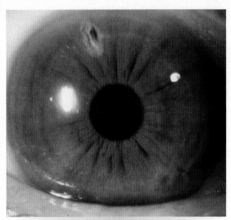

Figure A.15.1 Laser peripheral iridotomy.

8. Engage the laser. There will be a gush of posterior iris pigment when the iris is completely penetrated. If not penetrated, advance the

YAG beam to refocus on the newly created crater. Re-engage the laser until the iris is completely penetrated.

9. Administer one drop of prednisolone 1% and apraclonidine 1% after laser treatment.

10. Check post-LPI intraocular pressure.

11. Treat inflammation with prednisolone 1% q.i.d. for 4 to 7 days. If the LPI required a significant amount of power (e.g., more than six triple shots), taper the steroids before discontinuation to prevent rebound inflammation.

12. Have the patient return within 1 to 2 weeks for IOP measurement, iridotomy evaluation, and gonioscopy.

Ophthalmic Acronyms and Abbreviations

A

ABK Aphakic bullous keratopathy

ABMD or EBMD Anterior (or epithelial) basement membrane dystrophy

AC Anterior chamber

AC/A Accommodative convergence/accommodation angle

ACIOL Anterior chamber intraocular lens

AFB Acid-fast bacillus

AFGE Air-fluid gas exchange

AFX Air-fluid exchange

AGIS Advanced Glaucoma Intervention Study

AION Arteritic ischemic optic neuropathy

AK Astigmatic keratotomy

ALT Argon laser trabeculoplasty

AMD Age-related macular degeneration

AMT Amniotic membrane tissue or transplant

APMPPE Acute posterior multifocal placoid pigment epitheliopathy

Anti-VEGF Anti–vascular endothelial growth factor

APD or RAPD (Relative) afferent pupillary defect

ARC Abnormal retinal correspondence

ARN Acute retinal necrosis

ASC Anterior subcapsular cataract

ASP Anterior stromal puncture

AV Arteriovenous

AZOOR Acute zonal occult outer retinopathy

B

BCVA Best corrected visual acuity

BDR Background diabetic retinopathy

BRAO Branch retinal artery occlusion

BRVO or BVO Branch retinal vein occlusion

BSCL Bandage soft contact lens

BSS Balanced salt solution

Bx Biopsy

C

C$_3$F$_8$ Perfluoropropane

CACG Chronic angle closure glaucoma

CAI Carbonic anhydrase inhibitor

CAR Cancer-associated retinopathy

CB Ciliary body

CBC Complete blood count

CCF Carotid-cavernous (sinus) fistula

CCT Central corneal thickness

C/D Cup/disc ratio

CE Cataract extraction

C/F Cell/flare

CF Count fingers

CHED Congenital hereditary endothelial dystrophy

CHRPE Congenital hypertrophy of the retinal pigment epithelium

CIN Conjunctival intraepithelial neoplasia

CL Contact lens

CLW Contact lens wearer

CME Cystoid macular edema

CMV Cytomegalovirus

CN Cranial nerve

CNV or CNVM Choroidal neovascularization or choroidal neovascular membrane

CPA Cerebellopontine angle

CPC Cyclophotocoagulation

CPEO Chronic progressive external ophthalmoplegia

CRA Chorioretinal atrophy or central retinal artery

CRAO Central retinal artery occlusion

CRVO or CVO Central retinal vein occlusion

CSCR or CSR Central serous (chorio) retinopathy

CSM Central, steady, and maintained fixation

CSME Clinically significant macular edema

CSNB Congenital stationary night blindness

CVF Confrontation visual field

CVOS Central Vein Occlusion Study

CWS Cotton–wool spot

CXL Corneal crosslinking

D

DALK Deep anterior lamellar keratoplasty

DBD Diamond burr debridement

DCR Dacryocystorhinostomy

DDT Dye disappearance test

DD Disc diameter(s)

DES Dry eye syndrome

DFE Dilated fundus examination

DLK Diffuse lamellar keratitis

DM Diabetes mellitus

DMEK Descemet membrane endothelial keratoplasty

D/Q Deep and quiet

DR Diabetic retinopathy

DRS Diabetic Retinopathy Study

DS(A)EK Descemet stripping (automated) endothelial keratoplasty

DSO Descemet stripping only

DUSN Diffuse unilateral subacute neuroretinitis

DVD Dissociated vertical deviation

E

E Esophoria

EBMD Epithelial basement membrane dystrophy

ECCE Extracapsular cataract extraction

ECD Endothelial cell density

EDTA Ethylenediamine tetraacetic acid

EKC Epidemic keratoconjunctivitis

EL Endolaser

EOG Electrooculogram

EOM Extraocular muscles or motility

ERG Electroretinogram

ERM Epiretinal membrane

ESR Erythrocyte sedimentation rate

ET Esotropia

ETDRS Early Treatment Diabetic Retinopathy Study

EUA Examination under anesthesia

F

FA Fluorescein angiogram

FAF Fundus autofluorescence

FHIC Fuchs heterochromic iridocyclitis

FAZ Foveal avascular zone

FB Foreign body

FBS Fasting blood sugar or foreign body sensation

FEVR Familial exudative vitreoretinopathy

FNA Fine needle aspiration

FTA-ABS Fluorescent treponemal antibody absorption

FTFC Full to finger counting

FTN Finger tension normal

G

GA Geographic atrophy

GC Gonococcus

GCA Giant cell arteritis

GLT Glaucoma Laser Trial

GPC Giant papillary conjunctivitis

H

HA Headache

HM Hand motion

HSV Herpes simplex virus

HT Hypertropia

HVF Humphrey visual field

HZO Herpes zoster ophthalmicus

I

ICCE Intracapsular cataract extraction
ICE Iridocorneal endothelial syndrome
ICG Indocyanine green
IGRA Interferon-gamma release assay
IK Interstitial keratitis
ILM Internal limiting membrane
INO Internuclear ophthalmoplegia
IO Inferior oblique muscle
IOFB Intraocular foreign body
IOIS Idiopathic orbital inflammatory syndrome
IOL Intraocular lens
IOO Inferior oblique overaction
IOP Intraocular pressure
IR Inferior rectus muscle
IRMA Intraretinal microvascular abnormalities
IVFA Intravenous fluorescein angiography

J

JOAG Juvenile open angle glaucoma
JIA Juvenile idiopathic arthritis
JXG Juvenile xanthogranuloma

K

K Keratometry or cornea
K-pro Keratoprosthesis
KCN Keratoconus
KP Keratic precipitates

L

LASER Light amplification by stimulated emission of radiation
LASIK Laser in situ keratomileusis
LASEK Laser subepithelial keratomileusis
LL Lower eyelid
LF Levator function
LP Light perception
LPI Laser peripheral iridotomy
LR Lateral rectus muscle
LTG Low-tension glaucoma

M

MA Microaneurysm
MAR Melanoma-associated retinopathy

MCE Microcystic corneal edema
ME Macular edema
MEWDS Multiple evanescent white dot syndrome
MG Myasthenia gravis
MGD Meibomian gland dysfunction
MHA-TP Microhemagglutination assay for *Treponema pallidum*
MIGS Microinvasive glaucoma surgery
MM Malignant melanoma
MMC Mitomycin C
MMP Mucous membrane pemphigoid
MP Membrane peel
MPS Macular Photocoagulation Study
MR Medial rectus muscle
MRD Margin to reflex distance
MRSA Methicillin-resistant *Staphylococcus aureus*
MS Multiple sclerosis

N

NAION Nonarteritic ischemic optic neuropathy
Nd-YAG Neodymium-doped yttrium aluminum garnet (laser)
NFL Nerve fiber layer
NI No improvement
NK Neurotrophic keratopathy or keratitis
NLDO Nasolacrimal duct obstruction
NLP No light perception
NPA Near point of accommodation
NPC Near point of convergence
NPDR Nonproliferative diabetic retinopathy
NRC Normal retinal correspondence
NS Nuclear sclerosis
NTG Normal tension glaucoma
NV (A, D, E, or I) Neovascularization (angle, disc, elsewhere [in retina], or iris)
NVG Neovascular glaucoma

O

OCP Ocular cicatricial pemphigoid
OCS Orbital compartment syndrome
OCT Optical coherence tomography
OD Oculus dexter, or right eye
OHT Ocular hypertension

OIS Ocular ischemic syndrome

OKN Optokinetic nystagmus

ON Optic nerve

OS Oculus sinister, or left eye

OU Oculus uterque, or both eyes

P

P Pupils

PAM Primary acquired melanosis or potential acuity meter

PAS Peripheral anterior synechiae

PBK Pseudophakic bullous keratopathy

PC Posterior chamber

PCIOL Posterior chamber intraocular lens

PCO Posterior capsular opacity

PD Prism diopters or pupillary distance

PDR Proliferative diabetic retinopathy

PDS Pigment dispersion syndrome

PDT Photodynamic therapy

PE Phacoemulsification or physical examination

PED Pigment epithelial detachment

PERRL(A) Pupils equal, round, and reactive to light (and accommodation)

PF Palpebral fissure

PFAT Preservative-free artificial tear

PFV Persistent fetal vasculature

PH Pinhole

PI Peripheral iridectomy/iridotomy

PK Penetrating keratoplasty

PLE Pen light examination

PMD Pellucid marginal degeneration

PMMA Polymethylmethacrylate

POAG Primary open angle glaucoma

POHS Presumed ocular histoplasmosis syndrome

PORN Progressive outer retinal necrosis

PPCD Posterior polymorphous corneal dystrophy

PPD Purified protein derivative

PPL Pars plana lensectomy

PPV Pars plana vitrectomy

PRP Panretinal photocoagulation

PRK Photorefractive keratectomy

PSC Posterior subcapsular cataract

PTK Phototherapeutic keratectomy

PVD Posterior vitreous detachment

PVR Proliferative vitreoretinopathy

PXE Pseudoxanthoma elasticum

PXF Pseudoexfoliation

R

RA Rheumatoid arthritis

RAPD or APD Relative afferent pupillary defect

Rb Retinoblastoma

RCE Recurrent corneal erosion

(R)RD (Rhegmatogenous) retinal detachment

RGP Rigid gas permeable (contact lens)

RK Radial keratotomy

ROP Retinopathy of prematurity

RP Retinitis pigmentosa

RPR Rapid plasma reagin

RPE Retinal pigment epithelium

S

SB Scleral buckle

SCH Subconjunctival hemorrhage

SEI Subepithelial (anterior stromal) infiltrate

SF$_6$ Sulfur hexafluoride

SLE Slit lamp examination or systemic lupus erythematosus

SLK Superior limbic keratoconjunctivitis

SLT Selective laser trabeculoplasty

SMILE Small incision lenticule extraction

SO Superior oblique muscle or sympathetic ophthalmia or silicone oil

SPK Superficial punctate keratopathy or keratitis

SR Superior rectus muscle

SRF Subretinal fluid

SS Scleral spur

SVP Spontaneous venous pulsation

T

T (a,t) Tension or tonometry (applanation, Tonopen)

TBUT Tear break-up time

TED Thyroid eye disease

TIA Transient ischemic attack

TID Transillumination defect

TM Trabecular meshwork
TRD Tractional retinal detachment
TTT Transpupillary thermotherapy

U

UCVA Uncorrected visual acuity
UGH Uveitis–glaucoma–hyphema syndrome
UBM Ultrasound biomicroscopy
UL Upper eyelid

V

VA (cc or sc) Visual acuity (with correction or without correction)
VDRL Venereal Disease Research Laboratory
VER Visual-evoked response
VF Visual field

VH Vitreous hemorrhage
VKH Vogt–Koyanagi–Harada syndrome
VZV Varicella zoster virus

W

WEBOF White-eyed blowout fracture

X

X Exophoria
XT Exotropia

Y

YAG Yttrium aluminum garnet (laser)

Index

Note: Page numbers followed by "f" indicate figures and "t" indicate tables.